Molecular Neuropharmacology:
A Foundation for Clinical Neuroscience

Eric J. Nestler, MD, PhD

*Lou and Ellen McGinley Distinguished Professor
and Chairman*
Department of Psychiatry
The University of Texas Southwestern Medical Center at Dallas
Dallas, Texas

Steven E. Hyman, MD

National Institutes of Health
Bethesda, Maryland

Robert C. Malenka, MD, PhD

*Nancy Friend Pritzker Professor of Psychiatry
and Behavioral Sciences*
Director, Nancy Friend Pritzker Laboratory
Department of Psychiatry and Behavioral Sciences
Stanford University School of Medicine
Palo Alto, California

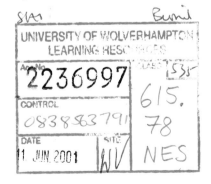

UNIVERSITY OF WOLVERHAMPTON
LEARNING RESOURCES

2236997

CONTROL
0838563791

DATE
11 JUN 2001

SITE
WV

535
615.
78
NES

The McGraw-Hill Companies, Inc.

Medical Publishing Division

*New York   Chicago   San Francisco   Lisbon   London   Madrid   Mexico City
Milan   New Delhi   San Juan   Seoul   Singapore   Sydney   Toronto*

McGraw-Hill

A Division of The McGraw-Hill Companies

MOLECULAR NEUROPHARMACOLOGY

Copyright © 2001 by the McGraw-Hill Companies, Inc.
All rights reserved. Printed in the United States of America.
Except as permitted under the United States
Copyright Act of 1976, no part of this publication may be
reproduced or distributed in any form or by any means,
or stored in a data base or retrieval system, without the
prior written permission of the publisher.

1234567890   KGP KGP   0987654321

ISBN 0-8385-6379-1 (domestic)

*Cover illustraton: Trafficking and Ca^{2+}—dependent exocytosis
of a norepinephrine-containing synaptic vesicle is depicted.*

This book was set in New Baskerville by V&M Graphics.
The editors were Janet Foltin, Harriet Lebowitz,
and Karen G. Edmonson.
The production supervisor was Catherine H. Saggese.
The index was prepared by Kathryn Unger.
The text was designed by Joan O'Connor.
The cover was designed by Eve Siegel.
The illustration manager was Charissa Baker.
Quebecor Printing/Kingsport was printer and binder.
This book is printed on acid-free paper.

LIBRARY OF CONGRESS
CATALOGING-IN-PUBLICATION DATA

Nestler, Eric J. (Eric Jonathan). 1954–
    Molecular neuropharmacology: a foundation for clinical neuro-
science / Eric J. Nestler, Steven E. Hyman, Robert C. Malenka.—
1st ed.
        p. ; cm.
    Includes bibliographical references and index.
    ISBN 0-8385-6379-1
    1. Neuropharmacology. 2. Molecular neurobiology. I. Hyman,
Steven E. II. Malenka, Robert C. III. Title.
    [DNLM: 1. Central Nervous System Agents—pharmacology.
2. Central Nervous System—drug effects. 3. Central Nervous
System—physiology. 4. Central Nervous System Diseases—drug
therapy. QV 76.5 N468m 2001]
RD315.N455 2001
617'.78—dc21
                                                            00–051549
ISBN: 0-07-112065-3 (international)
Exclusive rights by The McGraw-Hill Companies, Inc., for
manufacture and export. This book cannot be re-exported
from the country to which it is consigned by McGraw-Hill.
The International Edition is not available in North America.

Molecu
Neurop
A Foundatio

9/02

UNIVERSITY OF
WOLVERHAMPTON
ENTERPRISE LTD.

LR/LEND/001

Harrison Learning Centre
Wolverhampton Campus
University of Wolverhampton
St Peter's Square
Wolverhampton WV1 1RH
Wolverhampton (01902) 322305

2 5 MAR 2009 23/10/2009		

Telephone Renewals: 01902 321333
Please RETURN this item on or before the last date shown above.
Fines will be charged if items are returned late.
See tariff of fines displayed at the Counter.   (L2)

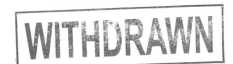

Notice

Medicine is an ever-changing science. As new research and clinical experience broaden our knowledge, changes in treatment and drug therapy are required. The editors and the publisher of this work have checked with sources believed to be reliable in their efforts to provide information that is complete and generally in accord with the standards accepted at the time of publication. However, in view of the possibility of human error or changes in medical sciences, neither the editors, authors, nor the publisher nor any other party who has been involved in the preparation or publication of this work warrants that the information contained herein is in every respect accurate or complete, and they disclaim all responsibility for any errors or omissions or for the results obtained from use of the information contained in this work. Readers are encouraged to confirm the information contained herein with other sources. For example and in particular, readers are advised to check the product information sheet included in the package of each drug they plan to administer to be certain that the information contained in this book is accurate and that changes have not been made in the recommended dose or in the contraindications for administration. This recommendation is of particular importance in connection with new or infrequently used drugs.

This book is dedicated

to our wives and children:

Susan, David, Matt, and Jane

Barbara, Emily, Julia, and Charlie

Pam, Nick, and Ben

CONTENTS

CONTRIBUTING AUTHORS

JOHN ALVARO, PhD

Yale University School of Medicine
New Haven, Connecticut

JENNIFER A. CUMMINGS, MA

University of California, San Francisco

CATHARINE DUMAN, PhD

Yale University School of Medicine
New Haven, Connecticut

CHARLES GLATT, MD, PhD

University of California, San Francisco

KELLY VAN KOUGHNET, PhD

Canadian Institutes of Health Research
Ottawa, Ontario

DAVID KRANTZ, MD, PhD

University of California, Los Angeles

CHRIS McBAIN, PhD

National Institute of Child Health & Development
Bethesda, Maryland

THOMAS NEYLAN, MD

University of California, San Francisco

HEATHER RIEFF, PhD

University of Virginia Medical Center
Charlottesville, Virginia

NICOLE ULLRICH, MD, PhD

Children's Hospital and Harvard Medical School
Boston, Massachusetts

DAN WOLF, MD, PhD

Yale University School of Medicine
New Haven, Connecticut

PREFACE

Neuropharmacology, the study of drug actions on the nervous system, comprises several areas of investigation of critical importance to science and medicine. Neuropharmacology involves studies aimed at understanding the mechanisms by which drugs alter brain function. These include medications used to treat a wide range of neurologic and psychiatric disorders as well as drugs of abuse. A primary goal of neuropharmacology is to use this information to develop new medications with ever-improving efficacy and safety for diseases of the nervous system. In addition, neuropharmacologic agents are valuable tools with which to probe the molecular and cellular basis of nervous system functioning. For example, the mechanisms of drugs that produce their clinically relevant effects only after repeated administration, agents such as antidepressants in treating depression or drugs of abuse in causing addiction, provide a means of learning about neural plasticity. Overall, much of what we now know about the nervous system—how individual neurons work, how neurons communicate with one another, and how neurons adapt over time to external stimuli—has come from studies using pharmacologic probes.

To comprehend the actions of a drug on the nervous system, a great deal more is needed than simply identifying the drug's initial target in the nervous system. Rather, one must understand the entire sequence of events that commences with the binding of a drug to an initial molecular target. The resulting alteration in the functioning of that target, the influence of that occurrence on the complex biochemical networks that exist within neurons, the subsequent changes in the output of the neuron, and their consequences for the functioning of circuits within which the targeted neuron exists are all important for gaining a real understanding of drug action. Only with an awareness of the many steps in the process can we grasp how a drug changes complex nervous system functions such as movement, cognition, pain, or mood. Thus, the action of a drug on the nervous system must be comprehended at many levels under both normal and pathologic conditions.

The organization of this textbook represents an attempt to build an understanding of drug action by adding the different levels of explanation layer by layer. As a result this book differs significantly from many other pharmacology texts, which are usually organized drug by drug or neurotransmitter by neurotransmitter. In this book, information on fundamental molecular and cellular building blocks is provided first so that it can serve as the basis for the material associated with neural functions. This permits the reader to relate fundamental neuropharmacology to neural systems and ultimately to clinical neuroscience.

The book is divided into three parts. Part 1 includes a brief discussion of general principles of neuropharmacology (Chapter 1), followed by a detailed presentation of nervous system function (Chapters 2–6), from electrical excitability to signal transduction to gene expression. Drugs that act on these basic components of neuronal function are mentioned in these early chapters.

In Part 2 information about the major neurotransmitter systems in the brain and spinal cord is presented (Chapters 7–10). Highlighted in these chapters are the molecular details of neurotransmitter synthetic and degradative enzymes, receptors, and transporter proteins. These proteins represent the initial targets for the large majority of known psychotropic drugs. Also included in Part 2 is a discussion of neurotrophic factors (Chapter 11), which over the last 10 years have been shown to profoundly influence the adult nervous system and to be potentially important in therapeutics.

Part 3 uses the basic information contained in Parts 1 and 2 to build a systems-level description of the major domains of complex nervous system function. Chapter 12 focuses on the autonomic nervous system; Chapter 13 on neuroendocrine function, Chapter 14 on movement, Chapter 15 on emotion and mood, Chapter 16 on reinforcement and addiction, Chapter 17 on higher cognitive function and psychosis, Chapter 18 on attention and sleep, Chapter 19 on pain, Chapter 20 on memory and dementia, and Chapter 21 on stroke and seizures. Each chapter begins with a description of the normal neural mechanisms underlying a particular domain of nervous system functioning, followed by a discussion of the diseases that affect that domain. Drugs are discussed within the context of their influence on the neural circuits involved in both normal function and specific disease states.

The organization of *Molecular Neuropharmacology: A Foundation for Clinical Neuroscience* allows individual drugs to be discussed in several contexts. A drug is first mentioned when its initial target is described in Parts 1 or 2. The drug is mentioned again in Part 3 in the context of its effect on complex neural functions. Many drugs are discussed in several chapters of Part 3 because they affect more than one domain; for example, first-generation antipsychotic drugs not only reduce psychosis (Chapter 17), but also affect motor function (Chapter 14) and sleep (Chapter 18).

The book's structure also permits the incorporation of a great deal of clinical information, much of it representing the integration of modern molecular genetics with neuropharmacology. New insights on the molecular mechanisms underlying such disorders as Parkinson disease, Huntington disease, depression, schizophrenia, Alzheimer disease, stroke, and epilepsy,

to name a few, are provided. Our knowledge of the molecular underpinnings of normal brain function and disease, particularly in cases that have been successfully investigated by genetics, may be in advance of developments in pharmacology. Consequently, the book includes many molecular insights, even though drugs may not yet exist that exploit such molecular knowledge. In this regard the book can be seen as presenting a template for the future in identifying molecular mechanisms for novel therapeutic approaches. We anticipate that subsequent editions of this book will describe the development of such novel medications and thereby gradually fill in these gaps in pharmacology.

The scientific and clinical explanations in *Molecular Neuropharmacology: A Foundation for Clinical Neuroscience* are written in a style that makes them accessible to a wide audience: undergraduate and graduate students as well as students in the medical and allied health professions. This book is also an excellent resource for residents in psychiatry, neurology, and anesthesiology, and practicing clinicians and scientists in these areas. As a concise treatise of clinical information that provides descriptions of basic mechanisms and their clinical relevance, this book is suitable for both scientists and clinicians.

We would like to acknowledge the contributing authors who were instrumental in the initial phases of the preparation of this book. We also would like to thank Harvey Shoolman who originally recruited us for this project; Georgia Miller, who was an enormous help in numerous ways; and the folks at McGraw-Hill—Harriet Lebowitz, Janet Foltin, Pam Carley, Eve Siegel, and Susan Worley—who whipped this book (and us) into shape.

Eric J. Nestler
Steven E. Hyman
Robert C. Malenka

Molecular
Neuropharmacology:
A Foundation for Clinical Neuroscience

PART 1

Fundamentals of Neuropharmacology

Chapter 1

Basic Principles of Neuropharmacology

KEY CONCEPTS

- An understanding of drug action in the brain must integrate knowledge of the molecular and cellular actions of a drug with their effects on brain circuitry.

- The clinical actions of a drug in the brain often are due to neural plasticity—the long-term adaptations of neurons to the short-term actions of a drug.

- The binding of a drug to its specific target(s) normally is saturable and stereoselective.

- The specific binding of a drug to its target is quantified according to its affinity for the target, expressed as a dissociation constant (K_d) and the total amount of binding (B_{max}).

- Potency of a drug describes the strength of binding between the drug and its target; efficacy describes the maximal biologic effects that the drug exerts by binding to its target.

- Drugs can be classified as agonists, partial agonists, inverse agonists, or antagonists.

- Because the actions of a drug are dose dependent, drugs must be studied at a range of concentrations.

- Modern neuropharmacology takes advantage of the tools of molecular biology, genetics, and cell biology as well as combinatorial chemistry, which is used to generate novel molecules that may function as new drugs.

- Functional genomics and proteomics will help identify novel drug targets.

Neuropharmacology is the scientific study of the effects of drugs on the nervous system. Its primary focus is the actions of medications for psychiatric and neurologic disorders as well as those of drugs of abuse. Neuropharmacology also uses drugs as tools to form a better understanding of normal nervous system functioning. The goal of neuropharmacology is to apply information about drugs and their mechanisms of action to develop safer, more effective treatment and eventually curative and preventive measures for a host of nervous system abnormalities.

The importance of neuropharmacology to medical practice, and to society at large, is difficult to overstate. Drugs that act on the nervous system, including antidepressant, antianxiety, anticonvulsant, and antipsychotic agents, are among the most widely prescribed medications. Moreover, commonly prescribed medications that act on other organ systems often are associated with side effects that involve the nervous system and in turn may limit their clinical utility. In addition, a substantial number of individuals use common substances, such as caffeine, alcohol, and nicotine, that are included in the domain of neuropharmacology because of their effects on the central nervous system (CNS). In a much smaller fraction of the population, these and other drugs are used compulsively, in a manner that constitutes an addiction. Drug abuse and addiction exact an astoundingly high financial and human toll on society through direct adverse effects, such as lung cancer and hepatic cirrhosis, and indirect adverse effects—for example, accidents and AIDS—on health and productivity.

A number of terms are commonly used in reference to the study of the effect of drugs on the nervous system. *Neuropsychopharmacology* is an all-encompassing term that typically is applied to all types of drug effects that influence nervous system functioning. The term *psychopharmacology* is often used to describe the effect of drugs on psychological parameters such as emotions and cognition. Drugs that exert an effect on aspects of behavior are known as *psychotropic* agents. In this book we use the term *neuropharmacology* to describe the study of all drugs that affect the nervous system, whether they affect sensory perception, motor function, seizure activity, mood, higher cognitive function, or other forms of nervous system functioning.

HOW DRUGS WORK

The actions of drugs that affect the nervous system are considerably more complicated than those of drugs that act on other organ systems. To understand how drugs act on the nervous system, it is critical to integrate information about the molecular and cellular actions of a drug with knowledge of how these actions affect brain circuitry—a circuitry that is constantly changing in structure and function in response to both pharmacologic and nonpharmacologic input from the environment. The complexity that underlies such actions can be illustrated by a description of the effects of **fluoxetine,** a widely prescribed antidepressant, and those of **furosemide,** a widely prescribed diuretic. The chemical actions of these drugs are fairly simple. Both drugs initially bind to their specific protein target: fluoxetine binds to and inhibits serotonin transporters, which in turn inactivate the actions of the neurotransmitter serotonin (see Chapter 9), and furosemide binds to and inhibits Cl^- channels located in the ascending loop of Henle in nephrons of the kidney. However, the relation between the chemical and clinical actions of these drugs—particularly those of fluoxetine—requires a more elaborate explanation.

The association between furosemide's chemical and clinical activity is relatively straightforward. By inhibiting Cl^- transport in Henle's loop, furosemide causes more Cl^- to remain in the lumen of the nephron tubule, which in turn requires more H_2O to remain in the tubule. Furosemide exerts this same effect on all nephrons in the kidney, and the increase in H_2O in individual nephron tubules combines to cause diuresis at the level of the kidney. Diuresis is achieved as soon as effective concentrations of the drug reach the kidney's extracellular fluid, and is maintained with repeated use of the drug—for example, in the treatment of chronic congestive heart failure.

The relationship between the chemical and clinical actions of fluoxetine on the nervous system is more intricate and also more speculative. Most drugs that act on the nervous system interact with only the minute subset of the brain's neurons that express the initial protein target of the drug. Fluoxetine directly affects only those neurons that use serotonin as a neurotransmitter—a few 100,000 out of approximately 100 billion neurons in the brain. Although it is known that fluoxetine affects serotonin neurons by inhibiting serotonin transport, relatively little is understood about the effects of the drug on the millions of other neurons that are influenced by serotonin or about the drug's effects on the neural circuits in which these innumerable neurons function. Moreover, the mood-elevating effects of fluoxetine are not evident after initial exposure to the drug but require continued use of the drug for several weeks. This delayed effect suggests that it is not the inhibition of serotonin transporters per se, but some adaptation to sustained inhibition of the transporters that mediates the clinical actions of fluoxetine. However, where the adaptations to fluoxetine occur—for example, whether they occur in the neurons that use serotonin as a transmitter, in the neurons that are influenced by serotonin, or in the neurons that are affected by those neurons, is not yet known. Relevant adaptations at the molecular level also have yet to be identified with certainty.

The clinical actions of fluoxetine, like those of many neuropharmacologic agents, reflect drug-induced *neural plasticity,* which is the process by which neurons adapt over time in response to chronic disturbance. Consequently, to understand fully the effects of a neuropharmacologic drug, we must determine not only the initial effects of the drug, but also the intraneuronal signals that control a neuron's adaptations over time, the interneuronal signals through which neurons communicate with one another, and the ways in which large groups of neurons operate in circuits to produce complex brain functions.

Parts I and II of this book explore the intraneuronal and interneuronal signals that enable communication among neurons, which are fairly well understood. Part III addresses the relationships between circuits of neurons and complex brain functions, about which much remains to be discovered.

DRUGS AS TOOLS TO PROBE BRAIN FUNCTION

Neuropharmacology has contributed to many important advances in the neurosciences during the past several decades. Most significantly, drugs have been used as tools to dissect the functions of the brain and of individual nerve cells under normal and pathophysiologic conditions.

Historically, neuropharmacology has involved the delineation of numerous chemical agents that are currently known to function as neurotransmitters in the nervous system, including monoamines, amino acids, purines, and peptides. The identification of many of these neurotransmitters and the elucidation of their synthesis, degradation, and receptors occurred in conjunction with studies of synthetic and plant substances that were known to exert profound effects on behavior. The neuropharmacology of **ergot** alkaloids, **cocaine,** and **reserpine,** for example, led to the discovery and characterization of monoamine neurotransmitter systems; **opiate** alkaloids such as **morphine** led to endogenous opioid systems; **nicotine, muscarine,** and cholinesterase inhibitors led to cholinergic systems; and **caffeine** and related substances led to purinergic systems.

Neuropharmacology also played a fundamental role in the delineation of the numerous receptor subtypes through which neurotransmitters elicit biologic responses. The early idea that one neurotransmitter acts on only one receptor was replaced decades ago with the recognition that for each neurotransmitter there are multiple receptors. This discovery led to the development of synthetic drugs that had an increasing selectivity for individual types of receptors, and the evolution of these neuropharmacologic agents has represented important advances in clinical medicine. These advances include the use of selective β_1-adrenergic antagonists for cardiovascular disease, selective β_2-adrenergic agonists for asthma, μ-opioid antagonists for opiate overdose, and $5HT_{1d}$-serotonin agonists for migraine.

The identification of multiple receptor subtypes for neurotransmitters also has contributed to the recognition of complex postreceptor signal transduction cascades through which receptors ultimately produce their biologic responses. From G proteins to second messengers to protein phosphorylation pathways, studies of the effects of drugs on the nervous system have provided crucial windows onto the functioning of intracellular signaling pathways. Accordingly, investigation of the mechanisms by which **organic nitrates** cause vasodilation in the treatment of angina led to the discovery of nitric oxide as a critical signaling molecule. Similarly, studies of the actions of **aspirin** and related nonsteroidal antiinflammatory agents led to the discovery of a host of signaling molecules derived from arachidonic acid, including prostaglandins and leukotrienes. Recognition of the efficacy of **cyclosporin** as an immunosuppressive agent led to the discovery of immunophilins—proteins that modulate a specific type of protein phosphatase in many tissues, including those of the brain. Moreover, drugs that specifically perturb certain intracellular signaling proteins—for example, **forskolin** as an activator of adenylyl cyclase, **phorbol esters** as activators of protein kinase C, and **pertussis toxin** as

an inhibitor of the G protein G_i—have been powerful tools for elucidating specific signaling pathways within cells in the nervous system.

Drugs are also used as prototypical external or environmental factors in determining how the brain and neuronal populations within the brain adapt or maladapt over time in response to repeated perturbations. Some of the adaptations that occur in response to repeated drug exposure are models for adaptations to other external exposures, including stress and experience.

PRINCIPLES OF GENERAL PHARMACOLOGY

The ability of a drug to produce an effect on an organism is dependent on many of its properties, from its absorption to its stability to its elimination. To briefly summarize these processes, the first factor to be considered is the *route of administration,* which can determine how rapidly a drug reaches its target organ and which organs it affects. *Oral* administration typically results in a relatively slow onset of action. *Parenteral* describes all other routes of administration, including *subcutaneous* (under the skin), *intraperitoneal* (into the peritoneal–abdominal cavity), *intravenous* (into the venous system), *intracerebroventricular* (into the cerebral ventricular system), and *intracerebral* (into the brain parenchyma) delivery. The *bioavailability* of a drug determines how much of the drug that is administered actually reaches its target. Bioavailability can be influenced by *absorption* of the drug from the gut if it is administered orally. It also can be affected by *binding* of the drug to plasma proteins, which makes the drug unavailable to bind to its target. Moreover, it can be influenced by a drug's ability to penetrate the *blood–brain barrier,* if the drug acts on the brain, or its ability to permeate cell membranes, if the drug acts on intracellular proteins.

Drug action also depends on the *stability* of the drug once it is absorbed—for example, how rapidly it is metabolized to inactive congeners or eliminated from the body through urine, bile, or exhaled air. Some drugs (prodrugs) must be converted into active metabolites before they can exert their biologic effects.

Each of these factors, which can be categorized as pharmacokinetic considerations, is a critical determinant of drug action and influences both the clinical use of drugs and the process of developing new agents. However, these pharmacokinetic properties are not discussed in detail in this book because they are not, strictly speaking, related to the underlying mechanisms of drug action—the pharmacodynamic features that are the primary concern of these chapters. As an introduction to this topic, a brief description of the process by which a drug interacts with its initial protein target follows.

DRUG BINDING

Neuropharmacology is changing rapidly in response to the molecular revolution. In previous decades neuropharmacology focused on the role of the synapse and, more particularly, on the effects of drugs on neurotransmitters or neurotransmitter receptors. The action of drugs on synaptic targets remains an important field of investigation. The initial target of a drug generally determines the particular cells and neural circuits on which the drug acts and at the same time the potential efficacy and side effects of the pharmacologic agent. However, the molecular revolution has made it clear that the initial binding of a drug to its target—for example, the binding of a drug to a neurotransmitter receptor—is only the beginning of a signaling cascade that affects the behavior of cells and ultimately complex circuits.

When a drug binds to a protein, it affects the functioning of that protein, thereby establishing a form of allosteric regulation. A drug can conceivably bind to any site on a protein. A simple site may involve just a few contiguous amino acid residues in a protein's primary structure, while a relatively complex site may involve discontinuous residues from the protein's primary structure that are brought near each other by the protein's secondary and tertiary structures. Ultimately, the three-dimensional shape, or conformation, of a binding site and the electrostatic charges distributed across the site must complement the shape and charge of the drug. The interaction of a drug with its binding site can influence the intrinsic activity of the target protein, for example, the catalytic activity of an enzyme or the conductance of an ion channel, or it can influence the ability of the protein to interact with some other molecule, such as the ability of a receptor to bind to its neurotransmitter.

In classic studies of drug mechanisms of action, a mechanism is defined by a drug's ability to bind to an unknown receptor in tissue homogenates or on tissue sections. In these studies the drug, which is the *ligand,* is radiolabeled and incubated with a tissue preparation, which is washed extensively to remove loosely bound drug. A radioactive atom, typically ^{3}H, ^{14}C, or ^{125}I, must be added to the drug without altering its ligand-binding properties, a process that can be exceedingly difficult. Three major criteria are used to assess the resulting ligand binding. First, the binding should be *specific;* that is, the ligand must bind to its specific target protein. Specific binding must be distinguished from binding to other proteins or even to the wall of a

plastic test tube. In many cases, binding is *stereoselective,* or specific for only one stereoisomer of a drug. Second, binding should be *saturable.* A limited amount of ligand binding occurs in the preparation because the amount of the specific target is limited. (A tissue preparation contains a finite amount of an individual receptor protein compared with a test tube wall, which is theoretically infinite.) Third, binding should attain a *steady state.* Time and other conditions, such as temperature, associated with incubation should enable the ligand binding to achieve a state of equilibrium.

The extent to which a ligand binds to a tissue preparation is a function of the concentration of the ligand (Figure 1–1). The total binding of a ligand to the tissue preparation comprises two components: 1) specific binding, which occurs in a theoretically finite number of specific receptor sites in the tissue preparation and is therefore saturable, and 2) nonspecific binding, which occurs in all other sites of drug interaction in the tissue preparation and may include binding to the wall of the test tube. In the ideal situation, in which binding to a specific receptor site is competitive and fully reversible in the steady state, specific binding can be defined as the fraction of total binding that can be displaced by incubating the radiolabeled ligand-tissue mixture with a large excess of unlabeled (cold) ligand. Conversely, the nondisplaceable radioactive portion of the preparation is considered nonspecific binding.

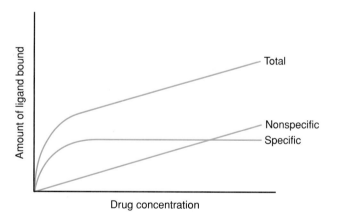

Figure 1–1. Radioligand binding assay. In this theoretical representation the amount of radioligand bound to a tissue preparation (e.g., homogenate, brain slice) is a function of the concentration of the radioligand. Total binding is the total amount of binding observed. Nonspecific binding represents the nonsaturable portion of binding that is presumably not associated with the specific binding site under investigation; it is often calculated as the binding of radioligand that persists in the presence of a large excess of nonradiolabeled ligand. Specific binding is calculated as the difference between total and nonspecific binding and reflects the amount of radioligand bound to the specific binding site.

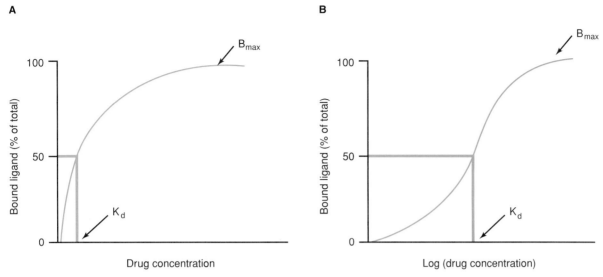

Figure 1–2. Determination of K_d and B_{max} from radioligand binding assays. The amount of specific radioligand binding to a specific site in a tissue preparation (determined in Figure 1–1) is plotted as a function of radioligand concentration, using a normal **(A)** or semi-logarithmic **(B)** plot. The K_d is calculated as the concentration of radioligand that results in 50% of maximal binding (B_{max}). The semi-logarithmic plot, which better illustrates the effects of low radioligand concentrations, places the K_d near the middle of the graph.

There are several discrepancies, however, between ideal and actual conditions. Not all binding to target proteins is truly reversible; the affinity of some ligand–receptor interactions is so high that resulting complexes are not readily dissociable. Moreover, artifactual sites may be present and may show striking apparent specificity. Some studies have even indicated that the binding of certain drugs to test tube walls may be stereoselective. While the ideal situation assumes that the tissue preparation contains just one specific target, in actuality many drugs can bind specifically to many related subtypes of a protein target; for example, serotonin can bind to numerous subtypes of serotonin receptors. Consequently, the resulting binding curves can be quite complicated and difficult to interpret.

The specific binding of a ligand to a tissue preparation is quantified according to two properties: the *affinity* of the binding, which is expressed as a dissociation constant (K_d), and the *total amount* of the binding (B_{max}) (Figure 1–2). These terms are analogous to those used in studies of enzyme kinetics—for example, the Michaelis–Menten equation—in which K_a is the activation constant for an enzyme and its cofactor, and V_{max} is the maximum catalytic activity of the enzyme. The K_d is defined as the concentration of ligand at which half of the specific binding sites are occupied; larger K_d values (e.g. 100 nM versus 1 nM) reflect lower affinities of the drug. When ligand binding is plotted as a function of the log of drug concentration, a sigmoidal curve is obtained (see Figure 1–2B). Such semi-logarithmic plots are typically used because they illustrate ligand

binding over a wide range of ligand concentrations and place the K_d roughly in the middle of the concentration curve.

Ligand binding data are often transformed mathematically to yield a *Scatchard plot,* in which the ratio of bound ligand to free ligand is plotted as a function of bound ligand (Figure 1–3). Because it is difficult to measure the amount of free (unbound) ligand, total ligand minus bound ligand is used. Under ideal conditions, and particularly in situations that involve a single binding site, binding data plotted in this manner yield a straight line: the K_d of ligand binding is the slope of the line and the B_{max} of ligand binding is the x-intercept (see Figure 1-3A). When more than one binding site is involved, convex curves are obtained (see Figure 1–3B), which can be resolved into multiple straight lines—and hence K_d and B_{max} values—for the individual sites.

Another method for studying ligand–target interactions makes use of *competition curves.* These curves describe the ability of a drug to compete with a radioligand in binding to a tissue preparation (Figure 1–4). The drug concentration at which half of the radioligand binding is displaced (K_i) is a measure of the affinity of the drug for a binding site in the context of a specific radioligand. Historically, such competition studies have played an important role in defining many subtypes of neurotransmitter receptors. Large numbers of norepinephrine analogs, for example, have been studied to evaluate their ability to compete with radiolabeled norepinephrine for binding to tissue prepara-

A

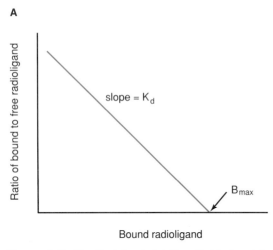

B

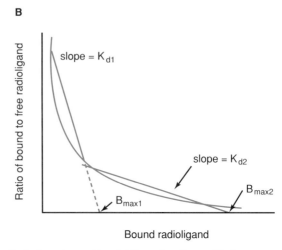

Figure 1–3. The Scatchard plot. Specific binding data are mathematically transformed to plot the ratio of bound to free radioligand as a function of bound radioligand. **A.** When one binding site is involved, the data follow a straight line. The slope of the line is the K_d and the x-intercept is the B_{max}. **B.** When more than one binding site is involved, the data follow convex curves, which can be converted into multiple straight lines. The slope of each line, and its x-intercept, represent the K_d and B_{max}, respectively, of each binding site.

tions, and as a result two populations of binding sites, which were termed α- and β-adrenergic receptors, have been delineated. In general, such pharmacologic distinctions of receptors accurately predicted broad categories of receptor proteins, which subsequently were identified with greater precision by means of molecular cloning techniques, as discussed later in this chapter.

In ideal situations, the competing drug and the radioligand bind to the same site of the target protein; such binding is termed *competitive*. In more complicated situ-

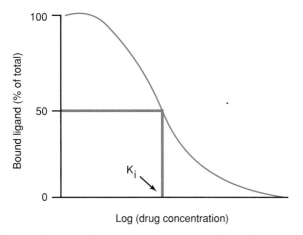

Figure 1–4. Radioligand competition curve. The ability of compounds to bind to a particular site in a tissue preparation can be compared by studying the ability of each to compete with a radioligand for a particular binding site. When the binding data are plotted on a semi-logarithmic graph, a sigmoidal curve results. The K_i represents the concentration of drug that results in a reduction of radioligand binding to 50% of maximal values.

ations, the drug and radioligand bind to different sites on the same protein; in such cases, the binding is *noncompetitive* and results in far more complicated competition curves.

These assessments of ligand binding can be performed in several different types of tissue preparation. The traditional preparation is a tissue homogenate or membrane fraction, although extracts of solubilized receptor or even samples of purified receptor may be used. An alternative approach, which provides critical data on the anatomic localization of a drug target, involves drug binding to tissue sections, a process termed *receptor autoradiography*. However, it is more difficult to obtain accurate measures of K_d and B_{max} from tissue sections than from solution assays.

As with any technique, the limitations of ligand binding assays, some of which have been presented in this chapter, must be appreciated. One of the most critical limitations is that binding assays, and the determination of K_d, K_i, and B_{max} values, are highly dependent on experimental conditions and therefore must be interpreted with considerable caution. The specific radioligand, the temperature of incubation, the salt and ionic content of the buffer, and the presence of different guanine nucleotides (see Chapter 5) are among the factors that can exert dramatic effects on ligand binding. The cloning of receptors and other target proteins and the ability to express them on cells without confounding background—for example, without endogenous expression of the target—have made at least some aspects of characterizing the binding properties of drugs more straightforward.

DRUG EFFICACY

Binding studies describe the physical relationship between a drug and its target but do not directly assess the biologic consequences of this association. Although drug binding and biologic effect are intricately related, they help define two distinct aspects of drug action: *potency* and *efficacy*. Potency (affinity, or K_d) describes the strength of the binding between a drug and its target. Efficacy describes the biologic effect exerted on the target by virtue of the drug binding. These properties can be understood by considering the effect of a drug on a neurotransmitter receptor. As previously explained, the drug must physically bind to the receptor, which requires a physical attraction between the two. Subsequently, that binding must elicit a change in the receptor that leads to a biologic response. For a G protein-coupled receptor, drug binding must trigger a conformational change in the receptor to enable it to interact with its G protein α subunit. For a ligand-gated channel (receptor ionophore), drug binding must trigger a conformational change that opens or closes the pore that is intrinsic to the receptor.

Drugs can differ dramatically with respect to their potency and efficacy. Traditionally, two categories of drug have been described: *agonist* and *antagonist*. When an agonist binds to a receptor, it mimics the endogenous neurotransmitter by producing the same conformational change and hence the same biologic response. According to this definition, all neurotransmitters are

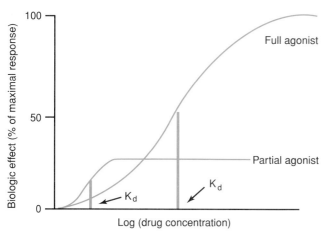

Figure 1–5. Drug efficacy versus drug potency. The biologic responses elicited by two drugs that bind to the same site are presented in this representation as a function of drug concentration. Efficacy refers to the maximal biologic response elicited by each drug. In this theoretical representation the partial agonist elicits a smaller maximal response than the full agonist. However, efficacy is independent of the potency (K_d) of the drug; the partial agonist is in fact more potent (possesses a higher affinity for the binding site) than the full agonist.

receptor agonists. When an antagonist binds to a receptor, it elicits no such change; thus, an antagonist is inherently inert and exerts a biologic effect only by interfering with an endogenous ligand. For opioid receptors, which are receptors for the endogenous opioid peptides, such as the enkephalins, **morphine** and **naloxone** are classic examples of an agonist and antagonist, respectively. The differences in efficacy associated with agonists and antagonists are independent of the affinity with which each binds to its receptor; both can exhibit high or low affinities. How can two molecules that bind to the same receptor site exert such different effects on the receptor? There are two possible explanations. An antagonist may share one moiety that is required for binding to the receptor with an agonist, but may lack a moiety required for efficacy. Alternatively, the antagonist and agonist may bind to overlapping but distinct sites on the receptor.

In addition to the actions of classic agonists and antagonists, an intermediate category of drug efficacy is exemplified by *partial agonists*. When a drug binds to a receptor and elicits only a partial biologic response, the drug presumably lacks a portion of the molecule required for full biologic effect or binds to a slightly different site on the receptor; such circumstances are indications of a partial agonist (Figure 1–5). An interesting situation arises when partial agonists possess high potency. At low drug doses, a mild agonist effect is obtained. At high doses, a similarly mild agonist effect is obtained because of limits in the intrinsic efficacy of the molecule. However, at high doses, the drug can antagonize the ability of a full agonist, including the endogenous neurotransmitter, to activate the receptor because its affinity is greater than that of the full agonist. For this reason, partial agonists are sometimes referred to as mixed agonists–antagonists. Partial agonists can be quite useful clinically; for example, **buprenorphine** is a partial agonist at opioid receptors and is used in the treatment of chronic pain. At low doses, buprenorphine elicits a mild analgesic effect. Higher doses not only fail to yield a stronger effect, which limits the abuse liability of this drug, but also antagonize the action of full opioid agonists and thereby discourage abuse of opiates such as **morphine**.

Inverse agonists achieve efficacy in still another way. When an inverse agonist binds to a receptor, it elicits the biologic response that is the opposite of that associated with an agonist. If an agonist opens an ion channel, an inverse agonist closes the channel. If an agonist facilitates receptor-to-G protein coupling, an inverse agonist attenuates such coupling. The action of an inverse agonist requires some basal activity on the part of the receptor, which means that the receptor is not quiescent in the absence of ligand but instead possesses some level of intrinsic biologic activity, such as channel conductance or G protein coupling. Indeed, considerable evidence currently suggests that most receptors do exhibit such intrinsic activity.

Very few drugs can be placed in discrete categories—agonist, antagonist, and inverse agonist. Many drugs that are classically described as agonists, such as **morphine,** are not full agonists but strong partial agonists. Conversely, many drugs that are classically categorized as antagonists—for example, **naloxone**—are not completely inert and thus can be very weak partial agonists. Moreover, some neurotransmitters show less efficacy than synthetic drugs, which indicates that they also are partial agonists. Consequently, drugs should be thought of as existing on a continuum ranging from full agonist to inert antagonist to full inverse agonist (Figure 1–6).

The complex nature of the interactions between drugs and their target receptors can be illustrated by a discussion of the γ-aminobutyric acid receptor (GABA$_A$)—an important receptor for the neurotransmitter GABA (see Chapter 7). This receptor is a heteropentamer that has two main types of subunits, α and β. GABA binds to a site on the β subunit and triggers the opening of a Cl$^-$ channel that is intrinsic to the receptor complex. **Muscimol** (an agonist) and **bicuculline** (an antagonist) also bind at this site and thus compete with GABA. The α subunit, and possibly the β subunit, of the GABA$_A$ receptor contains a binding site for a class of synthetic molecules known as **benzodiazepines.** Agonists that bind at this site, such as **diazepam,** are antianxiety agents that, when bound to the site, allosterically facilitate the ability of GABA to bind to and activate the GABA$_A$ receptor (see Chapters 7 and 15). Antagonists at this site, such as **flumazenil,** bind to the site but do not affect receptor function. Because this site lacks endogenous ligands, flumazenil is clinically inactive when bound to the GABA$_A$ receptor; however, it can be used to treat diazepam overdose because it displaces diazepam from the binding site. Inverse agonists, such as **β-carboline,** which intensify anxiety, bind very near the benzodiazepine agonist site and allosterically inhibit the ability of GABA to bind to and activate the receptor. Diazepam and β-carboline are a noncompetitive agonist and inverse agonist, respectively, of the GABA$_A$ receptor, in that they interact with a binding site distinct from the GABA site. Several other molecules that modulate GABA action also bind to the GABA$_A$ receptor complex; for example, **barbiturates,** a class of sedative-hypnotics (see Chapters 7 and 15), bind to a site within the pore of the receptor channel and, like benzodiazepine agonists, facilitate the ability of GABA to bind to and activate the receptor. Thus barbiturates

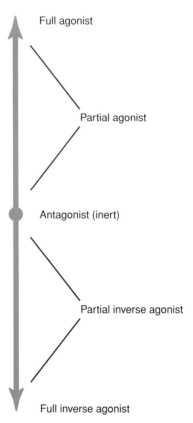

Figure 1–6. Drug efficacy as a continuum. Ligands for a receptor can be described as agonists (agents that activate the receptor), antagonists (agents that have no intrinsic effect on the receptor but can block the ability of agonists and inverse agonists to regulate the receptor), or inverse agonists (agents that regulate the receptor but produce effects opposite to those produced by agonists). However, ligands rarely can be placed into these discrete categories; instead they are distributed across a continuum. In strict pharmacologic terms, there are very few true antagonists, most being very weak partial agonists or inverse agonists, and very few full agonists or inverse agonists, most being strong partial agonists or inverse agonists.

are also considered noncompetitive agonists of the GABA$_A$ receptor.

Although this type of complex receptor pharmacology was first described for the GABA$_A$ receptor, it has been determined that a similar level of complexity can characterize drug interaction at virtually any type of receptor. This knowledge is contributing to the development of drugs with novel pharmacologic and hence clinical activity.

It must be emphasized that binding sites with a high affinity for drugs do not necessarily have an endogenous ligand. No evidence, for example, supports the existence of an endogenous ligand for the benzodiazepine binding site on the GABA$_A$ receptor. Rather, the discovery of this class of drugs and their binding site is testimony to the power and promise of medicinal chemistry to target distinctive features of proteins that are not exploited by nature.

DOSE-DEPENDENT DRUG RESPONSE

That the effect of a drug on a target protein is dependent on the concentration of a drug is implicit in the discussions of drug binding and efficacy presented in the preceding sections. This dose dependency of drug action is one of the principal tenets of neuropharmacology and illustrates the importance of studying the effects of a wide range of drug doses.

One application of dose-response curves is in determining whether a form of treatment—for example, chronic exposure to an antidepressant—increases or decreases the responsiveness of a particular receptor system. Hypothetical cases are illustrated in Figure 1–7, which shows that a reduction in receptor sensitivity in response to treatment is characterized by a rightward or downward shift in the dose-response curve, whereas an increase in receptor sensitivity is characterized by a leftward or upward shift in the dose-response curve.

Dose-response curves also can reveal that the biologic effects of a specific drug may not be a simple (monotonic) function of drug dose. The effects of some drugs vary in complex ways with respect to drug dose. When the effects of a drug are nonmonotonic, for example, they are represented by an inverted U-shaped curve (Figure 1–8). Such drugs elicit a progressively greater biologic response with greater drug dose up to a point, after which higher drug doses begin to

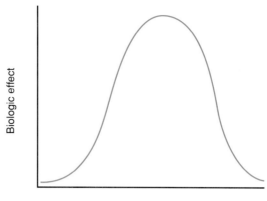

Log (drug concentration)

Figure 1–8. Inverted U-shaped dose-response curve. Dose-response curves that are placed on a semi-logarithmic plot often are not sigmoidal, such as those in previous figures, but instead form an inverted U shape. Such curves contain an ascending limb at lower drug doses and a descending limb at higher drug doses. These curves indicate that the biologic response elicited by a drug progressively increases as the drug dose increases and subsequently peaks at a moderate dose; higher doses elicit progressively smaller responses.

produce smaller effects. This shift in effect most likely occurs because the drug begins to act on a different target protein at higher drug doses, and action on the second target opposes the effects of the first. Alternatively, high doses may cause receptor desensitization.

The analysis of full dose-response curves is necessary to determine reliably whether a particular treatment causes an increase or decrease in drug responsiveness. Figure 1–9 shows a leftward shift in the dose-response curve for a drug whose biologic effects are an inverted U-shaped function of drug concentration. Without an analysis of the full dose-response curve, an investigator may incorrectly interpret effects of the drug; for example, depending on the concentration of drug used to activate the receptor, a shift in the curve may indicate a reduction, an increase, or a lack of change in drug response.

DRUG INTERACTION WITH NONRECEPTOR PROTEINS

Although most principles of drug action have been ascertained from studies of neurotransmitter and hormone receptors, the same general principles apply to interactions between drugs and nonreceptor proteins. A drug binds to a specific site on a protein, which can be determined by means of ligand binding assays. Drug binding influences the function of a protein by either facilitating or inhibiting that protein's normal functioning, including its interactions with other macro-

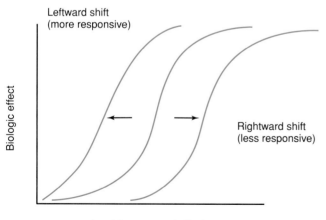

Log (drug concentration)

Figure 1–7. Rightward and leftward shifts in dose-response curves. A rightward, or downward, shift indicates a reduction in drug sensitivity: more drug is needed at all concentrations to elicit the same level of biologic response. A leftward, or upward, shift indicates an increase in drug sensitivity: less drug is needed at all concentrations to elicit the same level of biologic response.

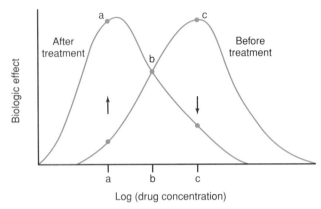

Figure 1–9. Analysis of a full dose-response curve. Because the biologic effects of many drugs are described by an inverted U-shaped dose-response curve, the effects of a drug should be analyzed over a wide range of doses. The graph shows a leftward shift in an inverted U-shaped dose-response curve occurring after an experimental treatment. With analysis of a single drug dose, it might be determined that the treatment causes (1) an increase in drug sensitivity (dose **a**); (2) no change in drug sensitivity (dose **b**); or (3) a decrease in drug sensitivity (dose **c**). The leftward shift in the dose-response curve becomes apparent only after a wide range of doses are analyzed.

molecules. Some drugs create a new function for the protein to which they bind; examples include **FK506** and related drugs that bind immunophilins (see Chapter 5). When such drugs bind to immunophilin proteins, the proteins become potent inhibitors of calcineurin, a protein phosphatase.

The conditions under which two proteins interact are conceptually similar to those for drug–target interactions. Protein–protein interactions have emerged as a central theme of cell regulation (see Chapters 5 and 6). The binding of proteins, such as transcription factors, to specific sequences of DNA—which is the major mechanism of gene expression in development and in neural plasticity in the adult—also operates according to principles like those of drug–target interactions.

NEUROPHARMACOLOGY IN THE MOLECULAR ERA

Neuropharmacology originally was a phenomenologic science. An investigator administered a drug to an animal or a cell preparation and examined the response. There were two major drawbacks to this black box approach (Figure 1–10A). First, it did not elucidate the mechanisms of drug action and thus did not enable investigators to relate the initial action of a drug on its protein target to the clinical effects of the drug. Earlier

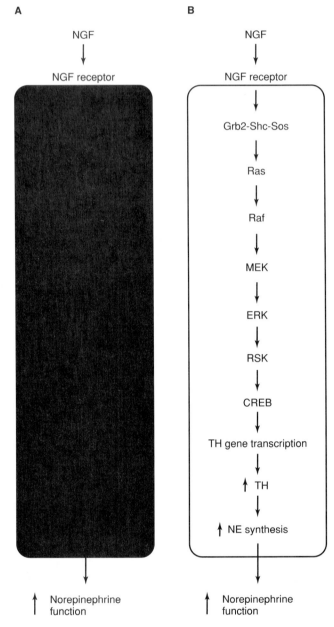

Figure 1–10. A comparison of black box and mechanistic approaches to neuropharmacology. The increased norepinephrine function in a sympathetic neuron caused by nerve growth factor (NGF) can be described in different ways. **A.** In classic studies, the effect of NGF was described in narrow, superficial terms—for example, NGF activates an NGF receptor—and insufficient attention was given to the detailed mechanisms by which drug-receptor interactions lead to a biologic response. **B.** In contrast, the tools of molecular and cell biology enable a detailed mechanistic description of NGF action, encompassing the delineation of the precise molecular steps by which activation of the NGF receptor leads to increased transcription of tyrosine hydroxylase (TH), the rate-limiting enzyme in norepinephrine synthesis. (See Chapters 5 and 11 for definitions of the various proteins shown in this figure.)

Box 1–1 Target Validation for CNS Drug Discovery

Neuropharmacologists are using the power of genetics, functional genomics, and proteomics to identify and validate new drug targets, including proteins and potentially even DNA sequences on which new drugs could act to produce important therapeutic effects. Functional genomics and proteomics, respectively, describe approaches to studying large-scale patterns of gene and protein expression or regulation. One type of functional genomics approach, for example, involves probing DNA microarrays containing many thousands of genes with cDNA samples from normal versus diseased tissue, or from control versus drug-treated tissue, to identify genes induced or suppressed by the experimental condition. These regulated genes or proteins are further studied to determine whether they might be promising drug targets.

Such new approaches are critically important for CNS therapeutics, especially for disorders in which the pathophysiology is not yet understood. To date, drug development for these disorders has largely depended on the clever exploitation of serendipitous findings. As described in later chapters, the initial antipsychotic drug **chlorpromazine** and the original antidepressant drugs **iproniazid** and **imipramine** were discovered during screening procedures for other types of treatment. Once their psychotropic effects were recognized, however, they became reference compounds that ultimately led to the improved drugs currently used. For example, working from existing drugs, the serotonin reuptake transporter was validated as a drug target for the development of antidepressants.

In some fields, the use of molecular genetic tools to develop drug targets is quite advanced. Recently, the entire genomes of several human pathogens, such as *Mycobacterium tuberculosis*, have been sequenced. Critical pathogen-specific proteins can now be identified and tested as targets for new antimicrobial agents. We will also be able to isolate the mutations that confer microbial resistance to current antibiotics, permitting even more sophisticated drug design.

Although the identification of valid drug targets in the nervous system is far more difficult, there are some exciting developments. As discussed in Chapter 20, certain rare familial forms of Alzheimer disease are caused by mutations in the gene that encodes amyloid precursor protein. These genetic findings, along with substantial biochemical evidence, have suggested that abnormal processing of this protein may cause Alzheimer disease not only in rare familial cases but also in more common forms of the illness. Pathways of amyloid processing have been investigated, and it appears that enzymes called β- and γ-secretases are involved in the production of pathogenic forms of amyloid (see Chapter 20). While much remains to be learned about the pathophysiology of Alzheimer disease, this brief description illustrates the impact of human genetic studies on the identification of drug targets. Thus, the recently identified secretase enzymes have become important targets for drug development.

The need for novel drug targets explains, in part, why it is so important to find genes that confer vulnerability to schizophrenia, manic-depressive illness, depression, autism, and many other CNS disorders about which we still know relatively little at the neurobiologic level. Such genes should provide clues to the pathogenic pathways involved in the disorders and as a result reveal fundamentally new targets for drug development.

---

in this chapter, it was pointed out that the actions of fluoxetine extend beyond inhibiting serotonin transporters or increasing serotonin function. To understand fully how fluoxetine works it is necessary to determine its action on the overall workings of the brain, from its effects on molecules and cells to its effects on neural systems and ultimately on behavior.

Second, traditional neuropharmacology depended on ligand binding studies to identify the protein targets of a drug and to understand its actions on brain function. Such protein targets were typically defined by potency series, which compared the ability of ligands to interact with different binding sites. Originally, α- and β-adrenergic receptors were defined as follows: α receptors show the potency series epinephrine $\geq$ norepinephrine $\gg$ isoproterenol, whereas β receptors show the potency series isoproterenol $>$ epinephrine $\geq$ norepinephrine.

However, many of the neurotransmitter receptors that were originally identified by ligand binding studies proved to be misleading once it became possible to identify individual proteins by molecular means with near-perfect precision. We now know, for example, that there are six distinct α-adrenergic receptor subtypes, and three distinct β-adrenergic receptor subtypes (see Chapter 8). Serotonin receptors provide still another example; pharmacologic studies determined that there are three major subtypes of serotonin receptors, which in turn have several variants (see Chapter 9). On the basis of receptor structure and function, we currently know that some of the receptors originally classified as type 1 are really type 2. The 5-HT$_{1C}$ receptor, for example, is currently referred to as 5-HT$_{2C}$. In addition, many receptor types, such as 5-HT$_{4-7}$, were not discovered with earlier pharmacologic techniques.

Box 1-2 The Search for Novel Receptor Ligands

Many therapeutic agents currently being used act as agonists or antagonists at receptors—particularly at G protein-coupled receptors, which are described in subsequent chapters. Yet many of these agents have undesirable side effects because they bind not only to their molecular targets, the receptors related to the symptoms of a disorder, but also to other receptors, producing unintended effects. The desire to reduce unwanted side effects has prompted researchers to engage in the process of rational drug design. Consequently, molecular targets have been cloned and their three-dimensional characteristics have been examined by powerful techniques, including crystallography, NMR spectroscopy, molecular biology, and computational modeling, to predict the exact structural features of ideal agonists and antagonists. Researchers hope that this process will enable them to discover and design highly selective agents that produce fewer side effects. However, this goal requires knowledge of the precise conformation of ligand binding sites on specific receptors, about which much remains to be known.

Modern drug research has supplemented rational drug design with the use of mass ligand screening, also called high throughput screening, to identify novel therapeutic agents. Such screening aims to determine the receptor binding properties of compounds—as many as possible and as rapidly and cost effectively as possible—that share a particular molecular target. Interactions between these compounds and the receptor, called "hits," are examined to determine each compound's potency at, and specificity for,

the target under consideration. Newer versions of high throughput screening go beyond the analysis of ligand binding and search for chemicals that act as functional agonists or antagonists at a particular receptor. Lead candidates are selected for subsequent analysis and structural optimization before they are tested in model systems, both in vitro and in vivo, and eventually examined in clinical trials.

High throughput screening draws from a chemical library of randomly synthesized proprietary compounds to create an infinite number of novel chemical structures. Combinatorial chemistry is the process by which large numbers of new chemicals are generated, many of which are virtual, existing only in computer form. Only chemicals determined by computer modeling to be a good fit for a receptor, or those for which a congener has shown promising properties for the receptor, are actually synthesized. Alternatively, natural product libraries, consisting of compounds extracted from microorganisms, amphibian or insect venom, or exotic plants, are used. Automated ligand screening allows the examination of several hundreds of thousands of compounds—entire chemical libraries—in less than a year, and typically results in the identification of 1 or 2 hits for every 10,000 compounds screened.

In recent years, many novel receptor ligands have been successfully identified by means of combinatorial chemistry and high throughput screening methods. Moreover, the general approach applied to receptors can be applied to almost any type of cellular protein that is a putative target for a drug.

Moreover, studies that focused on the binding of a drug to its receptor revealed only the simplest aspects of drug action. These studies did not account for the complex effects elicited by drugs on intracellular signaling cascades (Figure 1–10B) either after brief exposure, which results in rapid drug effects, or after long-term administration, which results in drug-induced neural plasticity.

Neuropharmacologists are currently using the penetrating tools of molecular biology and cellular physiology to extend their experimental repertoire. New research is aimed at defining the action of a drug on its cloned protein target in precise molecular terms and analyzing the protein target in various functional states—for example, in phosphorylated versus dephosphorylated states. Ultimately, investigators hope to delineate the crystal structure of these proteins before and after they are bound to a drug, so that they can better understand the ways in which a drug alters the shape and surface charges of a protein.

Neuropharmacologists are also using new approaches to identify and validate novel targets for drug develop-

ment (Box 1–1), so that novel drugs can be synthesized to interact with those targets. *Combinatorial chemistry* is enabling the development of a large number of drugs with unique and diverse chemical structures. It incorporates knowledge of drug–target interactions at the molecular level, or *structure–activity relationships,* to determine what types of chemical moieties can be added to a drug to alter its actions on a protein target. *High throughput screening* allows the analysis of a vast number of chemical agents to discover their abilities to influence cloned proteins of interest. Together, these tools may enable researchers to develop any desired types of drugs—for example, agonists, antagonists, weak partial agonists, or inverse agonists—for any targeted proteins (Box 1–2).

Neuropharmacologists also hope to learn how drug-induced molecular alteration in a target protein alters the functioning of the cell in which the protein is expressed. Consequently, we may discover the ways in which proteins function within a complex intracellular milieu and the changes that occur in response to drug–target interactions. Ultimately, we may understand how drugs alter the functioning of individual nerve cells and, in turn, how the altered functioning of neural circuits leads to changes in complex behavior.

MOLECULAR DIVERSITY OF THE BRAIN

Traditional neuropharmacology focused on a very narrow subset of cellular proteins, which included neurotransmitter receptors and transporters and proteins involved in the synthesis or degradation of neurotransmitters. Such proteins account for only a few thousand of perhaps hundreds of thousands of distinct gene products that are expressed in the brain once alternative splicing and protein processing are taken into account (see Chapter 6).

The concentration on neurotransmitter-based drugs excessively narrowed the scope of neuropharmacology and interfered with the development of drugs based on new mechanisms of action. Focusing on the 100,000 or more proteins expressed in the brain but not based on neurotransmitters is likely to lead to the identification of fundamentally novel classes of neuropharmacologic agents. Within the next few years, *functional genomics* and *proteomics*—the processes of sequencing, identifying, and characterizing individual gene products—will provide a template for exploring this vast array of proteins (see Box 1–1). Large numbers of proteins that

regulate receptor sensitivity already have been identified, as have large numbers of modulatory proteins that govern these regulatory proteins. Indeed, it is an exciting prospect that the completion of the various genome projects will allow us to know the full set of receptors and regulatory proteins expressed by nerve cells. Neuropharmacology in the postgenomics era will be involved with the development of drugs aimed at a new set of proteins and the clarification of the mechanisms by which these drugs regulate brain function. This potential transformation of current treatment of psychiatric and neurologic disorders holds great promise for the future.

SELECTED READING

Daeffler L, Landry Y. 2000. Inverse agonism at heptahelical receptors: concept, experimental approach and therapeutic potential. *Fundamentals Clin Pharmacol* 14:73–87.

Gura T. 2000. A chemistry set for life. *Nature* 407:282–284.

Hardman JG, Limbird LE. 1996. *Goodman and Gilman's The Pharmacological Basis of Therapeutics*, 9th ed. New York: McGraw-Hill.

Sweetnam PM, Rice CH, Ferkany JW. 1995. Mass ligand screening as a tool for drug discovery and development. In Wolff ME (ed). *Burger's Medicinal Chemistry and Drug Discovery*, 5th ed, pp. 697–731. New York: John Wiley and Sons.

Chapter 2
Neurons and Glia

KEY CONCEPTS

- The many different types of neurons in the brain communicate with one another at synapses.

- The nucleus and major cytoplasmic organelles in the cell body of neurons synthesize and process proteins, which are subsequently transported to their appropriate locations within the neuron.

- The axon transports molecules and conducts action potentials to presynaptic terminals to initiate communication with other neurons.

- Dendrites, multiple fine processes that extend from the neuronal cell body, together with the cell body, serve as the primary structure for the reception of synaptic contacts from other neurons.

- The cytoskeleton—the inner scaffold of a neuron formed by a system of interconnected protein filaments called microtubules, intermediate filaments, and actin filaments—plays a key role in the structure of neurons and in the transport of various proteins and organelles from the cell body to axonal and dendritic processes.

- Astrocytes, oligodendrocytes, and microglia are three major classes of glia that play important supporting roles in brain function.

- The blood–brain barrier, formed by tight junctions between endothelial cells of capillaries in cerebral vascular beds, allows only small lipophilic substances to enter the brain from the general circulation.

It has been estimated that there are at least 100 billion neurons in the human brain, although this number in itself reveals little of the brain's complexity. Unlike other organs, the brain contains an enormous diversity of cell types. Depending on the definition of a neuronal cell type, there may be thousands in the brain—each with their own structural, biochemical, and functional properties. A remarkable example of neuronal cell diversity has been provided by the systematic study of the amacrine cell, a type of interneuron in the retina. No fewer than 22 types of amacrine cells have been distinguished on the basis of their dendritic arborization and their stereotypic location within the layers of the retina. Yet the complexity of the brain as an information processing organ extends beyond its cellular diversity. Communication among neurons, which occurs through highly intricate and specific pathways, is so elaborate that any given neuron communicates with thousands of other neurons.

Communication among neurons occurs through a combination of electrical and chemical processes. The electrical process relies on the ability of each neuron to produce electrical signals under appropriate circumstances. However, the chemical process takes place because the vast majority of communicating neurons are not physically connected but are separated by a minute space, as small as 20–40 nm, called a synapse (the Greek word for *clasp;* Figure 2–1). The simplest synaptic arrangement involves an electrical impulse in one neuron, the presynaptic neuron, that triggers the release of a chemical substance, or neurotransmitter, which diffuses across the *synaptic cleft* and binds to specific receptors on another, the postsynaptic, neuron. The binding of a neurotransmitter to its appropriate receptors precipitates changes in the electrical activity of the postsynaptic neuron, which in turn leads to the release of a neurotransmitter and further interneuronal communication. In a small fraction of cases, neurons

Box 2-1 Seeing Is Believing: Neuroanatomic Visualization Techniques

Neuroanatomic visualization techniques are indispensable tools for exploring the mechanisms of nervous system functioning. They have allowed us to visualize and thereby categorize the widely varying morphologic and biochemical properties of cells in the nervous system and to delineate the detailed neural connectivity within the mammalian brain. Two of the most important methods for visualizing individual cells are the *Nissl* and *Golgi techniques* (named after Franz Nissl and Camillo Golgi, respectively).

The Nissl stain involves the application of cationic dyes, such as cresyl violet or toluidine blue, to nervous tissue, where they bind to the abundant aggregations of ribosomes (Nissl substance) in neurons and glia. Because these dyes stain virtually all neurons and astrocytes in exposed tissue samples, they are useful for surveying overall tissue architecture; for example, they can be used to distinguish different layers of the cerebral cortex or to gauge the integrity of brain tissue in response to injury. However, the Nissl stain is useful for visualizing only cell bodies; it does not reveal axonal and dendritic processes.

Use of the Golgi stain during the late nineteenth century initiated the modern era of neuroanatomy. This staining method involves several days of sequential application of potassium dichromate and silver nitrate to the tissue being examined. Such treatments result in the complete, dark staining of approximately 1% of cells in exposed tissue, including the soma, dendrites (as well as dendritic spines), and axon collaterals. The staining of such a small percent-

age of all cells is an important feature of the Golgi method because it allows detailed examination of individual cell morphology; if a higher proportion of cells were stained, the structural details of individual cells would be lost in the dense, overlapping array of neural processes (neuropil) found in most areas of the brain.

Intracellular filling techniques involve the use of sharp microelectrodes to provide images that are similar to those obtained with the Golgi stain. Stains that are injected directly into the cell's soma include *fluorescent dyes*, such as *Lucifer yellow*, and *enzymes*, such as *horseradish peroxidase*, that catalyze the oxidation of certain compounds to yield visible reaction products. Currently scientists are able to transfect neurons with genes that encode fluorescent proteins, such as *green fluorescent protein* (*GFP*), to achieve visualization of living neurons.

Modern visualization techniques also can provide important information about the biochemical characteristics of cells. *Histochemical*, or *cytochemical*, techniques are used to localize chemical substances in specific populations of neurons; *immunohistochemistry* involves the use of antibodies to recognize such substances. These substances include neurotransmitters and enzymes involved in the synthesis, uptake, or degradation of neurotransmitters. *In situ hybridization* is a modified histochemical technique that permits visualization of specific mRNA; short stretches of DNA (oligonucleotides) or stretches of RNA (riboprobes) that hybridize to specific mRNA are chemically or radioactively labeled and applied

---

physically connect with one another so that direct electrical transmission between the neurons can occur.

Neurons in the brain can form thousands of synapses with other neurons; for example, a Purkinje cell in the cerebellum or a monoamine-containing cell in the brain stem may form more than 100,000 synapses. Overall in a single human brain, there are likely to be more than 100 trillion synapses. Complex processes of brain development that are not fully understood result in connections among neurons that are both highly specific and highly plastic. Neurons form circuits with other neurons, some of which may be local and some of which may involve communication over long distances, such as interactions between the brain and spinal cord. Each neuron most likely functions in several overlapping circuits that work together to process input to and output from the brain (Box 2–1).

The overall patterns of neural connectivity in the mammalian central nervous system are dictated by a complicated set of genetically programmed interactions. Nevertheless, both spontaneous neural activity

and neural activity that occurs in response to experience during gestation and throughout life have profound influences on the fine-tuning of an individual's pattern of synaptic connections. Although there are critical periods of early postnatal development during which the pattern of neural connectivity in some brain regions is markedly influenced by experience, the adult brain is far more plastic than previously thought and synaptic connectivity is modified from birth until death. Thus, unlike computers, which are sometimes represented as artificial brains, the mammalian brain is not hard-wired but instead constantly reacts and adapts to an ever-changing environment.

Although the neuron is the critical cell type for communication in any neural network, essential supporting roles are played by glial cells. The brain contains three major classes of glia: astrocytes, oligodendrocytes, and microglia. Astrocytes have the most diverse functions, which include maintenance of the extracellular milieu (the composition of extracellular fluid in the brain) for healthy neuronal function, metabolism of certain neuro-

to tissue sections. *Electron microscopy* is used to reveal the internal, ultrastructural details of a cell; this technique can be combined with immunohistochemical or intracellular filling techniques to identify individual cells within a tissue section.

The visualization methods described thus far are used primarily to examine individual cells in the nervous system. Other equally important techniques permit analysis of the neural pathways that connect different regions of the brain. *Myelin stains* exploit the high phospholipid content of myelin to reveal large tracts of myelinated axons in low-power images of comprehensive sections of the brain, for example, for use in neuroanatomic atlases.

More detailed experimental analyses of neural connectivity rely on the use of *retrograde* and *anterograde tracers*. Nerve terminals can take up and retrogradely transport to the cell body a number of different substances, including horseradish peroxidase, various radioactive agents, and very small fluorescent latex beads. Small injections of such substances into a particular region of the brain allow investigators to trace the path taken by axons in the region and ultimately to localize their cell bodies. Indeed, several injections in different areas of a brain can reveal the collateral axon targets of small groups of neurons in a single brain nucleus. A current tool for retrograde tracing exploits neurotropic viruses. One example is *pseudorabies virus,* which is taken up by nerve terminals and subsequently transported to cell bodies. After it enters the cell bodies, the virus replicates and infects neighboring nerve terminals, which in turn transport it to their cell bodies, and the process continues. Because the virus can be detected by immunohistochemical staining for a viral protein, pseudorabies virus provides a time-dependent retrograde map of neural networks.

Anterograde tracers are taken up by cell bodies and transported anterogradely to nerve terminals. Radioactive amino acids, which are taken up by cell bodies and incorporated into proteins and some of these are transported to nerve terminals, are one type of anterograde tracer used. Autoradiography of treated tissue sections reveals a nearly precise distribution of the axons arising from the cells that have taken up the tracer.

The first retrograde and anterograde tracing techniques depended on neuronal response to injury. Experimental lesions of axon terminals caused retrograde reactions (chromatolysis) in the soma of the cells whose axons were damaged. Although such reactions could be revealed by the light microscope, they took two to three weeks to develop—a delay that limited the usefulness of this technique. Alternatively, the severing of axons from the cell bodies that emit them results in anterograde axonal degeneration, or wallerian degeneration, distal to the site of the cut. The degenerating axons can be stained by several techniques. Among the best known are the *Marchi stain,* which stains degenerating but not intact myelin, and various modifications of the *Nauta stain,* which exploits the tendency of degenerating fibers and nerve terminals to take up silver.

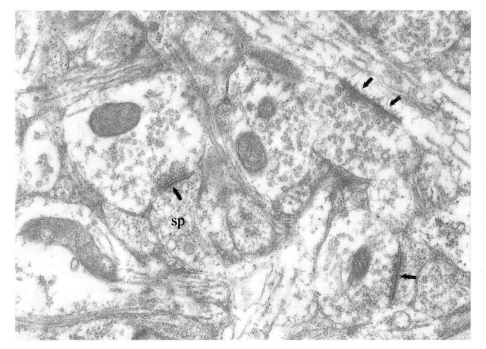

Figure 2–1. Electron micrograph of excitatory synapses. Each excitatory synapse forms an asymmetric junction, which exhibits a prominent postsynaptic thickening called the postsynaptic density (*arrows*). Axon terminals opposite the postsynaptic density contain small, spherical vesicles. One terminal can be seen making contact with a dendritic spine (sp). (Micrograph borrowed with permission from J. Buchanan, Stanford University School of Medicine.)

transmitters, and formation of the blood–brain barrier. Astrocytes also are critical in the CNS response to injury. Within the CNS, oligodendrocytes produce myelin sheaths that encase axons, facilitating the conduction of action potentials. Microglia, together with lymphocytes and macrophages that migrate to the CNS from the periphery, are the cellular components of the brain's immune system. All types of glia elaborate soluble factors, including neurotrophic factors and cytokines, which are involved in the maintenance of the nervous system and in its adaptation to changes in the environment. Glia also are key components in guiding the migration of growing neurons during development.

The basic features of neurons and glia are reviewed in this chapter. More detailed discussions of the electrical excitability of neurons and the molecular and cellular basis of synaptic transmission are provided in subsequent chapters.

THE NEURON

Neurons are highly asymmetric (polarized) cells that have three major components: a cell body (also known as a soma or perikaryon), a single long process called an axon, and a varying number of branching processes known as dendrites (Figure 2–2). Aggregations of neuronal cell bodies form the gray matter of the brain (named for its appearance on freshly cut sections), including the cerebral and cerebellar cortices and subcortical collections of cell bodies called nuclei. Axons make up the white matter, whose appearance results from the myelin sheaths that insulate many axons and facilitate the conduction of action potentials. Although most neurons share a common set of features, they have a variety of sizes and shapes (Figure 2–3) and serve very different functions within the networks in which they operate.

THE CELL BODY

The cell body contains the nucleus and major cytoplasmic organelles such as the rough and smooth endoplasmic reticulum (ER) and Golgi apparatus, or Golgi complex (Figure 2–4). It is primarily responsible for synthesizing and processing proteins, which are subsequently transported to their appropriate locations within the neuron. The nucleus contains genomic DNA that it transcribes to mRNA; mRNA is exported from the nucleus to the cytoplasm, where it is translated into protein (see Chapter 6). Although most mRNA remains in the cell body, some of it is transported to dendrites and axon terminals. The translation of mRNA to protein occurs on ribosomes, some of which are attached to the rough ER and some of which exist

freely in the cytosol. Proteins that are soluble are formed on free ribosomes, and membrane and secretory proteins are formed on rough ER. After they are synthesized, secretory and membrane proteins are transported to the Golgi apparatus, where they are further modified by the addition of sugar chains, the

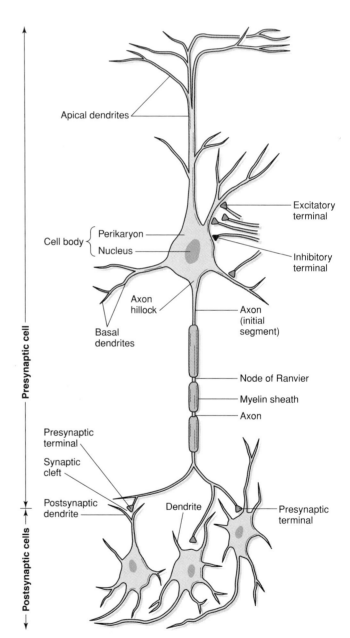

Figure 2–2. Principal features of a typical vertebrate neuron. Dendrites, which are the primary sites of synaptic contact, receive most of the incoming synaptic communication. The cell body contains the nucleus and is the site of gene transcription. The axon transmits information and often has multiple branches, the terminals of which form synapses with the dendrites of other neurons. (Reproduced with permission from Kandel ER, Schwartz JH, Jessell TM. 2000. *Principles of Neuroscience*, p. 22. New York: McGraw-Hill.)

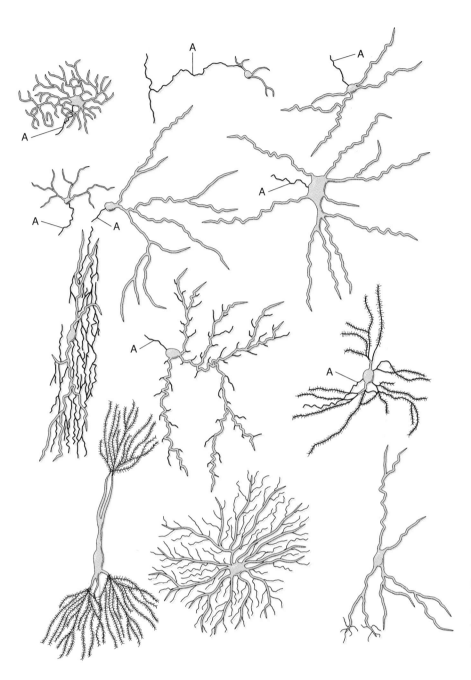

Figure 2–3. Drawings of typical neurons in the CNS. (A) marks the axons of some of these neurons. (Adapted with permission from Carpenter MB. 1996. *Carpenter's Human Neuroanatomy,* 9th ed., p. 143. Baltimore: Williams and Wilkins.)

attachment of fatty acids, or the sulfation of tyrosine residues. Modified proteins are packaged into vesicles that are conveyed along the neuronal cytoskeleton by various forms of axoplasmic transport and are directed to their appropriate locations in axons or dendrites. Axonal transport not only has a constitutive component to replace inactivated or degraded proteins but also can be regulated in response to changes in the neuronal environment. Likewise, it enables breakdown products within axons, and signaling molecules taken up from the extracellular space, to be transported to the cell body.

Proteins are transported to highly specific locations within neurons; some proteins are found only in axons or axonal terminals and others are found only in dendrites. Moreover, although most protein synthesis occurs in the cell body, ribosomes involved in protein synthesis and processing can be found elsewhere. Polyribosomes, which are multiple ribosomes arrayed on mRNA, and ER are found in dendrites, often right beneath synapses, where they presumably permit localized protein synthesis. However, the conveyance of mRNA to dendritic regions is a highly regulated process and only a small percentage of mRNA undergoes this process. Small

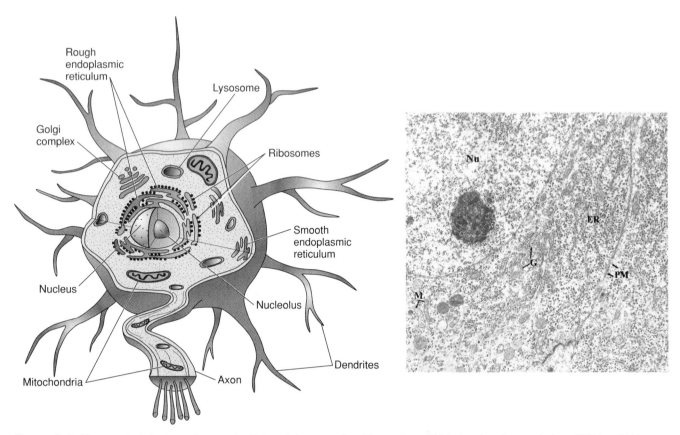

Figure 2–4. Diagram and electron micrograph of intracellular organelles. The nucleus (Nu) is the site of transcription of DNA to RNA. Proteins are synthesized in the endoplasmic reticulum (ER) and subsequently transported to the Golgi complex (G) where they undergo further modifications before they are transported to their final destination. Also shown are mitochondria (M), the energy storehouses for the cell, and the plasma membrane (PM). (Micrograph borrowed with permission from J. Buchanan, Stanford University School of Medicine.)

amounts of specific mRNA also are transported to axon terminals, most likely to enable more rapid changes in protein synthesis in response to synaptic activity.

The cell body is the smallest part of the neuron; the bulk of cytoplasmic volume is distributed throughout the axon and the dendritic arbor, or tree, which may be very large. Yet because it must produce components that sustain the rest of the neuron, the metabolic and synthetic demands upon the neuronal cell body are immense. Thus, the cell body contains large numbers of mitochondria, which are the sites of oxidative phosphorylation and thus provide the form of energy (adenosine triphosphatase [ATP]) used by all major eukaryotic cells.

THE AXON

The axon is a fine tubular process that extends from the neuronal cell body; it conducts electrical impulses from the cell body to the axon terminals (presynaptic boutons) that form the presynaptic component of a synapse. Projection neurons are those that send axons to another region of the CNS or to the periphery, as opposed to interneurons whose axons remain within the CNS region of origin. Neurons generally have a single axon, the length of which varies from less than a millimeter for interneurons to more than a meter for motor neurons that innervate the extremities. The axons of long projection neurons typically are myelinated; those of local circuit neurons usually do not have myelin sheaths. The axon normally emerges from a region of the cell body called the axon hillock (see Figure 2–2), the region of the neuron from which an action potential is most often generated (see Chapter 3). As it approaches its terminal field of innervation, an axon may branch to varying degrees, depending upon the number of neurons with which it makes synaptic contact. Axons also may give rise to recurrent collaterals that often serve feedback regulatory functions. Some neurons make very restricted synaptic contacts and thus have fairly limited axonal arbors. Other neurons have axons that arborize extensively, contacting millions of neurons in their terminal fields of innervation.

The axon is considered the simplest component of the neuron. Generally devoid of ribosomes or other intracellular organelles, except mitochondria, it is responsible for transporting molecules and conducting action potentials to presynaptic terminals to initiate communication with other neurons. The presynaptic terminal typically forms one side of a synapse and is responsible for the release (or secretion) of neurotransmitter (see Figure 2–2); however, not all synapses are formed at axon terminals. As they course through the dendritic arborizations of the postsynaptic neurons they innervate, some axons express small expansions, termed *en passant* boutons, that contain all the machinery necessary for neurotransmitter release and form functional synapses. In fact, the terms presynaptic terminal and presynaptic bouton are often used interchangeably, despite their different origins.

DENDRITES

Dendrites are multiple fine processes that extend from the neuronal cell body and, together with the cell body, serve as the primary structure for the reception of synaptic contacts from other neurons. The geometry of dendritic arbors can be very complex and indeed beautiful (see Figure 2–3). The precise location and extent of a dendritic arbor determine the role of a cell in a network. Many types of neurons, especially those with a pyramidal shape, have discrete spines protruding from their dendrites (Figure 2–5). Such spines typically receive the major excitatory inputs directed to their respective cells; however, they also may receive additional synaptic input. Moreover, the spines may structurally and biochemically isolate synapses so that each synapse serves as a small, individual unit of information processing (see Chapter 4). Investigations of neuronal plasticity have revealed that dendritic spines are not immutable; rather neuronal cells can regulate the number and morphology of their spines in response to neural activity and other cues from the environment.

Although it can be difficult to distinguish the axonal arbors of a neuron from its dendritic tree, dendrites have several distinct morphologic features that differ from those of axons. The diameter of an axon is relatively constant throughout its length, but the diameter of a dendrite decreases along its branches; the dendritic branch emanating from the soma is much thicker than secondary or tertiary branches. Dendrites also contain organelles that are not found in axons, and several proteins are dendrite- or axon-specific.

The main functions of the dendritic tree include the reception, processing, and integration of incoming synaptic communications. Initially dendrites were believed to be rather passive structures that integrated synaptic

inputs simply by means of their basic electrical properties (see Chapter 3). Currently we know that dendrites are both electrically and biochemically quite complex. Dendrites, like axons, contain voltage-dependent ion channels and thus can fire action potentials and actively propagate information to the soma. They also contain a wide variety of intracellular signaling molecules (see Chapter 5) that are activated during synaptic communication and can profoundly influence neuronal functioning.

THE CYTOSKELETON AND THE TRANSPORT OF PROTEINS

The *cytoskeleton*, which represents the inner structure, or scaffold of a neuron, is formed by a system of interconnected molecular filaments termed *microtubules*,

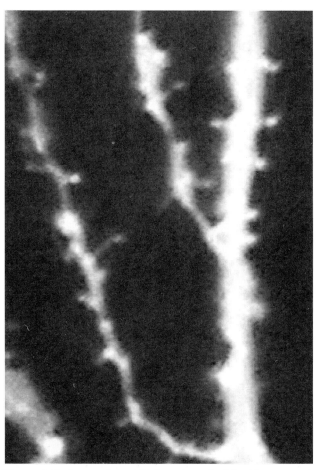

Figure 2–5. Image of dendritic branches of a living hippocampal pyramidal neuron reveals a high density of dendritic spines. This cell was stained with a fluorescent dye and imaged using 3D laser confocal fluorescence microscopy. (Image borrowed with permission from M. E. Dailey and S. J. Smith, Stanford University School of Medicine.)

intermediate filaments, and *actin filaments.* Microtubules are made of polymers of tubulin, a globular protein that forms a heterodimer between α and β tubulin. Microtubules copurify with several microtubule-associated proteins (MAPs), which have significant roles in the assembly of microtubules, in cross-linking them to other filaments, and in transport functions. Intermediate filaments of neurons, called neurofilaments, are formed by three polypeptide subunits with different molecular masses: 200 kDa (NF-H; high), 160 kDa (NF-M; middle), and 68 kDa (NF-L; low). Actin filaments (also called microfilaments) are made of actin, a globular protein that self-assembles into a linear polymer. Microtubules and intermediate filaments are cross-linked to form a longitudinal scaffold for axons and dendrites. Actin microfilaments form a network underneath the entire surface membrane of the neuron; in dendrites and axons they are connected to microtubules and intermediate filaments. Interestingly, actin microfilaments are heavily concentrated in dendritic spines and growth cones, both of which are dynamic structures that can respond to extracellular signals by changing shape.

Among the various drugs that act on these cytoskeletal components is **colchicine,** a potent antiinflammatory drug used primarily in the treatment of **gout arthritis.** It disrupts microtubule function by binding directly to tubulin; consequently it disrupts the ability of leukocytes to migrate to a location of inflammation. Experimentally, it is often used to study processes that depend on microtubular function.

Colchicine

Cytochalasin D, which disrupts actin filaments, is used experimentally to study the role of actin in cellular processes.

The cytoskeleton, which is specialized according to the distinct cellular compartments of the neuron in which it is found, not only has important structural functions but also plays a key role in the transport of proteins from the cell body to axonal and dendritic processes. This discovery was first made in 1948, when investigators ligated a nerve with a thread and found that axons were grossly distended proximal to the ligature and narrowed distal to it. They determined that

cellular material must be able to flow in an anterograde (cell body to terminals) direction. Currently we know that both fast anterograde and retrograde transport of proteins (100–400 mm/day) and slow anterograde transport (0.1–3.0 mm/day) occurs in axons. Fast anterograde axonal transport involves the movement of transport vesicles, derived from the Golgi, along axonal microtubules. As previously mentioned, these vesicles contain many of the proteins necessary for the functioning of the presynaptic terminal.

The power to move vesicles along microtubules by fast axonal transport is derived from two force-generating proteins, *kinesin* and *dynein.* These proteins are ATPases that, by binding to microtubules, are stimulated to transport vesicles. Because microtubules have an intrinsic polarity, with plus ends pointing toward presynaptic terminals and minus ends pointing toward the cell body, they can serve as a compass to direct vesicle traffic. Kinesin and dynein also have an intrinsic polarity; kinesin moves vesicles only toward the plus end of microtubules and therefore is the motor protein for anterograde fast transport, and dynein moves them only toward the minus end and thus is the motor protein for retrograde fast transport. Retrograde axonal transport functions to return various membrane molecules to the soma for elimination and may also be important for communicating information from nerve terminals to the soma. This form of transport enables the trophic factor known as nerve growth factor (NGF; see Chapter 11) to be taken up by presynaptic terminals and, together with its receptor and, in some cases, its postreceptor signaling proteins, to be transported to the cell body, where it can influence gene expression in the nucleus.

The molecular mechanisms responsible for slow axonal transport and for the transport of proteins to dendrites are not well understood. Slow axonal transport appears to utilize the proteins that comprise the cytoskeleton itself—a dynamic rather than a static structure that is continually renewed. Proteins that are specifically directed toward dendrites rather than axons must be guided by molecular recognition signals that dictate the direction of transport. We know that the cytoskeleton of dendrites is different from that of axons. Unlike axons, in which the polarity of microtubules is fixed, dendrites have microtubules whose polarity varies because equal numbers of microtubules are oriented in each direction. The proteins associated with dendritic microtubules also differ from those of axonal microtubules; MAP2 is found only in dendrites and in the cell body, whereas the protein tau is found almost exclusively in axons. Perhaps these differences play a role in guiding the transport of specific proteins toward dendrites.

Box 2–2 Identification of Neurotransmitters in the Brain

Our understanding of the molecular basis of neuropharmacology is significantly dependent upon our ability to identify neurotransmitters in the mammalian brain. Although the definition of a neurotransmitter has become more complicated with the discovery that intercellular messengers in the brain can communicate across a substantial distance, are not restricted to communication across a synaptic cleft, and also may not require transport in presynaptic vesicles, criteria can be established for the purpose of classifying a chemical substance as a neurotransmitter. Theoretically, a substance that is released in response to stimulation of a specific neural pathway and that is sufficient to generate a measurable postsynaptic response, electrophysiologic or biochemical, should be classified as a neurotransmitter. However, the overwhelming complexity of the mammalian brain and its relative inaccessibility requires more indirect criteria.

Localization

A putative neurotransmitter must be localized to presynaptic terminals (or in some cases to dendrites or somas) in specific neural pathways (see Box 2–3). Techniques for such localization include immunohistochemical staining and biochemical analysis of regional concentrations of the substance under study. Often these techniques can be combined with the placement of lesions that cause the degeneration of specific neural pathways. The localization of enzymes required for the synthesis, degradation, or uptake of the substance helps to confirm the identification of a neurotransmitter.

Release

To determine whether stimulation of a particular brain region or pathway causes the release of a substance, extra-cellular fluid can be collected with a technique such as microdialysis. The electrochemical detection of substances, for example, by means of voltametry, may be possible in some cases. The release of a substance is relevant to classic synaptic transmission only if it is dependent on extracellular Ca^{2+}; thus such dependency must be confirmed (see Chapter 4).

Synaptic Mimicry

The action of a suspected neurotransmitter should be mimicked by exogenous application of the substance. Such mimicry can be accomplished in vitro by application of the substance to reduced brain preparations, or in vivo by means of microiontophoresis. The substance's actions can be evaluated by means of electrophysiologic, biochemical, or behavioral measurements.

Synaptic Pharmacology

Neurotransmitters act on receptors for which there are often a plethora of pharmacologic antagonists and agonists. Thus, if the action of a synaptically released substance is blocked by a known receptor antagonist, the identity of the neurotransmitter is strongly suggested. Of course, the antagonists and agonists used to identify neurotransmitters should produce the same effects when they are exogenously applied to neurons; exogenous confirmation of these effects offers the most convincing criteria for establishing the identity of neurotransmitter. Receptor agonists also may be used to demonstrate synaptic mimicry but may provide inaccurate results because various receptor subtypes often can be coupled to the same postsynaptic effector mechanisms.

THE SYNAPSE

A synapse is a specialized structure involved in the transmission of information from one neuron to another. Synapses typically are composed of a single presynaptic element—the presynaptic terminal or bouton of an axon—and a postsynaptic element, which for excitatory synapses is often a dendritic spine. Although the *synaptic cleft* lies between these two elements, it is incorrect to think of the cleft as empty space that separates two independent structures. Instead the presynaptic and postsynaptic elements of a synapse are tightly bound to one another and to the extracellular matrix by means of a number of proteins, such as cell adhesion molecules (CAMs), cadherins, and integrins. Thus the synapse, both functionally and structurally, should be considered an individual unit whose sole purpose is to transmit and process information.

Most synapses in the brain involve chemical messengers called neurotransmitters (Box 2–2), which typically are released from presynaptic terminals. Neurotransmitters diffuse across synaptic clefts and attach to specialized receptor proteins on postsynaptic cells (see Chapter 4). The presynaptic terminal contains a number of cellular structures that allow it to remain, to a certain extent, metabolically and functionally independent from the neuronal cell body. It contains large numbers of mitochondria to provide energy in a rapid and efficient fashion, enzymes to synthesize and degrade neurotransmitters, and synaptic vesicles to store substantial concentrations of neurotransmitter in a protected state while they wait for the signal to be released. In contrast,

Box 2–3 The Many Faces of Synaptic Transmission

A synapse was initially defined as a postsynaptic dendrite or cell body undergoing innervation by a presynaptic nerve terminal (**A**). This classic definition described a synapse both structurally and functionally in terms of presynaptic and postsynaptic elements. Although such synapses, which can be termed *axodendritic* or *axosomatic*, are widespread in the CNS and may represent the predominant mode of synaptic transmission involving excitatory and inhibitory amino acids, we have learned that many additional types of synaptic transmission occur in the brain.

Research has determined that axoaxonic synapses also occur throughout the CNS. An axoaxonic synapse occurs when neurotransmitter released from one nerve terminal acts on receptors located on other nearby nerve terminals (**B**). Such nerve terminals may be functionally presynaptic in one synapse but functionally postsynaptic in another. Although axoaxonic synapses lack the specializations typical of many axodendritic synapses, it is likely that axoaxonic synapses contribute an essential dimension to the integration of complex interneuronal communication that occurs in functioning neural circuits. Neurotransmitters also can act by means of autoreceptors located on the same terminals that release them (**C**). In a few cases, a neurotransmitter released from cell bodies or dendrites may act on neighboring nerve terminals (**D**), resulting in a *dendroaxonic* synapse.

It is likely that various types of synaptic relationship coexist in most regions of the brain. Consider a hypothetical situation in which an excitatory amino acid nerve terminal innervates a dendritic spine by means of a classic axodendritic synapse (**E**). In addition to acting on the dendritic spine, the released glutamate can affect further glutamate release by acting on autoreceptors at its own nerve terminals. Glutamate release is further modulated by nearby γ-aminobutyric acid (GABA)-ergic nerve terminals, which function as axoaxonic synapses with the glutamatergic terminals. More extensive modulation occurs at monoaminergic terminals; released monoamine modifies glutamate release from glutamatergic nerve terminals by means of actions on presynaptic receptors and modifies postsynaptic responses to glutamate through actions on receptors on the dendritic spines. Although this description of a synapse is hypothetical and represents a simplification of the complex local circuits in the CNS, similar relationships have been experimentally confirmed in many brain regions.

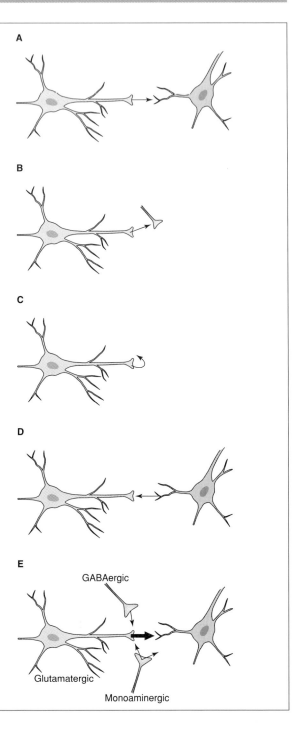

the postsynaptic dendritic membrane at the synapse is markedly enriched with appropriate neurotransmitter receptors and intracellular signaling machinery, which together complete the transmission of the message delivered by the released neurotransmitter.

Synapses that involve the innervation of a postsynaptic dendrite by a presynaptic nerve terminal represent just one anatomic arrangement of chemical synapses. Other arrangements are described in Box 2–3. Overall, chemical synapses are predominant in the CNS but do not represent the only form of synaptic transmission. In far less frequent instances, neurons are connected by means of a gap junction rather than separated by an intervening space. Gap junctions, which are formed by a large number of tightly packed proteins (connexons), produce so-called electrical synapses that permit electrical currents to flow directly between cells. Research regarding the structure of the synapse and the process of synaptic transmission has been critical to our understanding of the nervous system and the actions of drugs in the brain (see Chapter 4).

GLIA

ASTROCTYES

One of the three main types of glial cells in the brain, astrocytes constitute between 25% and 50% of the cellular volume of most brain regions. Although a subset of these cells is morphologically reminiscent of stars as their name implies, their form varies widely. In gray matter the predominant form is the protoplasmic astrocyte, whereas in white matter the predominant

form is the fibrous astrocyte. In addition to their shape, astrocytes can be identified by the unique intermediate filaments composed of glial fibrillary acidic protein (GFAP) that fill their processes. Accordingly, antibodies to GFAP robustly stain astrocytes but not neurons.

Partly because of their high concentration of filaments, astrocytes give structure to the brain. Their processes extend to the pia mater, one of the membranes that cover the brain, to the ependyma, which lines the brain's ventricular system, and to the serosal surface of capillaries that penetrate the brain parenchyma. Moreover, astrocytes extend processes to the cell bodies of neurons and form sheaths around breaks in myelin (nodes of Ranvier) and around many synapses as well (Figure 2–6; see also Chapter 3). Astrocytes also help to keep the brain isolated from the general circulation. They play a central role in building and maintaining the blood–brain barrier by inducing endothelial cells that line capillaries in the brain to form tight junctions between cells.

Astrocytes serve many functions in the mature brain in addition to providing structure (Table 2–1). Radial glia, which are the embryonic precursors of astrocytes,

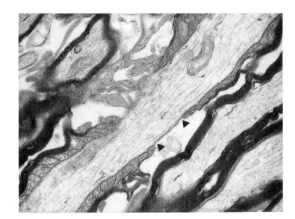

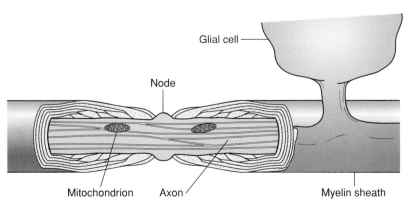

Figure 2–6. Electron micrograph and diagram of a single node of Ranvier. A break in the myelin sheath at the node (*between arrowheads in photomicrograph*) exposes the axonal plasma membrane to the extracellular space (see Chapter 3). (Image borrowed with permission from J. Kocsis, Yale University.)

Table 2–1 Functions of Astrocytes

Neuronal survival
Secretion of neurotrophic factors
Regulation of apoptosis
Regulation of the extracellular milieu, including K⁺, glutamate,
γ-aminobutyric acid (GABA)
Glycogen storage

Neuronal differentiation
Regulation of neuronal migration
Regulation of axon and dendrite outgrowth

provide a scaffolding, or path, for the migration of neurons—a critical event in the development of the mature architecture of the brain. Astrocytes also synthesize adhesion molecules and extracellular matrix proteins, including CAMs, fibronectin, and laminin. These proteins are involved in neuronal migration and may play a role in axonal pathfinding. As previously mentioned, astrocytes also elaborate neurotrophic factors and cytokines throughout life—molecules that are involved in the development and maintenance of both neurons and glia (see Chapter 11).

Because astrocytes take up excess neurotransmitters and ions, including K⁺, that are a product of neurotransmitter release and receptor activation, they help maintain the extracellular milieu that surrounds neurons during synaptic transmission (see Chapter 3). Among transporters that are known to promote the reuptake of excitatory amino acid neurotransmitters, the highest density are found on astrocytes. Astrocytes also may play a heretofore unappreciated role in neuronal communication because they can be coupled to each other by means of gap junctions and can generate intracellular Ca^{2+} waves in response to activity in neurons. Moreover, some astrocytes express proteins normally considered neuronal, such as ion channels and neurotransmitter receptors. Although the physiologic significance of these properties remains unclear, they suggest that astrocytes can alter their function in response to neuronal activity in their vicinity.

Research indicates that astrocytes also may be involved in disease. After **brain injury,** inflammation, and some types of infection, and in response to neurodegenerative processes such as **Alzheimer disease,** astrocytes hypertrophy and may proliferate. Such reactive gliosis is accompanied by alterations in gene expression in the reactive glia and the elaboration of cytokines and other soluble factors. Some of these factors may recruit additional glia to respond to injury, which under extreme circumstances can result in damage to large numbers of nearby neurons.

OLIGODENDROCYTES AND SCHWANN CELLS

Oligodendrocytes in the CNS and Schwann cells in the peripheral nervous system produce and ensheathe axons with myelin. By forming a relatively thick layer of insulation, myelin plays a critical role in permitting rapid electrical conduction down axons by markedly diminishing the capacitance of the neuronal membrane and increasing its resistance (see Chapter 3). Whereas Schwann cells can produce only one myelin sheath, oligodendrocytes can produce several of them. This is accomplished by the oligodendrocyte membrane wrapping itself in multiple layers around the axon (see Figure 2–6). A small gap in myelin, called a node of Ranvier, exists between each myelinated segment of an axon. Within these nodes, the axon expresses a high level of voltage-gated Na⁺ channels, which permit the regeneration of an action potential (see Chapter 3).

Although the major chemical components of myelin in the CNS differ from those of myelin in the peripheral nervous system, both types contain hydrophobic proteolipids that function as insulators. Thus the destruction of myelin sheaths can lead to marked deficits in nerve conduction velocity and a variety of sensory and motor deficits. Such deficits are characteristic of **multiple sclerosis,** a disease caused by the destruction of oligodendrocytes and the subsequent loss of myelin, presumably in response to an autoimmune mechanism (see Chapter 11).

MICROGLIA

Microglia, which subserve immunologic functions in the brain and spinal cord, are among the defense mechanisms against infectious diseases of the CNS. Although the source of microglial cells remains controversial, it is believed that they are derived primarily from monocytic progenitor cells of bone marrow that enter the brain and undergo differentiation; thus many microglia appear to be related to peripheral macrophages. Evidence suggests that some microglia also may be derived from glial lineages, although this pathway remains incompletely characterized. Like astrocytes, microglia respond to insult and injury with alterations in their morphology and number and thereby play a critical role in tissue defense and repair. However, as with immune cells in other tissues, excessive activation of microglia can be deleterious and may contribute to inflammatory, and perhaps neurodegenerative, disorders of the CNS. Microglia are, for example, major mediators of the CNS effects of **human immunodeficiency virus (HIV) infection** (Box 2–4).

Box 2–4 Microglia and HIV Infection

Microglia and peripheral macrophages are the primary targets of human immunodeficiency virus (HIV) infection in the CNS, sometimes called neuro-AIDS. At different stages in their development, microglia express chemokine receptors—CCR_3, CCR_5, and $CXCR_4$ (see Chapter 11)—that belong to the G protein-coupled receptor superfamily (see Chapter 5) and are essential coreceptors for HIV. In vitro, for example, HIV requires the presence of one of these receptors on vulnerable lymphocytes to penetrate and infect the cells.

Most likely, infection of the CNS begins in perivascular cells, although infected microglia can be found deep in the brain parenchyma. HIV is transmitted to microglia primarily by means of infected lymphocytes, or infected cells of the monocyte–macrophage lineage, in the peripheral blood circulation. These cells most likely cross the blood–brain barrier

as a result of local inflammation and changes in endothelial adhesion molecules. In severe cases of HIV infection, there may be an overwhelming loss of blood–brain barrier integrity.

The link between HIV-infected microglia and the cognitive and motor dysfunction associated with neuro-AIDS most likely can be attributed to disruption of normal microglial–neuronal interactions. Elevated levels of certain cytokines, which are secreted by microglia and other glial cells (see Chapter 11), are believed to be important mediators of neural dysfunction and damage. Toxic viral products and other regulatory immune factors—for example, platelet-activating factor and arachidonic acid metabolites—also appear to be involved. A more complete understanding of these pathologic processes at the molecular level should facilitate the development of improved treatment and preventive measures for neuro-AIDS.

CEREBRAL BLOOD FLOW

Compared with other organs in the human body, the brain consumes a disproportionate share of energy and oxygen and consequently is richly vascularized. Its vascular bed is supplied by perforating arteries that branch into the subarachnoid space and subsequently enter the brain parenchyma. These arterioles in the brain's gray matter, which is more densely vascularized than the white matter, give rise to a large number of capillary beds. These in turn drain into a venous network that terminates in large venous sinuses before returning blood to the general circulation.

The strict local control of cerebral circulation correlates well with neural activity. This correlation is the basis of current brain imaging techniques that utilize cerebral blood flow, such as positron emission tomography with ^{15}O water, or that rely on blood oxygenation, such as magnetic resonance imaging with endogenous blood oxygen level-dependent contrast (BOLD), as a surrogate to gauge neural activity. The chemical signals that couple neural activity to regulation of the vasculature remain an important matter of investigation.

Because presynaptic nerve terminals exhibit tremendous metabolic activity and contain a large fraction of the mitochondria in the brain, imaging signals related to blood flow or to the use of oxygen or glucose tend to reflect the functioning of nerve terminals rather than the activity of cell bodies or dendrites. This tendency greatly complicates the interpretation of brain imaging studies; for example, strong imaging signals that result

from increased activity of inhibitory nerve terminals may reflect a decrease in the activity of postsynaptic cell bodies. This type of problem challenges scientists to better understand the biologic processes that underlie images of the living human brain and to develop markers that more closely approximate the firing of neurons.

BLOOD–BRAIN BARRIER

The blood–brain barrier isolates the homeostatic milieu of the CNS from the rest of the body. This barrier is formed by tight junctions between endothelial cells of capillaries in cerebral vascular beds, which restrict the passage of soluble molecules (Figure 2–7). The endothelial cells line the lumen of the vessels and are surrounded by a continuous basal lamina. Potential space around the capillaries is taken up by pericytes that surround the capillary walls (see Figure 2–7); these cells are involved in secretion of proteins that contribute to the basement membrane. Because the end feet (terminal processes) of perivascular astrocytes intercalate between the pericytes and contact the basal lamina, they are believed to be involved in the formation and maintenance of the tight junctions between the cerebral endothelial cells. In contrast, small spaces between endothelial cells in the general circulation permit blood solutes to enter the surrounding tissues.

The blood–brain barrier can be thought of as a continuous lipid bilayer that quarantines the brain's extracellular fluid from the general circulation. Only highly lipophilic molecules can diffuse passively through the

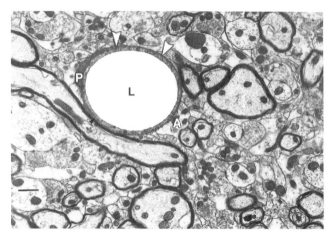

Figure 2–7. Electron micrograph of a capillary that forms part of the blood–brain barrier. In contrast to peripheral tissues, where small gaps (fenestrations) between endothelial cells of capillary walls allow small substances to pass freely, endothelial cells in the CNS form tight junctions without fenestrations, which occlude passive diffusion. These tight junctions, together with pericytes (P), the associated basement membrane, and astrocyte foot processes (A), form the blood–brain barrier. The exterior wall of the capillary is marked by arrowheads. L, lumen. (Reproduced with permission from Zigmond MJ, Bloom FE, Landis SC, et al. (eds.) 1999. *Fundamental Neuroscience.* New York: Academic Press.)

membranes of vascular cells to enter the brain; thus any peripherally administered drug that targets the CNS must be relatively lipophilic. In contrast, hydrophilic molecules are generally excluded from the brain; only water-soluble molecules that are recognized by ATP-dependent transport processes, such as glucose, amino acids, and nucleosides, can enter the CNS (Figure 2–8). However, some substances gain access to the brain by means of receptor-mediated processes (e.g., iron-transferrin, insulin, and lipoproteins; Box 2–5).

Signaling in the nervous system depends on precise concentrations of extracellular ions in the brain (see Chapter 3) and on the carefully controlled release, re-uptake, and metabolism of neurotransmitters. If the brain were not isolated from the general circulation, changes in ion concentration related to diet or hydration status would routinely disrupt neural function in profound ways. Without the blood–brain barrier, ingestion of dietary nutrients that serve as neurotransmitters or precursors of neurotransmitters, such as glutamate, or the release of peripheral hormones, would likewise regularly disrupt normal brain function.

Some areas of the brain that surround the cerebral ventricles, including the area postrema of the medulla, the circumventricular organs, and regions of hypothalamus, lack a blood–brain barrier. These regions exhibit fenestrated capillaries that, unlike the cerebral vasculature in other parts of the brain, have endothelia whose

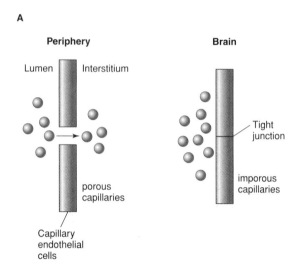

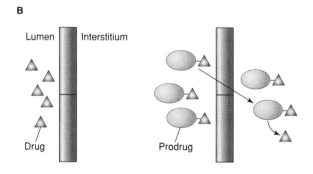

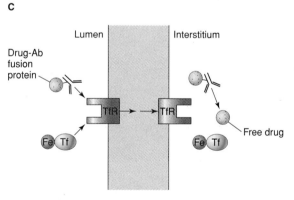

Figure 2–8. Schematic illustrations of the blood–brain barrier. **A.** The blood–brain barrier shown in Figure 2–7 is depicted. **B.** *Left,* A hydrophilic drug that cannot penetrate the blood–brain barrier. *Right,* The drug is converted into a hypothetical prodrug after it is coupled to a large lipophilic entity. The resulting prodrug is able to cross the blood–brain barrier; after it enters the brain, it is cleaved into free drug. **C.** Hypothetical use of the transferrin receptor (TfR) to transport a drug into the CNS. Fe-transferrin (Fe-Tf) complexes bind to the TfR. An anti-TfR antibody (Ab), to which a peptide drug is fused, also binds to the receptor. The entire Fe-Tf-TfR-Ab-drug complex is internalized by the endothelial cell, transported across the cell, and incorporated into the opposing cell membrane, where Fe-Tf and Ab-drug are released into the interstitial fluid. Free drug is subsequently cleaved from the Ab-drug complex.

Box 2–5 Overcoming the Blood–Brain Barrier

Although the blood–brain barrier provides essential protection for the brain by maintaining constant composition of the interstitial fluid and preventing the entry of potentially toxic substances, it also impedes the delivery of drugs for the treatment of neuropsychiatric disorders. Because only highly lipophilic drugs can gain access to the brain, the development of drugs that affect the CNS is restricted in profound ways. Many small molecules with potentially useful biologic activities are hydrophilic and thus unable to penetrate the brain. Moreover, many of the brain's intercellular messengers are neuropeptides and even, in the case of neurotrophic factors, relatively large proteins. These substances, as well as their structural analogs with antagonist functions, are almost completely excluded from the CNS by the blood–brain barrier. Consequently, CNS-related drug research is focused on devising novel ways to penetrate the blood–brain barrier to deliver agents to the brain. Some current approaches include the use of invasive (surgical) procedures, transient disruption, prodrugs, and receptor-mediated transport.

Invasive methods are perhaps the most straightforward. The introduction of a shunt into the cerebrospinal fluid (CSF), through intracerebroventricular or intrathecal cannulae, enables most substances to be administered to the CNS. Such shunts can be introduced by means of a relatively benign surgical procedure and are most commonly used in the treatment of hydrocephalus (excessive CSF pressure) to allow the flow of CSF into the abdominal cavity. The placement of a cannula in a region of the brain entails far greater risk of neural damage and infection. Moreover, drug delivered into the CSF may not penetrate very far from the ventricular system: drug might reach neural tissue immediately surrounding the CSF, but not deeper nuclei. Such surgical procedures are not undertaken except when severe neuropsychiatric or neurodegenerative disorders justify the risk involved. In these cases surgical shunts may be the only feasible way of administering potentially palliative growth factors into the CNS; however, the efficacy of such treatment remains unproven (see Chapter 11).

Another general approach to penetrating the blood–brain barrier is to administer a substance that disrupts the barrier temporarily; **mannitol's** osmotic properties, for example, are able to force apart the tight junctions on endothelial cells. Such disruption is followed by peripheral administration of a drug, which would be able to penetrate the compromised barrier. However, substances such as mannitol have a transient effect; the tight junctions that help form the barrier typically are restored within a couple of hours. Recently it has been possible to temporarily open the blood–brain barrier with selective agents that open tight junctions, including **cereport,** which activates bradykinin B_2 receptors. (Bradykinin is a peptide that serves transmitter functions in the brain and periphery; see Chapter 10.)

A drug also can be delivered into the brain when it is coupled with a large lipophilic moiety; such coupling enables the drug to passively cross the blood–brain barrier. After it enters the brain, the lipophilic moiety is cleaved, resulting in the release of free drug. This prodrug concept (see Figure 2–8) is appealing but requires a great deal of chemical modification that cannot yet be applied to most drugs. A related approach involves the packaging of a drug into lipid vesicles. After peripheral administration, the lipid microcells penetrate the blood–brain barrier and the drug is subsequently able to diffuse into brain tissue. Although this approach is conceptually quite simple, it has not yielded much success.

Another strategy for penetrating the blood–brain barrier exploits several receptor-mediated processes that normally transport needed substances into the CNS. The best understood receptor-mediated transport process involves the transferrin receptor. Related processes may exist for insulin and other peptides and for some lipoproteins. The transferrin receptor, located on the luminal surface of capillary endothelial cells, binds to Fe-transferrin complexes since transferrin is an iron-binding protein. The Fe-transferrin-transferrin receptor complex is subsequently internalized into the endothelial cells and transported to the opposite or basal aspect of the cell where it is incorporated into the cell membrane. When it faces the interstitial side of the capillary wall, Fe-transferrin is free to diffuse into the brain's extracellular fluid. Investigators are currently attempting to construct antibodies that bind to the transferrin receptor in a way that does not disrupt the receptor's ability to bind Fe-transferrin. Neuropeptides and larger proteins, such as neurotrophic factors, could then be linked to these antibodies. Evidence suggests that the entire complex (Fe-transferrin-transferrin receptor-antibody-neuropeptide) may be effectively transported across the capillary wall.

---

many vesicles move solutes from the lumen of the capillary into the brain. At these regions the brain is able to sample the general homeostatic milieu, including hormones and cytokines, and subsequently direct adaptive responses to important signals. The area postrema, for example, contains chemoreceptors that trigger vomiting in response to circulating toxins.

Because the blood–brain barrier excludes all but small, highly lipophilic substances from the CNS, many potential pharmacotherapeutic agents cannot be used successfully. Thus neuropharmacologic research continues to focus on developing strategies for penetrating the blood–brain barrier to improve drug delivery (see Box 2–5).

Another limitation to achieving effective drug concentrations in the CNS comes from transmembrane pumps that can rapidly transport drugs from cells, even after the drugs penetrate the blood–brain barrier. One such family of pumps, the P-glycoproteins, was first investigated as a cause of resistance to cancer chemotherapy agents; P-glycoproteins are expressed in cells at the blood–brain barrier. Moreover, some drugs, such as **L-type Ca^{2+} channel blockers** (see Chapter 3), can inhibit the function of P-glycoproteins and thereby increase levels of other drugs in the brain, causing side effects. Learning how to manipulate P-glycoproteins is therefore another important goal of research in neuropharmacology.

SELECTED READING

Compston A, Zajicek J, Sussman J, et al. 1997. Glial lineages and myelination in the central nervous system. *J Anat* 190:161–200.

Cowan WM, Sudhof TC, Stevens CF. 2000. *Synapses.* Baltimore: Johns Hopkins University Press.

Edelman GM, Jones FS. 1998. Gene regulation of cell adhesion: A key step in neural morphogenesis. *Brain Res Rev* 26:337–352.

Goldowitz D, Hamre K. 1998. The cells and molecules that make a cerebellum. *Trends Neurosci* 21:375–382.

Goldstein LSB, Yang Z. 2000. Microtubule-based transport systems in neurons: the roles of kinesins and dyneins. *Annu Rev Neurosci* 23:39–71.

Granholm AC, Albeck D, Backman C, et al. 1998. A non-invasive system for delivering neural growth factors across the blood-brain barrier: A review. *Rev Neurosci* 9:31–55.

Ibrahim S, Peggins J, Knapton A, et al. 2000. Influence of antipsychotic, antiemetic, and Ca^{2+} channel blocker drugs on the cellular accumulation of the anticancer drug daunorubicin: P-glycoprotein modulation. *J Pharmacol Exp Ther* 295:1276–1283.

Janzer RC, Raff MC. 1987. Astrocytes induce blood-brain barrier properties in endothelial cells. *Nature* 325:253–257.

Kandel ER, Schwartz JH, Jessell TM. 2000. *Principles of Neural Science,* 4th ed. New York: McGraw-Hill.

Kelley MS, Steward O. 1997. Injury-induced physiologic events that may modulate gene expression in neurons and glia. *Rev Neurosci* 8:147–177.

Kettenman H, Ransom BR (eds). 1995. *Neuroglia.* Oxford: Oxford University Press.

Kroll RA, Neuwelt EA. 1998. Outwitting the blood-brain barrier for therapeutic purposes: Osmotic opening and other means. *Neurosurgery* 42:1083–1099.

Lindgren M, Hallbrink M, Prochiantz A, Langel U. 2000. Cell-penetrating peptides. *Trends Pharmacol Sci* 21:99–103.

MacNeil MA, Masland RH. 1998. Extreme diversity among amacrine cells: Implications for function. *Neuron* 20:971–982.

Pardridge WM. 1998. CNS drug design based on principles of blood-brain barrier transport. *J Neurochem* 70: 1781–1782.

Seal RP, Amara SG. 1999. Excitatory amino acid transporters: A family in flux. *Annu Rev Pharmacol Toxicol* 39: 431–456.

Shen Q, Qian X, Capela A, Temple S. 1998. Stem cells in the embryonic cerebral cortex: Their role in histogenesis and patterning. *J Neurobiol* 36:162–174.

Smith SJ. 1998. Glia help synapses form and function. *Curr Biol* 8:R158–160.

Chapter 3
Electrical Excitability of Neurons

KEY CONCEPTS

- In their resting state neurons maintain a negative electrical potential in relation to the extracellular milieu because their membranes are relatively permeable to potassium and relatively impermeable to sodium, chloride, and calcium.

- The generation of all-or-none action potentials is due to voltage-dependent ion channels, highly specialized proteins that in response to changes in a neuron's electrical potential allow the flow of a specific ion (K^+, Na^+, or Ca^{2+}) across a neuron's membranes.

- Sodium channels are the targets of many important drugs including local anesthetics and some antiseizure medications.

- The 5 general classes of potassium channels include delayed rectifiers, A channels, calcium-activated potassium channels, anomalous rectifiers, and ATP-gated potassium channels.

- Entry of calcium into neurons through voltage-dependent calcium channels, of which there are 4 major classes, L-type, N-type, T-type, and P-type, plays an important role in neurotransmitter release and activation of intracellular signaling cascades.

- Mutations in ion channels are the cause of a number of neurologic disorders, most notably several inherited neuromuscular disorders.

Every heartbeat, every nerve impulse, every movement, and every thought is critically dependent on the tightly controlled and precisely timed flow of ions across cell membranes. A disruption of this flow, for example, by the puffer fish poison **tetrodotoxin,** can be fatal; and mutations of ion channels can result in severe deficits in neuromuscular functioning, including episodic ataxias and paralyses, myotonia, and long QT syndrome of the heart (Table 3–1), in humans and animal models. Ion channel abnormalities are responsible for many human diseases and also are the targets of widely used and efficacious pharmacologic agents. **Phenytoin** and **carbamazepine,** which are used to treat **epilepsy,** act by altering Na^+ channel kinetics. **Lidocaine,** a common local anesthetic, blocks voltage-gated Na^+ channels and prevents the conduction of nerve impulses that signal the occurrence of tissue damage and therefore pain. An awareness of ion channel structure and function is crucial to the understanding of pharmacology and disease processes.

This chapter begins with a brief review of the fundamental physiology that underlies ion channel function. It describes how cells maintain an electrical potential across their membranes through selective ionic permeability and ionic pumping and explains how the activity of ion channels results in neuronal signaling through graded potentials and action potentials. The second half of the chapter is devoted to a detailed examination of the molecular structure and function of ion channels. It explores how the mutation of ion channel structures and the binding of pharmaceutical agents or toxins alter the functional properties of ion channels and, in turn, the health and behavior of the affected organism.

Table 3–1 Heritable Diseases of Ion Channels

Disease	Mode of Inheritance	Ion-Channel Gene (Type)	Chromosome Location	Number of Amino Acids	Common Mutations[1]
Cystic fibrosis	AR	CFTR (epithelial chloride channel)	7q	1480	ΔF508 (70% of cases) and >450 other defined mutations
Familial persistent hyperinsulinemic hypoglycemia of infancy	AR	SUR1 (subunit of ATP-sensitive pancreatic potassium channel)	11p15.1	1582	Truncation of NBD2 (nucleotide-binding domain 2)
Hypercalciuric nephrolithiasis (Dent disease)	X-linked	CLCN5 (renal chloride channel)	Xp11.22	746	1 intragenic deletion, 3 nonsense, 4 missense, 2 donor slice, 1 microdeletion
Liddle syndrome (hereditary hypertension; pseudoaldosteronism)	AR	ENaC (epithelial sodium channel)			R564stop, P616L, Y618H (all in β subunit); premature stop codon in β and γ subunits; C-terminal truncation
		α subunit	12p	1420	
		β subunit	16p	640	
		γ subunit	16p	649	
Long-QT syndrome (cardiac arrhythmia)	AD				
LQT1		KVLQT1 (cardiac potassium channel)	11p15.5	581	1 intragenic deletion, 10 missense
LQT2		HERG (cardiac potassium channel)	7q35–36	1159	2 intragenic deletions, 5 missense
LQT3		SCN5A (cardiac sodium channel)	3p21–24	2016	ΔKPQ1505–1507, N1325S, R1644H
Benign familial neonatal convulsions	AD	KCNQ2/3 (neuronal potassium channels)	20q13.3/8q24	844/872	Y284C, A306T, G310V
Myopathies					
Becker generalized myotonia	AR	CLCN1 (skeletal-muscle chloride channel)	7q35	988	D136G, F413C, R496S
Central core storage disease	?	RYR1 (ryanodine calcium channel)	19q13.1	5032	R163C, I403M, Y522S, R2434H
Congenital myasthenic syndrome	?	nAChR (nicotinic acetylcholine receptor)			
		ε subunit	17p	473	T264P, L269F
		α subunit (slow channel)	2q	457	G153S
Hyperkalemic periodic paralysis	AD	SCN4A (skeletal-muscle sodium channel)	17q23–25	1836	T698M, T704M, M1585V, M1592V
Hypokalemic periodic paralysis	AD	CACNL1A3 (dihydropine-sensitive calcium channel)	1q31–32	1873	R528H, R1239H
Malignant hyperthermia	AD	RYR1	19q13.1	5032	G341R, G2433R
Masseter-muscle rigidity (succinylcholine-induced)	?	SCN4A	17q23–25	1836	G1306A
Myotonia levior	AD	CLCN1	7q35	988	Q552R
Paramyotonia congenita	AD	SCN4A	17q23–25	1836	V1293I, G1306V, T1313M, L1433R, L1448C, R1448H, V1589M
Pure myotonias (fluctuations, permanins, acetazolamide-responsive)	AD	SCN4A	17q23–25	1836	S804F, G1306A, G1306E, I1160V
Thomsen myotonia congenita	AD	CLCN1	7q35	988	D136G, G230E, I290M, P480L

[1]Missense mutations are represented by standard nomenclature (AxxxB, means that at amino acid position xxx, amino acid A has been replaced by amino acid B).
AR, autosomal recessive; AD, autosomal dominant.
Reproduced with permission from Ackerman MJ, Clapham DE. 1997. *N Engl J Med* 366:1575.

ELECTRICAL POTENTIAL IN CELLS

An animal's nervous system receives information from the environment, integrates this information with past experience, and creates a behavioral response that promotes the survival of the organism. Sensory neurons receive information from both the external environment—for example, sounds and sights—and the internal environment, such as the sensation of hunger or the stretch of a muscle, and relay messages to other neurons. Neurons that receive these messages are responsible for directing appropriate signals to various locations that may include muscles, internal organs, glands, or other neurons. The swift communication of these signals typically benefits an organism. It can, for example, enable a prey's rapid response to the appearance of a predator, or produce a reflexive postural correction that is necessary to prevent a fall.

A neuron is able to convey signals rapidly by alternately maintaining and varying its electrical potential in relation to the extracellular milieu. All neurons maintain a negative electrical potential relative to their extracellular environment. This negative potential provides a driving force for charged particles: in the absence of other forces, positive charges tend to be drawn into the cell, and negative charges tend to be repelled from the cell. When a neuron is activated by a chemical or electrical signal from another neuron, or by an event in the environment, it may *depolarize;* that is, its electrical potential may become less negative relative to the extracellular milieu. A neuron may, for example, depolarize from −70 mV to −50 mV. If a neuron undergoes significant depolarization, it may generate an action potential—a brief, all-or-none depolarization and repolarizaton of the membrane potential (Figure 3–1). Such substantial, rapid depolarization may stimulate a neuron to release neurotransmitter and thus convey a signal to other cells; for example, a signal conveyed to muscle cells may cause the contraction of a muscle, and a signal conveyed to an internal organ may stimulate or attenuate its activity.

HOW NEURONS MAINTAIN ELECTRICAL POTENTIAL

Two characteristics of nerve cells contribute to their ability to maintain an electrical potential. First, the neuronal cell membrane is differentially permeable to ions. In the resting state, most neurons are highly permeable to K^+, somewhat permeable to Cl^-, and very slightly permeable to Na^+ and Ca^{2+}. Because the cell membrane is a lipid bilayer, it would be completely impermeable to ions if it did not contain specialized proteins for ion transit. Ions move slowly across lipid

bilayers because they strongly prefer interaction with the polar water molecules in intracellular and extracellular spaces to interaction with the hydrophobic lipid groups that comprise the bulk of the cell membrane. The selective permeability of the cell membrane, which is discussed later in this chapter, depends on the numbers, states, and structures of its various ion channels.

Second, different types of ions are unequally distributed across the neuronal cell membrane. Generally, the neuron's interior contains a higher concentration of K^+ and lower concentrations of Na^+, Ca^{2+}, and Cl^- than does the extracellular space. These ionic gradients, which occur not only in neurons but in most cell

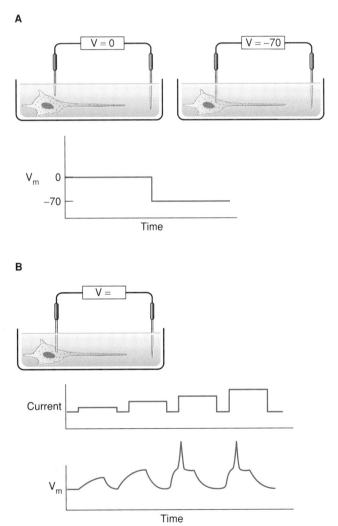

Figure 3–1. Membrane potential. **A.** As a sharp electrode penetrates a neuron, the difference in potential between the recording electrode and the bath drops from 0 to −70 mV. **B.** When small currents pass through the electrode, the potential of the cell changes in a passive manner. Larger currents elicit an all-or-none action potential.

types,[1] are maintained through ion-specific pumps that require energy in the form of adenosine triphosphate (ATP) hydrolysis. Moreover, the neuron's interior contains many negatively charged, membrane-impermeable proteins that do not exist in the extracellular milieu. These neuronal properties—unequal permeability of ions across the cell membrane and unequal distribution of ions—are theoretically sufficient to maintain an electrical potential in a cell.

A SIMPLE CELL MODEL

Consider a very simple model of a cell. The interior of the cell (*I*) contains 100 mM K^+A^-, where A^- is an impermeant anion such as a negatively charged protein. Exterior to the cell (*O*), the concentration of K^+A^- is 5 mM (Figure 3–2). To simplify this model, the effects of osmosis are ignored.

If the cell's lipid bilayer is impermeable to both K^+ and A^-, no movement of ions occurs across the bilayer, and the concentration of ions on each side of the bilayer remains constant. However, if the lipid bilayer of this cell became permeable to K^+, and only to K^+—for example, from the opening of K^+-specific ion channels in the lipid bilayer—K^+ ions but not A^- ions would be free to move from *I* to *O* or from *O* to *I*. Because *I* contains twenty times more K^+ than *O*, many more K^+ ions would be likely to contact the membrane and travel from *I* to *O* than from *O* to *I*. Consequently, a net efflux of K^+ from *I* to *O* would be likely to occur; because A^- would remain impermeable, it would not cross the membrane.

As soon as K^+ ions begin to move to *O*, however, an electrical potential develops across the cell membrane. Although more K^+ tends to travel from *I* to *O* than from *O* to *I*, a net positive charge develops in *O* because K^+ has left the cell without accompanying A^-. This net positive charge *repels* K^+ from *O*. Thus, two tendencies act in opposition to one another: (1) the tendency of K^+ to move out of *I* because more K^+ is present in *I* than in *O*, and (2) the tendency of K^+ to be drawn into *I* because of its relative negative potential.

Eventually, these two tendencies reach an equilibrium whereby the net efflux of K^+ from *I* (favored by the concentration gradient) is equal to the net efflux of K^+ from *O* (promoted by the electrical potential). Only a minuscule fraction of K^+ must venture from *I* to *O* to create an electrical potential strong enough to balance the tendency of K^+ to leave *I* along its concentration

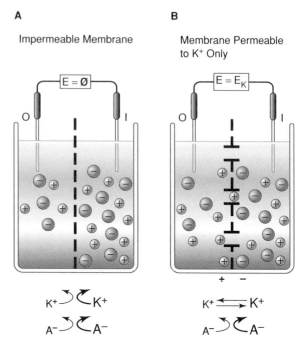

Figure 3–2. A cell model. **A.** If an impermeable membrane is placed between two compartments that contain different concentrations of the ionic solution K^+A^-, no movement of electrical charge can occur and the difference in potential between the two compartments (E) is zero. **B.** If the membrane becomes permeable to K^+, K^+ initially flows down its concentration gradient from I to O, creating an electrical potential that opposes the movement of K^+. The net movement of K^+ between I and O stops when the electrical force repelling K^+ equals the force of the concentration gradient; at this point K^+ has reached its equilibrium potential (E_K), which can be estimated with the Nernst equation.

gradient. The electrical potential at which this balance occurs can be determined by the *Nernst equation*[2]:

$$Em = 58 \log \left(K_o / K_i \right)$$

According to this equation, the greater the concentration difference across the membrane, the greater the electrical potential that is needed to balance the tendency of K^+ ions to move from *I* to *O*. Because so few K^+ ions leave *I*, the original concentrations can be used in the equation. The net number of K^+ ions that shift to create the membrane potential is approximately 10^{-12} moles per cm^2 of membrane, which has a negligible effect on the millimolar concentrations of ions in the intracellular and extracellular solutions.

---

[1]Evolutionarily, the maintenance of ionic gradients may have developed from a drive to maintain an extracellular environment similar to that of seawater, where it is speculated that life began and which, though higher in osmolarity than mammalian extracellular fluid, possesses a similar K^+ to Na^+ to Cl^- ratio.

[2]The factor of 58 in the Nernst equation is derived from several chemical values—gas constant, temperature in °K, valence of each ion, and Faraday constant—and involves the conversion of natural logarithms to base 10 logarithms.

The following equation describes the electrical potential at which equilibrium occurs in the previously described simple cell model:

$$58 \log \left(5/100\right) = -75 \text{ mV}$$

In this model a minuscule fraction of the A^- ions in I exist without accompanying K^+ ions because the latter traveled down the concentration gradient to the outside of the cell membrane. This tiny separation of charge creates a negative potential of -75 mV on the inside of the cell membrane (I) relative to the outside of the cell membrane (O). This negative charge within the cell exerts just enough force on the K^+ ions that the net flow of K^+ ions across the membrane is zero, despite the existing concentration gradient of K^+. The transmembrane potential at which this equilibrium occurs (-75 mV) is termed the *equilibrium potential* (or the *Nernst potential*) for K^+.

Because the cell membrane in this theoretical model is permeable to K^+ and only to K^+, no energy must be supplied to the system to maintain either the electrical potential or the concentration gradient. In real cells, ion pumps are required to maintain the differential concentration of ions inside and outside the cell.

A MORE COMPLICATED CELL MODEL

A basic understanding of membrane potential drawn from the previous cell model can assist in understanding a model that more closely resembles a mammalian nerve cell. This more complicated model involves (1) a more complete complement of extracellular and intracellular ions, and (2) more realistic ionic permeabilities.

Table 3–2 describes several features of this cell model. First, the net total charge on each side of the cell is zero, a condition that is necessary for electrical neutrality.[3]

Second, the cell membrane is far more permeable to K^+ than to any other ion, which is the case for most neurons at rest. All other permeabilities are described relative to the permeability of K^+.

What is the electrical potential at which the net flux of charge across the cell membrane equals zero? If the cell were *only* permeable to K^+, we could determine this equilibrium potential using the Nernst equation

---

Table 3–2 Idealized Free Ion Concentrations Inside and Outside a Nerve Cell

Ion	Concentration Inside Cell (mM)	Concentration Outside Cell (mM)	Relative Permeability
K^+	100	5	1
Na^+	10	100	0.01
Cl^-	10	105	0.2
A^- (large anions)	100	0	0

because all other ions would be trapped on one side of the cell and could not migrate to contribute to the generation of an electrical potential. However, the cell *is* permeable to other ions, although to a much lesser degree than it is to K^+. If the membrane were permeable *only* to Na^+, the resting potential also could be determined by means of the Nernst equation, as follows:

$$\text{Em} = 58 \log \left(K_o/K_i\right)$$

In this case the cell interior would develop a *positive* potential relative to the exterior of the cell. Subsequently the positive potential in the cell interior would repel Na^+ ions and balance the statistical tendency of these ions to flow down their concentration gradient and into the cell.

The true equilibrium potential for this cell model, which would be expected to lie somewhere between the equilibrium potentials for the various ions, can be calculated using the Goldman–Hodgkin–Katz equation[4]:

$$E = 58 \cdot \log \left(\frac{PK\left[K^+\right]_{out} + PNa\left[Na^+\right]_{out} + PCl\left[Cl^-\right]_{in}}{PK\left[K^+\right]_{in} + PNa\left[Na^+\right]_{in} + PCl\left[Cl^-\right]_{out}}\right)$$

Note that this equation is similar to the Nernst equation: the equilibrium potential is proportional to the relative concentrations of ions on the inside and outside of the membrane. In fact, when the permeabilities of Na^+ and Cl^- are zero, the Goldman–Hodgkin–Katz equation is reduced to the Nernst equation.

The values for the cell model are applied to this equation as follows:

$$E = 58 \cdot \log \left(\frac{PK\left[K^+\right]_{out} + PNa\left[Na^+\right]_{out} + PCl\left[Cl^-\right]_{in}}{PK\left[K^+\right]_{in} + PNa\left[Na^+\right]_{in} + PCl\left[Cl^-\right]_{out}}\right)$$

$$= 58 \cdot \log \left(\frac{(1)[5]_{out} + (.01)[100]_{out} + (0.2)[10]_{in}}{(1)[100]_{in} + (.01)[10]_{in} + (0.2)[105]_{out}}\right)$$

Thus the equilibrium potential for this cell is -68 mV. Note that, as expected, this membrane potential lies

---

[3]Note that electrical neutrality cannot be achieved because a separation of charge persists across the cell membrane. It is also important to note that ionic concentrations in this table are given in millimolar values, although a resting potential in a normal cell of -75 mV can be produced by a femtomolar net separation of charge. Moreover, both the cytoplasm of the cell and the extracellular milieu are electrically neutral, having an equal number of positive and negative charges; the difference in charge exists across the cell membrane, which acts as a capacitor.

[4]For the derivation of this equation, see Hille 1992.

between the equilibrium potentials estimated for K^+, Na^+, and Cl^-. Because the membrane's permeability to K^+ is so much greater than its permeability to the other ions, the neuron's resulting membrane potential is much closer to the equilibrium potential of K^+ (-75 mV) than to that of Na^+ ($+58$ mV) or Cl^- (-59 mV).

If many of the Na^+ channels in this cell model were suddenly opened, causing Na^+ to be three times more permeable than K^+, the membrane potential would change as follows:

$$E = 58 \cdot \log\left(\frac{PK[K^+]_{out} + PNa[Na^+]_{out} + PCl[Cl^-]_{in}}{PK[K^+]_{in} + PNa[Na^+]_{in} + PCl[Cl^-]_{out}}\right)$$

$$= 58 \cdot \log\left(\frac{(1)[5]_{out} + (3)[100]_{out} + (0.2)[10]_{in}}{(1)[100]_{in} + (3)[10]_{in} + (0.2)[105]_{out}}\right)$$

The resulting membrane potential in this case ($+19.6$ mV) would be much closer to the equilibrium potential for Na^+. If the Na^+ channels were to close suddenly, bringing the permeability ratio of Na^+ to K^+ back to its original value of 0.01, the membrane potential would return to -68 mV in response to the efflux of K^+ through the many open K^+ channels.

Many electrophysiologic concepts, and the roles of ion channels and ion channel-targeting drugs in physiologic processes, can be understood intuitively by recalling the Nernst potentials of the four major ions that surround the plasma membranes of cells. When only one type of ion channel opens, it drives the membrane potential of the cell toward the Nernst potential of that ion. If, for example, a Na^+ channel opens in a cell in which all other types of ion channels are closed, the transmembrane potential of the cell becomes E_{Na}. If an ion channel were equally permeable to K^+ and to Na^+, its opening would tend to drive the cell toward a potential of approximately 0 mV, which is halfway between the Nernst potentials for Na^+ and K^+. It also is important to emphasize that the Nernst potential for a particular ion depends on the relative concentrations of that ion inside and outside the cell, which can vary considerably among different cell types and tissues. For example, the Nernst potential for Cl^- can range from -60 to -90 mV.

MAINTENANCE OF RESTING POTENTIAL BY ATP-DEPENDENT PUMPS

The equilibrium potential predicted by the Goldman–Hodgkin–Katz equation provides for an equal exchange of cations back and forth across the cell membrane: for every excess Na^+ ion that sneaks across the membrane, a K^+ ion moves out, holding the membrane stable at the predicted potential. This exchange occurs slowly enough that the ionic concentrations may be considered constant for short periods of time. However, if a slow exchange of Na^+ for K^+ were allowed to continue for hours or days, the concentration gradients would eventually degenerate and the membrane potential would slowly begin to dissipate.

Na^+–K^+ pumps maintain the ionic gradients across a cell membrane by extruding Na^+ from and pumping K^+ into the cell against their respective concentration gradients (Figure 3–3). Each pump is a multimeric integral membrane protein consisting of transmembrane α subunits, which possess the catalytic and iontophoretic (ion pore-containing) domains of the pump, and accessory transmembrane β subunits. Although the exact function of the β subunits is poorly understood, several studies have demonstrated that the α subunit is not functional and does not insert into plasma membranes when expressed in the absence of the β subunit. Moreover, the identity of the β subunit seems to alter the affinity of the pump for K^+. The likely structure of the pump complex is $\alpha_2\beta_2$, although more complex oligomeric structures are possible.

The catalytic subunit of each pump has binding sites for K^+ on its extracellular face and binding sites for Na^+ and ATP on its intracellular face. ATP transfers its terminal phosphate to the catalytic subunit in a Na^+-dependent manner; because the pump is a protein that cleaves ATP by means of ion-dependent enzymatic activity, it often is referred to as Na^+/K^+-ATPase. This phosphorylation of the catalytic subunit triggers a conformational change; for every molecule of ATP that is hydrolyzed, 3 Na^+ ions typically are transported out of the cell and 2 extracellular K^+ ions are transported in. Thus, the pump is *electrogenic*: it exports more positive charge than it imports. The phosphorylated catalytic subunit is subsequently hydrolyzed in the presence of K^+ ions, returning the catalytic subunit to its resting state. The resting potential of a cell with active Na^+–K^+ pumps is usually a few mV more negative than would be predicted on the basis of ion distribution and relative permeabilities alone.

The importance of Na^+–K^+ pumps in the maintenance of cellular membrane potential becomes quite evident when they are inhibited by pharmacologic agents. Cardiac glycosides such as **ouabain** and **digoxin,** which increase the contractile force of cardiac muscle and are used in the treatment of **congestive heart failure** and some cardiac **dysrhythmias,** are the best known inhibitors of the Na^+–K^+ pump. Normally, cardiac myocytes maintain low levels of intracellular Ca^{2+}, partly through a Na^+–Ca^{2+} pump that uses energy from the

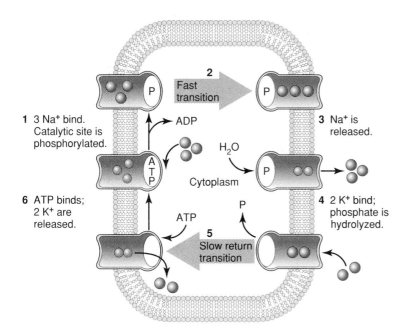

Figure 3–3. The adenosine triphosphate (ATP)-dependent Na⁺–K⁺ pump. The pump removes three Na⁺ ions from the cell and introduces two K⁺ ions. **1,** Three Na⁺ ions bind to the interior face of the catalytic subunit, which subsequently is phosphorylated; **2,** through a conformational transition Na⁺ ions become less tightly bound to the pump and obtain access to the extracellular space; **3,** Na⁺ ions dissociate from the pump; **4,** when two K⁺ ions bind to the pump it undergoes dephosphorylation; **5,** the pump changes conformation, providing the two bound K⁺ ions with access to the cytoplasm; **6,** after ATP binds to the catalytic subunit, the two K⁺ ions are released into the cytoplasm. ADP, adenosine diphosphate; P, phosphorylation. (Adapted with permission from Siegel GJ, Agranoff BW, Albers RW, et al. (eds). 1999. *Basic Neurochemistry,* p. 102. New York: Raven Press.)

movement of Na⁺ down its concentration gradient to transport Ca²⁺ out of the cell. Because cardiac glycosides inhibit Na⁺–K⁺ pumps and increase intracellular Na⁺ concentrations, they make Na⁺–Ca²⁺ pumps less effective. Consequently, intracellular Ca²⁺ concentrations increase, which results in the increased contractile force of cardiac muscle. These drugs also can slowly reduce the resting potential of neurons eventually to zero; in large neurons, this decline in potential occurs after several hours. This action of the drugs in the CNS accounts for common side effects of cardiac glycosides, including disturbed vision, confusion, and delirium.

Digoxin

BIOPHYSICAL PROPERTIES OF THE CELL MEMBRANE

In the cell model described previously, it was possible to create a potential across the membrane by making it selectively permeable to the ions distributed unequally across it. It also was possible to alter the potential of the membrane by changing the relative permeabilities of various ions, for example, by increasing the permeability of Na⁺ relative to K⁺; likewise the membrane's original potential could be restored by reinstating the original permeabilities. Real neurons also transmit electrical signals by transiently changing their ionic permeabilities; however, they have two biophysical properties that affect the movement of charge and the development of potential across a neuronal membrane.

First, unlike the movement of charge in the cell model, charge is not transferred instantaneously from one neuronal compartment to another. Real ions require a finite amount of time to come into contact with and pass through the ion channels in a cell membrane. Electrically, the membrane can be thought of as a *resistor,* a material through which ions can pass, but with some difficulty.

Second, unlike the membrane in the cell model, the neuronal cell membrane acts as a *capacitor,* a device that stores charge. The separation of charge that develops in a real cell consists of thin layers of positive and negative ions that extend across the inner and outer surfaces of the membrane (Figure 3–4). Because electrical fields composed of excess cations outside the cell and leftover anions inside the cell exert attractive forces on one another, cations and anions are drawn together as closely as possible by lining up along the membrane, which is a layer of nonconductive material. This close separation of positive and negative charges causes a potential to develop across the membrane.

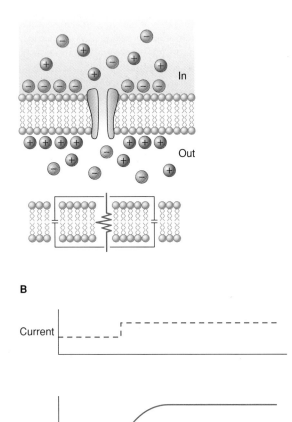

A

B

Current

Voltage

Time

Figure 3–4. The cell as a resistor-capacitor circuit. **A.** The lipid bilayer of the cell's membrane separates charge and thus can be represented as a simple electrical circuit comprising resistance and capacitance. The number and state of the various ion channels in a cell membrane determine that membrane's *resistance,* or the ease with which ions can cross the membrane. Cell membranes with many open ion channels have low resistance; cell membranes with only a few open ion channels have high resistance. The *capacitance* of a membrane, or its ability to store charge, is determined by factors such as the area and thickness of the membrane. **B.** The opening of ion channels and the subsequent flow of current do not result in an instantaneous change in membrane potential. High-resistance and high-capacitance membranes require more time to develop a charge than low-resistance and low-capacitance membranes.

The amount of charge needed to create a particular potential is determined by the equation $V = Q/C$, whereby V is the potential, Q is the transferred charge, and C is a property termed *capacitance.* The capacitance describes a membrane's ability to store charge; the more charge required to raise a membrane's potential, the better the membrane's capacitance. Several properties, such as size and, most significantly, thickness, can affect a membrane's capacitance. A very large membrane area requires more stored charge to bring it to a given potential, or in other words it has a greater capacitance, than does a small membrane area because the same number of charges are less tightly packed in a larger membrane, resulting in less potential energy. In contrast, very thick membranes are poor capacitors: because ions separated across a greater distance possess greater potential energy, fewer ions are required to reach a certain membrane potential. Because a myelin sheath increases a membrane's thickness, a myelinated axonal membrane is a poor capacitor compared with a nonmyelinated membrane. Therefore, a myelinated axonal membrane is easy to "charge up": very few charges must move across it to produce a large difference in potential.

SENSORY, SYNAPTIC, AND ACTION POTENTIALS

Neurons exploit their ability to rapidly change their transmembrane potentials in order to receive information from the environment and to relay messages. Input from a variety of sources, including other neurons, can cause a neuron's membrane potential to fluctuate. If a neuron depolarizes enough, or reaches threshold, it produces an *action potential*: a rapid, all-or-none depolarization that propagates down its axon. The firing of an axon generally leads to the release of neurotransmitter from the axon's terminals, which in turn conveys the neuron's signal to muscle cells, to effector organs such as glands, or to other neurons.

Receiving information   Some neurons are equipped with specialized systems that enable them to receive information from the environment. Hair cells in the cochlea, for example, are sensitive to vibrational energy: vibrations cause the movement of tiny cilia on the surface of these cells. Such movement activates mechanosensitive ion channels that increase the membrane's permeability to Na^+, which in turn leads to depolarization of the hair cell. If enough of these ion channels are activated, the hair cell may reach threshold and fire an action potential. Photoreceptor cells in the retina can respond to light because photons activate a series of chemical reactions (Box 3–1) that cause

Box 3-1 Seeing and Smelling: The Role of Cyclic Nucleotide-Gated Channels

The transduction of visual and olfactory stimuli into signals that the nervous system can decipher depends on the operation of ion channels that are gated by the binding of cyclic nucleotides. Photoreception in the retina, for example, depends on cyclic guanosine monophosphate (cGMP)-gated channels, and the transduction of odorant signals by the olfactory epithelium depends on channels gated by cyclic adenosine monophosphate (cAMP).

These channels have been cloned and appear to be structurally homologous to the voltage-gated channels discussed in this chapter. Although their exact stoichiometry is unknown, they are believed to be tetramers of α and β subunits. The expression of only α subunits results in a functional channel, but the properties of these channels are most similar to naturally occurring channels when the two subunits are coexpressed. Each subunit binds a single molecule of cAMP or cGMP. Although the binding of only one subunit can cause a channel to open, maximum activation of the channel requires the binding of all four subunits to cyclic nucleotide.

The role that cGMP-gated channels play in converting light energy, in the form of photons, to an electrical signal that the nervous system can interpret is well understood. Photons activate the light-sensing pigment rhodopsin in the outer segments of rods in the retina. Photoactivated rhodopsin in turn activates a phosphodiesterase that causes the breakdown of cGMP (see Chapter 5). This transient fall in the cytosolic concentration of cGMP results in the closure of tonically activated cGMP-gated channels, which causes hyperpolarization of the photoreceptor cell. Rods respond to this hyperpolarization by releasing less transmitter, thereby informing other cells in the retina that a light signal has been received.

The transduction of odorant signals is also well understood. Odorant receptors are G protein-coupled receptors whose activation results in the stimulation of adenylyl cyclase and the production of cAMP (see Chapter 5). The increase in cAMP activates cAMP-gated channels, which causes depolarization of the olfactory neurons. Resulting action potentials in these neurons signal efferent neurons that an olfactory stimulus has been received. In contrast to the channels involved in photoreception, which are activated preferentially by cGMP, olfactory channels can be opened by either cAMP or cGMP.

A distinct family of channels regulated by cyclic nucleotides operate in both the heart and the brain, where they play an important role in generating pacemaker activity. Such channels, which have been variously termed I_h channels, hyperpolarization-activated channels (HAC), and brain cyclic nucleotide-gated (BCNG) channels, are unusual in that they are activated by hyperpolarization and are permeable to both Na^+ and K^+. Thus, these channels are activated when a cell is hyperpolarized, after a burst of action potentials, due to the activation of several types of K^+ channels. Because their activation causes the cell to depolarize, often beyond spike threshold, these pacemaker channels help drive a repetitive cycle of rhythmic firing.

An increase in cAMP modifies the function of these channels by causing their voltage dependence to shift in a positive direction. As a result, when cAMP binds directly to these channels, they activate more rapidly and completely upon repolarization of the cell to a fixed negative potential. The effect of cAMP on these channels is exploited by several common drugs used to modify heart rate; for example, **propranolol,** a β-adrenergic antagonist, reduces cellular cAMP levels, which decreases heart rate in part by inhibiting I_h channels. Because the rhythmic activity of neurons is integral to functions such as arousal, maintenance of the sleep-wake cycle, and respiratory rate, these pacemaker channels are important targets for future drug development. Indeed, antagonists of these channels are currently undergoing evaluation for use in the treatment of cardiovascular and neuropsychiatric disorders.

changes in the ionic permeability of the cell membrane, which in turn leads to changes in the membrane potential of the cell.

Neurons generally receive signals from other neurons through chemical neurotransmitters. Signaling neurons typically release neurotransmitter into a specialized synapse, some of which binds to receptors on an adjacent neuron's cell membrane. The binding of neurotransmitter to a receptor leads to changes in the receiving neuron's ion permeability. This change in permeability may occur directly; many neurotransmitter receptors contain intrinsic ion channels. However, changes in permeability also take place indirectly; many types of neurotransmitter receptors activate second messenger systems within a cell that in turn modify ion channels, causing changes in membrane potential.

Integrating information   The opening of ion channels in a localized area, such as a synapse, produces a transmembrane current that changes the membrane potential of a cell. However, this change in potential does not occur instantaneously or remain localized to the narrow region of membrane in which the current was generated. The integration of local changes in the transmembrane voltage of a neuron is affected by two basic types of summation: *spatial summation* and *temporal summation* (Figure 3-5). Spatial summation occurs because a current that alters the membrane potential in one region of a cell, for example, in one synapse, does not remain localized to that particular region, but passively diffuses over the cell. However, the magnitude of depolarization, which is greatest in the vicinity of the synapse, attenuates as it spreads throughout the cell; thus, synapses close to the cell body may have a greater impact on membrane potential than those located on distal dendrites. Temporal summation occurs because the neuronal membrane requires time to charge and to discharge. Thus two excitatory inputs separated in time by 100 ms may not be sufficient to cause a neuron to fire. The same two inputs, separated by only 5 ms, may

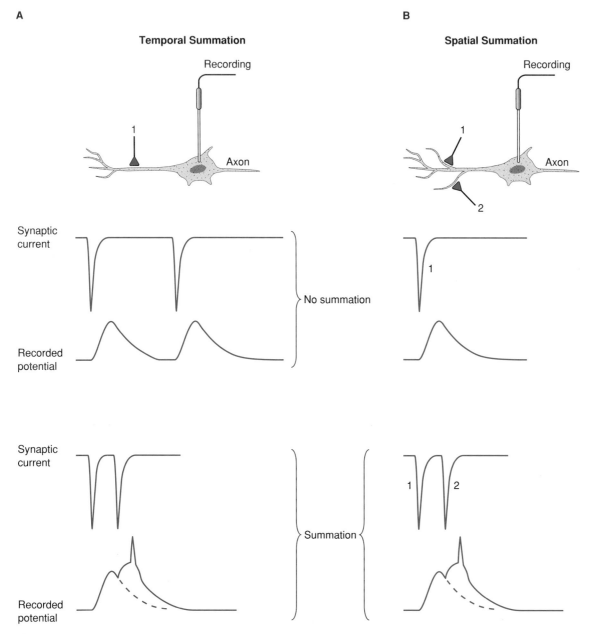

Figure 3–5. Temporal and spatial summation of synaptic inputs. **A.** Temporal summation occurs when repetitive synaptic input transpires so swiftly that synaptic potentials do not have time to decay. **B.** Spatial summation occurs when two independent inputs are activated within a finite window. Because of the passive electrical properties of the cell's membrane, they summate even though they were generated in different locations. (Adapted with permission from Kandel ER, Schwartz JH, Jessell TM. 2000. *Principles of Neural Science,* 4th ed, pp. 224. New York: McGraw-Hill.)

be sufficient to elicit an action potential if the second stimulus arrives before the charges from the first stimulus have completely dissipated.

Neurons are decision makers—they must repeatedly decide whether to respond to particular sets of stimuli by firing action potentials and in turn communicating with fellow neurons or with effector organs. A motor neuron in the spinal cord, for example, receives thousands of excitatory and inhibitory inputs from pathways that descend from the brain. These descending pathways deliver enormous amounts of information integrated from many areas of the brain, including motor planning, vestibular, and visual centers. The currents produced by excitatory and inhibitory inputs continually undergo summation to produce membrane potentials that fluctuate in time and space. A neuron reads fluctuating potentials at the base of its axon, called the *axon hillock*, where it has a high concentration of voltage-dependent Na^+ channels. If the sum of these potentials produces a sufficient level of depolarization, an action potential is triggered.

Action potential and neurotransmitter release

An action potential is a rapidly propagating depolarization of the axonal membrane that can lead to the release of neurotransmitter from axon terminals. This phenomenon is best understood in terms of the responses of Na^+ channels to changes in voltage. In this section the Na^+ channel is discussed as an abstract entity; its molecular structure is described in detail in the next section.

Because the depolarization of a cell membrane causes Na^+ channels to open transiently, they are termed *voltage-dependent,* or *voltage-gated,* channels. The opening of Na^+ channels leads to an inward current that in turn causes further depolarization because the equilibrium potential of Na^+ is positive compared with the resting potential of the cell membrane. Depolarization-activated Na^+ channels continue to open and to permit further depolarization in a repetitive, self-perpetuating manner. In response to this positive feedback loop, the membrane of the cell's axon is quickly driven toward the equilibrium potential for Na^+.

However, two phenomena quickly return the membrane potential to its resting, hyperpolarized state (Figure 3–6). First, Na^+ channels spontaneously close, or inactivate, after a brief period of time (1–2 ms), thus reducing the membrane's permeability to Na^+ and minimizing the contribution of the Na^+ gradient to the membrane's potential. Second, voltage-activated K^+ channels open, their response to membrane depolarization being similar to but slower than that of Na^+ channels. Subsequently, the transient influx of Na^+ is rapidly overwhelmed by an outflow of K^+ along its concentration gradient, and the membrane responds by resuming its resting potential near the K^+ equilibrium potential. Although the activation of K^+ channels is not required for the repolarization of the membrane because the automatic closing of the Na^+ channels and the membrane's high resting conductance to K^+ is sufficient to return the membrane to its resting potential, it does serve to accelerate the process. In fact, the amount and properties of the various K^+ channels in a neuron play a critical role in determining the duration of a neuron's action potentials and the neuron's rate of firing.

An action potential typically is triggered at the axon hillock, or initial segment. This point at which the axon leaves the cell body has, as mentioned previously, a high density of Na^+ channels and thus the lowest threshold for the initiation of action potentials. Because of Na^+ channels along the length of the axon, the action potential propagates down the axon and invades the presynaptic nerve terminals, where it triggers the influx of Ca^{2+} by activating voltage-dependent Ca^{2+} channels and subsequently leads to the Ca^{2+}-dependent release of neurotransmitter (see Chapter 4).

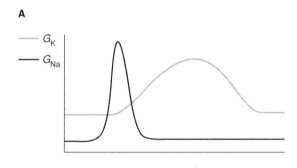

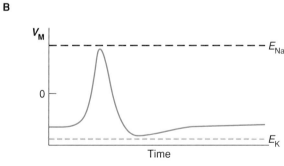

Figure 3–6. Changes in membrane conductance during an action potential. **A.** The first change is a rapid increase in Na^+ conductance; this is followed by a slower, longer-lasting increase in K^+ conductance. **B.** These changes result in a characteristic action potential: a sharp depolarization, from Na^+ current moving inward, followed by a repolarization, from K^+ current moving outward.

In nonmyelinated, small-diameter axons, action potential propagation is fairly slow because propagation is continuous and each segment of membrane must be depolarized to threshold. In myelinated axons, action potential propagation is *saltatory*: action potentials appear to jump from one node of Ranvier, a small gap in the myelin sheath, to the next at a much faster rate (Figure 3–7; see also Chapter 2). Because myelin increases the resistance and decreases the capacitance of the axonal membrane, current entering the axon at one node does not leak out of the internodal membrane but instead travels rapidly down the axon to depolarize the adjacent node until it reaches threshold. Moreover, thick, myelinated portions of the axon require less charge to reach threshold because of their lower capacitance.

Dendrites, the recipients of most incoming synaptic activity, are not electrically passive during this process; they contain a constellation of voltage-dependent Na^+, Ca^{2+}, and K^+ channels and are capable of generating action potentials. Dendritic action potentials presumably amplify incoming synaptic signals so that they can be heard at the soma. Investigators are currently attempting to elucidate the detailed biophysical and molecular properties of these dendritic channels and to determine their spatial distribution.

MOLECULAR PROPERTIES OF ION CHANNELS

The Na^+ and K^+ channels have been elevated from the status of mythical creatures in the minds of electrophysiologists to a position where they are in danger of being crystallized.

KT Wann

Thus far, ion channels have been discussed only in the most abstract sense. However, modern advances in molecular biology, such as the isolation, cloning, and mutagenesis of ion channels, and in cell physiology, such as patch clamping techniques that allow the observation of single ion channels, have provided scientists with remarkably detailed knowledge of the operation of ion channels. The crystallization of bacterial ion pores and channels, including KcsA, a bacterial K^+ channel that is homologous to some human K^+ channels, also has yielded important information. Consequently we know the exact amino acid composition of hundreds of ion channels, have detailed models about how these channels assemble in cellular membranes, and understand which amino acids are responsible for features of ion channels such as selective permeability and the binding of pharmaceutical agents.

This chapter focuses on several molecular properties of voltage-gated cation channels. Although each type of

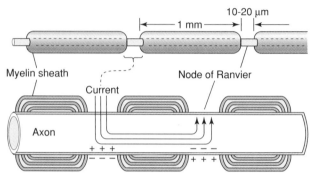

Figure 3–7. Myelin and saltatory conduction along axons. Current enters a myelinated axon at one node and exits at the next node, unlike the continuous exit of current that occurs in nonmyelinated axons. The myelin sheath greatly increases the resistance of the axonal membrane and decreases its capacitance.

channel has distinctive features, such as cellular location and permeability to specific ions, all of these channels must meet similar challenges. They must selectively allow some ions but not others to pass through the hydrophobic cell membrane, and they must sense changes in transmembrane voltage and transmute them into conformational adjustments that result in increased ionic permeability. Thus it is not surprising that voltage-gated Na^+, K^+, and Ca^2 channels share many structural similarities and are widely believed to have evolved from a single ancestral channel.

THE PROTOTYPIC VOLTAGE-GATED CHANNEL

The Na^+ channel was the first voltage-gated ion channel to be cloned. It was isolated with the use of binding assays based on the high affinity and specificity of Na^+ channel neurotoxins such as **tetrodotoxin,** a Na^+ current antagonist that has been used in electrophysiologic experiments for decades. Denaturing of the isolated channel protein with detergent and separation of its constituents by gel electrophoresis revealed that the channel was most likely a multimer of several distinct subunits. The α subunit is the largest of these proteins and is considered the principal subunit of the Na^+ channel; when it functions by itself in an independent system, for example, a *Xenopus* oocyte, it is able to carry out all of the basic functions of the channel.

The primary structure of the α subunit consists of 2400 amino acid residues and comprises four internally homologous domains, each of which contains 300 to 400 amino acids (Figure 3–8). Within each of the four domains are six membrane-spanning α helices. The transmembrane regions are believed to aggregate, as shown in Figure 3–8, with each of the four major domains forming a pillar of the channel. Interestingly, the aqueous pore of the channel is believed to be formed not by one of the transmembrane domains, but by the amino acids between transmembrane segments S5 and S6. This chain of amino acids, called SS1–SS2, is believed to form a hairpin loop that dips down into the channel and forms the lining of the ion pore. This belief is consistent with the crystalline structure of the KcsA K$^+$ channel, which shares many similarities with the Na$^+$ channel. Moreover, mutations in the SS1–SS2 region greatly affect the conductance properties of the channel.

Other voltage-gated channels display structures remarkably similar to those of the Na$^+$ channel. Most similar are the principal α subunits of Ca^{2+} channels, which also contain four internally homologous domains, each of which possesses six putative membrane-spanning regions (Figure 3–9). In contrast, the extensively characterized Shaker K$^+$ channel, named after the mutant strain of *Drosophila* from which it was cloned, appears to be composed of subunits that correspond to only one of the four internally homologous domains of the Na$^+$

A

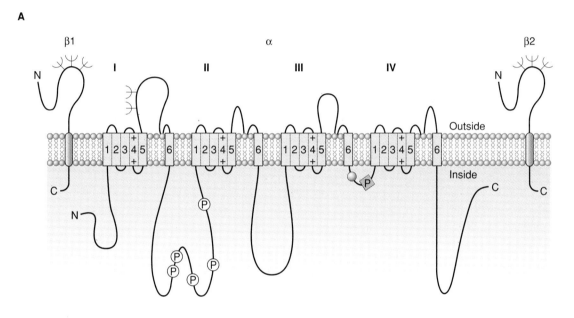

B

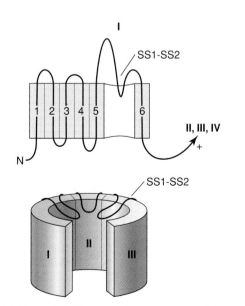

Figure 3–8. Structure of the Na$^+$ channel. **A.** Transmembrane structure of the α subunit. Domains I–IV each contain six segments that span the membrane in the form of an α helix. **B.** Each domain contains a sequence (SS1–SS2) that connects segments 5 and 6; these sequences are believed to form the pore of the ion channel.

Na⁺ channels

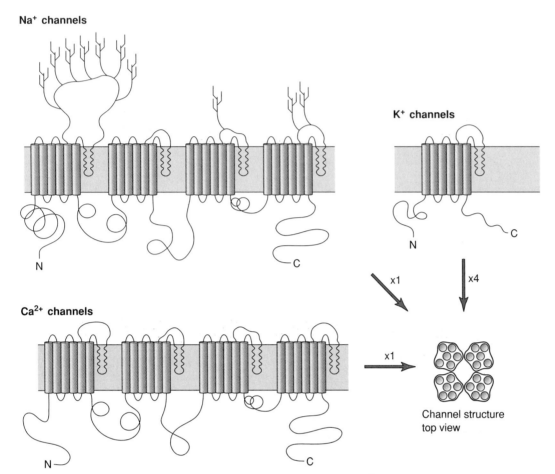

K⁺ channels

Ca²⁺ channels

Channel structure
top view

Figure 3–9. Structural similarities shared by voltage-dependent Na⁺, Ca²⁺, and K⁺ channels. Each channel has subunits whose domains contain six membrane-spanning segments. The α subunit in both Ca²⁺ and Na⁺ channels contains four domains. The subunit of the Shaker K⁺ channel contains only one domain. The region that connects segments 5 and 6 in each domain (SS1–SS2) is believed to form the pore of each channel. (Adapted with permission from Barchi RL. 1992. Sodium channel gene defects in the periodic paralyses. *Curr Opin Neurobiol* 2:633.)

and Ca²⁺ channels. It is believed that four of these smaller subunits in the Shaker K⁺ channel multimerize in the plasma membrane to form a channel that is similar in structure to the Na⁺ and Ca²⁺ channels. Despite their structural similarity, Na⁺, K⁺, and Ca²⁺ channels each exhibit exquisite selectivity for a unique subset of ions. The molecular basis of this selectivity is reviewed in Box 3–2. In mammalian cells, each of these voltage-gated channels are composed of several subunits in addition to their primary α subunits; the role of these accessory proteins is discussed in Box 3–3.

VOLTAGE-ACTIVATED OPENING OF ION CHANNELS

Na⁺ channels responsible for propagating action potentials, K⁺ channels responsible for terminating action potentials, and Ca²⁺ channels that admit Ca²⁺ to

nerve terminals in response to action potentials are all voltage-activated: they open when a membrane is depolarized. How can this be explained on a molecular basis? Before ion channels could be studied on a molecular level, Hodgkin and Huxley proposed that the steep voltage dependence of Na⁺ conductance involved the actions of three or four *gating particles*. Accordingly, they believed that changes in membrane voltage caused a movement or conformational change of each gating particle, whose movement ultimately allowed Na⁺ ions to cross the cell membrane. Indeed, sophisticated electrophysiologic techniques reveal that voltage-activated ion channels display a gating charge, or a shift in the distribution of charge across the membrane, that occurs concomitantly with channel activation and is believed to result from the movement of a putative voltage sensor.

Molecular studies of voltage-dependent ion channels have revealed that the S4 transmembrane domain may

Box 3–2 Selectivity of Ion Channels

Na^+ channels are 12 times more selective for Na^+ than for any other ion, and some Ca^{2+} channels are a thousand times more selective for Ca^{2+} than for other cations. Although it is relatively easy to understand how an ion channel discriminates between cations (ions that carry a positive electrical charge) and anions (ions that carry a negative electrical charge), a channel's ability to select one cation over another suggests remarkably sophisticated protein design and has been the focus of intense investigation.

Investigators have learned that the SS1–SS2 region of a channel (the extracellular region between transmembrane domains S5 and S6), which is believed to dip into the channel to form the lining of the channel pore (see Figure 3–8), is at least partly responsible for ion selectivity. Studies involving the transfer of the SS1–SS2 region between channel types, such as between chimeric K^+ channels, have indicated that this region determines both single-channel conductance and affinity for a particular blocking ion, such as **tetraethylammonium** (**TEA**); other channel regions have little effect on these properties. Mutagenesis studies also have determined the key amino acid residues that impart various permeability properties. Although these experiments are informative, they do not explain the process by which an ion channel becomes permeable to one ion and not to another. An explanation of selective permeability requires a model of ionic interactions with waters of hydration (bound water molecules) and channel pore amino acids that is consistent with current molecular, electrophysiologic, and structural data.

Ions do not flow through ion channels like water through a pipe; such a model cannot explain how some channel pores are selective for Na^+ and others are selective for K^+. Instead an ion most likely binds transiently to one or more sites in a channel. Presumably its permeability is determined by the amount of energy released during its binding to amino acid residues and by the energy required for its dissociation from some or all surrounding water molecules. The speed with which an ion can dissociate from a pore and escape from a channel is also likely to play a role in selectivity.

Crystallization of the bacterial KcsA K^+ channel has provided great insight into how ionic selectivity may be accomplished. When a K^+ ion enters this channel from the intracellular side, it first passes through a hydrophobic pore that is wide enough to permit the ion to travel with its waters of hydration. Subsequently the ion reaches a water-filled vestibule of uncertain significance. To reach the extracellular side of the membrane, it must pass from this vestibule through a selectivity filter formed by the SS1–SS2-like region of the KcsA channel. This filter, which is so narrow that only fully dehydrated ions can pass through it, with bound water molecules being denied entry, consists of four or five main chain carbonyl oxygen molecules from each of the channel's four subunits. These oxygen molecules form a stack of four or five oxygen rings that make the filter selective because (1) K^+ can accept these rings as a substitute for its waters of hydration, and (2) the position of oxygen in the rings is such that only the binding of K^+ can compensate for the energy lost during dehydration. Na^+, a smaller ion, does not bind to the oxygen cylinder well enough to offset the energy it expends during dehydration. Thus, only K^+ ions can pass through the filter.

---

in fact behave as a gating particle. S4 segments are marked by positively charged amino acids, arginine or lysine, at every third or fourth position, in a pattern that is unique to ion channels. Neutralization, by site-directed mutagenesis, of the positively charged residues in the S4 segment of the Na^+ channel has profound effects on the voltage dependence of channel activation; moreover, these mutations change the gating charge of the channels. Mutations of hydrophobic residues in the S4 region also can cause dramatic changes in the voltage dependence of channel activation, presumably because energy is required to move these residues past hydrophilic residues. However, the exact conformational change that results from movement of the S4 domain and causes the opening of a channel remains unknown.

VOLTAGE-ACTIVATED CLOSING OF ION CHANNELS

In some cases the closing of a voltage-gated ion channel is simply the opposite of its opening; that is, the channel undergoes conformational changes in response to a particular membrane voltage and subsequently returns to its resting conformation when the membrane voltage subsides. The closure of voltage-gated ion channels such as the delayed rectifier K^+ channel, which restores an axon's resting potential after an action potential, does not appear to require additional regulatory mechanisms. (Note that the term *rectifier* describes a channel that passes current much more efficiently in one direction; for example, an inward rectifier preferentially passes current into a cell, and an outward rectifier preferentially passes current out of a cell.)

In response to depolarization, however, a voltage-gated Na^+ channel closes immediately after it is activated, even if the depolarization is maintained, such as during an action potential. Biophysical experiments indicate that this process of *inactivation* is distinctly different from that of *deactivation*, the return of the Na^+ channel to its resting state. The "ball and chain" model of inactivation postulates the movement of a positively charged segment of a channel protein into an open ion

Box 3–3 Accessory Subunits of Channels

The major α subunits of Na^+, K^+, and Ca^{2+} channels are capable of conducting their own voltage-dependent, ion-selective current, such as in *Xenopus* oocytes. However, channels formed by these subunits activate and inactivate much more slowly than do voltage-dependent ion channels found in their native cells. This difference is partly explained by the fact that α subunits do not exist in isolation but are complexed with several accessory proteins that are not required for channel function. For example, investigators have demonstrated biochemically that antibodies directed against the α subunit coprecipitate specific accessory proteins, also called accessory subunits.

Studies that have examined the systematic coexpression of α subunits and accessory proteins, as well as the biochemical characteristics of these proteins, in *Xenopus* oocytes have led to the following speculations about the impact of the accessory subunit on ion channel properties:

- A large number of functional channels seem to be inserted into the plasma membrane when accessory subunits are coexpressed with α subunits. Thus accessory subunits may play a role in channel trafficking or in the stabilization of membrane channels.
- Coexpression of accessory subunits with α subunits speeds the kinetics of a channel; both activation and inactivation become more rapid, approaching those observed in naturally occurring channels. The exact mechanism by which these subunits affect channel kinetics is uncertain but their presence may stabilize the main subunit, allowing the channel to change states more rapidly.
- Coexpression of accessory subunits increases voltage dependence; thus less depolarization is required for channel activation.
- Some accessory subunits contain phosphorylation consensus sequences; thus they may be involved in channel regulation (see Box 3–4).
- Some toxins and pharmacologic agents bind specifically to accessory subunits or bind more tightly to channels that contain them.

channel, which prevents further conductance (Figure 3–10). This model is supported by a great deal of experimental evidence. Perfusion of the inside of an axon with the protease trypsin, for example, abolishes the inactivation of Na^+ channels but leaves the voltage-dependence of Na^+ channels intact; presumably the protease selectively cleaves the ball and chain segment of the Na^+ channel. Site-directed mutagenesis indicates that the ball and chain portion of the Shaker K^+ channel is most likely the N terminus, and that of the Na^+ channel is in the cytoplasmic domain between S3 and S4. Mutations at these sites abolish the inactivation of these respective channels but leave the other properties of the channels relatively intact.

Several toxins and pharmaceutical agents act by modulating the process of inactivation. Some toxins selectively slow Na^+ channel inactivation, causing these channels to remain open for a longer period of time; a class of **scorpion toxins** that act in this manner can lead to spastic paralysis, seizures, and death. Other substances, including some drugs used in the treatment of **epilepsy,** selectively stabilize the inactivated state of the Na^+ channel, thereby decreasing neuronal excitability (see Chapter 21).

TYPES OF ION CHANNELS

The voltage-dependent cation channels are similar enough in general architecture that it is possible to discuss their basic properties as a group. However, rapid advances in molecular biology, pharmacology, and electrophysiology have made it possible to distinguish hundreds of variations of ion channels. Distinct channels arise from different gene products, splice variants of the same gene transcript, posttranslational modifications, and combinations of individual channel subunits. Most of these channels are poorly named. The common designation of "P" or "Q," for example, gives little information about the function of a Ca^{2+} channel. Likewise, the title "inward rectifier K^+ channel" reflects this channel's activity only in experimental situations in which K^+ is artificially high on both sides of the membrane. In vivo, a neuron's potential is almost never more negative than the equilibrium potential of K^+; thus, K^+ channels almost never carry inward K^+ current. The following sections of this chapter serve as a catalogue of the various types and subtypes of voltage-dependent cation channels. The properties, medical relevance, and molecular composition of each are summarized in the most general terms; more information about each channel type can be found in the references listed at the end of the chapter.

SODIUM CHANNELS

Na^+ channels are a relatively homogeneous group of ion channels. Variations do exist: several different Na^+ channels have been cloned, and organisms express tissue-specific Na^+ channel genes. However, across

A

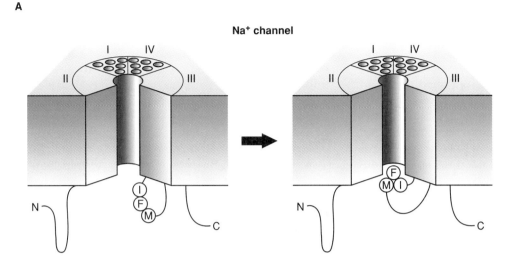

B

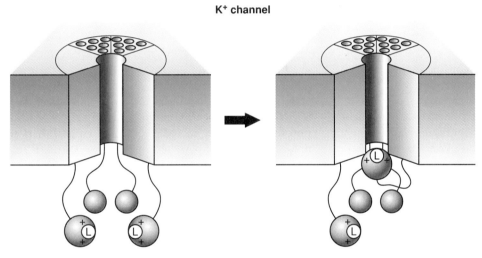

Figure 3–10. Ball and chain inactivation of K^+ and Na^+ channels. **A.** In the Na^+ channel, the intracellular loop between domains III and IV is believed to occlude the mouth of the pore during inactivation. **B.** In the K^+ channel, any one of the N termini may occlude the channel pore. (Adapted with permission from Catterall WA. 1993. Structure and function of voltage-gated ion channels. *TINS* 16:500.)

species and tissue types, Na^+ channel properties are remarkably similar; for example, Na^+ currents in human heart cells display voltage dependence and activation-inactivation kinetics that are comparable to those of Na^+ currents observed in the axons of frogs.

Pharmacology and toxicology of sodium channels Toxins that bind to Na^+ channels are uncommon, but their effects can be dramatic. As mentioned previously, the isolation of the Na^+ channel was initially possible because it binds tightly and specifically to toxins such as **tetrodotoxin,** a heterocyclic compound

found in many marine species, including the Japanese puffer fish, the globe fish, and the blue-ringed octopus. How the same toxin evolved in so many different species is something of a mystery; some scientists speculate that tetrodotoxin is produced by a bacterium that lives symbiotically within these organisms. Approximately 200 humans experience tetrodotoxin poisoning each year, in most cases after consuming improperly prepared puffer fish. The musculature of the puffer fish is safe for consumption and is considered a culinary delicacy in Japan; the toxin resides only in the fish's innards, which must be properly removed to prevent poisoning. Symptoms of tetrodotoxin poisoning include facial numbness, headache, and increasing paralysis and respiratory distress. Although victims are completely paralyzed, they may be conscious and lucid until shortly before death, which generally occurs within 4 to 6 hours. Among those poisoned, the mortality rate is approximately 50%; survival is usually attributed to rapid treatment (gastric lavage) or the victim's ingestion of only a small amount of toxin. Because tetrodotoxin binds to the outside of the Na^+ channel at the S5–S6 loop of the α subunit, site-directed mutagenesis of amino acids in this region greatly reduces its ability to bind to the channel (see Figure 3–8).

Other Na^+ channel toxins act not by blocking the channel but by activating it, usually by slowing or eliminating its voltage-dependent inactivation, which leads to the hyperexcitability of neurons and muscle tissue. Victims of these toxins, which have been isolated from scorpion and sea anemone species, may undergo convulsions and spastic paralysis.

Substances used to treat human disease generally have less dramatic effects on the Na^+ channel. **Phenytoin** and **carbamazepine,** which are used to treat **epilepsy,** act on Na^+ channels by slowing their recovery from an inactivated state. Because prolonged inactivation of these channels limits the firing rates of affected neurons, these drugs can prevent seizures. **Local anesthetics,** such as **cocaine,** and synthetic derivatives such as **lidocaine** and **procaine,** which are membrane permeable in their nonionized form, bind to the cytoplasmic side of the Na^+ channel and also cause Na^+ to bind to the inactivated state of the Na^+ channel, creating a use-dependent blockade of the channel.

Lidocaine

Procaine

The sodium channel in disease   Some inherited neurologic disorders, including certain **myotonias** and **periodic paralyses,** are linked to SkM1, the Na^+ channel in adult skeletal muscle. The myotonias are a group of disorders that involve impaired muscle relaxation. Affected individuals complain of muscle stiffness and may report difficulty in movements such as releasing the grip of a handshake. Myotonic muscle is characterized by an abnormality known as the myotonic run—a series of repetitive discharges that persist for several seconds after a voluntary contraction. Individuals who undergo periodic paralysis experience episodes of extreme muscle weakness. During these episodes, the muscle membrane is depolarized from its resting potential, action potentials cannot be generated, and an electromyogram (EMG) records an absence of activity.

Although myotonia, which is characterized by muscle excitability, and periodic paralysis, which is characterized by muscle hypoexcitability, seem to be diametrically opposed, the underlying Na^+ channel defects are similar. Electrophysiologic studies indicate that both disorders involve slowed or impaired inactivation of the Na^+ channel. In individuals who experience periodic paralysis, the defect in Na^+ channel inactivation is severe enough that muscle remains at a depolarized potential and becomes refractory to further action potentials; in those who experience myotonia, the defect is less severe and results in repetitive firing (Figure 3–11).

POTASSIUM CHANNELS

K^+ channels generally act as a stabilizing force. Their diverse functions include setting a cell's resting potential, repolarizing the cell after an action potential, and controlling an action potential's rate of firing and shape, as seen with an oscilloscope. Proper K^+ channel functioning is critical not only to neuronal activity but also to the operation of many organ systems; mutations in K^+ channels lead to a variety of disorders, ranging from ataxia to cardiac arrhythmias (see Table 3–1). A malfunctioning K^+ channel generally causes some form of hyperexcitability in affected tissue; for example, the **long QT syndrome,** a delay in ventricular repolarization that can cause heart arrhythmias, results from a malfunction of the HERG K^+ channel, which is responsible for repolarizing the ventricle after contraction. Mutations of the related KCNQ2/3 K^+ channel cause **benign familial neonatal convulsions,** which resolve as the affected child grows. Mutation of another K^+ channel—a human Shaker-like channel that is expressed at high levels in the cerebellum—is linked to a type of **episodic ataxia** believed to be caused by an abnormal increase in the firing of cerebellar cells.

Potassium channel classifications   The K^+ channels can be placed into five broad classes based on strikingly different molecular structures, voltage-dependent properties, and functions (Table 3–3). The differences in these channels reflect the variety of ways that they can affect the firing properties of a neuron.

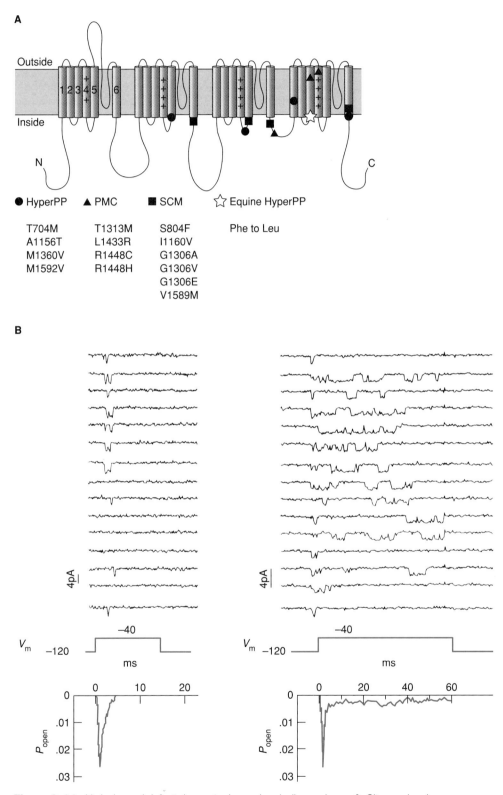

A

Outside

Inside

N

C

● HyperPP   ▲ PMC   ■ SCM   ☆ Equine HyperPP

T704M	T1313M	S804F	Phe to Leu
A1156T	L1433R	I1160V	
M1360V	R1448C	G1306A	
M1592V	R1448H	G1306V	
		G1306E	
		V1589M	

B

Figure 3–11. Na⁺ channel defects in myotonias and periodic paralyses. **A.** Sites and amino acid substitutions of missense mutations that cause hyperkalemic periodic paralysis (HyperPP), paramyotonia congenita (PMC), sodium channel myotonia (SCM), and equine HyperPP. **B.** Recorded activity of single mutant sodium channels indicates a failure to inactivate, which is characteristic of HyperPP. (Adapted with permission from Cannon SC. 1996. Ion-channel defects and aberrant excitability in myotonia and the periodic paralyses. *TINS* 19:5.)

Delayed rectifiers are referred to as classic K^+ channels. They undergo delayed activation after depolarization and inactivate slowly; thus they facilitate repolarization by remaining open for a prolonged period of time. These channels also shape action potentials; blocking their activity increases the duration of action potentials, which in turn depend solely on the inactivation of Na^+ channels for repolarization. *A channels,* also referred to as *Shaker-related* or *Kv channels,* are transiently activated when a cell is depolarized after a period of hyperpolarization. They can function to decrease the frequency of action potential firing by prolonging the interspike interval. *Ca^{2+}-gated K^+ channels* open, as their name implies, in response to the binding of Ca^{2+}, which usually occurs after a depolarization-induced influx of Ca^{2+}. Generally, these channels can remain open for prolonged periods, such as a few seconds, and are responsible for several different types of long *after hyperpolarization* (AHP), which is a hyperpolarization of the membrane that occurs after an action potential

or series of action potentials. A long AHP can profoundly affect the firing pattern of a neuron; for example, when a steady stimulus produces a train of action potentials, an AHP that can gradually slow the rate of firing often is generated in response. However, an AHP is not generated if Ca^{2+} is blocked from entering the cell. This phenomenon, known as spike-frequency adaptation, occurs throughout the nervous system and has many functional consequences.

Anomalous rectifiers (*inward rectifiers*) structurally resemble truncated Shaker-type channels that are missing S1–S4 segments; that is, they comprise only the putative pore-lining segments S5, S6, and SS1–SS2. As with the Shaker-type channels, four of these subunits are believed to multimerize to form a functional channel. Such rectifiers are described as anomalous because they open when the membrane is hyperpolarized and close as the membrane depolarizes. They most likely stabilize a membrane's potential when the potential is near rest, without inhibiting depolarization. By con-

Table 3–3 The Potassium Channels

Channel Name	Activation	Pharmacologic Blockers	Structure
Delayed rectifiers		TEA; Cs^+; H^+; Ba^{2+}; dendrotoxins (from green mamba venom); noxiustoxin; quaternary amines; 4-AP; strychnine; quinidine	
A Channels *Shaker (Kv1.1–1.7)* *Shab (Kv2.1.2.2)* *Shaw (Kv3.1–3.4)* *Shal (Kv4.1–4.3)* *eag (HERG)* *slow (MaxiK)*	Rapidly inactivating delayed rectifiers	TEA; dendrotoxins; 4-AP; quinidine	
K(Ca)	Activated by calcium	TEA; Cs^+; apamin; charybdotoxin; Na^+; Ba^{2+}; quinidine	
Inward rectifier (Kirl–5)	Kir3 family activated by $G\beta\gamma$ subunits of G proteins	TEA; Cs^+; Rb^+; Na^+; Ba^{2+}; Sr^{2+}; H^+; Mg^{2+}	
K(ATP) (Kir3,4)	Inactivated by ATP (activated in the absence of ATP)	TEA; Cs^+; Ba^{2+} sulfonylurea drugs (e.g., tolbutamide, glibenclamide, quinidine; used to enhance insulin secretion from islet cells)	

AP, aminopyridine; TEA, tetraethylammonium.

ducting outward current in the voltage range just slightly positive to E_K, they maintain a resting potential near E_K; however, if the cell is sufficiently depolarized they shut off, freeing the membrane to undergo further depolarization. Anomalous rectifiers are metabolically efficient: by shutting down at more positive potentials, they prevent the outflow of K^+ ions that would otherwise occur during depolarization, sparing the Na^+–K^+-ATPase unnecessary work. This type of K^+ channel is found in many tissues located in the heart, in striated muscle, and in neurons.

Five subfamilies of anomalous rectifiers—Kir1 through Kir5—have been identified. Channels formed by members of the Kir3 subfamily are especially noteworthy because of the role that G proteins play in their regulation (see Chapter 5). G protein-coupled Kir3 channels, termed GIRKs, are critical to many physiologic functions; for example, they mediate the slowing of heart rate by acetylcholine. The binding of acetylcholine to muscarinic acetylcholine receptors in the atrium activates a G protein and liberates its βγ complex, which in turn leads to the activation of a GIRK. The K^+ current produced by this activation slows the depolarization of sinoatrial cells to their firing threshold. This process explains the positive ionotropic and chronotropic effects of muscarinic cholinergic antagonists such as **atropine**. GIRKs are also expressed in the brain, where, among other functions, they mediate a neuron's electrical responses to the activation of many types of G protein-coupled neurotransmitter receptors, especially those coupled with G proteins from the G_i family (see Chapter 5). GIRK knockout mice demonstrate the importance of this action; neurons from these mice exhibit dramatically reduced inhibitory currents to these neurotransmitters.

K(ATP) channels, which are similar to Kir3.4 channels, play an important role in cellular and systemic metabolic regulation. Structurally, each of these ATP-sensitive K^+ channels is a multimeric complex comprising inwardly rectifying K^+ channel subunits and the so-called **sulfonylurea** receptor protein. Sulfonylureas such as **tolbutamide** are used to treat adult-onset **diabetes** and act by increasing insulin secretion from pancreatic β cells. Studies of their mechanisms of action led to the discovery of novel binding proteins, which are currently known to be regulatory subunits of K(ATP) channels. Functionally, these channels are voltage-insensitive; they close in the presence of high (100 μM–1 mM) intracellular ATP concentrations, and open when these concentrations are low, resulting in a more hyperpolarized membrane potential. They may serve a protective function in neurons by reducing neural firing when neural energy reserves are depleted.

CALCIUM CHANNELS

Ca^{2+} is an important signaling molecule that is present in low concentrations in extracellular fluid (1–5 mM) and in minute concentrations in most cell interiors (approximately 0.1–0.2 μM). The opening of Ca^{2+} channels is the critical link between cell depolarization and Ca^{2+} entry, which can result in local intracellular Ca^{2+} concentrations as great as 100 μM. The subsequent binding of Ca^{2+} to intracellular molecules can lead to many significant responses, including the detachment of troponin from actin, which enables muscle contraction; the triggering of neurotransmitter release from nerve terminals (see Chapter 4); the activation of second messenger systems that cause many changes, including alterations in gene expression (see Chapters 5 and 6); and in extreme cases neuronal self-destruction (see Chapter 21). Some Ca^{2+} channels also impart electrical properties to the cells in which they are expressed; for example, such cells may show Ca^{2+} spikes—action potentials in which the depolarizing current is carried predominantly by Ca^{2+}.

Ca^{2+} channels are categorized in terms of their voltage dependence, kinetics (speed of activation and inactivation), and pharmacology. Multiple Ca^{2+} channel genes have been isolated, many of which correspond to Ca^{2+} channel types that were originally classified according to their electrophysiologic properties (Table 3–4).

L channels L-type (*l*arge current or "*l*ong open time") Ca^{2+} channels are activated by large depolarizations (approximately −20 mV), can remain open for a long time before inactivating (500 ms or more), and are blocked by **dihydropyridines.** Three major L-channel subunits have been cloned: α1S, α1C, and α1D. The α1S subunit resides exclusively in skeletal muscle, where it is abundant in transverse tubules; α1C subunits are found in cardiac muscle, smooth muscle, and the brain; and α1D subunits predominate in endocrine and kidney cells but also reside in the brain.

Clinically, these channels are targets for **antianginal** and **antihypertensive** drugs. Dihydropyridine L-type Ca^{2+} channel blockers such as **verapamil, nifedipine,** and **diltiazem** decrease myocardial contractile force, thereby reducing myocardial oxygen requirements, or reduce smooth muscle contractility, thereby decreasing arterial and intraventricular pressure. L-type Ca^{2+} channels are located primarily on the cell bodies and proximal dendrites of neurons. Their role in these neurons is not fully known; however, they admit Ca^{2+} to the cell body during periods of strong depolarization, and this influx causes second messenger activation and changes in gene transcription. Yet substances that

Table 3–4 The Calcium Channels

Channel Name	Activation	Pharmacologic Blockers	Pore-Forming Subunits	Comments
L (*Large* current; *Long* open time)	High-voltage activated (HVA); very slow inactivation ($\tau > 500$ ms)	Blocked by dihydropyridines and related drugs (e.g., veroprine, nifedipine, nitrendipine) and Cd^{2+}; potentiated by BayK	$\alpha 1C, \alpha 1D$	Present in many tissues (e.g., nerve, heart, muscle). In neurons, are preferentially located in cell bodies and proximal dendrites.
N (*Neuronal*)	HVA; inactivation ($\tau \simeq 50$–80 msec)	Blocked by ω-conotoxin GVIA and Cd^{2+}	$\alpha 1B$	Located in neurons only, preferentially in dendritic shafts and nerve terminals.
P (*Purkinje*)	HVA	Blocked by ω-agatoxin IVA (in low concentrations) and ω-conotoxin MVIIC	$\alpha 1A$	Located in neurons only; predominately in synaptic regions and dendritic shafts. High density in cerebellar Purkinje cells.
T (*Transient*)	Low-voltage activated (LVA); rapidly inactivating ($\tau \simeq 20$–50 msec)	Blocked (nonspecifically) by Ni^{2+}, ethosuximide	$\alpha 1G$	Blockers useful in the treatment of petit mal seizures.

block these channels rarely have noticeable neurologic side effects, despite the fact that some—for example, **nimodipine**—can cross the blood–brain barrier.

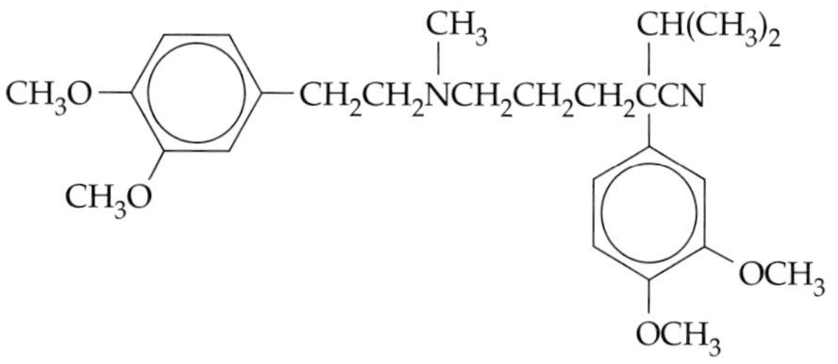

Verapamil

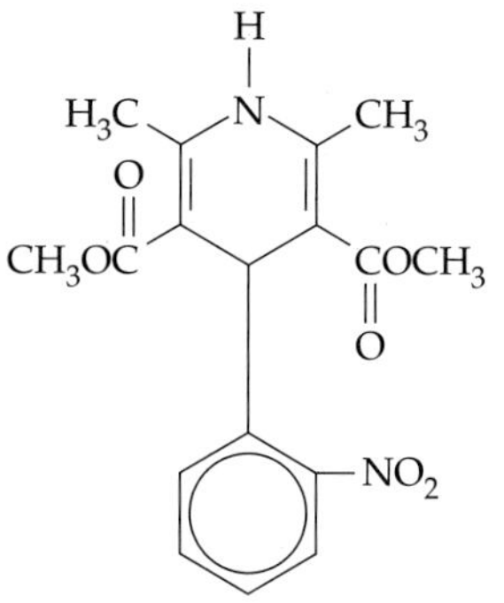

Nifedipine

T channels   T-type (*tiny* current or *transient*) Ca^{2+} channels are activated by depolarizations near resting potential; half-maximal activation of these channels occurs at approximately -40 mV. They exhibit voltage-dependent inactivation such that depolarization produced by their activation ultimately triggers their inactivation. Because of this self-limiting property,

these channels are excellent oscillators; in fact, they are believed to provide a pacemaker current in thalamic neurons that generate the rhythmic cortical discharge associated with **absence seizures (petit mal)**. **Ethosuximide,** which blocks T-type current, is an effective therapy for these seizures (see Chapter 21). The recent cloning of a T-type channel subunit ($\alpha 1G$) should facilitate the development of drugs that interact more specifically with this important Ca^{2+} channel subtype.

N channels   N-type (*n*euronal or "*n*either L nor T") Ca^{2+} channels are activated by large depolarizations, activate and inactivate with moderate kinetics (inactivation $\tau = 50$–80 ms), and are blocked by **ω-conotoxin GVIA**. One major subunit of these channels, known as $\alpha 1B$, has been cloned. These channels are best known for their regulation of neurotransmitter release: Ca^{2+} flows into nerve terminals through N channels in a voltage-dependent manner that triggers this release. However, N-type channels are not solely responsible for such regulation. In the mammalian CNS, blockade of these channels reduces neurotransmission by only 20–30%; blockade of both N and P channels further reduces neurotransmitter release but does not eliminate it completely. A Ca^{2+} channel that has yet to be characterized most likely assists in neurotransmission.

P channels   P-type Ca^{2+} channels, which were first described in cerebellar (*P*urkinje) cells, have single-channel conductances similar to those of N-type channels yet are characterized by minimal inactivation. Like N-type channels, they are involved in triggering neurotransmitter release in some neurons.

The principal subunit of these channels has been cloned and termed α1A. Mutations of the human α1A gene have been linked to two disorders: **familial hemiplegic migraine** and **episodic ataxia.** Although this gene is richly expressed in Purkinje cells, how the mutant P channels cause the abnormalities seen in these disorders remains unknown.

CHLORIDE CHANNELS

Thus far, this chapter has focused on the molecular properties of cation channels, yet muscle cells, neurons, and most other cells are also permeable to Cl^-. Cl^- channels are critical for many physiologic processes, and mutations of these channels have been implicated in a variety of diseases (see Table 3–1).

These channels serve two primary functions. First, they dampen electrical excitability. In most cells, including neurons and myocytes, the intracellular concentration of Cl^- is close to, but below, its electrochemical equilibrium. In a manner similar to that of K^+ channels, Cl^- channels provide a force—the concentration gradient of Cl^-—that pulls the cell toward the equilibrium potential of Cl^-, which is generally a

hyperpolarized value. Thus the inactivation of Cl^- channels can lead to hyperexcitability; for example, mutations in the Cl^- channel protein CLC-1 in skeletal muscle lead to muscle hyperexcitability, which results in **myotonia.** Similarly, the binding of **strychnine** to Cl^--conducting glycine receptors on, among other cells, motor neurons of the spinal cord can lead to violent convulsions and death (see Chapter 7).

Cl^- channels also control the osmotic flow of water across the cell membrane. Some Cl^- channels that regulate osmotic balance are in fact activated by the swelling of a cell; activation of these channels allows Cl^- to exit the swollen cell, accompanied by cations and water. These channels play an important role in secretory cells, such as those of the mucosal epithelium, and in the functioning of the kidney. Indeed, the so-called **loop diuretics,** such as **furosemide,** block Cl^- channels in the ascending loop of Henle and are widely used in the treatment of **congestive heart failure.**

As might be expected, the channels that permit Cl^- to cross plasma membranes differ in molecular composition from the voltage-gated cation channels. Cl^- channels comprise three molecular varieties (Figure 3–12). *Ligand-gated Cl^- channels are among the most*

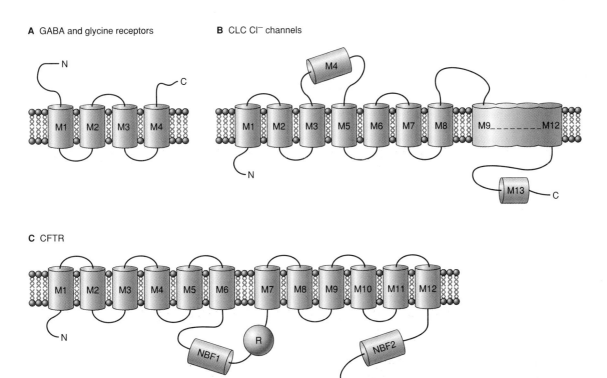

Figure 3–12. Structural models of three Cl^- channel families. **A.** Topological model of γ-aminobutyric acid (GABA) and glycine receptor channels (see Chapter 7). **B.** CLC channel. **C.** CFTR channel. M, transmembrane domains; NBF, nucleotide-binding fold; R, regulatory (phosphorylation) domain. (Adapted with permission from Jentsch TJ. 1996. Chloride channels: A molecular perspective. *Curr Opin Neurobiol* 6:304.)

Box 3–4 Phosphorylation of Ion Channels

Changes in the electrical properties of neurons, which are directly related to modifications of their ion channels, often play a role in the survival of an organism. In a threatening situation, for example, neurons that typically fire only a single action potential may respond by firing long trains of action potentials. The increased firing of such neurons can heighten awareness, provoke a stronger or more rapid behavioral response, or assist in forming a potent memory about a dangerous situation.

Among the most common means by which the excitability of neurons is altered is through the phosphorylation of ion channels, which involves the addition of free phosphate ($-PO^{4-}$) groups to particular amino acid residues of a channel protein. This process changes the stable conformational state of a channel and in turn alters the magnitude and time course of the ionic currents it conducts. Thus phosphorylation provides an excellent basis for ion channel flexibility (see Chapter 5); in seconds or less, the activation of second messenger systems in a neuron can lead to the phosphorylation of channel proteins and to equally swift changes in the electrical properties of the neuron. Depending on the channel, the phosphorylation site, the location of the phosphorylated amino acid residue, and the internal milieu of the cell, this process can alter the following biophysical properties:

- *Inactivation kinetics.* Protein kinase C phosphorylation of a single residue of a Na^+ channel's α subunit—serine 1506 on the intracellular loop between transmembrane domains III and IV—can slow the channel's inactivation. Similarly, phosphorylation of the rapidly inactivating K^+ channel known as Kv3.4 by protein kinase C causes the channel's inactivation to abate. Interestingly, the phosphorylation sites in both of these channels are believed to reside in their "ball and chain" regions.
- *Current amplitude.* Activation of protein kinase A increases the amplitude of K^+ channel Kv1.2 currents; activation of protein kinase C decreases the amplitude of currents through Na^+ channels; and activation of protein kinase A increases the amplitude of currents in KCN2 K^+ channels (mutations of this latter channel cause **benign familial neonatal convulsions;** see Table 3–1). However, investigators have yet to discover how phosphorylation causes these changes.

- *Voltage dependence of channel responses.* Phosphorylation of L-type Ca^{2+} channels by protein kinase A not only slows channel inactivation but also shifts the channel's voltage dependence to more negative potentials.
- *Accumulation of channel protein in the plasma membrane.* Long-term protein kinase A treatment of oocytes expressing Kv1.1 potassium channels increases the amplitude of currents expressed by these channels. Studies indicate that this response is most likely caused by increased amounts of channel protein in the plasma membrane.

The effect of norepinephrine (NE) on hippocampal pyramidal cells illustrates how the phosphorylation of an ion channel protein can affect the behavior of a neuron, as shown in the figure. In the absence of norepinephrine, depolarization of a pyramidal cell results in a small number of action potentials. The activation of a Ca^{2+}-activated K^+ channel causes an after hyperpolarization (AHP), which limits the number of action potentials that occur in response to a depolarizing stimulus. In the presence of norepinephrine, depolarization of the pyramidal cell leads to a much more prolonged train of action potentials. Because norepinephrine binds to the β-adrenergic receptor, which activates adenylyl cyclase, it leads to an accumulation of cAMP and activation of protein kinase A. Protein kinase A in turn phosphorylates Ca^{2+}-activated K^+ channels and blocks their activity. Thus norepinephrine increases the firing of a neuron by removing the hyperpolarizing currents, or AHP, that inhibit its activity.

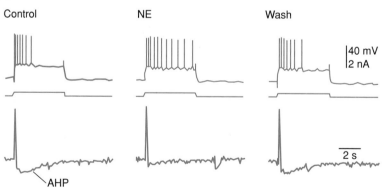

(Adapted with permission from Madison DV, Nicoll RA. 1986. Actions of noradrenaline recorded intracellularly in rat hippocampal CA1 pyramidal neurons in vitro. *J Physiol* 372:221.)

important in the brain; they act as signaling proteins for the inhibitory neurotransmitters γ-aminobutyric (GABA) and glycine (see Chapter 7). *CLC chan*which are believed to function as multimers of teins, are a family of homologous proteins ed by twelve presumptive transmembrane

domains (see Figure 3–12). Eight CLCs have been cloned, among them the previously mentioned CLC-1 in skeletal muscle, and CLC-5, which is highly expressed in the kidney. **Dent disease,** an X-linked kidney disorder associated with an unusually high incidence of kidney stones, is caused by loss-of-function mutations in CLC-5.

Cystic fibrosis transmembrane conductance regulator (*CFTR*) *channels* are activated by the binding of ATP to two nucleotide-binding domains and by the phosphorylation of key serine residues on the regulatory domain (see Figure 3–12; also see Box 3–4 for a discussion of ion channel phosphorylation). Like CLC channels, CFTRs are believed to possess twelve transmembrane domains; however, CFTR channels are distinguished from CLC channels by features such as their nucleotide binding domains. The CFTR is among the most intensively studied ion channels because mutations of this channel cause **cystic fibrosis,** a relatively common hereditary disease that affects one in 3000 Caucasian newborns. In individuals with cystic fibrosis, the loss of CFTR Cl^- channels in several types of epithelial cells limits the egress of Cl^- ions into the lumen. Through mechanisms that are not completely understood, the disease also affects epithelial Na^+ channels, whose malfunctioning causes the production of a thick, desiccated mucus. This abnormal secretion leads to obstruction of the biliary and pancreatic tracts and to a greatly increased incidence of pulmonary disease.

SELECTED READING

Ackerman MJ, Clapham DE. 1997. Ion channels: Basic science and clinical disease. *N Engl J Med* 336:1575–1586.

Beaumont V, Zucker RS. 2000. Enhancement of synaptic transmission by cyclic AMP modulation of presynaptic I_h channels. *Nature Neurosci* 3:133–141.

Catterall WA. 2000. From ionic currents to molecular mechanisms: the structure and function of voltage-gated sodium channels. *Neuron* 26:13–25.

Choe S, Kreusch A, Pfaffinger PJ. 1999. Toward the three-dimensional structure of voltage-gated potassium channels. *Trends Biochem Sci* 24:345–349.

Cooper EC, Jan LY. 1999. Ion channel genes and human neurological disease: recent progress, prospects, and challenges. *Proc Natl Acad Sci USA* 96:4759–4766.

Doyle DA, Cabral JM, Pfuetzner RA, et al. 1998. The structure of the potassium channel: molecular basis of K^+ conduction and selectivity. *Science* 180:69–77.

Dunlap K, Luebke JL, Turner TJ. 1995. Exocytotic Ca^{2+} channels in mammalian central neurons. *Trends Neurosci* 18: 89–98.

Hausser M. Spruston N, Stuart GJ. 2000. Diversity and dynamics of dendritic signaling. *Science* 290:739–744.

Hille B. 1992. *Ionic Channels of Excitable Membranes.* Sunderland, MA: Sinauer Press.

Hille B, Catterall WA. 1999. Electrical excitability and ion channels. In: Siegel GJ, Agranoff BW, Albers RW, et al (eds). *Basic Neurochemistry,* 6th ed., pp. 119–137. Raven Press.

Jan LY, Jan YN. 1989. Voltage-sensitive ion channels. *Cell* 56: 13–25.

Jentsch TJ. 1996. Chloride channels: A molecular perspective. *Curr Opin Neurobiol* 6:303–310.

Jentsch TJ. 2000. Neuronal KCNQ potassium channels: physiology and role in disease. *Nature Rev Neurosci* 1:21–30.

Johnston D, Wu SM-S. 1995. *Foundations of Cellular Neurophysiology.* MIT Press.

Noda M, Shimizu S, Tanabe T, et al. 1984. Primary structure of electrophorus electricus sodium channel deduced from cDNA sequence. *Nature* 312:121–127.

Papazian DM, Schwarz TL, Tempel BL, et al. 1987. Cloning of genomic and complementary DNA from Shaker, a putative potassium channel gene from *Drosophila. Science* 237: 749–753.

Sargent PB. 1992. Electrical signaling. In: Hall Z (ed). *An Introduction to Molecular Neurobiology.* Sunderland, MA: Sinauer Press.

Schroeder BC, Kubisch C, Stein V, Jentsch TJ. 1998. Moderate loss of function of cyclic-AMP-modulated KCNQ2/KCNQ3 K^+ channels causes epilepsy. *Nature* 396:687–690.

Schwiebert EM, Egan ME, Hwang TH, et al. 1995. CFTR regulates outwardly rectifying chloride channels through an autocrine mechanism involving ATP. *Cell* 81:1063–1073.

Tempel BL, Papazian DM, Schwarz TL, et al. 1987. Sequence of a probable potassium channel component encoded at Shaker locus of *Drosophila. Science* 237:770–775.

Timpe LC, Schwarz TL, Tempel BL, et al. 1988. Expression of functional potassium channels from Shaker cDNA in *Xenopus* oocytes. *Nature* 331:143–145.

Vassilev PM, Scheuer T, Catterall WA. 1988. Identification of an intracellular peptide segment involved in sodium channel inactivation. *Science* 241:1658–1661.

Wann KT. 1993. Neuronal sodium and potassium channels: Structure and function. *Br J Anaesth* 71:2–14.

Chapter 4

Synaptic Transmission

KEY CONCEPTS

- Synaptic transmission is a signal transduction process that begins with the action potential-dependent release of neurotransmitter from a presynaptic terminal. The neurotransmitter then binds to and activates postsynaptic receptors that modify the electrical and biochemical properties of the postsynaptic cell.

- The major classes of neurotransmitters are amino acid transmitters, such as glutamate and GABA; biogenic amines, including dopamine and norepinephrine; peptides; diffusible gases, such as nitric oxide; and nucleosides, such as adenosine.

- Neurotransmitters are stored in small organelles called synaptic vesicles that fuse with the presynaptic terminal membrane and release their contents when an action potential invades the terminal and causes a rise in calcium due to activation of voltage-dependent calcium channels.

- A single neurotransmitter typically activates several different subtypes of receptors.

- Neurotransmitter receptors are classified as ligand-gated ion channels or G protein-coupled receptors.

- After being released, most neurotransmitters are transported back into the presynaptic terminal or into glia by specialized proteins called plasma membrane transporters. A different family of transporters is responsible for pumping neurotransmitter into synaptic vesicles.

- Neurotransmitter transporters are important targets of many antidepressant medications and psychostimulant drugs such as cocaine.

- The proteins that are responsible for the fusion of synaptic vesicles with the presynaptic plasma membrane, a process known as exocytosis, have been identified and extensively characterized. Some of these proteins are the targets of bacterial toxins, such as tetanus and botulinum toxin.

- After exocytosis, synaptic vesicles are recycled and used again by repackaging them with neurotransmitter.

- Many of the proteins responsible for synaptic vesicle exocytosis and recycling also play a role in other cellular processes that require the transport of proteins in vesicles or membrane fusion.

When we think, feel, or move, information passes rapidly among neurons across specialized gaps called synapses. Like other cellular events, synaptic communication requires highly regulated interaction among a complex set of proteins. Activity-dependent changes in synaptic transmission are the basis of learning and memory, and abnormal synaptic function underlies many neuropsychiatric illnesses. This chapter explores the biochemical basis of synaptic transmission and explains how this process is regulated.

NEURONAL MORPHOLOGY

DENDRITES AND AXONS

Nerve cell components are morphologically specialized to receive, process, and send information (Figure 4–1; see Chapter 2). The reception of chemical information from both neighboring and distant cells occurs primarily in dendrites, which extend from neuronal cell bodies (soma) in complex patterns resembling the branches of a tree. These processes may reach a length several times that of a soma and in some cells contain numerous small spines on which excitatory synaptic transmission is focused. Here chemical information is converted into electrical information, which is integrated in both the dendrites and the soma before passing from these sites to the morphologic specialization known as the axon. Axons are single processes that complete the cycle of synaptic transmission by converting electrical impulses into chemical signals, which mediate communication with other neurons. Axons vary greatly in length: some extend only a few microns, while others, such as those that innervate spinal motor neurons, must travel a distance of nearly one meter. Yet remarkable electrical properties enable even the longest axons to retain the speed and accuracy of the impulses that pass through them (see Chapter 3). At the ends of axons are morphologic specializations called nerve terminals or presynaptic boutons. Electrical impulses that travel through an axon terminate here, triggering the release of one or more chemical signals from the nerve terminal. A single axon typically branches to form many of these terminals, which in turn innervate one or more cells.

Thus synaptic transmission is a signal transduction process that occurs in three steps: (1) electrical information in the axon of a presynaptic cell is converted to a chemical signal in its nerve terminal, (2) this chemical signal is transmitted to another cell, and (3) the chemical message received by the postsynaptic cell is converted into an electrical signal. This process occurs at the interface between presynaptic and post-

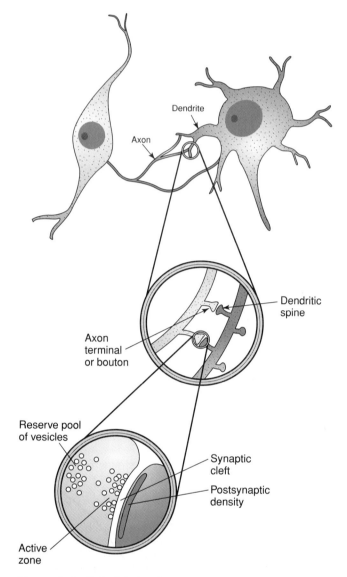

Figure 4–1. At the interface between an axon and a postsynaptic cell, known as the synaptic cleft, an axon terminal, or synaptic bouton, innervates a dendritic spine. In the active zone of the presynaptic terminal, synaptic vesicles cluster against the plasma membrane. A reserve pool of synaptic vesicles lies nearby, and the postsynaptic density lies opposite the active zone within the dendritic spine.

synaptic cells at a subcellular structure called the synapse. A small fraction of synapses are referred to as gap junctions; these are electrical junctions that are morphologically distinct from chemical synapses (see Chapter 2). Because virtually all pharmacologic agents act at chemical synapses rather than at gap junctions, only chemical synapses are addressed in this chapter.

THE SYNAPSE

Communication between neurons must be precise, and the accuracy of this exchange of information is partly ensured by its restriction to the site of the synapse (a term coined by Charles Sherrington in 1897). The anatomist Ramón y Cajal was the first to determine that the synapse is composed of three distinct elements: a presynaptic nerve terminal or bouton, its postsynaptic target, and the space between these two elements, known as the synaptic cleft. Since Cajal's time, extensive morphologic analyses have revealed additional details, including specialized presynaptic structures that release chemical signals known as neurotransmitters from the nerve terminal, and postsynaptic structures involved in processing the signals (Figures 4–1 and 4–2). On the presynaptic side of the synapse, in the active zone of the nerve terminal, neurotransmitter is released from vesicles that cluster near the plasma membrane. On the other side of the synapse are postsynaptic specializations, the composition of which varies with the type of neurotransmitter released from the presynaptic terminal. The postsynaptic density, which is detected at excitatory synapses, is the best-characterized postsynaptic specialization. It is easily identified in electron micro-

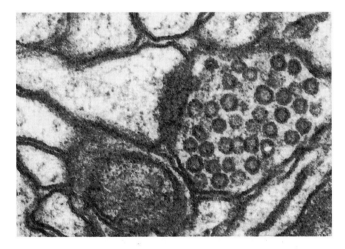

Figure 4–2. Electron micrograph of an excitatory synapse. Two primary components are evident: a presynaptic terminal (*right*) and the postsynaptic target, with a dendritic spine to the left. A depolarization-dependent influx of Ca^{2+} into the terminal causes synaptic vesicles, visible as uniform spherical organelles, to fuse with the plasma membrane, thereby releasing neurotransmitter into the synaptic cleft. Released transmitter subsequently binds to postsynaptic receptors. The postsynaptic density, the site at which receptors are located, is visible as the dark, electron-dense region adjacent to the plasma membrane at the end of the dendritic spine. (Image provided by D. K. Selig and K. M. Harris, Boston University).

graphs (see Figure 4–2) as a proteinaceous matrix of fine filaments just under the plasma membrane of postsynaptic dendritic spines. The proteins that comprise this structure, such as postsynaptic density protein 95 (PSD95), act as a scaffold to cluster and organize molecules involved in postsynaptic signaling. The synaptic cleft itself is bound by extracellular matrix proteins and cell adhesion molecules that may function to strengthen or weaken synaptic contacts.

CHEMICAL SYNAPTIC TRANSMISSION

Classes of neurotransmitters Information is passed across the synapse by neurotransmitters. There are several categories of neurotransmitters (Table 4–1), including amino acid transmitters, such as glutamate and γ-aminobutyric acid (GABA); biogenic amines, including dopamine and norepinephrine; peptides; diffusible gases, such as nitric oxide; and nucleosides, such as adenosine. Historically, it was believed that only one type of transmitter could be synthesized and released from a cell—a principle that became known as Dale's Law in honor of Sir Henry Dale. Ironically, Dale never made this strict assertion. However, more recent evidence suggests that a single cell may co-release two or perhaps more neurotransmitters. The co-release of monoamines with peptides, and of several transmitters with adenosine, is particularly well documented. Moreover, some spinal interneurons release both GABA and glycine, and some midbrain dopaminergic cells may release both glutamate and dopamine. The biosynthesis, metabolism, and functions of the different types of neurotransmitters, as well as the receptors that mediate their signaling, are discussed extensively in subsequent chapters. This chapter focuses on the mechanisms underlying transmitter release.

STORAGE AND RELEASE OF NEUROTRANSMITTERS

With the exception of the diffusible gases, all chemical transmitters are stored in secretory vesicles. Like other cellular organelles, these vesicles have a limiting membrane composed of phospholipids (Box 4–1) and an aqueous lumen. The lumen is filled with thousands of transmitter molecules that sometimes reach near-molar concentrations. During synaptic transmission, secretory vesicles fuse with the plasma membrane, allowing communication between the aqueous interior of the vesicle and the extracellular space. The most abundant form of secretory vesicle in the CNS is the so-called small synaptic vesicle. These vesicles cluster in the active zone of the nerve terminal and are released rapidly when the nerve terminal depolarizes.

Table 4–1 Chemical Neurotransmitters

Transmitter Type	Representative Example	Structure
Biogenic amines	Monoamines: Dopamine	
	Acetylcholine	
Amino acids	γ-aminobutyric acid (GABA)	
	Glutamate	
Peptides	Leu-enkephalin	Tyr–Gly–Gly–Phe–Leu
Nucleosides	Adenosine	
Gases	Nitric oxide	$\cdot N{=}O$

The amount of transmitter in each vesicle is called a quantum. Because transmitter release proceeds through the fusion of individual vesicles with the presynaptic terminal plasma membrane, the release process is known as quantal release. The biochemical processes that are responsible for quantal release of transmitter are addressed in detail later in this chapter.

POSTSYNAPTIC SIGNALING

After a neurotransmitter diffuses across the synaptic cleft to the postsynaptic neuron, receptors embedded in the postsynaptic membrane bind to the neurotransmitter and cause an electrical or biochemical alteration in the postsynaptic cell. **Excitatory** signals cause the membrane to *depolarize* so that positive charge flows into the cell, and **inhibitory** signals cause the membrane to *hyperpolarize,* whereby positive charge flows out of the cell or negative charge flows into the cell. These electrical signals are integrated in the dendrites and cell body and, if depolarization is sufficient, an all-or-none action potential fires and transmits an electrical impulse along the axon (see Chapter 3). Whether synaptic transmission is fast, occurring within several

Box 4–1 Oil and Water: Lipid Membranes and Aqueous Cytoplasm

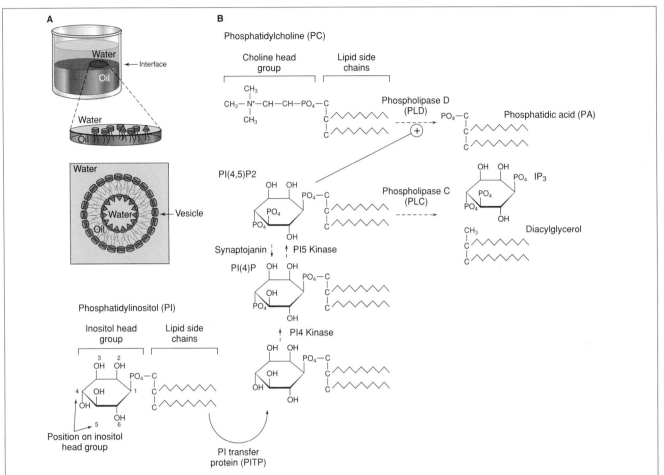

Oil and water are incapable of mixing because hydrophobic and hydrophilic molecules form separate phases. A similar principle enables cells to maintain the compartmentalization of their contents; aqueous contents of one compartment are unable to mix with aqueous contents of another compartment because they are separated by lipids (i.e., a membrane bilayer).

The generation of a lipid bilayer occurs naturally from the separation between hydrophobic and hydrophilic phases. This is because most membrane lipids are amphiphiles, which means that they contain both hydrophilic and hydrophobic parts. The hydrophilic part prefers to associate with an aqueous phase such as water, whereas the hydrophobic part prefers a hydrophobic phase such as lipid. As a result, amphiphiles are found at the interface between lipid and water. When the concentration of amphiphiles in an aqueous solution is sufficiently high, a distinctive phenomenon occurs. The hydrophobic parts face outward toward the hydrophilic phase, for example, water (Figure A). This fundamental property of amphiphilic lipids results in the formation of lipid bilayers, which form the boundaries of all cellular compartments including synaptic vesicles.

Although such bilayers serve to compartmentalize cells, they are both fluid and flexible; thus vesicles can fuse with a plasma membrane and can form by budding from parent organelles. Furthermore, the lipid bilayers surrounding organelles vary in terms of their phospholipid composition, and the head groups of the component lipids are sometimes altered enzymatically. The 3, 4, and 5 positions of the inositol head groups may be linked to phosphate groups by reactions that are catalyzed by different lipid kinases, depending on the position (Figure B). In addition, lipid phosphatases may remove phosphate from the inositol ring. A growing number of observations link phosphotidylinositol (PI) phosphorylation to membrane fusion events.

Because phospholipases can cleave chemical bonds in phospholipids, they play an important role in cell signaling and membrane trafficking events. Two products of phospholipase C and D are shown in Figure B. The products of PLC, IP_3 and DAG, are important second messengers and play a role in cell signaling as discussed in Chapter 5. In contrast, the product of PLD, phosphatidic acid (PA), appears to be involved in membrane trafficking (see Box 4–6). Studies have revealed that IP_3 can activate PLD, thus indicating the complex functional interaction between these pathways.

milliseconds, or slow—taking place in seconds or minutes—depends on the type of receptor targeted by the neurotransmitter (Figure 4–3).

FAST SYNAPTIC TRANSMISSION

Fast synaptic transmission is mediated by transmitter- or ligand-gated ion channels, also called receptor ionophores. The most extensively studied of these is the nicotinic acetylcholine receptor, which is composed of five subunits that enclose a central aqueous pore. When acetylcholine binds to this receptor, the pore opens transiently (1 to 10 ms) and allows the passage of approximately 20,000 positively charged Na^+ ions. Molecular cloning has revealed that the basic design of

most if not all ligand-gated channels is similar to that of voltage-gated channels (see Chapters 3 and 7).

SLOW SYNAPTIC TRANSMISSION

Many of the neurotransmitters involved in fast synaptic transmission induce slower synaptic responses when they activate receptors coupled to heterotrimeric guanine nucleotide-binding proteins (G proteins). When a neurotransmitter binds to a G protein-coupled receptor, the receptor activates a nearby G protein. The α subunit of the G protein subsequently dissociates from its βγ subunits. Both α and βγ subunits can activate downstream molecules, including specific types of ion channels (see Chapter 5). These various biochemi-

Ligand-gated ion channel

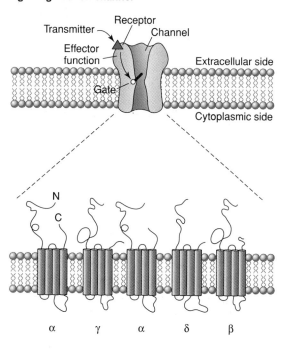

G protein-coupled receptor

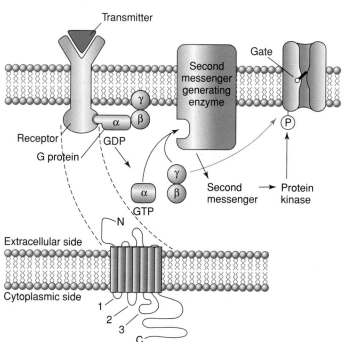

Figure 4–3. Ligand-gated channels and G protein-coupled receptors. Ligand-gated ion channels, which mediate fast synaptic transmission, are composed of one or more proteins embedded in the plasma membrane that form a central, gated pore. In response to the binding of transmitter, this type of receptor undergoes a conformational change, opening the gate and allowing ions to diffuse passively along concentration gradients through a hydrophilic opening in an otherwise hydrophobic bilayer. G protein-coupled receptors, which mediate slow synaptic transmission, transduce neurotransmitter signals through a different mechanism. These proteins do not form gated pores in the membrane; rather, the binding of transmitter induces a conformational change that allows the receptor to activate a heterotrimeric G protein (see Chapter 5). The activated G protein dissociates into a free α subunit bound to GTP and a free βγ subunit dimer. Both can activate enzymes that synthesize second messengers; in addition, βγ dimers directly regulate certain ion channels. Second messengers also regulate ion channels, most often by activating protein kinases, which subsequently phosphorylate such channels (P). 1 2 3, cytoplasmic domains of G protein-coupled receptor. (Adapted with permission from Kandel ER, Schwartz JH, Jessell TM. 2000. *Principles of Neural Science,* 4th ed, p. 184. New York: McGraw-Hill.)

cal steps mediate slow synaptic transmission because they generally require more time to develop compared with the opening of a ligand-gated channel. Stimulation of G protein-coupled receptors does not always produce excitatory or inhibitory transmission; in some cases it modulates the actions of other neurotransmitters, such as glutamate.

In addition to regulating ion channels, G proteins activate several enzymes that regulate the formation of second messengers such as cAMP, cGMP, and diacylglycerol (DAG). G proteins also regulate the flow of the second messenger Ca^{2+} into neurons. Once formed, second messengers stimulate or inhibit protein kinases or protein phosphatases, whose subsequent phosphorylation or dephosphorylation of ion channels results in the generation of postsynaptic electrical signals. Some second messengers, such as cAMP and cGMP, and G protein subunits (α and $\beta\gamma$) can directly bind to and modify the activity of specific ion channels. Moreover, each step in an intracellular signaling cascade typically undergoes additional regulation (see Chapter 5). Thus the involvement of G protein-coupled receptors greatly increases the complexity and flexibility of the types of electrical signals that can be generated by neurotransmitters.

Neurotransmitter receptors influence neurons in many ways beyond modifying their electrical properties. Their activation or inhibition of second messenger-protein phosphorylation cascades can profoundly change the intracellular milieu of a cell by regulating the activity of its enzymes—including metabolic or degradative enzymes, or those involved in the synthesis of neurotransmitter—and its other proteins, including those that form the cytoskeleton or direct synaptic vesicle traffic. Moreover, these cascades regulate gene transcription and protein synthesis and can activate multiple downstream effectors. Such activities can have long-lasting effects on neuronal function (see Chapters 5 and 6).

RECEPTOR SUBTYPES

Ligand-gated ion channels and G protein-coupled receptors each comprise multiple subtypes. A single neurotransmitter can activate a variety of these receptor subtypes, and several members of the same receptor family can co-localize at a single synapse; thus the signal received by a postsynaptic neuron can vary considerably and may be quite complex. Moreover, the actions of any individual transmitter are in fact dictated by the receptor subtype to which it binds and by the subsynaptic localization of that receptor.

Before the advent of molecular cloning techniques, receptor subtypes were grouped according to their pharmacologic profiles, including their responses to particular agonists and antagonists. More recently,

cloned receptors have been grouped more precisely on the basis of structural and functional similarities and according to their cellular localization. Some receptor subtypes tend to be located in particular cell types or subcellular regions. Presynaptic localization does not exclude postsynaptic localization, and the presence of some receptor subtypes—for example, the serotonin 5-HT$_{1a}$ receptor—in both presynaptic terminals and postsynaptic cells further increases the complexity of synaptic communication. The activation of receptors located in the presynaptic bouton typically modifies the release of neurotransmitter. Presynaptic receptors that respond to the transmitter released by that terminal are called *autoreceptors;* presynaptic receptors that respond to other transmitters are sometimes called *heteroreceptors.* Variations in signaling pathway activation among receptor subtypes underscore the role of receptors in dictating the actions of the transmitters that bind to them.

NEUROTRANSMITTER STORAGE, REUPTAKE, AND RELEASE

THE ROLE OF CALCIUM IONS

Much of our current understanding of synaptic transmission is based on the pioneering work of Bernard Katz and his colleagues. In the 1950s, Katz uncovered the role of Ca^{2+} in neurotransmitter release through his investigation of the neuromuscular junction (NMJ). The NMJ comprises a presynaptic motor nerve terminal and a postsynaptic specialization on the muscle cell known as an end plate. Although the NMJ differs significantly from a synapse in the CNS, it is similar enough to serve as a model. When the motor nerve of the NMJ is electrically stimulated, it releases a chemical message that produces an electrical signal in the muscle cell, called the excitatory postsynaptic current, which in turn causes contraction of the muscle. When this contractile process is paralyzed, the relationship between chemical transmission and the electrical response can be studied in isolation. The chemical transmitter at the vertebrate NMJ is acetylcholine, identified by Otto Loewi in 1921 as the first known chemical neurotransmitter.

To understand the relationship between the action potential of the motor nerve and neurotransmitter release, Katz had to determine how electrical information was converted into chemical information. He and his colleagues demonstrated that the action potential per se was not required for acetylcholine release. Rather, the action potential caused the nerve terminal to depolarize, which in turn caused the release of transmitter. They demonstrated this by eliminating the action potential with the Na^{2+} channel-blocking neurotoxin known as **tetrodotoxin** (see Chapter 3) and changing the voltage in the nerve terminal with an electrode, which allowed them to depolarize the terminal and induce transmitter release directly. Next they sought to explain how depolarization caused the release of transmitter. During their investigations, Katz and his coworkers discovered that they could prevent the release of neurotransmitter by eliminating extracellular Ca^{2+}; thus they concluded that the entry of Ca^{2+} into the nerve terminal triggered transmitter release. We now know that the opening of voltage-gated Ca^{2+} channels in response to depolarization (see Chapter 3) causes a rapid increase in the intracellular concentration of Ca^{2+}, which in turn causes the release of neurotransmitter.

QUANTAL RELEASE

Katz and colleagues subsequently addressed the process of neurotransmitter release. They studied the electrical response of the muscle cell in the absence of presynaptic stimulation and discovered that the post-synaptic cell exhibited small, spontaneous electrical responses even when the nerve terminal was not stimulated. Equally important was the discovery that these miniature end plate potentials (MEPPs or *minis*) were all approximately the same size. Indeed, when the nerve was stimulated to evoke larger postsynaptic currents, the resulting end plate potentials were always integral sums of the MEPPs (Figure 4–4). Consequently Katz postulated that a single MEPP represents the postsynaptic response to the smallest amount of transmitter released by a presynaptic cell, thus giving birth to the idea of quantal release.

The precise physical equivalent of a quantum remained to be determined, but two pieces of evidence suggested that this elemental unit represented the transmitter contained in a single synaptic vesicle. First, electron micrographs revealed clusters of regular round vesicles lined up at the presynaptic membrane (see Figure 4–2). Second, these vesicles sometimes appeared

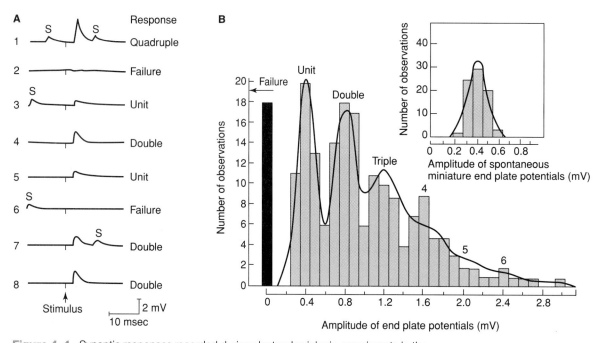

Figure 4–4. Synaptic responses recorded during electrophysiologic experiments in the 1950s and 1960s. These experiments demonstrated that neurotransmitter is released from presynaptic terminals in discrete packages or quanta. Moreover, they determined that the postsynaptic response does not have a fixed amplitude but occurs in discrete steps, each of which represents the response to transmitter released from a single vesicle. **A.** Spontaneous miniature end plate potentials (S), which are electrical recordings of postsynaptic electrical activity in the absence of an external stimulus, and synaptic responses (end plate potentials) evoked by a weak stimulus. The recorded end plate potentials are generated by the release of 1 to 4 quanta of neurotransmitter; occasionally a weak stimulus fails to trigger such a release. **B.** A histogram that indicates the amplitude of the end plate potentials reveals peaks that are multiple integrals of the miniature end plate potentials (*inset*). (Reproduced with permission from Kandel ER, Schwartz JH, Jessell TM. 2000. *Principles of Neural Science*, 4th ed, p. 260. New York: McGraw-Hill.)

to be fused with the plasma membrane, and in the process of opening their lumen to the extracellular space, such vesicles look like the Greek letter Ω and are called omega profiles. Thus small vesicles at the site of transmitter release appeared capable of releasing their contents into the synaptic cleft by fusing with the plasma membrane. Whether these synaptic vesicles contained neurotransmitter was unclear; however, biochemical studies demonstrated that synaptic vesicles at the NMJ contained acetylcholine. These findings validated the theory that a synaptic vesicle represents the anatomic equivalent of electrophysiologically defined quanta. Fittingly, the process of transmitter release was subsequently referred to as *exocytosis.*

Although morphologic studies indicate that there are tens to hundreds of synaptic vesicles in each nerve terminal, neurotransmitter is not released every time an action potential invades this structure. Instead, neurotransmitter release is a stochastic or probabilistic process: in response to an action potential it sometimes occurs and sometimes fails to occur. The probability of transmitter release can vary widely from synapse to synapse and can be modified by the activation of presynaptic neurotransmitter receptors, by drugs, and by recent synaptic activity.

The quantal hypothesis has stood the test of time. With few exceptions, studies have confirmed that neurotransmitter is released from the nerve terminal in synaptic vesicles. Whether these packets of neurotransmitter are always the same size has been technically difficult to determine; however, variations among quanta most likely exist. Indeed, some of the first synaptic vesicles isolated from the NMJ revealed cholinergic vesicles that contained varying amounts of transmitter. In the CNS, quantal size may vary even more than it does at the NMJ. Variations in the postsynaptic response to each quantum and evidence indicating that different populations of synaptic vesicles may differ in the amount of neurotransmitter they store strongly support this theory. Although investigators have yet to determine the mechanisms underlying variations in synaptic vesicle content, they most likely involve the proteins that synthesize neurotransmitters and transport them into synaptic vesicles.

PACKAGING AND TRANSPORT OF NEUROTRANSMITTERS

Small-molecule neurotransmitters such as the biogenic amines and amino acid transmitters are synthesized in the cytoplasm of the neuron; the enzymes that convert precursors into mature neurotransmitters are discussed in subsequent chapters on individual neurotransmitters. Because they are synthesized in the cytoplasm, these neurotransmitters must be transported

across the synaptic vesicle membrane into its lumen. The process of vesicular transport serves to package neurotransmitters for regulated exocytotic release.

Purified secretory vesicles express distinct proteins called transporters that mediate the pumping or transport of monoamines, such as serotonin, dopamine, and norepinephrine; acetylcholine; GABA and glycine; and glutamate into the vesicles (Figure 4–5; Table 4–2). The active transport of monoamines and acetylcholine is driven by the pH gradient (ΔpH) across these vesicle membranes, which propels the exchange of two luminal protons for one cytoplasmic amine. In contrast, glutamate transport depends primarily on an electrochemical gradient ($\Delta\Psi$), and GABA transport depends on both ΔpH and $\Delta\Psi$. The transporter for purine transmitters such as adenosine has not been identified. Drugs that inhibit such vesicular transport have signifi-

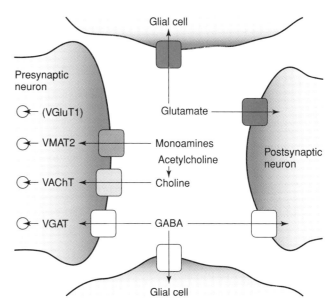

Figure 4–5. Transmitter fates. Mechanisms for terminating the action of transmitters include transport into the presynaptic terminal, uptake by glia or postsynaptic cells, enzymatic degradation, and passive diffusion away from the synapse. For monoamines, neurotransmission is terminated by transport across the plasma membrane. In contrast, acetylcholine is degraded in the synaptic cleft by acetylcholinesterase and transported into the presynaptic terminal as choline. The actions of the amino acid transmitters glutamate and γ-aminobutyric acid (GABA) are terminated by active transport into postsynaptic neurons or glia; GABA also can be transported into presynaptic terminals. After reaching a presynaptic terminal, a neurotransmitter may be degraded (not shown) or recycled into synaptic vesicles. Vesicular transporters include proteins specific for GABA (VGAT), acetylcholine (VAChT), and monoamines (VMAT2). A vesicular transporter for glutamate (VGlutT1) has recently been cloned. Acetylcholine must be resynthesized from choline and acetylCoA before it is transported by VAChT.

Table 4–2 Molecularly Cloned Plasma Membrane Transporters

Amine/GABA Family

Transporter	Transmitter	Localization
GAT-1	GABA	Neurons (presynaptic and postsynaptic); glia
GAT-2	GABA	Glia
GAT-3	GABA	Glia
GAT-4	GABA	Glia
DAT	Dopamine	Dopaminergic neurons
SERT	Serotonin	Serotonergic neurons
NET	Norepinephrine	Noradrenergic and adrenergic neurons

Glutamate Family

Animal Homologs of Human Transporters	Transmitter[1]	Localization
EAAT1 (GLAST1, rat)	Glutamate	Neurons
EAAT2 (GLT-1, rat)	Glutamate	Astrocytes
EAAT3 (EAAC1, rabbit)	Glutamate	Astrocytes; Bergmann glia
EAAT4	Glutamate	Purkinje cells
EAAT5	Glutamate	Retina

Vesicular Transporters

Transporters	Transmitter	Localization
VGAT	GABA; glycine	Synaptic vesicles
VMAT1	Monoamines	Non-neuronal vesicles
VMAT2	Monoamines	Synaptic vesicles; dense core vesicles
VAChT	Acetylcholine	Synaptic vesicles
VGluT1	Glutamate	Synaptic vesicles

[1]All known glutamate transporters also transport aspartate. However, aspartate's role as a neurotransmitter is not well established (see Chapter 7). The plasma membrane transporter for choline has not yet been cloned.

cant behavioral effects. **Reserpine** inhibits the vesicular transport of monoamines and causes their depletion at the synapse (see Chapter 8). In a small subset of patients this can produce **clinical depression. Amphetamines,** which act in part by releasing vesicular monoamine stores, first into the cytoplasm and then into the synapse, have profound psychostimulant effects and in high doses may induce psychosis. Because of their central role in synaptic transmission, vesicular transporters are likely to be important targets for the development of novel psychotropic drugs.

TERMINATION OF NEUROTRANSMITTER ACTION

After exocytosis, neurotransmitter is inactivated, either by enzymatic degradation or by active transport out of the synaptic cleft. The latter process may include transport across the plasma membrane of the presynaptic terminal, postsynaptic neurons, or neighboring glia (see Figure 4–5). Like vesicular transport, plasma membrane transport requires specific transport proteins. However, unlike vesicular transport, it depends

on energy provided by the Na^+ gradient across the plasma membrane. These transport activities have been important targets of therapeutic drugs since the early 1960s, when Julius Axelrod and his colleagues discovered that **cocaine** and many **antidepressants** act initially by inhibiting the plasma membrane transport of monoamines such as dopamine, norepinephrine, and serotonin (see Chapters 8 and 9).

Many of the proteins responsible for plasma membrane transport have been identified through molecular cloning and belong to one of two families (see Table 4–2). One family includes transporters for GABA and for monoamine transmitters, which are structurally similar (see Chapters 7–9). Transporters of dopamine, serotonin, or norepinephrine are expressed only in their specific aminergic cell populations. In contrast, vesicular amine transport depends on a single widely expressed protein (VMAT2) to transport all CNS monoamines. Plasma membrane transporters of both monoamines and GABA use the cotransport of Na^+ and Cl^- ions to drive transmitter into the cytosol. A second family of plasma membrane transporters includes at least four structurally related glutamate transporters (see Table 4–2). In contrast to monoamine and GABA transporters, glutamate transporters drive transmitter uptake through cotransport of Na^+ and H^+ into the cell and the countertransport of K^+ out of the cell. In addition, glutamate transporters may function as Cl^- channels, an activity that appears to be uncoupled from transmitter transport.

Differences in the subcellular localization of plasma membrane transporters have important functional ramifications (see Figure 4–5). The monoamine transporters are concentrated in the plasma membranes of presynaptic terminals; thus in addition to terminating synaptic transmission, plasma membrane transport of monoamines also serves to recycle them for another round of exocytosis. Four isoforms of the GABA transporter have been identified, and at least one (GAT-1) is found in the presynaptic terminals of GABAergic neurons. However, other GAT isoforms are located on glia and possibly postsynaptic neurons, which suggests that a portion of exocytosed GABA is not recycled. Likewise, glutamate transporters are located primarily on glia and to a lesser extent on postsynaptic neurons; thus the bulk of exocytosed glutamate also does not appear to be recycled—rather, each round of glutamatergic transmission uses transmitter synthesized de novo.

Degradative enzymes also play an important role in the termination of synaptic transmission. Enzymes that inactivate monoamines in this manner are located in the extracellular space of the synaptic cleft, as well as intracellularly. At the NMJ and in the CNS, acetylcholine is rapidly inactivated by acetylcholinesterases in the synaptic cleft; the metabolite choline is subsequently transported into the presynaptic terminal for recycling. Acetylcholine itself does not appear to undergo transport across the plasma membrane (see Figure 4–5).

The fate of exocytosed transmitter also may include diffusion out of the synaptic cleft. Electrophysiologic studies suggest that glutamate may diffuse out of the synaptic cleft and bind to receptors at adjacent synapses, in a process that may serve to alter the spatial specificity of synaptic transmission. In contrast, monoamine plasma membrane transporters can be concentrated at the boundaries of the active zone of a presynaptic nerve terminal and may act to restrict diffusion of transmitter to adjacent synapses.

SYNAPTIC VESICLES AND LARGE DENSE CORE VESICLES

Many neurons express a distinct class of secretory vesicles called large dense core vesicles (LDCVs), which release neurotransmitter but differ from small synaptic vesicles (Table 4–3). Synaptic vesicles are smaller (approximately 40 nm in diameter) and more abundant and cluster at active zones in the nerve terminal. In contrast, LDCVs are slightly larger (80–120 nm) and contain peptides as well as monoamine transmitters in their lumen. LDCVs also contain aggregates of soluble proteins that appear as a dense core in electron micrographs—hence their name. Unlike synaptic vesicles, LDCVs are not closely linked to the active zone and are released from other sites in the cell.

Although both types of vesicles use similar machinery for exocytosis, the release of neurotransmitter from LDCVs occurs in response to different concentrations of intracellular Ca^{2+} and to different patterns of presynaptic activity compared with release from small synaptic vesicles. Synaptic vesicles cluster near Ca^{2+} channels at active zones, most likely because these channels bind directly to components of the exocytotic machinery, and exocytose in response to high Ca^{2+} concentrations (200 μM). In contrast, LDCVs do not cluster at active zones, and the local Ca^{2+} concentrations required for their release are likely to be much lower (5–10 μM). However, because LDCVs are much farther from the Ca^{2+} channels, which is the site of Ca^{2+} entry into the nerve terminal, repetitive presynaptic activity is generally required to achieve the requisite Ca^{2+} level for release. These features of LDCVs are consistent with a modulatory role of peptide neurotransmitters.

Compared with small-molecule transmitters, peptide transmitters are synthesized and packaged differently (see Chapter 10). Like larger proteins, peptide transmitters are synthesized on ribosomes docked at the

Table 4–3 Characteristics of Neurotransmitter Vesicles

	Size (nm)	Location	Contents	Ca^{2+} Required for Release (μM)
Small synaptic vesicles	40	At or near active zone	Small molecules	200
Large dense core vesicles	80–120	Ectopic	Peptides[1]; chromogranins	5–10

[1]In adrenal medulla chromaffin cells, large dense core vesicles contain epinephrine.

endoplasmic reticulum. Peptide precursors leave the endoplasmic reticulum to receive further processing in the Golgi apparatus, from which LDCVs emerge. The mechanism by which peptide transmitters target LDCVs vesicles is not completely clear but may involve self-aggregation or binding to proteins that help make up the dense core of LDCVs.

VESICLE BIOSYNTHESIS AND TRANSPORT

Synaptic vesicles and LDCVs are synthesized through two distinct biosynthetic pathways. Most evidence suggests that synaptic vesicles mature in two steps. First, proteins destined for synaptic vesicles sort to so-called constitutive secretory vesicles at the trans-Golgi network (TGN). These vesicles subsequently travel by way of the cell's constitutive secretory pathway to the nerve terminal, where they fuse with the plasma membrane. The endocytosis of the vesicle proteins from the plasma membrane produces mature synaptic vesicles. In contrast, LDCVs bud directly from the TGN as part of the cell's regulated secretory pathway.

Synaptic transmission at the nerve terminal requires that synaptic vesicles be transported out of the cell body and along the axon. Because the length of an axon can be greater than one meter, passive diffusion over such a distance would take weeks. However, early light microscopy studies of living cells revealed rapid anterograde and retrograde transport of vesicular organelles along axons, which suggested the existence of transport engines operating at different speeds and orientations (see Chapter 2). Indeed more recent studies suggest that vesicle transport occurs with the assistance of molecular motors. Vesicles are transported along cytoskeletal tracks, or microtubules, composed of a protein called tubulin. Electron micrographs have revealed that movement along these paths is made possible by short cross bridges that link vesicles to these microtubules. Because these cross bridges vary in shape and size, initially they were believed to represent physical correlates of the varying speeds of axonal transport.

During the past ten years investigators have determined that the cross bridges are related to the protein motors **kinesin** and **dynein.** Kinesin and dynein are well-known agents of intracellular movements, including the migration of chromosomes during mitosis. Molecular cloning studies have identified dozens of similar axonal protein motors whose variations in structure and function account for the different speeds and modes of organelle transport. One of these motors, KIF1A, appears to be responsible for the transport of some immature synaptic vesicles. KIF1A knock-out mice show a decrease in vesicles at the nerve terminal, and vesicles bound to KIF1A in the axon contain some

but not all of the proteins found on mature synaptic vesicles. These observations are consistent with the hypothesis that synaptic vesicles mature in the nerve terminal. Moreover, they indicate that other motors, yet to be identified, transport vesicles containing the remaining synaptic vesicle proteins.

SEGREGATION OF VESICLES

All synaptic vesicles appear to be created equal, but class differences develop in the nerve terminal, where vesicles segregate into pools that are more or less likely to be released. Readily releasable pools of vesicles, which are defined as vesicles that may be released at a regular rate in response to electrical stimulation of the terminal, have been distinguished from storage pools of vesicles by physiologic methods. Another operational definition of releasable pool includes vesicles that may be released in response to hypertonic sucrose, although the mechanism for this form of release is not clear.

However, the distinction between these two types of pools is not rigid. Fluorescent dyes such as **FM1-43** have been used to visualize trafficking between different pools of vesicles. Because FM1-43 is lipid soluble it reversibly intercalates into plasma membranes when added to media of cultured cells. Synaptic vesicles that recycle from the plasma membrane retain the dye; thus their intracellular movements can be followed microscopically. In stained cultures, recycled vesicles appear to traffic freely in the nerve terminal. More recently, investigators studying the *Drosophila* NMJ determined that a series of depolarizing pulses at the nerve terminal depleted a pool of vesicles close to the plasma membrane; however, a distinct pool in the center of the bouton was not depleted. These results suggest that the depleted pool may be equivalent to the readily releasable pool defined in earlier functional studies, and the central pool may represent the storage pool.

BIOCHEMISTRY OF NEUROTRANSMITTER RELEASE: THE EXOCYTOTIC CYCLE

The cornerstone of presynaptic function is the quantal release of transmitter through exocytosis. As outlined by Katz, the quantal release of transmitter must be localized and rapid, repeatable at high frequencies, and amenable to up- or down-regulation over time. Rapid release is necessary to allow communication between neurons within milliseconds, and temporal precision is necessary to preserve the timing of the electrical information encoded in an action potential. Thus exocytosis must be precisely coordinated with the influx of Ca^{2+} induced by depolarization of the nerve terminal. Terminals must be capable of sustained firing and neurotransmitter release because communication between neurons often involves repeated trains of stimuli. Finally, exocytosis must be a highly regulated process to accommodate the neural plasticity that underlies learning and memory. These requirements are satisfied by the following five steps in the cycle of exocytotic release (Figure 4–6).

1. *Docking.* Synaptic vesicles release neurotransmitter only at the active zone of a nerve terminal, exactly opposite the signal transduction machinery of the postsynaptic cell. This arrangement minimizes the time required for transmitter to reach the postsynaptic cell and also enhances the precision of communication between the two cells. Because the active zone occupies a relatively restricted area along the plasma membrane of the nerve terminal, vesicles must be specifically targeted to this region through a process referred to as docking. Although the mechanisms that underlie this targeting event have yet to be elucidated, they are likely to be similar to those that direct other types of intracellular organelles to specific membranes.

2. *Priming.* Morphologic analyses indicate that approximately 10 to 30 vesicles are docked at the active zone

of CNS synapses. However, most of these vesicles are not capable of Ca^{2+}-induced release and must undergo an active maturation process known as priming, which requires adenosine triphosphate (ATP) hydrolysis. Primed vesicles release neurotransmitter within a millisecond of Ca^{2+} influx into the cell. The speed of this release suggests that priming may initiate a partial fusion of the synaptic vesicle with the plasma membrane. Moreover, the energy obtained from ATP hydrolysis may be used to alter the conformation of proteins involved in exocytosis.

3. *Fusion/Exocytosis.* Fusion of the synaptic vesicle with the presynaptic plasma membrane requires deformation of the two apposing membranes. Because this event is tightly linked to the influx of Ca^{2+}, the underlying protein machinery is believed to involve a Ca^{2+} sensor. Fusion of the membranes allows exocytosis: extrusion of vesicle contents into the synaptic cleft.

4. *Endocytosis.* After the synaptic vesicle fuses with the plasma membrane and releases its contents, the vesicle membrane is recycled by a process of internalization known as endocytosis. Similar membrane-budding events have been characterized in a variety of organisms ranging from yeast to human. As with other endocytotic processes, the internalization of

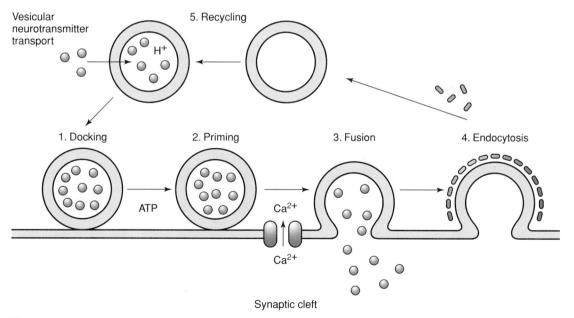

Figure 4–6. The exocytotic cycle consists of several distinct steps: (**1**) docking of synaptic vesicles at the plasma membrane of the active zone; (**2**) priming, an ATP-dependent step that prepares each vesicle for release; (**3**) fusion/exocytosis, the release of neurotransmitter triggered by the influx of Ca^{2+} through voltage-gated channels in the plasma membrane; (**4**) endocytosis, retrieval of vesicle membrane facilitated by a protein coat (*dashed line*) that subsequently dissociates from each vesicle; and (**5**) recycling, whereby vesicles move through an endosome intermediate (not shown) or invaginations from the plasma membrane.

synaptic vesicles is facilitated by a protein lattice that coats the internal face of the plasma membrane.

5. *Recycling.* This mechanism conserves synaptic vesicle membrane and helps to maintain a pool of release-competent vesicles. Two major models of synaptic vesicle recycling have been proposed. In the first, vesicles fuse with larger endosomes after endocytosis; subsequently, synaptic vesicles bud from these endosomes to engage in another round of exocytosis. According to the second model, synaptic vesicles bud directly from deep invaginations of the plasma membrane that are distinct from endosomes. Although synaptic vesicles clearly recycle according to the first model in some neuroendocrine cells in culture, the latter process is believed to predominate in the CNS. Two other models of recycling are noteworthy. One of these, based on experiments in which lipid-permeable dyes and microscopy were used to follow synaptic vesicles in real time, proposes that synaptic vesicles recycle intact without a transition involving either endosomes or plasma membrane invagination. The "kiss and run" model is also characterized by vesicles that never completely fuse with the plasma membrane; in this model transmitter leaks out through a pore that opens between the lumen of the vesicle and the extracellular space.

The entire exocytotic cycle lasts approximately 1 minute. Exocytosis occurs within 1 ms and endocytosis occurs within 5 seconds; the other steps of the cycle occupy the remaining time. The speed of exocytosis, which is truly breathtaking, is required for the overall efficiency of information processing in the nervous system.

PROTEINS INVOLVED IN THE EXOCYTOTIC CYCLE

Until the 1990s, the mechanisms underlying vesicle release and recycling remained obscure, partly because the proteins involved in these processes were not known. During the past 10 years many of these proteins have been identified. Thus the component of synaptic transmission that was for decades represented by a black box, namely the triggering of exocytosis by Ca^{2+} entry, is gradually being replaced by a series of precisely defined molecular events.

Determining the characteristics of proteins involved in the exocytotic cycle has required several lines of investigation, including the use of: (1) in vitro biochemical purification and binding assays to determine how identified proteins functionally interact; (2) **bacterial neurotoxins** and **black widow spider venom,** which have been proven to inactivate or activate specific pro-

teins involved in exocytosis (Box 4–2); (3) mutant mice in which genes postulated to be involved in synaptic transmission have been inactivated through gene knockout technology; (4) genetic mutations in model organisms such as yeast, *Caenorhabditis elegans,* and *Drosophila* that exhibit disrupted vesicle traffic or exocytosis (Box 4–3); and (5) model neuroendocrine cell lines, such as pheochromocytoma, or PC12, cells, in biochemical experiments.

The function of SNAREs: targeting or fusion? The morphologic differences between vesicles docked at the active zone of a nerve terminal and those that are undocked suggest that neurons contain mechanisms for segregating these pools and for targeting vesicles to the active zone. Initial experiments suggested that a group of proteins known as SNAREs might be involved in this process. SNAREs include three synaptic proteins that were first isolated biochemically and have since become integral to our understanding of vesicle fusion and transmitter release: synaptobrevin, also known as vesicle-associated membrane protein (VAMP); syntaxin; and synaptosomal associated protein of 25 kDa (SNAP 25), each of which have several similar isoforms. Synaptobrevins are 18 kDa and span the vesicle membrane, with one transmembrane domain near the C terminus. Syntaxins are 35 kDa and are also integral membrane proteins. In contrast, SNAP-25 is anchored to the membrane by lipid groups (long-chain fatty acids) attached to central cysteine residues (Box 4–4). At the active zone, syntaxin and SNAP-25 localize in the plasma membrane and are known as t-SNAREs (*t* for target membranes). In contrast, synaptobrevin is localized primarily in the vesicular membrane and thus has been labeled a v-SNARE, or vesicle SNARE. However, such localization is not universal; varying quantities of all three proteins have been found on vesicle membranes.

Three important findings led to the hypothesis that these proteins are involved in exocytosis at the presynaptic terminal. First, several **bacterial toxins** known to cause neurologic symptoms were proven to inhibit exocytosis and to cleave specific SNARE proteins (see Box 4–2). Likewise, the **black widow spider toxin (α-latrotoxin)** affects transmitter release by acting on proteins in the presynaptic nerve terminal. Second, mutation of yeast homologs of the SNAREs causes defects in membrane trafficking (see Box 4–3). These two lines of investigation implicated the SNAREs in synaptic transmission, but did not address the mechanism through which they might promote exocytosis. The third finding, which emerged from in vitro biochemical studies, was that syntaxin, synaptobrevin, and SNAP-25 spontaneously form a thermodynamically stable 1:1:1 com-

Box 4–2 Bacterial and Spider Toxins Influence Exocytosis

Botulism and tetanus are neurologic disorders caused by toxins from pathogenic bacteria. **Botulism,** which occurs after the ingestion of contaminated food, is caused by *Clostridium botulinum.* This strain secretes an armamentarium of seven potent neurotoxins (A, B, C1, D, E, F, and G), each of which affects exocytosis by acting on specific synaptic vesicle proteins (see table). The toxins thereby induce an asymmetric descending paralysis due to inactivation of cranial and peripheral nerves. Because of its ability to cause paralysis in muscle, localized injections of botulinum toxin are used therapeutically to treat **blepherospasm,** spasms of the muscle surrounding the tear duct, and **dystonia,** abnormal skeletal muscle tone. **Tetanus** is caused when *Clostridium tetanus* contaminates a wound. Tetanus toxin also targets synaptic vesicle proteins and affects exocytosis. The result is a poisoning of both motor neurons and inhibitory neurons, which causes increased muscle tone and spasms; it often strikes the masseter muscles first, resulting in **lockjaw.**

Black widow spider venom contains **α-latrotoxin,** which induces a profound paralysis by causing a massive release and subsequent depletion of acetylcholine at the neuromuscular junction. The targets of α-latrotoxin are shown in the table, and the effect of the toxin on nerve terminals is discussed in Chapter 9.

Each of these toxins functions as a protease that breaks apart its specific protein target and thus prevents its normal functioning. The discovery of targets for these toxins was a major breakthrough in our understanding of the molecular basis of exocytosis because it led to the identification of several proteins that play a key role in this process.

Toxin	Neural Target[1]
Botulinum neurotoxin	
A	SNAP-25
B	Synaptobrevin
C1	Syntaxin
D	Synaptobrevin
E	SNAP-25
F	Synaptobrevin
G	Synaptobrevin
Tetanus toxin	Synaptobrevin
α-Latrotoxin	Neurexin1; CIRL/latrophilin

[1]Some clostridial toxins also cleave a non-neuronal form of synaptobrevin known as cellulobrevin.

plex. Indeed, the complex is resistant to dissociation by sodium dodecylsulfate (SDS), a powerful ionic detergent that denatures most proteins and lyses most protein–protein interactions. Because syntaxin and SNAP-25 are located primarily in the plasma membrane and synaptobrevin is located primarily in the vesicle membrane, it was proposed that the association of these proteins might serve to target synaptic vesicles to the plasma membrane during the docking step of the exocytotic cycle. This postulate, known as the SNARE hypothesis, has been a major focus of investigations into the molecular mechanisms underlying synaptic transmission.

However, current data suggest that SNAREs may also play a role in membrane fusion and that additional molecules may facilitate docking. Genetic deletions of syntaxin in *Drosophila* decrease exocytosis but do not decrease the number of docked vesicles in nerve terminals. Similarly, the injection of **tetanus toxin** (see Box 4–2) or fragments of SNARE proteins into the presynaptic terminal of the giant axon of the squid lead to an increased number of docked vesicles. A decrease in the number of docked vesicles would be expected if the SNAREs were required for docking; thus the increase suggests that the SNAREs may function predominantly at a later step in the exocytotic cycle, perhaps during fusion.

Recent evidence strongly supports the participation of the SNAREs in the fusion of vesicle and plasma membranes. SNAREs that have been reconstituted into lipid vesicles have been assayed for vesicle fusion with the use of fluorescent dyes. Vesicles containing equimolar amounts of syntaxin and SNAP-25 fused with vesicles containing synaptobrevin, indicating that v- and t-SNAREs alone can generate fusion between lipid bilayers. The mechanism for fusion has been suggested by in vitro biophysical experiments in which SNAREs bind to each other in parallel with the C terminus of each SNARE similarly oriented. Thus, like viral hairpin proteins, which mediate the entry of viruses into cells, the SNAREs (or SNAREpins) may change their conformation or binding properties to allow fusion between opposing bilayers (Figures 4–7 and 4–8). The favorable thermodynamics of SNARE complex formation may drive the fusion of two such bilayers over the energy barrier that normally prevents the intermingling of bilayers.

Disassembly of the SNAREs by NSF   Because association of the SNAREs appears to drive fusion of the vesicle membrane with the plasma membrane, dissociation of the SNAREs must occur before the vesicle can be reclaimed from the plasma membrane to

Box 4–3 Invertebrate Homologs: Keeping the Names Straight

Vertebrates and invertebrates possess strikingly similar machinery for membrane trafficking and membrane fusion. Cell biologists investigating such events in yeast, *Caenorhabditis elegans,* and *Drosophila* have exploited these similarities to improve our understanding of the exocytotic cycle. Such studies have led to a nomenclature that can be quite confusing. For a guide to the names of associated protein homologs, see table.

Mammalian Protein	Yeast Homologs[1,2]	*Caenorhabditis elegans* Homologs	*Drosophila* Homologs
Exocyst complex	SEC3/5/6/9 EXO		
Syntaxin	SED5/SSO1/SSO2		
VAMP/Synaptobrevin	SNC1/SNC2/BOS1		
SNAP-25	SEC9		
NSF	SEC18		
SNAPs	SEC17		
Munc18[3]	SEC1/SLY1/SLP1	unc-18[4]	rop
Munc13		unc-13	
Doc2			
Rabs	YPT proteins		
Dynamin			shibere
AP-2	(APs)		stoned
CAPS		unc-31	
AP-3[5]	(APs)		garnet
ARF[5]	SAR1		

[1]SECs are yeast proteins whose mutations cause a decrease in secretion. Many of these proteins are similar to those involved in secretion and synaptic transmission in vertebrates.

[2]Note that some of these homologs are involved in membrane trafficking for organelles other than vesicles at the plasma membrane. For example, many are involved in endoplasmic reticulum to Golgi or Golgi to endoplasmic reticulum traffic. They are included here because vesicular traffic between different compartments often involved similar principles.

[3]Muncs are mouse homologs of *C. elegans* unc proteins (*mouse uncs*).

[4]Unc denotes a class of *C. elegans* mutants that were isolated because the worms were visibly uncoordinated. Some of these are involved in secretion (e.g., unc-18). The protein unc-18 is homologous to the yeast protein SEC1.

[5]The formation of synaptic vesicles from endosomes involves a small G protein known as ADP-ribosylation factor (ARF). Like other small G proteins, ARF cycles through activated and inactivated states, based on the binding and hydrolysis of GTP. Moreover, it appears to control the recruitment of AP-3 coats to budding vesicles. ARF also controls coat recruitment in other membrane trafficking events, including the constitutive transport of vesicles to and from the Golgi.

embark on a new exocytotic cycle. *N*-ethylmaleamide sensitive factor (NSF) and the soluble NSF attachment proteins (SNAPs) may perform this function (see Figure 4–7).[1] NSF is a soluble tetramer composed of 76-kDa subunits and requires SNAPs to bind to vesicle membranes and participate in exocytosis. A key finding in the search for the molecular composition of the exocytotic apparatus was the discovery that both NSF and the SNAPs also bind with high affinity to the SNAREs, including syntaxin, synaptobrevin, and SNAP-25. The aggregate composed of these proteins is commonly referred to as a 20S complex because it sediments by differential centrifugation as a 20S particle.[2] Remark-

ably, this 20S complex can be dissociated into its component proteins by the addition of ATP, even though the three SNAREs alone form a 7S complex that is SDS resistant.

Disassembly of the 20S complex occurs because NSF is an ATPase; by hydrolyzing ATP, NSF generates the energy to dissociate the thermodynamically stable core complex. Experiments involving yeast and cultured cell lines suggest that disassembly is likely to occur when SNAREs occupy the same membrane, possibly before donor and acceptor membranes are in contact. Indeed, t-SNAREs and v-SNAREs have been found to coexist on synaptic vesicle membranes. These observations suggest the following model: SNAREs induce fusion between a vesicle membrane and a plasma membrane by fastening together in parallel; to allow another round of exocytosis, NSF uses energy obtained from ATP hydrolysis to unzip the stable SNAREs (see Figure 4–7).

[1]Note that SNAPs are not related to SNAP-25. Indeed, the name SNAREs reflects that SNAP receptors and SNAREs were originally identified based on their ability to bind SNAPs.

[2]S denotes Svedberg units, which are used to measure the size of relatively large microscopic particles by use of high-speed centrifugation.

Box 4–4 Association of Proteins with Cell Membranes: Role in Fusion

There are two general types of membrane proteins (see figure). Integral membrane proteins contain transmembrane domains that span the hydrophobic core of the lipid bilayer. Examples include ion channels and transporters that pass aqueous material across the membrane or G protein-coupled receptors that transduce information across the membrane. Peripheral membrane proteins associate with the surface of a membrane or with other proteins in the membrane and are less likely to affect the lipid structure of a membrane.

Proteins also bind to membranes by attaching themselves covalently to lipids embedded in the bilayer. Such attachment may involve glycolipid anchors on the extracellular surface; palmitoylation on cysteine residues, required for the attachment of the SNARE protein SNAP-25; or the addition of geranylgeranylate to cysteine residues, required for attachment of Rab3a. Palmitoyl and geranylgeranyl

groups represent types of long-chain fatty acids, which insert into the hydrophobic core of the lipid bilayer and thereby anchor the proteins to the membrane. Lipid-anchored proteins do not contain transmembrane domains but behave biochemically like integral membrane proteins. One important difference between proteins anchored by lipids and proteins attached by transmembrane domains is that lipid-anchored proteins may be reversibly removed from the membrane (see Box 4–5).

It is believed that these various types of membrane-bound proteins (see Figure 4–9) are intimately involved in the process by which synaptic vesicles fuse with the nerve terminal plasma membrane. Although the details are incomplete, proteins involved in membrane fusion, like those that allow viral entry through a plasma membrane, likely require the ability to disrupt the structure of the lipid bilayer (see Figure 4–8).

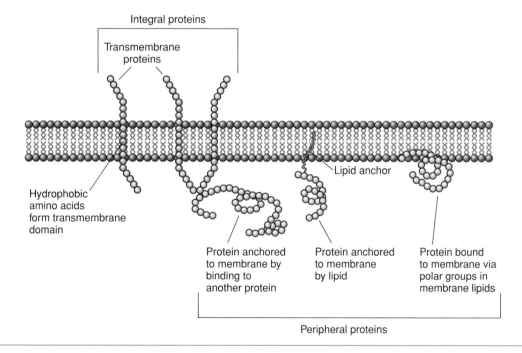

According to this model the SNAREs are responsible for membrane fusion. The SNAREs may also participate in targeting vesicles to membranes and in docking, although other candidates for these roles are currently under investigation, including homologs of proteins responsible for targeting in other vertebrate and invertebrate systems (see Box 4–3).

Synaptotagmin: A Ca²⁺ Sensor? Unlike most membrane trafficking events, which appear to proceed constitutively, neurotransmitter release is triggered by

Ca^{2+}. Thus an important goal in the study of synaptic transmission has been to identify the mechanism by which exocytotic machinery senses Ca^{2+} influx. Several lines of evidence suggest that the 65-kDa protein synaptotagmin plays a primary role in this process. Investigators first proposed this possibility after the elucidation of synaptotagmin's primary structure revealed so-called C2 domains similar to those found in protein kinase C, a Ca^{2+}- and phospholipid-dependent kinase (see Chapter 5). Synaptotagmin contains two C2 domains, C2A and C2B (Figure 4–9), each of which is

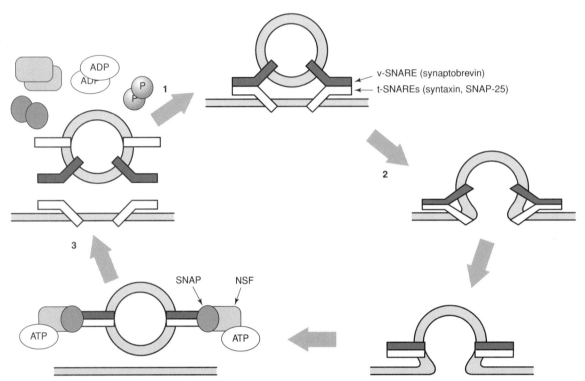

Figure 4–7. Model of the cycle whereby SNAREs induce membrane fusion and *N*-ethylmaleamide factor (NSF) dissociates the SNARE complex to initiate another round of fusion. This cycle includes the following steps: (**1**) SNAREs form a stable complex. v- and t-SNAREs engage partners on opposite membranes in a parallel fashion with respect to their membrane anchors. (**2**) SNAREs induce fusion. This fusion of the vesicle with the plasma membrane may be homologous to membrane fusion by viral hairpin proteins that assist the entry of viruses into cells. (**3**) NSF dissociates the SNARE complex. After binding to the SNAREs with the aid of a SNAP, NSF dissociates the complex with energy derived from adenosine triphosphate (ATP) hydrolysis into adenosine diphosphate (ADP) and free phosphate (P).

believed to bind two Ca^{2+} atoms to voluntarily conserved negatively charged aspartate residues. Extensive NMR and crystallographic analyses reveal that these domains form a novel Ca^{2+}-binding motif composed primarily of β sheets. Such binding does not induce a conformational change but is believed to induce a significant shift in electrostatic potential, or charge, in the Ca^{2+} binding domain, which may function to regulate the interaction of synaptotagmin with other molecules, such as SNAREs.

Because there are several different forms of synaptotagmin, a variety of methods have been used to determine whether the predominant form, synaptotagmin I, is a Ca^{2+} sensor in vivo. Experiments involving microinjection into the giant synapse of the squid, and studies of synaptotagmin mutations in *Drosophila, C. elegans,* and mice, have confirmed that synaptotagmin I plays an important role in exocytosis. Knockout mice have provided particularly useful corroborative information. In synaptotagmin I knockouts, fast Ca^{2+}-dependent transmitter release is strongly suppressed, but a second,

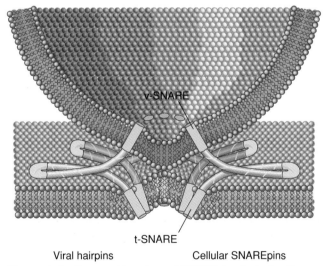

Figure 4–8. Proposed topology of SNAREpins, including the v-SNARE synaptobrevin and the t-SNAREs syntaxin and SNAP-25. Viral hairpin proteins are proposed to form similar structures to induce the fusion of apposing lipid membranes. (Reproduced with permission from Weber T et al. 1998. *Cell* 92:759.)

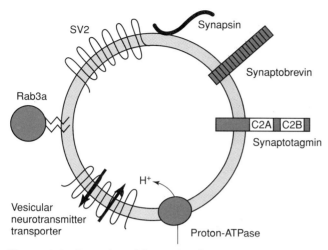

Figure 4–9. Synaptic vesicle proteins. Proteins involved in transmitter packaging and exocytosis include the proton-ATPase, which generates a proton gradient across the vesicle membrane, and vesicular transporters, which use the proton gradient to actively transport neurotransmitter into the lumen of vesicles. Synaptobrevin is involved in vesicle fusion and possibly targeting, and synaptotagmin functions as a Ca^{2+} sensor, binding Ca^{2+} ion with C2 domains encoded in the primary structure of the protein. The small G protein Rab3a, which is bound to vesicles by a lipid anchor, functions to regulate the exocytotic cycle (see Box 4–5). Synapsins associate peripherally with vesicles and may segregate them into storage pools. The function of SV2, a 12-transmembrane-domain protein that resembles a transporter, is not known.

slower phase of transmitter release, which is also Ca^{2+}-dependent, is not affected. A theory that remains unproved suggests that this second phase may be mediated by other synaptotagmin isoforms, such as synaptotagmin III. Other parameters of transmitter release also remain unchanged in these mice, thus verifying that synaptotagmin I regulates only one step of the exocytotic cycle: fast Ca^{2+}-triggered fusion.

The mechanism by which synaptotagmin I triggers fusion most likely involves the SNAREs. Although synaptotagmin I requires high concentrations of Ca^{2+} (>100 μM) to bind syntaxin, it binds phospholipids at much lower Ca^{2+} concentrations (approximately 5 μM). Thus it has been hypothesized that rapid changes in Ca^{2+} concentration mediate changes in the binding of synaptotagmin to the SNAREs and thereby induce fusion. It is likely that Ca^{2+} entry triggers rapid fusion of synaptic vesicles with the plasma membrane because of a tight physical association between Ca^{2+} channels in the nerve terminal plasma membrane and the complex of proteins that mediate fusion. Indeed, morphologic studies of plasma membrane show synaptic vesicles lined up near Ca^{2+} channels. Furthermore, syntaxin binds to Ca^{2+} channels in vitro, thus providing

a molecular mechanism for ensuring the presence of high concentrations of Ca^{2+} near the fusion machinery during exocytosis.

Regulating SNAREs: SECs and Muncs SNAREs also bind to proteins that may perform regulatory roles during membrane fusion and exocytosis. The functions of these proteins have been investigated primarily in invertebrate systems, including yeast, *C. elegans,* and *Drosophila;* for example, a genetic screen for secretory mutants in yeast led to the initial isolation of SEC1, a regulatory protein with homologs that were later identified in *C. elegans* (unc18), *Drosophila* (rop), and mammals (Munc18/n-SEC1). The nomenclature for these proteins, which can be quite confusing, is summarized in Box 4–3.

A functionally important relationship between the t-SNARE syntaxin and the SEC1 family was first suggested by genetic interactions between yeast SEC1 and a yeast homolog of syntaxin. Moreover, the vertebrate homolog of yeast SEC1, known as Munc18, was first identified based on its in vitro binding to vertebrate syntaxin. To determine how the binding of SEC1 family members to syntaxin might affect the function of the fusion complex, investigators examined rop, the *Drosophila* homolog of SEC1. Overexpression of rop in flies inhibits transmitter release, suggesting that interactions between SEC1 family members and syntaxins inhibit exocytosis. Interestingly, phosphorylation of Munc18 (the vertebrate SEC1) inhibits its binding to syntaxin in vitro, suggesting a potential mechanism for regulating interactions between Munc18 and syntaxin.

Other presynaptic proteins may facilitate SNARE function. These include Munc13, the vertebrate homolog of the *C. elegans* paralytic mutant unc-13. Three isoforms of Munc13 have been identified: Munc13-1, Munc13-2, and Munc13-3. Each of these is a large protein (1400 amino acids) whose primary structure, like that of synaptotagmin, includes C2 domains. Munc13-1 is located in presynaptic nerve terminals, and its overexpression in motor neurons increases transmitter release; thus Munc13-1 may play a role in the presynaptic regulation of neurotransmission. Furthermore, Munc13-1 binds to the t-SNARE syntaxin in vitro, suggesting that Munc13-1 influences transmitter release by facilitating SNARE function.

The actions of Munc13-1 appear to involve another protein, known as Doc2. Doc2 also contains C2 domains and, when overexpressed, enhances transmitter release. In vitro, Doc2 binds to Munc13 in a manner such that the overexpression of a Munc13 fragment in a cell abolishes the effect of Doc2 on transmitter release. These findings indicate that Munc13 and Doc2 may function together as a complex to up-regulate synaptic transmis-

Box 4–5 The Rab Cycle

Rabs are proposed to cycle through discrete stages of activation and inactivation that are regulated by their association with guanine nucleotides (GTP and GDP) and by their association with membranes. Like other G proteins (see Chapter 5), Rabs are believed to be active when bound to GTP (Rab-GTP), and inactive when bound to GDP (Rab-GDP); they are also believed to possess a GTPase activity that controls the cycling between these forms. Additional proteins regulate the binding of Rabs with GDP or GTP and their anchoring to lipid membranes.

In their active state, small G proteins are postulated to activate downstream effector molecules. For example, when a prototypical member of the Ras family is bound to GTP, it activates a downstream cascade of protein kinases (see Chapter 5). The downstream effectors activated by Rabs have not been determined, and the precise mechanism by which Rabs influence membrane trafficking is not known. Nonetheless, the process by which Rab3 hydrolyzes GTP and associates with membranes coincides with the exocytotic cycle and may play a role in the regulation of synaptic transmission.

To cycle on and off of lipid membranes, Rabs require the covalent attachment of lipid anchors. For example, geranylgeranyltransferase (GGT) attaches two chains of isoprenylate or geranylgeranylate to cysteine residues in Rab3. The addition of geranylgeranylate is facilitated by the protein known as REP (Rab escort protein), which binds to free Rab-GDP. After the addition of geranylgeranylate, Rab-GDP cycles through the following steps (see figure):

1. **GDI binding and presentation to vesicles.** In the cytosol, geranylgeranylated Rab-GDP binds to a protein called GDI (GDP-dissociation inhibitor), which chaperones Rab-GDP to synaptic vesicles. (REP appears to function as one type of GDI.) There, the geranylgeranylate tail inserts into the outer lipid leaflet of the vesicle bilayer.
2. **Displacement of GDI.** After Rab is attached to vesicles, GDI is displaced by a GDI displacement factor (GDF). Unmasked Rab-GDP is now free to undergo GTP–GDP exchange.
3. **GTP–GDP exchange.** To convert Rab from an inactive to an active state, GDP is removed in exchange for GTP. The exchange is facilitated by a guanine nucleotide exchange factor (GEF). Because exchange occurs only when Rab is attached to membranes, the spatial and temporal specificity of Rab activation is ensured.
4. **Downstream effectors.** Activated Rabs in turn activate downstream effector molecules. Two candidates for Rab3a effectors, rabphilin and RIM, are described in this chapter.
5. **Inactivation.** GTP hydrolysis inactivates Rab. The intrinsic rate of GTP hydrolysis by Rabs is very slow, and the GTPase activity is enhanced by a regulatory protein known as GTPase-activating protein (GAP).
6. **Removal from the membrane.** GDI transports Rab-GDP from the membrane to the cytoplasm, where the complex may initiate another cycle of membrane association and activation.

sion. Interestingly, the regulation of transmitter release by these two proteins is influenced by **phorbol esters,** pharmacologic agents that activate protein kinase C and thereby mimic some of the actions of the second messenger DAG (see Chapter 5). DAG and phorbol esters both bind to a regulatory domain, called C1, in protein kinase C, which is believed to form a zinc-finger-like structure. Like protein kinase C, Munc13 contains a C1 domain and, in vitro, binds with high affinity to phorbol esters. The binding of phorbol esters to Munc13 both stimulates the interaction of Munc13 with Doc2 and appears to induce translocation of Munc13 to the plasma membrane. Moreover, phorbol esters stimulate the ability of Munc13 and Doc2 to up-regulate transmitter release. Thus, because Munc13 binds to syntaxin, the Munc13/Doc2 complex may stimulate transmitter release at the plasma membrane through interactions with the SNARE complex.

Regulation of storage pools   Additional mechanisms exist for regulating features of exocytosis. It is believed, for example, that a regulatory mechanism

limits the number of vesicles docked at the active zone of a nerve terminal by anchoring some vesicles in storage pools. This process may involve interactions between synaptic vesicles and the cytoskeleton; quick-freeze etch microscopy indicates that vesicles that remain undocked at the active zone are associated in the cytoplasm with a cytoskeletal actin matrix and a variety of nonactin filaments. One candidate for regulating interactions between vesicles and the cytoskeleton is synapsin I, a synaptic vesicle-associated protein first described by Greengard and colleagues (see Figure 4–9). This protein is a substrate for the Ca^{2+}-dependent protein kinase CaMKII and for the cAMP-dependent protein kinase, protein kinase A (see Chapter 5; a homologous protein, synapsin II, is also associated with synaptic vesicles but is not a substrate for CaMKII). Phosphorylation of synapsin I by these kinases has been postulated to regulate its association with synaptic vesicles and the cytoskeleton. Moreover, the phenotype of knockout mice lacking synapsin I, synapsin II, or both isoforms is consistent with the involvement of synapsins in maintaining a pool of fusion-competent vesicles at the active

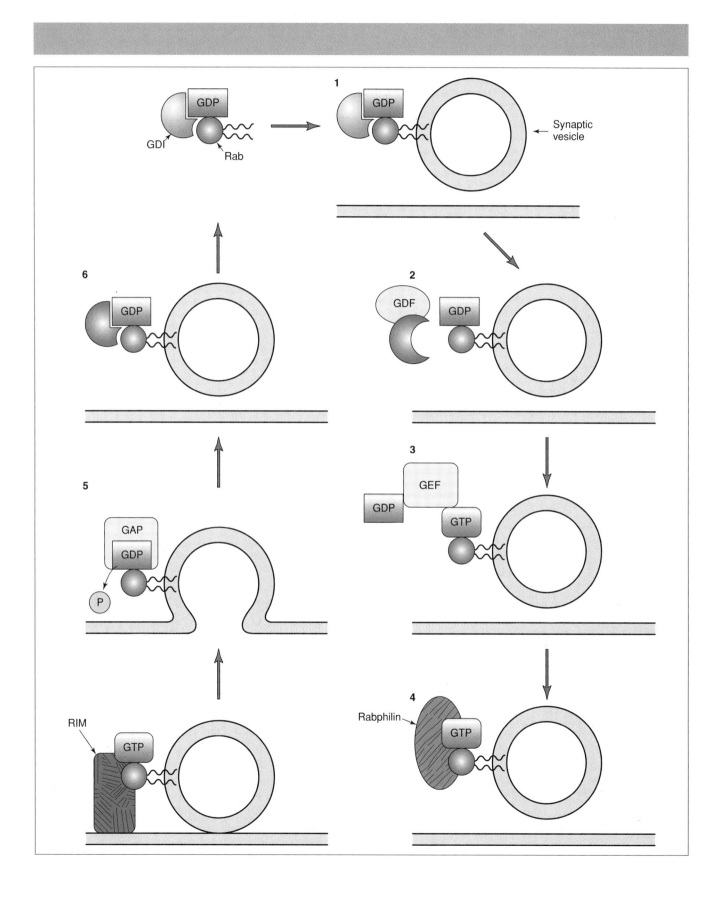

zone during periods of accelerated neurotransmitter release. Thus synapsin phosphorylation by CaMKII and other kinases could mediate regulation of the size of this pool in response to Ca^{2+} influx at the nerve terminal or to activation of presynaptic transmitter receptors.

Regulation of vesicle exocytosis by Rab3a   The exocytotic cycle is also regulated by members of the Ras superfamily of small G proteins, which are known to influence a variety of cellular processes (see Chapter 5). Small G proteins are structurally distinct from the family of heterotrimeric G proteins through which many neurotransmitter receptors signal. The largest group of small G proteins, including more than 40 mammalian members, is represented by the Rab subfamily. Rabs regulate the biogenesis, targeting, and fusion of membrane vesicles, and Rab3 in particular has been implicated in the regulation of synaptic vesicle trafficking and exocytosis (Box 4–5). Four isoforms of Rab3 (Rab3a, b, c, and d) have been described. Rab3a is most abundant in the brain and is located primarily in synaptic vesicles. Functional studies of cultured neuroendocrine cells implicate both Rab3a and Rab3b in the regulation of exocytosis but suggest that they may perform opposing tasks. Inhibition of Rab3a function stimulates neurotransmitter release, indicating that this isoform normally limits release. In contrast, inhibition of Rab3b inhibits release, implicating Rab3b in the facilitation of exocytosis.

In vivo models also suggest that Rab3a assists in regulating exocytosis. In Rab3a knockout mice, an excessive number of synaptic vesicles are likely to be released from the active zone when the presynaptic cell is stimulated. Moreover, these mice show defects in presynaptic long-term potentiation, which is hypothesized to be a cellular correlate of learning and memory (see Chapter 20). These findings confirm that Rab3a restricts the number of synaptic vesicles released during exocytosis and that this function is important for synaptic plasticity.

The mechanisms underlying the regulation of exocytosis by Rab3a are unclear. All Rabs cycle between membrane-bound and soluble forms and, like other small G proteins, are active when bound to GTP. Rab3s in particular cycle on and off of synaptic vesicles during the exocytotic cycle; other regulatory proteins ensure that they bind GTP and are activated only when bound to membranes. In their GTP-bound state, Rab3s also activate downstream effector proteins (see Box 4–5). One downstream effector activated by Rab3a is rabphilin, which appears to bind to Rab3a on synaptic vesicles before the vesicles have docked. Functional studies of rabphilin suggest that it regulates the bundling of cytoskeletal elements and that this activity may be further regulated by the binding of rabphilin to Rab3a. These

findings suggest that the Rab3a–rabphilin complex may regulate synaptic transmission by reducing the association of synaptic vesicles with the cytoskeleton. Another downstream effector activated by Rab3a is a protein called RIM. In contrast to rabphilin, RIM localizes in the plasma membrane and most likely binds to Rab3a only after vesicles move close to the active zone to dock. Thus the Rab3a–RIM complex may assist in binding synaptic vesicles to proteins at the active zone.

ENDOCYTOSIS AND RECYCLING

Clathrin-mediated endocytosis   After fusion and exocytosis, synaptic vesicles are reclaimed from the plasma membrane through clathrin-mediated endocytosis (Figure 4–10). Clathrin is composed of two highly conserved subunits that self-assemble into structures called triskelions, each of which consists of three light-chain and three heavy-chain subunits. It forms a proteinaceous coat that helps shape the membrane into a bud that is subsequently pulled away from the inner surface of the plasma membrane. Electron micrographs of clathrin-mediated endocytosis reveal shallow invaginations of the plasma membrane coated on the cytoplasmic side with polyhedral cups of assembled triskelions, which are clathrin-coated pits.

Clathrin is linked to membranes through heteromeric adapter proteins (APs), each of which comprises a large central domain and two projecting ears. The two sides of the central domain and both ears are composed of α and β subunits; two smaller σ and μ subunits also bind to the central domain. At least four types of adapters are known to exist, and each localizes in a different subcellular organelle; the adapter at the plasma membrane is called AP-2. Each type of adapter protein may contain cell type-specific subunits. A neuron-specific subunit known as β3b, or β-NAP, was originally isolated as the antigen responsible for a so-called paraneoplastic syndrome, or **tumor-induced autoimmunity syndrome,** which results in cerebellar degeneration.

To ensure that other types of proteins are not mistakenly recruited into synaptic vesicles, adapters bind to highly specific proteins at the plasma membrane. The only synaptic vesicle protein known to bind AP-2 is synaptotagmin. Thus this protein may play a dual role: it may serve as a Ca^{2+} sensor during exocytosis and as a tag during endocytosis. However, different isoforms of synaptotagmin may be involved in these processes.

After endocytosis, the clathrin coat is removed from the membrane to allow further trafficking and recycling to the existing pool of synaptic vesicles. The molecular chaperone hsp70c likely plays a role in disassembling clathrin, with the assistance of additional tissue-specific cofactors.

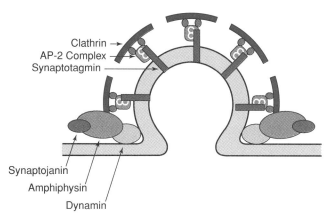

Clathrin →
AP-2 Complex →
Synaptotagmin →

Synaptojanin
Amphiphysin
Dynamin

Figure 4–10. The endocytotic machinery. Clathrin-mediated endocytosis allows synaptic vesicles to be retrieved from the nerve terminal. Because the protein machinery required for this process is complex, only a few of the major components are shown in this figure. Clathrin and the heteromeric AP-2 adaptor complex form the coat around the budding vesicle, which may be linked to the vesicle membrane by synaptotagmin. Dynamin is a pinchase that pinches or severs the neck of the budding vesicle. Amphiphysin, which plays a central role in the coordination of endocytosis, binds to several proteins, including dynamin, AP-2, clathrin, and the phospholipid phosphatase synaptojanin. The locations of both synaptojanin and amphiphysin may differ from those in this figure, which primarily serves to show protein–protein interactions.

Endocytotic machinery An important component of the biochemical machinery underlying endocytosis is the protein dynamin. This protein, which was identified biochemically and previously known as dephosphin, cycles between phosphorylated and dephosphorylated states during the exocytotic cycle. Biochemical assays have revealed that dynamin also encodes a GTPase activity that was linked to endocytosis after the discovery of a mutation in the *Drosophila dynamin* gene known as *shibere*. Flies containing this mutation were isolated more than 25 years ago and display defects in cell signaling. Electron micrographs of the nerve terminals of mutant flies revealed hundreds of vesicles attached to each plasma membrane by short ring-coated necks. Discovery of the shibere phenotype suggested that these rings, which are oligomers of *shibere* protein, may function to pinch off the neck of a vesicle as it buds from the plasma membrane.

The relationship between dynamin's GTPase activity and the mutant phenotype of *shibere* was further elucidated when cells undergoing endocytosis were incubated in GTP-γ-S, a GTP homolog in which the terminal (γ) phosphate has been replaced by a sulfate group. Because GTP-γ-S cannot be hydrolyzed by

GTPases such as dynamin, its presence causes the latter to remain in an activated state. Micrographs of plasma membranes from these incubated cells reveal vesicles linked to the membranes by short ring-coated necks that are strikingly similar to those seen in micrographs of *shibere* flies. These findings indicate that dynamin is intimately involved in the endocytosis of synaptic vesicles and that GTP hydrolysis helps to drive this process. Thus, as originally suggested by the *shibere* mutant, current evidence supports a scheme wherein dynamin, with the assistance of proteins that are located in the necks of budding vesicles, may function as a "pinchase" to sever or pinch off the necks of coated vesicles as they bud from the plasma membrane.

Regulation of endocytosis Dynamin encodes the interactions of several proteins that may in turn regulate endocytosis. These include DAP 160, which may act as a scaffold to anchor the endocytotic machinery, and amphiphysin, which binds to the coat proteins AP-2 and clathrin and also binds dynamin to other proteins. The injection of amphiphysin into cells blocks the recruitment of dynamin to sites of endocytosis, thereby confirming amphiphysin's central role in the coordination of endocytotic machinery.

Protein phosphorylation may underlie several phases of endocytotic regulation. Dynamin's oscillation between phosphorylated and dephosphorylated forms may regulate its binding to amphiphysin. Moreover, the phosphorylation of amphiphysin may influence its binding to AP-2 and clathrin. In vitro, dynamin and amphiphysin dissociate from their binding partners when they are phosphorylated and reassociate when they are dephosphorylated. Interestingly, the dephosphorylation of these proteins may be catalyzed by the Ca^{2+}-activated protein phosphatase calcineurin (see Chapter 5). It is tempting to speculate that the same pool of Ca^{2+} that triggers exocytosis also initiates endocytosis.

Endocytosis also appears to be regulated by membrane phospholipids, although many of the mechanistic details remain poorly understood (Box 4–6).

Vesicle recycling After endocytosis, synaptic vesicles are recycled. As mentioned previously, the biogenesis and recycling of synaptic vesicles may involve budding from both plasma membrane invaginations and endosomal compartments discrete from the plasma membrane. Although the contribution of each pathway to vesicle formation in neurons remains unclear, some of the molecular components of the endosomal pathway have been determined with the use of model neuroendocrine cells. Like endocytosis at the plasma membrane, the budding of synaptic vesicles from endosomes involves protein coats formed from heteromeric APs.

Box 4–6 The Role of Lipids in Exocytosis and Endocytosis

Membrane-bound lipids are integrally involved in regulating exocytosis and endocytosis. Among these are phosphoinositides (PIs) and phosphatidic acid (PA), both of which contain acidic, negatively charged head groups that are critical for their functioning (see Box 4–1).

The isolation of several enzymes during a biochemical screen for soluble factors involved in priming led to the demonstration that the metabolism of PIs is involved in priming vesicles for exocytosis. Among the enzymes isolated were two PI kinases and a PI transfer protein responsible for shuttling PI between membranes. The mechanism by which these proteins prime vesicles for exocytosis remains unknown; however, because priming requires PI kinases, the phosphorylation of PIs and changes in the charge of the head groups may be important for exocytosis. Conversely, a decrease in the charge of the inositol group may be involved in endocytosis. Among the proteins that bind amphiphysin, which is an important component of the

endocytotic machinery, is an inositol 5-phosphatase called synaptojanin (see Figure 4–10), which cleaves the phosphate moiety from position 5 of several PIs. Because this protein is associated with endocytosis, the dephosphorylation of PIs also may be involved in this process.

The biophysical properties of PIs and PA also may influence exocytosis and endocytosis. Changes in the charge of their head groups can alter the electrostatic properties of a membrane surface. Furthermore, the shape and saturation of their side chains can alter properties that are important in membrane fusion, such as the flexibility of the membrane and its ability to bend. Lipids also may act as specific protein receptors. PIs are known to bind several proteins involved in the exocytotic cycle, including synaptotagmin and AP-2. Such lipid binding may induce changes in protein conformation or link together proteins localized in lipid bilayers.

However, endosomal budding employs a different AP protein (AP-3) and does not require clathrin. Interestingly, mutations in one of the large subunits of AP-3 (δ3) may disrupt vesicle trafficking in both mice and humans. The phenotypes of *mocha*, a δ3 mutation in mice, include an increase in baseline electrical activity in the brain and a unique hypersynchronized 6- to 7-Hz EEG pattern. In humans, a similar mutation results in a form of **Hermansky–Pudlak syndrome** (**HPS**), which is notable for defects in storage granules. Moreover, tumor-related antibodies to a neuronally expressed β subunit of AP-3 (known as β3B or β-NAP) induce **cerebellar degeneration**. Such findings suggest that defects in secretory vesicle biogenesis and its regulation may underlie other neuropsychiatric syndromes.

COMPLEXITY AND SPECIALIZATION

The molecular processes involved in the exocytotic cycle may seem quite complex, yet this chapter presents a simplified view. Neurons express multiple isoforms of many of the proteins described here; for example, more than ten isoforms of synaptotagmin have been isolated, and each may regulate a different aspect of synaptic transmission. Moreover, isoforms of some synaptic proteins exhibit striking cell type-specific distributions in the brain.

During the past two decades, many of the molecules responsible for the quantal release of transmitter have been identified, and some of the protein–protein interactions underlying this complex process and its intricate regulation have been teased apart. As we move

beyond the identification of these proteins and their binding partners, many important questions remain. How are lipids involved in neurotransmitter release? What changes in protein structure occur? How is the regulation of synaptic transmission linked to development, to learning and memory, and to disease?

This book explores such topics in depth because details of the mechanisms underlying neurotransmitter release are likely to reveal a great deal about the pathophysiology, and perhaps even the pathogenesis, of neuropsychiatric disorders. Furthermore, it is anticipated that several proteins involved in this process will be important targets of therapeutic agents, and the many isoforms of these proteins should facilitate the design of drugs that act on specific neuronal cell types or synaptic processes. Indeed, nature has already exploited such mechanisms. Further study of the **bacterial** and **spider toxins** that target specific synaptic vesicle proteins may lead to promising breakthroughs in the treatment of neuropsychiatric disorders.

SELECTED READING

Bellocchio EE, Reimer RJ, Fremeau RT, Edwards RH. 2000. Uptake of glutamate into synaptic vesicles by an inorganic phosphate transporter. *Science* 289:957–960.

Bennett MK, Scheller RH. 1994. A molecular description of synaptic vesicle membrane trafficking. *Annu Rev Biochem* 63:63–100.

Chaudhry FA, Reimer RJ, Krizaj D, et al. 1999. Molecular analysis of system N suggests novel physiological roles in nitrogen metabolism and synaptic transmission. *Cell* 99:769–780.

Cowan WM, Sudhof TC, Stevens CF. 2000. *Synapses*. Baltimore: Johns Hopkins University Press.

Cremona O, De Camilli P. 1997. Synaptic vesicle endocytosis. *Curr Opin Neurobiol* 7:323–330.

Fernandez-Chacon R, Sudhof TC. 1999. Genetics of synaptic vesicle function: Toward the complete functional anatomy of an organelle. *Annu Rev Physiol* 61:753–776.

Geppert M, Sudhof TC. 1998. RAB3 and synaptotagmin: The yin and yang of synaptic membrane fusion. *Annu Rev Neurosci* 21:75–95.

Hamm HE. 1998. The many faces of G protein signaling. *J Biol Chem* 273:669–672.

Hilfiker S, Pieribone VA, Czernik AJ, et al. 1999. Synapsins as regulators of neurotransmitter release. *Phil Trans Royal Soc London Biol Sci* 354:269–279.

Jessell TM, Kandel ER. 1993. Synaptic transmission: A bidirectional and self-modifiable form of cell–cell communication. *Cell* 72(suppl):1–30.

Katz B. 1969. *The Release of Neural Transmitter Substances*. Liverpool: Liverpool University Press.

Kelly RB. 1993. Storage and release of neurotransmitters. *Cell* 72(suppl):43–53.

Kennedy MB. 2000. Signal processing machines at the postsynaptic density. *Science* 290:750–754.

Kuromi H, Kidokoro Y. 1998. Two distinct pools of synaptic vesicles in single presynaptic boutons in a temperature-sensitive *Drosophila* mutant, shibere. *Neuron* 20:917–925.

Li L, Chin LS, Shupliakov O, et al. 1995. Impairment of synaptic vesicle clustering and of synaptic transmission, and increased seizure propensity, in synapsin I-deficient mice. *Proc Natl Acad Sci USA* 92:9235–9239.

Liu Y, Edwards RH. 1997. The role of vesicular transport proteins in synaptic transmission and neural degeneration. *Annu Rev Neurosci* 20:125–156.

Martin TFJ. 1997. Phosphoinositides as spatial regulators of membrane traffic. *Curr Opin Neurobiol* 7:331–338.

Neher E. 1998. Vesicle pools and Ca^{2+} microdomains: New tools for understanding their roles in neurotransmitter release. *Neuron* 20:389–399.

Prior C, Tian L. 1995. The heterogeneity of vesicular acetylcholine storage in cholinergic nerve terminals. *Pharmacol Res* 32:345–353.

Scales SJ, Scheller RH. 1999. Lipid membranes shape up. *Nature* 401:123–124.

Seal RP, Amara SG. 1999. Excitatory amino acid transporters: A family in flux. *Annu Rev Pharmacol Toxicol* 39:431–456.

Sollner T, Whiteheart SW, Brunner M, et al. 1993. SNAP receptors implicated in vesicle targeting and fusion. *Nature* 362:318–324.

Takamori S, Rhee JS, Rosenmund C, Jahn R. 2000. Identification of a vesicular glutamate transporter that defines a glutamatergic phenotype in neurons. *Nature* 407:189–194.

Verhage M, Maia AS, Plomp JJ, et al. 2000. Synaptic assembly of the brain in the absence of neurotransmitter secretion. *Science* 287:864–869.

Weber T, Zemelman BV, McNew JA, et al. 1998. SNAREpins: Minimal machinery for membrane fusion. *Cell* 92:759–772.

Chapter 5

Signal Transduction Pathways in the Brain

KEY CONCEPTS

- Signal transduction refers to the processes by which signals between cells carried by neurotransmitters, hormones, trophic factors, and cytokines are converted into biochemical signals within cells.

- Neurotransmitter receptors can be divided into two classes by their signal transduction mechanism—one class involving activation of an ion channel that is intrinsic to the receptor and the other involving activation of G proteins.

- Signal transduction can alter neuronal function on vastly different time scales ranging from very rapid (millisecond) changes in membrane potential produced by ligand-gated channels to changes over seconds produced by intracellular second messengers and protein kinases.

- Many critical drugs that act on the nervous system are agonists or antagonists at G protein-coupled receptors.

- Although second messengers such as cyclic nucleotides and Ca^{2+} may directly gate ion channels, their major role in intracellular signaling systems is to regulate protein kinases that phosphorylate other proteins.

- Second messenger-regulated protein kinases have separate regulatory domains that interact with the second messenger and catalytic domains involved in phosphorylation.

- Protein kinases are localized in distinct regions of the cell by specific anchoring proteins; the best characterized are the A kinase-anchoring proteins that tether the cyclic-AMP-dependent protein kinase to microtubules.

- The brain contains four major serine–threonine protein phosphatases, which reverse the actions of second messenger-dependent protein kinases, known as protein phosphatases 1, 2A, 2B, and 2C.

- Neurotrophins, such as nerve growth factor, brain-derived neurotrophic, and NT3, interact with a family of receptors—receptor tyrosine kinases (Trks).

- Certain cytokines, such as ciliary neurotrophic factor and leukemia inhibitory factor, act on receptors that activate tyrosine kinases called Janus kinases, which in turn activate a family of transcription factors called signal transducers and activators of transcription.

Signal transduction refers to the processes by which intercellular signals such as neurotransmitters, neurotrophic factors, circulating hormones, and cytokines produce intracellular biochemical alterations that in turn modify neuronal functioning. Indeed, intercellular signals and their receptors, generally located in the neuronal plasma membrane, represent only a small amount of all information processing in the brain. An understanding of the complex biochemical mechanisms that operate inside neurons and ultimately mediate the actions of all intercellular signals is required to appreciate not only the ways in which the brain responds to specific stimuli but also the ways in which it continuously adapts to a host of environmental changes.

OVERVIEW OF SIGNAL TRANSDUCTION PATHWAYS

Four general patterns of signal transduction occur in the brain (Figure 5–1). One pattern (see Figure 5–1A), discussed briefly in Chapters 3 and 4, involves the binding of neurotransmitter to a multimeric plasma membrane receptor complex that contains a ligand-gated ion channel. Protein–protein interactions tether such ion channels, or receptor ionophores, at proper subcellular locations and often to other signaling proteins. This mechanism of signal transduction is used primarily by the amino acid neurotransmitters at their ionotropic receptors (see Chapter 7) and by acetylcholine at nicotinic receptors (see Chapter 9), as well as by serotonin at 5-HT$_3$ receptors (see Chapter 9), adenosine triphosphate (ATP) at certain purinergic receptors (see Chapter 10), and heat at certain vanilloid receptors (see Chapter 19). The structural features of ligand-gated ion channels are discussed in detail in the chapters devoted to these transmitters.

A second pattern, also briefly described in Chapter 4, is characterized by the binding of neurotransmitters to plasma membrane receptors that couple with guanine nucleotide-binding proteins or G proteins (see Figure 5–1B). As explained in later chapters, most neurotransmitters bind to this superfamily of G protein-coupled receptors, as do several cytokines, including interleukin-8. All such receptors have a seven-transmembrane domain structure, whose N terminus faces the extracellular space and whose C terminus faces the cytoplasm; other structural features of these receptors are discussed in detail in Chapter 8, wherein the β-adrenergic receptor is presented as a prototype. Coupling between these receptors and their G proteins occurs primarily through the receptor's third cytoplasmic loop, although other domains most likely support this process. The

binding of ligands to these receptors initiates receptor–G protein interactions that produce a range of biologic effects on target neurons. These effects include direct G protein regulation of certain ion channels (see Figure 5–1B, *left*) and the triggering of complex cascades of intracellular messengers. Activation of intracellular messenger pathways lead to the generation of second messengers and the regulation of protein phosphorylation, and ultimately to diverse physiologic responses to extracellular stimuli (Figure 5–2), including regulation of ion channels (see Figure 5–1B, *right*). As will be become evident, protein phosphorylation is the major molecular currency of intracellular signal transduction pathways. Protein phosphorylation describes a process by which enzymes called protein kinases add phosphate groups to specific target proteins, and enzymes called protein phosphatases remove these phosphate groups. Phosphate groups, because of their large size and negative charge, alter the conformation and overall charge of a protein and hence its function.

A third pattern of signal transduction involves the direct activation of a class of protein kinases, called protein tyrosine kinases, which phosphorylate proteins on tyrosine residues (see Figure 5–1C). This type of signaling is used by most types of neurotrophic factors and cytokines. In some cases the neurotrophic factor receptor and the protein tyrosine kinase reside in a single protein; in other cases the receptor must recruit cytoplasmic protein tyrosine kinases to effect their signaling. Activation of the protein tyrosine kinase triggers cascades of further protein phosphorylation that ultimately lead to the many effects of neurotrophic factors on brain function, including the regulation of ion channels. Knowledge of these additional protein phosphorylation pathways, which are discussed in detail and illustrated later in the chapter, has added new layers of complexity to current models of synaptic transmission (see Figure 5–2).

A fourth pattern, which characterizes transduction by all known steroid hormones, thyroid hormone, retinoic acid, and vitamin D, involves lipophilic extracellular signals that cross the plasma membrane and activate receptors in the neuronal cytoplasm (see Figure 5–1D). After they are bound to hormone, cytoplasmic receptors translocate to the nucleus, where they bind DNA and function as transcription factors (see Chapter 6). Thus these receptors can be considered ligand-activated transcription factors.

Intracellular signaling pathways may be viewed as subserving three major functions in the nervous system. First, they mediate some short-term aspects of synaptic transmission; for example, the rapid actions of neurotransmitters and neurotrophic factors on ion channels, with the exception of ligand-gated channels, are achieved through intracellular messengers. Second,

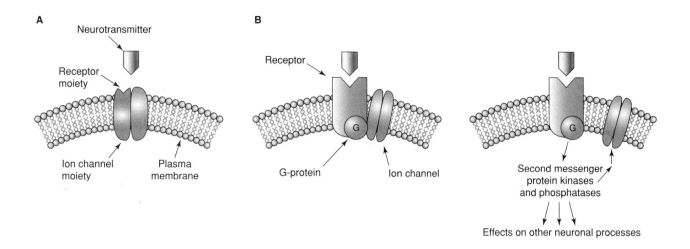

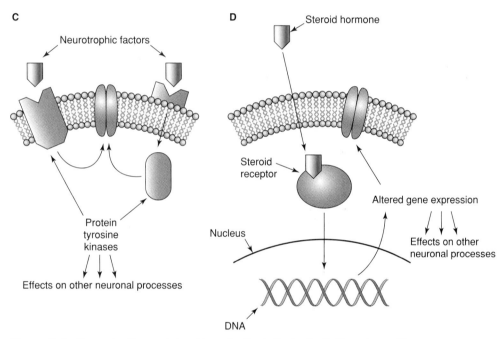

Figure 5-1. General patterns of signal transduction in the brain. **A.** Neurotransmitter activation of a receptor that contains an ion channel. **B.** Neurotransmitter activation of a G protein-coupled receptor. After it is activated, the G protein can directly regulate an ion channel (*left*). Activation of the G protein also triggers the regulation of second messenger-dependent protein kinases and protein phosphatases, which can in turn regulate other ion channels and many neuronal processes (*right*). **C.** Neurotrophic factor activation of a receptor that contains protein tyrosine kinase activity or activates such a kinase indirectly. **D.** Steroid hormone activation of a cytoplasmic receptor. After the receptor is bound by hormone, it translocates to the nucleus and either regulates the expression of genes directly as shown or binds other transcription factors (not shown) (see Chapter 6).

virtually all slower actions that are yet short-term consequences of synaptic transmission are mediated by intracellular messenger pathways. Finally, all of the long-term consequences of synaptic transmission are achieved through intracellular messengers; these include phosphorylation of diverse types of proteins and alterations in neuronal gene expression (see Chapter 6). It is

important to emphasize that neurotransmitters that activate ligand-gated ion channels, for example, glutamate and γ-aminobutyric acid (GABA), also trigger intracellular messenger cascades. Although activation of ligand-gated ion channels leads to initial changes in the electrical activity of neurons without the involvement of intracellular messengers, such activation also

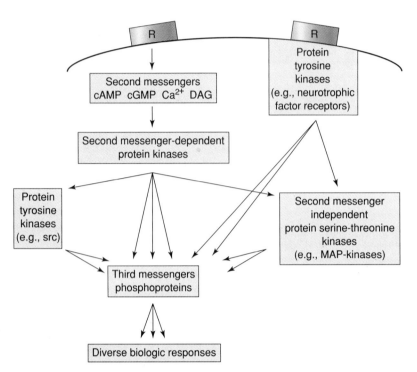

Figure 5–2. Signal transduction pathways in neurons. Extracellular signals, or first messengers, produce biologic responses in target neurons through a series of intracellular signals. Many activate second messenger pathways resulting in the phosphorylation of diverse types of proteins that can be considered third messengers. Such phosphorylation mediates the biologic responses of the first messengers. First messengers also produce biologic responses through the activation of protein tyrosine kinases, some of which are physically linked to plasma membrane receptors (R), whereas others are cytoplasmic.

results in numerous other, albeit somewhat slower, effects—for example, changes in gene expression—that are mediated by these messengers. Third, interactions among the various intracellular messenger pathways are responsible for adjusting neuronal response to diverse types of synaptic inputs and environmental cues, thereby enabling neurons to coordinate a myriad of neuronal processes.

G PROTEINS AND SECOND MESSENGERS

G PROTEINS

As previously mentioned, G proteins perform a central function in the process of transmembrane signaling in the nervous system. These proteins, first identified and characterized by Gilman, Rodbell, and colleagues, were named because of their ability to bind the guanine nucleotides, guanosine triphosphate (GTP) and guanosine diphosphate (GDP). G proteins couple receptors to specific intracellular effector systems (see Figure 5–1). Three major types of G protein are involved in the transduction of signals produced by neurotransmitter binding: G_s, $G_{i/o}$, and G_q (Table 5–1). A fourth type of G protein, called transducin (G_t), regulates the electrical properties of photoreceptor cells in conjunction with rhodopsin, a light-sensitive molecule in the retina that can be viewed as a G protein-linked receptor. Gustducin (G_g), which represents a fifth type of G protein, plays an analogous role in taste transduc-

tion in the tongue. A sixth type of G protein (G_{12}) exists in diverse cell types, including those in the brain, but its role in the control of cellular signaling events remains poorly understood. All eukaryotic cells also contain a distinct class of guanine nucleotide-binding proteins that subserve a variety of roles in the regulation of cell function; these are termed *small-molecular-weight G proteins* and are described in Box 5–1.

Each type of G protein is a heterotrimer composed of single α, β, and γ subunits. Because different types of G protein appear to have common β and γ subunits, it is tempting to conclude that distinctive α subunits confer specific functional activity on these proteins. Thus individual $α_s$, $α_i$ and $α_o$, $α_q$, $α_t$, $α_g$, and $α_{11}$ subunits most likely are responsible for the unique functions of the G proteins that contain them; moreover, multiple subtypes of most of these α subunits have been identified (Table 5–1). However, several types of β and γ subunits also have been identified, and increasing evidence indicates that these subtypes complex with one another and associate with subtypes of α subunits to confer still greater degrees of specificity on intracellular signaling proteins.

The functional cycle of G proteins is shown schematically in Figure 5–3. In their resting state, G proteins exist as heterotrimers that are bound to GDP and are not functionally associated with extracellular receptors or intracellular effector proteins (see Figure 5–3A). When a receptor is activated by ligand binding, a conformational change in the receptor causes it to associate with the α subunit of a G protein (see Figure 5–3B).

Table 5–1 Heterotrimeric G Protein α Subunits in Brain

Class	Molecular Mass (kDa)	Toxin-Mediated ADP-Ribosylation	Effector Protein(s)
G_s family			
$G_{\alpha s1}$	52	Cholera	Adenylyl cyclase (activation)
$G_{\alpha s2}$	52		
$G_{\alpha s3}$	45		
$G_{\alpha s4}$	45		
$G_{\alpha olf}$	45		
G_i family			
$G_{\alpha i1}$	41	Pertussis	Adenylyl cyclase (inhibition)
$G_{\alpha i2}$	40		?K^+ channel (inhibition)
$G_{\alpha i3}$	41		?Ca^{2+} channel (activation)
			?Phospholipase C (activation)
			?Phospholipase A_2
$G_{\alpha o1}$	39	Pertussis	?K^+ channel (inhibition)
$G_{\alpha o2}$	39		?Ca^{2+} channel (activation)
$G_{\alpha t1}$	39	Cholera and	Phosphodiesterase in rods and cones (activation)
$G_{\alpha t2}$	40	pertussis	
$G_{\alpha gust}$	41	Unknown	Phosphodiesterase in taste epithelium (activation)
$G_{\alpha z}$	41	None	?Adenylyl cyclase (inhibition)
G_q family	41–43		
$G_{\alpha q}$		None	Phospholipase C (activation)
$G_{\alpha 11}$			Unknown
$G_{\alpha 14}$			
$G_{\alpha 15}$			
$G_{\alpha 16}$			
G_{12} family	44	None	Unknown
$G_{\alpha 12}$			
$G_{\alpha 13}$			

This association, in turn, alters the conformation of the α subunit and leads to (1) reduced affinity of the α subunit for GDP, resulting in the binding of GTP—a much greater concentration of which is present in cells than is GDP—to the subunit, (2) the dissociation of the β and γ subunits from the α subunit, and (3) the release of the receptor from the G protein (see Figure 5–3B and C). The union of a free α subunit with GTP results in a biologically active entity that regulates the functional activity of many effector proteins in the cell. Free β and γ subunits also form biologically active complexes that regulate specific effector proteins. The system returns to its resting state when the ligand is released from the receptor and the GTPase that resides in the α subunit hydrolyzes GTP to GDP (see Figure 5–3D). The latter action leads to the reassociation of the free α subunit with the βγ complex and thus to the restoration of the original heterotrimer.

Several bacterial toxins produce their pathogenic effects by regulating the activity of specific α subunits of G proteins through a process termed *ADP-ribosylation* (see Table 5–1). This process involves the addition of

an ADP-ribose group from nicotinamide adenine dinucleotide (NAD) to an amino acid residue in the α subunit. **Cholera toxin** ADP-ribosylates and irreversibly activates $G_{\alpha s}$ by inhibiting its GTPase activity, whereas **pertussis toxin** ADP-ribosylates and inactivates $G_{\alpha i}$ and $G_{\alpha o}$ by stabilizing their association with βγ subunits. **Diphtheria toxin** ADP-ribosylates and inactivates a small G protein, known as eukaryotic elongation factor 2, which is distinct from the heterotrimeric G proteins and regulates ribosomal function (see Box 5–1). Evidence suggests that the brain contains cholera toxin-like enzymes, implying that certain G proteins and perhaps other proteins may be physiologically regulated in this manner.

G proteins also are the targets of certain insect venoms. The best characterized is **mastoparan,** a 10–amino acid-long peptide contained in wasp venom. The peptide stimulates the GTPase activity of $G_{\alpha i}$ subunits, thereby shortening the duration of the GTP-bound activated subunits. Mastoparan appears to produce this effect by forming an α-helix that inserts into the plasma membrane where it binds to $G_{\alpha i}$.

Box 5-1 Small G Proteins

Two general classes of guanine nucleotide-binding proteins are critical to the functioning of neurons and other cells. These are the heterotrimeric G proteins and a large superfamily typically referred to as small G proteins because of their low molecular mass (20–35 kDa). Like the α subunits of heterotrimeric G proteins, small G proteins bind guanine nucleotides, possess intrinsic GTPase activity, and cycle through GDP- and GTP-bound forms (see Figure 5–3). All classes of G protein undergo a change in their affinity for target molecules as they shift from GDP- to GTP-bound forms, most likely because such a shift causes them to undergo a large conformational change. However, small G proteins are unique in that they appear to function as molecular switches that control several cellular processes (see table).

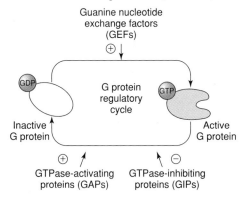

Among the best characterized small G proteins are those that comprise the Ras family, a series of related proteins of approximately 21 kDa. Their activity is highly regulated by a variety of associated proteins (see figure). Guanine nucleotide exchange factors (GEFs) increase the activity of Ras proteins by stimulating the release of GDP from their inactive forms and facilitating their binding to GTP. In contrast, GTPase-activating proteins (GAPs) bind to Ras proteins, thereby stimulating their intrinsic GTPase activity and reducing their functional activity. A mutation in one type of GAP results in **neurofibromatosis,** a disease characterized by the uncontrolled growth of glial cells that express myelin. It is proposed that GTPase inhibitory proteins (GIPs) also may bind to Ras proteins and inhibit their GTPase activity.

Ras proteins and heterotrimeric G proteins interact with their related proteins in strikingly analogous ways. For example, G protein-coupled receptors provide essentially the same function for heterotrimeric G proteins that GEFs perform for Ras proteins. Likewise, GTPase-activating and -inhibiting proteins modify Ras proteins in much the same way that RGS proteins and βγ subunits regulate heterotrimeric G proteins. However, there are important differences as well. Because Ras proteins are characterized by far less intrinsic GTPase activity than heterotrimeric G protein α subunits, GAPs exert a more profound effect on the functioning of the Ras system and are essentially responsible for turning it on and off.

Numerous types of cell signals, including most neurotrophic factors, converge on Ras and related proteins to regulate MAP-kinase pathways, which in turn produce diverse effects on cell function. The mechanisms involved in these cascades are presented in greater detail in the text.

Rab proteins, which are involved in membrane vesicle trafficking, represent another small G protein family. Rab subtypes, particularly Rab3, have been implicated in the regulation of exocytosis and neurotransmitter release at nerve terminals (see Chapter 4). ARF is a small G protein involved in functioning of the Golgi apparatus. It appears to control the binding of a protein coat to budding vesicles, including synaptic vesicles that mediate neurotransmitter release at the synapse.

Examples of Small G Proteins

Class	Proposed Cellular Function
Ras	Signal transduction (control of growth factor and MAP-kinase pathways)
Rac, Cdc42	Signal transduction (control of cellular stress responses and MAP-kinase pathways)
Rab	Vesicle trafficking and exocytosis in synaptic vesicles
Rho	Assembly of cytoskeletal structures (e.g., actin microfilaments)
ARF	Assembly and function of Golgi complex ADP-ribosylation of $G_{\alpha s}$
EF-2	Regulation of protein synthesis at ribosomes
Ran	Nuclear-cytoplasmic trafficking of RNA and protein

CdC42, cell division cycle 42; ARF, ADP-ribosylation factor; EF-2, eukaryotic elongation factor 2.

Naturally occurring mutations in the α subunits of G proteins are known to cause **endocrinopathies** and other hereditary diseases in humans. Examples of these disorders include **pseudohypoparathyroidism** and **hereditary osteodystrophy** (Box 5–2).

G protein function can be regulated by several modulatory proteins. A neurotransmitter receptor may be seen as one type of modulatory protein, specifically a guanine nucleotide exchange factor, because it triggers the release of GDP from the α subunit. Recently characterized *regulators of G protein signaling* (RGS proteins) activate the GTPase activity intrinsic to the α subunits of G proteins; thus, these proteins inhibit G protein function by shortening the duration of the signals from both the activated GTP-α subunit and the free βγ subunits. All G protein α subunits, except for $G_{\alpha s}$, are known to be reg-

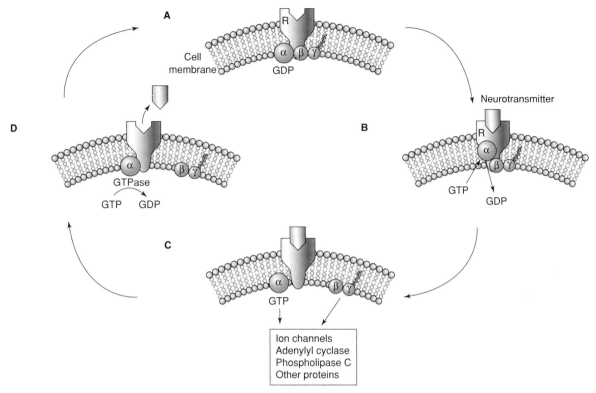

Figure 5–3. G protein function. **A.** Under basal conditions, G proteins exist in cell membranes as heterotrimers composed of single α, β, and γ subunits. The α subunits are bound to GDP, and the G protein heterotrimer is anchored to the plasma membrane by an isoprenyl (acyl) group attached to C-terminal cysteine residues of the γ subunit. **B.** After the receptor (R) is activated by its ligand (e.g., neurotransmitter), it physically associates with the α subunit, causing the latter to release GDP. Subsequently GTP binds to the α subunit. **C.** GTP binding causes the dissociation of the α subunit from its βγ subunits and from the receptor. Free α subunits, bound to GTP, are functionally active and directly regulate a number of effector proteins, such as ion channels, adenylyl cyclase, and phospholipase C. Free βγ subunits are also biologically active and directly regulate some of the same effector proteins. **D.** GTPase activity intrinsic to the α subunit degrades GTP to form GDP, and in turn causes the reassociation of the α and βγ subunits. This reassociation, in conjunction with the dissociation of the ligand from the receptor, restores the basal state.

ulated in this manner. More than 20 subtypes of RGS proteins have been identified, most of which are located in specific neuronal cell types. Phosducin is another modulatory protein that binds to βγ subunits and thereby competes with these subunits for binding to α subunits and possibly to effector proteins.

As previously indicated, G proteins couple neurotransmitter receptors to two general types of effector proteins (see Figure 5–1): ion channels and enzymes that regulate the generation of second messengers.

G PROTEIN REGULATION OF ION CHANNELS

Many types of neurotransmitter receptors regulate ion channels by means of G proteins. The process by which this regulation occurs is best established for neurotransmitter receptors that couple to $G_{\alpha i}$ or $G_{\alpha o}$, including opioid, α_2-adrenergic, D_2-dopaminergic, muscarinic cholinergic, 5-HT_{1a}-serotonergic, and $GABA_B$ receptors. When coupled to G proteins, these receptors activate specific inwardly rectifying K^+ channels (GIRKs) or inhibit voltage-gated Ca^{2+} channels, depending on the cell type involved. The regulation of both types of channel most likely occurs primarily through the βγ subunits of G proteins, which directly open, or gate, GIRKs and limit the opening of Ca^{2+} channels in response to membrane depolarization. Ion channels also may couple to neurotransmitter receptors in an analogous fashion by means of other G protein subunits. Some evidence suggests, for example,

Box 5-2 Genetic Mutations of G Proteins and Disease

All proteins involved in G protein-coupled signal transduction are subject to genetic mutation in humans, including associated receptors, heterotrimeric G proteins, and downstream effector molecules. The genetic defects underlying **hypoparathyroidism** serve as examples. Parathyroid hormone (PTH) signals target cells by binding to the G protein-coupled PTH receptor; subsequently the ligand-bound PTH receptor signals target cells through G_s. Although true hypoparathyroidism is caused by a decrease in the secretion of PTH, defects in the PTH signaling cascade can lead to **pseudohypoparathyroidism** (PHP), a disease that produces hypoparathyroid symptoms in individuals with normal levels of PTH. One type of PHP (PTP1b) is believed to result from a defect in the PTH receptor. Another form, PTP1a, is caused by mutations in $G_{\alpha s}$.

Patients with PTP1a, which is commonly referred to **as Albright syndrome** or **hereditary osteodystrophy,** exhibit dysmorphic features characteristic of congenital hypoparathyroidism, including short stature, a round face, shortened metacarpal and metatarsal bones, and subcutaneous ossifications. Both our understanding of the defects involved in PTP1a and the nomenclature of hypoparathyroidism were complicated by the discovery of a syndrome known as **pseudopseudohypoparathyroidism.** Some patients with this syndrome exhibit the phenotype that is characteristic of Albright syndrome but do not manifest inborn errors of PTH metabolism and in fact have normal levels of PTH. Some of these latter cases are also caused by $G_{\alpha s}$ mutations, although mutations in other proteins involved in $G_{\alpha s}$ signaling may be involved in other cases.

Mutations in $G_{\alpha s}$ also may underlie hereditary endocrine tumors such as those that occur in patients with **McCune-Albright syndrome** (MAS). MAS, which occurs sporadically, is characterized by the clinical triad of fibrous dysplasia, cafe au lait spots, and precocious puberty—often in conjunction with other endocrinopathies. The mutated subunits act in a dominant manner, causing heterozygous cells that express the mutation to resist hormones that signal by means of $G_{\alpha s}$. Interestingly, mutated subunits are detected in a mosaic pattern in adult tissues. This means that the defect is seen in some cells of an individual but not others. This pattern is consistent with a somatic mutation early in embryogenesis, which is not carried in the germline.

that $G_{\alpha s}$ can potentiate the voltage-dependent gating of certain Ca^{2+} channels; however, whether this effect is mediated by α or $\beta\gamma$ subunits is not yet known.

SECOND MESSENGERS

G proteins also transduce the activation of neurotransmitter receptors by neurotransmitter binding to altered intracellular levels of second messengers in target neurons. Prominent second messengers in the brain include cyclic adenosine monophosphate (cAMP), cyclic guanosine monophosphate (cGMP), Ca^{2+}, nitric oxide (NO), and the major metabolites of both phosphatidylinositol—inositol triphosphate (IP_3) and diacylglycerol (DAG)—and arachidonic acid, such as prostaglandins. Altered levels of second messengers mediate the effects of receptor activation on many types of ion channels and on numerous physiologic responses.

Cyclic nucleotides   cAMP and cGMP are classified as cyclic nucleotides because they are synthesized from ATP and GTP, respectively, through the formation of a cyclic phosphodiester ring (Figure 5–4). The molecular mechanisms by which neurotransmitters regulate cAMP levels are well-established (Figure 5–5). When G_s couples receptors, such as β-adrenergic, D_1-dopamine, VIP, and CRF receptors, to adenylyl cyclase, the enzyme responsible for the synthesis of cAMP, the enzyme is stimulated by receptor activation. In contrast, when G_i couples receptors, such as opioid, α_2-adrenergic, and D_2-dopamine receptors, to adenylyl cyclase, the enzyme is inhibited by receptor activation. The mechanisms by which neurotransmitters, for example, substance P, or acetylcholine at muscarinic receptors, typically stimulate cGMP levels are more complex and involve increases in intracellular levels of Ca^{2+} and of nitric oxide.

Adenylyl cyclases   Based on molecular cloning, nine forms of adenylyl cyclase (types I–IX) have been identified, each of which exhibits a distinctive pattern of expression in brain and peripheral tissues. All adenylyl cyclases are activated directly by binding to GTP-bound αs subunits and also are activated by the plant diterpene **forskolin;** however, they differ in their regulation by $G_{\alpha i}$, $\beta\gamma$ subunits, Ca^{2+}, and phosphorylation. Three general categories of adenylyl cyclase can be delineated based on regulatory properties: (1) types I, III, and VIII, which are activated synergistically by $G_{\alpha s}$ and by Ca^{2+} and calmodulin and are sometimes inhibited by $\beta\gamma$ subunits; (2) types II and IV and perhaps VII, which are activated synergistically by $G_{\alpha s}$ and by $\beta\gamma$ subunits; and (3) types V and VI, which are inhibited by free Ca^{2+} and by $G_{\alpha i}$ (Figure 5–6). Although many features of these categories remain hypothetical, they suggest that regulation of cAMP formation varies depending on the form of adenylyl cyclase expressed in neuronal cells.

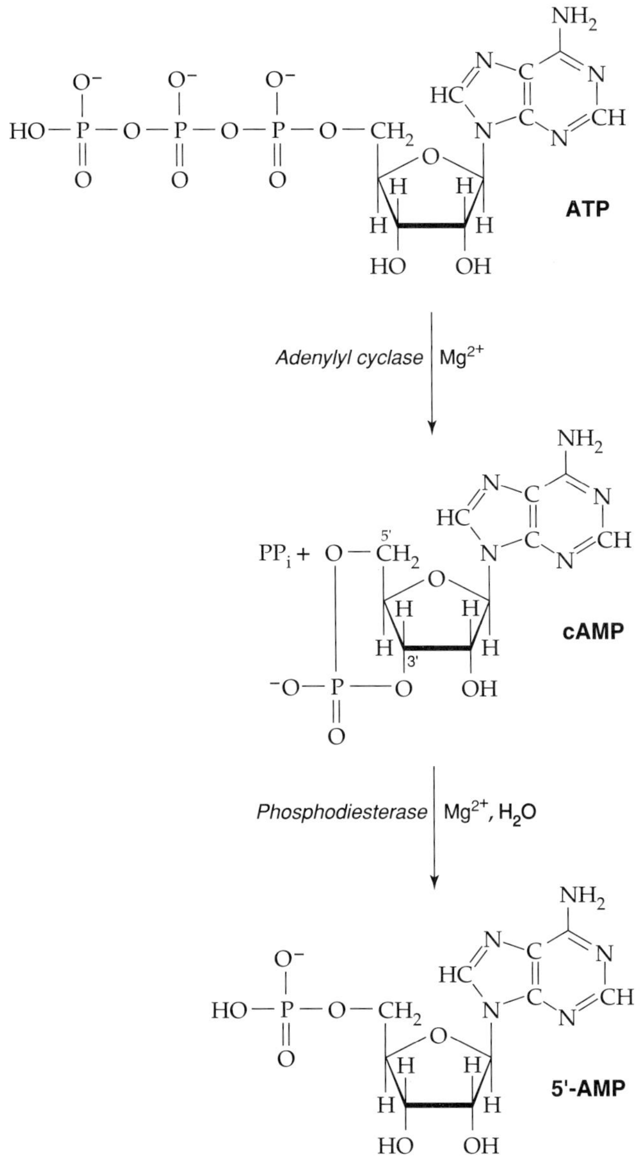

Figure 5–4. Cyclic AMP (cAMP) synthesis and degradation. The metabolism of cGMP is analogous to that shown for cAMP: guanylyl cyclase catalyzes the synthesis of cGMP from GTP, and phosphodiesterase hydrolyzes cGMP into 5'-GMP.

Guanylyl cyclases Neurotransmitters regulate cGMP levels by means of two mechanisms. A very small number of plasma membrane receptors, such as atrial natriuretic peptide receptors, contain guanylyl cyclase that is activated when a ligand binds to the receptor. In most cases, however, guanylyl cyclase is a cytosolic enzyme that is activated by nitric oxide (see Figure 5–5). Three major subtypes of nitric oxide synthase (NOS) are known; the names of two of these, neural NOS and endothelial NOS, indicate the tissue in which each was first found, and the name of the third, inducible NOS, indicates that it is induced by acute stimuli. All three

forms are widely distributed in brain and peripheral tissues. When NOS is activated by Ca^{2+}, in conjunction with the Ca^{2+}-binding protein calmodulin, it generates nitric oxide from the amino acid arginine. Accordingly, neurotransmitters that increase intracellular Ca^{2+} levels typically increase cGMP levels by generating nitric oxide. **Organic nitrates** that are used as vasodilators in the treatment of **ischemic heart disease,** such as angina pectoris, work by generating free nitric oxide in vascular smooth muscle, which increases cellular cGMP levels and in turn leads to muscle relaxation.

Because nitric oxide is a soluble gas, it can diffuse out of the neuron in which it is synthesized and stimulate guanylyl cyclase in neighboring cells, thereby increasing cGMP levels. Thus nitric oxide may function as an intercellular messenger as well as an intracellular messenger in brain. Indeed it has been hypothesized that nitric oxide functions as a retrograde messenger. According to this scheme, it is synthesized in a neuron in response to a neurotransmitter that increases cellular Ca^{2+} levels; subsequently it diffuses out of the neuron and influences the presynaptic nerve terminal that released the neurotransmitter. This series of events is plausible but has not yet been established with certainty.

Nitric oxide also has been implicated as a mediator of cell injury and cell death under certain circumstances (see Chapters 11 and 21).

Phosphodiesterases cAMP and cGMP are enzymatically degraded by phosphodiesterases (PDEs), which are expressed in numerous forms in brain and other tissues. As outlined in Table 5–2, these enzymes differ in their relative selectivity for cAMP and cGMP. They also differ in their regulation by other cellular signals: one form of phosphodiesterase expressed at high levels in retina is activated by $G_{\alpha t}$, whereas other forms are regulated by the cyclic nucleotides themselves or by Ca^{2+}/calmodulin. At high concentrations, **caffeine** and related **methylxanthines** inhibit phosphodiesterase activity, which may contribute to some of the pharmacologic effects of these drugs, particularly at higher doses.

The potential clinical utility of PDE inhibitors is currently under investigation. Nonselective PDE inhibitors, which affect many forms of the enzyme, are associated with pervasive side effects, but progress has been made in the development of selective PDE inhibitors. **Sildenafil** (Viagra), a specific inhibitor of PDE type V, is widely prescribed for the treatment of **penile impotence.** PDE type V is concentrated in vascular smooth muscle and especially, but not exclusively, in the vasculature of the penis. Interestingly, sildenafil was a byproduct of research aimed at enhancing the vasodilation of coronary arteries.

Considerable effort also has been made toward developing PDE inhibitors that are selective for isoforms

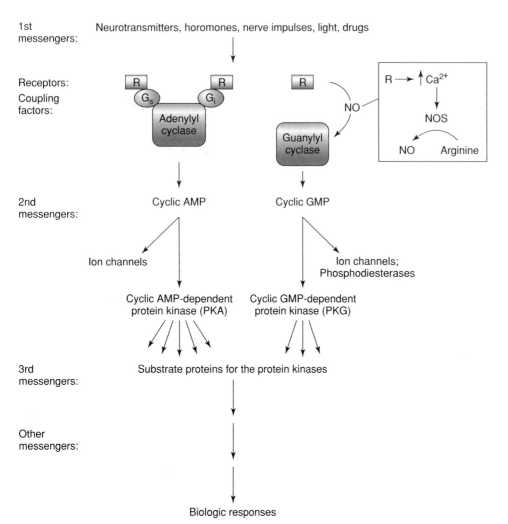

1st
messengers: Neurotransmitters, horomones, nerve impulses, light, drugs

Receptors:
Coupling
factors:

2nd
messengers: Cyclic AMP   Cyclic GMP

                  Ion channels   Ion channels;
                                                  Phosphodiesterases

                  Cyclic AMP-dependent   Cyclic GMP-dependent
                  protein kinase (PKA)   protein kinase (PKG)

3rd
messengers: Substrate proteins for the protein kinases

Other
messengers:

                            Biologic responses

Figure 5–5. Cyclic AMP (cAMP) and cyclic GMP (cGMP) second messenger systems. Most extracellular messengers influence these systems through interactions with neurotransmitter receptors (R); others, including many drugs, such as phosphodiesterase inhibitors that inhibit the breakdown of cAMP and cGMP, influence these second messenger systems directly. G proteins (G_s or $G_{i/o}$) are coupling factors that mediate the ability of neurotransmitter receptors to activate or inhibit adenylyl cyclase, the enzyme that catalyzes the synthesis of cAMP. Neurotransmitters typically increase cGMP levels by elevating cellular Ca^{2+} levels (see Figure 5–7). Increased Ca^{2+} levels trigger the activation of nitric oxide synthase (NOS), which converts arginine to nitric oxide (NO). NO subsequently activates guanylyl cyclase, which catalyzes the synthesis of cGMP.

After they are synthesized, the second messengers activate cAMP-dependent protein kinase and cGMP-dependent protein kinase, respectively. PKA and PKG phosphorylate an array of substrate proteins termed third messengers, whose altered physiologic activity provokes biologic responses to extracellular messengers, either directly or indirectly (e.g., through intervening fourth, fifth, or sixth messengers). Alternatively, cAMP and cGMP directly gate certain types of ion channels, and cGMP can directly activate phosphodiesterases, for example, in the retina.

of the enzyme expressed only in the brain. **Rolipram,** for example, inhibits all isoforms of PDE type IV; this drug initially showed promise as an **antidepressant,** but its clinical utility was limited by side effects such as nausea. However, because the type-IV enzyme comprises many subtypes (see Table 5–2), an inhibitor of one sub-

type may lead to the development of an effective antidepressant without rolipram's side effects.

Calcium   The regulation of intracellular Ca^{2+} levels by neurotransmitter receptors is highly complex, but two major types of mechanisms operate to varying

A

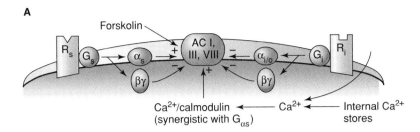

B

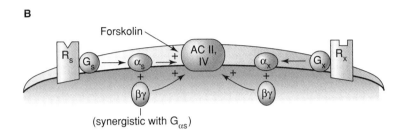

C

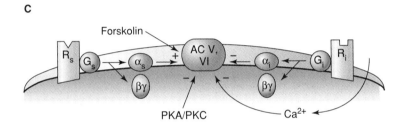

Figure 5–6. Regulation of adenylyl cyclase (AC) activity. Although all forms of the enzyme are activated by $G_{\alpha s}$ and forskolin, they vary in their regulation by Ca^{2+} and G protein $\beta\gamma$ subunits. **A.** Because adenylyl cyclase types I, III, and VIII are stimulated by Ca^{2+}/calmodulin, these enzymes typically are activated by an increase in cellular Ca^{2+} levels. $G_{\alpha s}$ interacts synergistically with Ca^{2+}/calmodulin, and in the presence of activated $G_{\alpha s}$, type I adenylyl cyclase is inhibited by $\beta\gamma$ subunits. $G_{\alpha i}$ has been proven to mediate neurotransmitter inhibition of these adenylyl cyclases. **B.** Adenylyl cyclase types II and IV are not sensitive to Ca^{2+}/calmodulin and, in the presence of activated $G_{\alpha s}$, are stimulated synergistically by $\beta\gamma$ complexes. The source of the $\beta\gamma$ complexes could be $G_{\alpha s}$ itself or any of several other types of G proteins (e.g., G_i, G_o, G_q), depicted as G_x in the figure. **C.** Types V and VI are inhibited in response to phosphorylation by cAMP-dependent protein kinase (PKA) or protein kinase C (PKC). They are also inhibited by free Ca^{2+} and by $G_{\alpha i}$, but are not influenced by $\beta\gamma$ subunits.

Table 5–2 Classification and Selected Properties of Cyclic Nucleotide Phosphodiesterases

Family	Regulatory and Kinetic Characteristics	Genes Described	Selective Inhibitors[1]
I	Ca^{2+}/calmodulin-stimulated; regulated by Ca^{2+}/calmodulin and phosphorylation; have a low affinity for cAMP and cGMP except for PDE1C gene product, which has high affinity for cAMP	PDE1A (59-61 kDa) PDE1B (63 kDa) PDE1C (67 kDa, 75 kDa in brain)	Trifluoperazine Vinpocetine 8-methoxymethyl-3-isobutyl-1-methylxanthine
II	cGMP-stimulated; regulated by cGMP; have low affinity for cAMP and cGMP	PDE2 (105 kDa, soluble and particulate)	EHNA
III	cGMP-inhibited; regulated by phosphorylation and cGMP; high affinity, cGMP > cAMP	PDE3A PDE3B (110-135 kDa)	Milrinone Enoximone Amrinone[2]
IV	cAMP-specific; regulated by phosphorylation and cAMP; high affinity, cAMP >>> cGMP	PDE4A PDE4B PDE4C PDE4D (short and long forms of each)	Rolipram Ro20-1724
V	cGMP-binding; cGMP-specific	PDE5 (smooth muscle)	Sildenafil Zaprinast
VI	Retina cGMP specific; regulated by transducin; high affinity, cGMP >>> cAMP	PDE6A (α subtype) PDE6B (rod β subtype) PDE6C (cone β subtype)	–
VII	cAMP-specific; rolipram insensitive	PDE7A	–

[1]A number of compounds, particularly the methylxanthines (e.g., theophylline, isobutylmethylxanthine, caffeine) also inhibit most major forms of PDE.
[2]These compounds represent a small portion of the known specific inhibitors of PDE III.
PDE, phosphodiesterase

degrees in every cell (Figure 5–7). Through one mechanism neurotransmitter receptor activation alters the flux of extracellular Ca^{2+} into neurons. Such alteration can occur in a number of ways: (1) Ca^{2+} may pass directly through certain subtypes of ligand-gated channels, such as activated nicotinic cholinergic and N-

methyl-D-aspartate (NMDA) glutamate receptors (see Chapter 7); (2) the properties of specific voltage-gated Ca^{2+} channels may be altered by G proteins that directly couple receptors to these channels—for example, opioid receptors in some cell types, as previously outlined; (3) the depolarization of a neuron, which causes

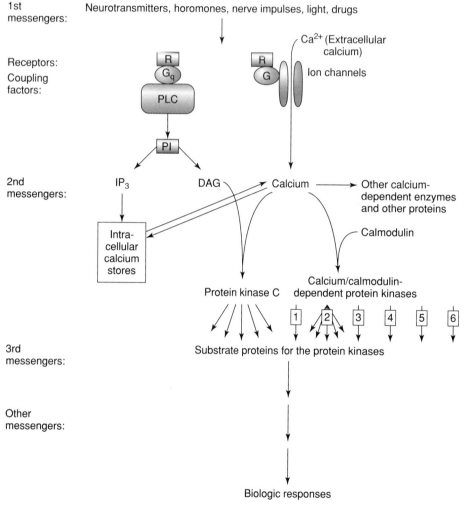

Figure 5–7. Ca^{2+} and phosphatidylinositol second messenger systems. Most extracellular messengers act on these systems, as they do on the cAMP and cGMP systems, through interactions with neurotransmitter receptors (R). However, some drugs, such as Ca^{2+} channel blockers and lithium, can influence these systems directly. G proteins (typically G_q) are coupling factors that mediate the ability of neurotransmitter receptors to regulate phospholipase C (PLC), which metabolizes phosphatidylinositol (PI) to form inositol triphosphate (IP_3) and diacylglycerol (DAG). IP_3 acts to increase intracellular levels of free Ca^{2+}, also a second messenger in the brain, by releasing Ca^{2+} from internal stores. Increased levels of intracellular Ca^{2+} also result from the flux of Ca^{2+} across the plasma membrane stimulated by nerve impulses and certain neurotransmitters. The brain contains two major classes of Ca^{2+}-dependent protein kinases. One is activated by Ca^{2+} in conjunction with the Ca^{2+}-binding protein calmodulin (CaM-kinase), and the other, protein kinase C, is activated by Ca^{2+} in conjunction with diacylglycerol and various phospholipids. Many of these kinases have broad substrate specificities (as indicated by the multiple arrows in the figure). Phosphorylation of substrate proteins, or third messengers, by these various Ca^{2+}-dependent protein kinases, alters their physiologic activity and either directly or indirectly triggers biologic responses to extracellular messengers.

the activation of voltage-gated Ca^{2+} channels, may lead to large increases in intracellular Ca^{2+} levels (see Chapter 3); or (4) the activation of other second messenger systems may alter Ca^{2+} channel properties; for example, cAMP and neurotransmitters that act through cAMP can modulate voltage-gated Ca^{2+} channels by regulating their phosphorylation.

The second major type of mechanism by which neurotransmitters can increase intracellular levels of free Ca^{2+} is through regulation of the phosphatidylinositol system and subsequent actions on intracellular Ca^{2+} stores (see Figure 5–7). Such regulation is possible because many types of neurotransmitter receptors are coupled through G proteins to an enzyme termed *phospholipase C (PLC)*. Receptor activation of phospholipase C is mediated most often by subtypes of G_q, although mediation by G_i and G_o also has been implicated. Whether the α or the βγ subunits of G_q govern this process remains unclear.

Phospholipase C and the phosphatidylinositol pathway

As discussed in Chapter 4, phospholipase C catalyzes the breakdown of phosphatidylinositol, which results in the generation of two lipid molecules that function as second messengers in the brain: inositol triphosphate (IP_3) and diacylglycerol (DAG) (Figure 5–8). The two major forms of phospholipase C in the brain are designated β and γ (Figure 5–9). The β form is predominantly responsible for mediating the effects of neurotransmitters that are coupled to G_q, and the γ form is predominantly responsible for mediating the effects of neurotrophic factors on this enzyme.

Phosphatidylinositol is a membrane phospholipid whose fatty acid chains typically consist of stearate and arachidonate (see Figure 5–8). Phospholipase C action on this phospholipid results in the generation of free inositol-1-phosphate, which, through a series of lipid phosphorylation events, is converted into active IP_3 or inositol-1,4,5-triphosphate. IP_3 is subsequently recycled by means of successive dephosphorylation into inositol, which cells use to replenish phosphatidylinositol in their membranes. **Lithium,** which remains an important drug in the treatment of **mania** and is used to enhance the actions of antidepressants in **depression,** inhibits several of these inositol phosphatases. Because inositol does not freely pass the blood–brain barrier, the therapeutic effectiveness of lithium may be explained by depletion of free inositol within neurons after prolonged treatment. Whether such depletion is responsible for lithium's clinical effects remains unknown; indeed, lithium also is known to inhibit several adenylyl cyclases, G proteins, and protein kinases (see Chapter 15). IP_3 acts on an IP_3 receptor, which functions to release Ca^{2+} from intracellular organelles such as the endoplasmic reticulum. **Thapsigargan** is a small molecule known to inhibit this effect. Some organelles also contain a related **ryanodine** receptor, which triggers the release of Ca^{2+} from intracellular stores in response to a rise in Ca^{2+} itself. DAG, the other metabolite of phosphatidylinositol, functions as a second messenger in cells by activating protein kinase C, as will be discussed below.

Arachidonic acid metabolites

The prostaglandin and leukotriene family of intracellular messengers appears to play an important role in the regulation of signal transduction in the brain and elsewhere. Many of the effects of these major metabolites of arachidonic acid are achieved by modulating the generation of second messengers.

Prostaglandins and leukotrienes are generated by a complex biochemical cascade. An enzyme termed phospholipase A_2 cleaves membrane phospholipids to yield free arachidonic acid. The activity of phospholipase A_2 is regulated by neurotransmitter–receptor interactions. In some cases, a receptor causes an increase in intracellular Ca^{2+} levels, which in turn activates phospholipase A_2; alternatively, G proteins may be responsible for activating the enzyme, although this remains speculative. Next, arachidonic acid is cleaved by cyclooxygenase to yield, after numerous enzymatic steps, several types of prostaglandins and other cyclic endoperoxides, such as prostacyclins and thromboxanes, or it is cleaved by lipoxygenase to yield the leukotrienes (Figure 5–10).

The varied biologic activities of these endoperoxides and leukotrienes serve to regulate adenylyl cyclase, guanylyl cyclase, ion channels, protein kinases, and other cellular proteins. The arachidonic acid metabolites appear to bind directly to some of these signaling proteins, including protein kinases and ion channels, and to allosterically modulate their function. More often, the metabolites appear to serve as the endogenous ligands for G protein-coupled receptors. In the latter scenario, metabolites generated intracellularly diffuse out of the neuron because of their lipophilic properties and act on its extracellular receptors (autocrine effect) or on those of a neighboring neuron (paracrine effect).

Receptors for the leukotrienes are termed BLT or LT receptors, and those for prostaglandins and thromboxanes are termed prostanoid receptors. Several prostanoid receptors are known, and each is named for the arachidonic acid metabolite with the highest affinity for that receptor. EP receptors, for example, are activated preferentially by prostaglandin E_2 (PGE_2), the DP receptor is activated preferentially by PGD_2, the FP receptor by PGF_{2a}, the IP receptor by PGI_2, and the TP receptor by thromboxane A_2.

All LT receptors are coupled by G_q and presumably act by stimulating the PLC pathway. In contrast, the numerous subtypes of prostanoid receptors are coupled by either G_q, G_s, or G_i. Indeed, it has been well estab-

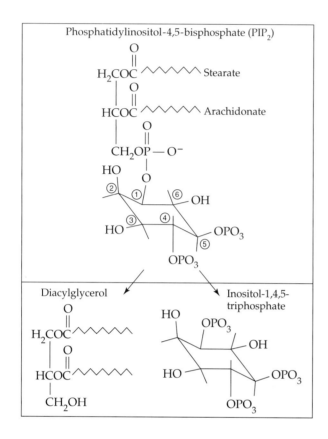

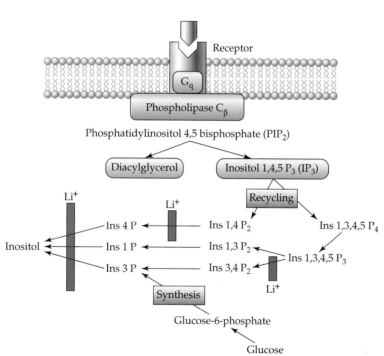

Figure 5–8. The phosphatidylinositol cycle: actions of lithium. Many neurotransmitter receptors are linked by G_q (or another G protein) to phospholipase Cβ, which hydrolyzes phosphatidylinositol-4,5–bisphosphate (PIP_2) to generate two second messengers: diacylglycerol and inositol 1,4,5–triphosphate (IP_3). IP_3 acts to release Ca^{2+} from intracellular stores and subsequently is metabolized to forms that may not participate in neural signal transduction, including inositol 1,3,4,5 tetraphosphate (Ins 1,3,4,5 P_4). These forms are eventually metabolized to produce three inositol monophosphates, which differ only in terms of the carbon atom to which the phosphate group is linked. Synthesis of inositol from glucose-6-phosphate also must pass through an inositol monophosphate intermediate. All inositol monophosphates are metabolized by inositol monophosphate phosphatase, an enzyme that is inhibited by therapeutic concentrations of lithium (Li^+). Thus in the presence of lithium, these monophosphates cannot be dephosphorylated to yield free inositol, which is required to regenerate phosphatidylinositol-4,5 bisphosphate. Lithium also inhibits inositol polyphosphate-1-phosphatase, an enzyme required for other metabolic steps in the recycling pathway.

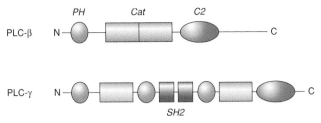

Figure 5–9. Structure of phospholipase C (PLC). The two major forms of PLC in the brain are termed PLCβ and PLCγ. PLCβ mediates the ability of G protein-coupled receptors (linked by G_q) to stimulate the phosphatidylinositol pathway (see Figure 5–7). PLCγ mediates the ability of neurotrophic factor pathways to stimulate the pathway (see Figure 5–13). Both forms contain a pleckstrin homology domain (PH) on the N terminus that anchors the enyzme to the plasma membrane, a catalytic domain (Cat) composed of two homologous units, and a C2 domain that binds to and is activated by Ca^{2+}. PLCβ contains a larger C-terminal domain, which enables it to couple to G proteins, whereas PLCγ contains two additional PH domains and two SH2 domains, which enable it to couple to neurotrophin receptors (see Figure 5–13).

lished that prostaglandins regulate cellular cAMP levels in part by coupling to G_s and G_i.

Aspirin, acetaminophen, and all nonsteroidal antiinflammatory drugs (**NSAIDs**) such as **ibuprofen** exert their antipyretic, analgesic, and antiinflammatory effects by inhibiting cyclooxygenase, which has both constitutive (COX_1) and inducible (COX_2) forms. COX_1 is expressed in many locations, including the upper gastrointestinal tract, where nonselective COX inhibitors block the protective functions of prostaglandins. Such interference increases the risk of peptic ulceration, a common side effect of these drugs. Selective COX_2 inhibitors, such as **rofecoxib**, that are analgesic and antiinflammatory but do not disturb the gastrointestinal tract are currently in wide use (see Chapter 19).

Therapeutic uses of various arachidonic acid metabolites have been considered for the treatment of **asthma,** the induction of **labor,** the inhibition of **platelet aggregation,** and in the case of **misoprostol,** which is a preparation of PGE_1, the reduction of stomach acid. However, none of these applications is currently in routine clinical use. A rich pharmacology of specific agonists and antagonists for various LT and prostanoid receptors also has been developed, but such drugs are not yet used clinically.

PROTEIN PHOSPHORYLATION: A FINAL COMMON PATHWAY IN THE REGULATION OF NEURONAL FUNCTION

Although a large number of second messengers can be activated in neurons, the signaling pathways of these messengers are relatively uniform. Some second messenger molecules act directly as effectors; for example, cAMP and cGMP bind to and directly gate ion channels in some neurons, Ca^{2+} binds to and directly regulates the activity of several enzymes, and cGMP binds to and directly activates phosphodiesterase in the retina. However, most of the known effects of intracellular second messengers are produced through their regulation of protein phosphorylation. As previously explained, the addition or removal of phosphate groups from specific amino acid residues in target proteins alters the function of such proteins. Accordingly, protein phosphorylation may inactivate a neurotransmitter receptor, cause an ion channel to open more or less readily, or enable the synthesis of a neurotransmitter much more rapidly.

Protein phosphorylation is regulated by neurotransmitters, typically through the second messengermediated activation of protein kinases. Kinases catalyze the transfer of phosphate groups from ATP to serine, threonine, or tyrosine residues in specific substrate proteins (see Figure 5–2). Neurotransmitters also regulate protein phosphorylation through second messengermediated regulation of protein phosphatases, which catalyze the removal of phosphate groups from proteins through hydrolysis.

SECOND MESSENGER-DEPENDENT PROTEIN PHOSPHORYLATION CASCADES

Among the best characterized protein kinases in the brain are those activated by the second messengers cAMP, cGMP, Ca^{2+}, and diacylglycerol. All of these protein kinases, which are named for the second messengers that activate them, phosphorylate substrate proteins on serine or threonine residues, and thus are referred to as protein serine–threonine kinases.

cAMP-dependent protein kinases The brain contains one major type of cAMP-dependent protein kinase, termed protein kinase A (PKA), which consists of catalytic and regulatory subunits. In the absence of cAMP, the enzyme exists as an inactive holoenzyme composed of a dimer of identical catalytic subunits, each approximately 40 kDa and bound, at its active site, to a regulatory subunit of approximately 50 kDa (Figure 5–11). By binding to the regulatory subunits, cAMP activates the enzyme. Two molecules of cAMP bind to each regulatory subunit, thereby causing its dissociation from the catalytic subunits. Three forms of catalytic (C) subunit (Cα, Cβ, and Cγ) and four forms of regulatory (R) subunit (RIα, RIβ, RIIα, and RIIβ) have been identified. Although they differ in their tissue and cellular distributions, the various C and R subtypes are homologous and can be considered isoforms.

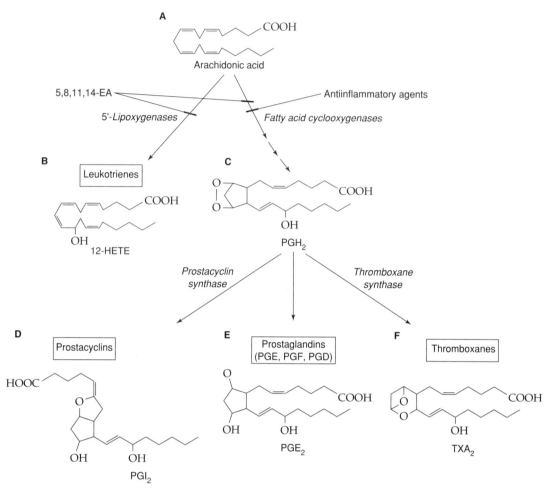

Figure 5–10. Arachidonic acid signaling pathways. **A.** Arachidonic acid gives rise to many important signaling molecules, which are products of two main pathways. **B.** One involves 5′-lipoxygenase and gives rise to the leukotrienes. **C.** The other involves the action of cyclooxygenase and gives rise to three families of signals: prostacyclins (**D**), prostaglandins (**E**), and thromboxanes (**F**). Cyclooxygenases are inhibited by nonsteroidal antiinflammatory agents. 5,8,11,14-Eicosatetraenoic acid (EA) is a lipoxygenase inhibitor that also inhibits cyclooxygenases.

However, an important difference exists between the RI and RII subunits: RII, but not RI, isoforms undergo autophosphorylation by C subunits in the presence of cAMP. This serves to promote the dissociation of RII and C subunits and hence prolongs the duration of the activated PKA signal.

Virtually all cellular actions of cAMP in eukaryotic cells, except for those related to cyclic nucleotide-gated channels (see Chapter 3), are mediated by the activation of PKA (see Figure 5–5). PKA's integral role in these cellular processes stems from its ability to phosphorylate a wide array of substrate proteins, including many types of ion channels, receptors, cytoskeletal proteins, and nuclear transcription factors.

cGMP-dependent protein kinases   The brain also contains one major type of cGMP-dependent protein

kinase, termed protein kinase G (PKG). PKG is homologous to PKA, although the catalytic and regulatory functions of the enzyme reside within a single polypeptide of approximately 75 kDa, which exists as a homodimer (see Figure 5–11). PKG is activated by cGMP, which binds to the regulatory domain of the protein and thereby causes a conformational change that relieves inhibition of the catalytic domain. Several isoforms of PKG have been identified by molecular cloning.

Based on the relationship between cAMP and PKA, it is believed that many of the cellular actions of cGMP are mediated by the activation of PKG (see Figure 5–5). However, less is known about the function of PKG, in part because it is not as widely expressed as PKA. Thus it has been difficult to identify physiologic substrates for PKG, although certain ion channels appear to be regulated by this kinase.

Ca²⁺-dependent protein kinases   There are two major classes of Ca²⁺-dependent protein kinases (see Figure 5–7). One class is activated by Ca²⁺ in conjunction with calmodulin and is referred to as Ca²⁺/calmodulin-dependent protein kinase or CaM-kinase. The other is activated by Ca²⁺ in conjunction with diacylglycerol and other lipids and is referred to as Ca²⁺/

diacylglycerol-dependent protein kinase or protein kinase C (PKC). The brain contains several forms of each of these enzymes, which exhibit very different regulatory properties and are expressed in distinct neuronal cell types throughout the nervous system.

Six forms of CaM-kinase are known. Two subtypes, CaM-kinase II and IV, appear to be multifunctional en-

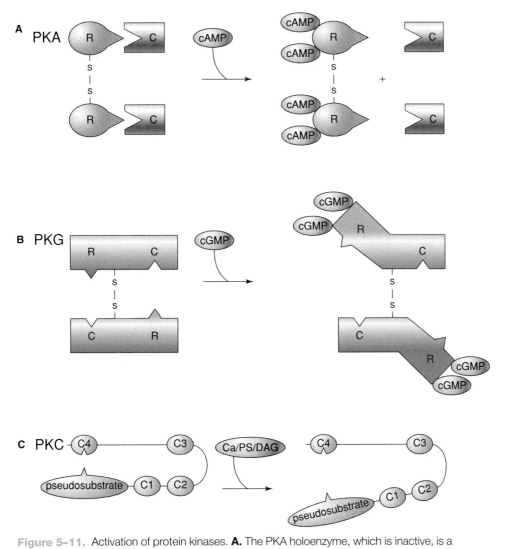

Figure 5–11. Activation of protein kinases. **A.** The PKA holoenzyme, which is inactive, is a dimer composed of two regulatory subunits (R) joined by disulfide bonds, each of which is associated with a catalytic subunit (C). Two molecules of cAMP bind to each regulatory subunit, causing it to dissociate from the catalytic subunit, which in turn becomes active. **B.** PKG is activated in a similar manner, although its regulatory and catalytic domains exist within a single polypeptide chain. Receptor subunits of PKA and receptor domains of PKG may be autophosphorylated in response to activation by cAMP or cGMP, respectively; such autophosphorylation promotes further dissociation and activation of the enzymes. **C.** PKC is a single polypeptide chain that comprises several identifiable domains. C1 binds diacylglycerol (DAG) and phorbol esters, C2 binds Ca²⁺ and phosphatidylserine (PS), C3 binds ATP, and C4 contains the active, or catalytic, site. The pseudosubstrate site is functionally analogous to the regulatory domain of PKA and PKG in that it inhibits catalytic activity of the enzyme. In response to the binding of Ca²⁺, PS, and DAG, this inhibition is relieved, and PKC is activated.

zymes; like PKA, each phosphorylates a large number of substrate proteins and in turn influences diverse neuronal processes. The other forms of CaM-kinase act in a more restricted manner. Myosin light chain kinase specifically phosphorylates myosin light chain and regulates myosin–actin function. Phosphorylase kinase is selective for the enzyme phosphorylase and thereby regulates glycogenolysis. CaM-kinase I is best known for its ability to phosphorylate the synaptic vesicle-associated protein called synapsin and thereby regulate neurotransmitter release, although additional substrates for this kinase may exist. CaM-kinase III, currently referred to as eukaryotic elongation factor-2 kinase (eEF2 kinase), selectively phosphorylates EF2 and in turn regulates protein synthesis at the level of the ribosome. In hippocampal neurons, and presumably in many other cell types, CaM-kinase IV is found in the nucleus, where it phosphorylates the transcription factor CREB (see Chapter 6) and thereby mediates some of the effects of Ca^{2+} on gene expression.

The molecular structure of these CaM-kinases, including the number and size of their constituent subunits, varies considerably. CaM-kinase II, for example, is composed of distinct 50-kDa α and 60-kDa β subunits, which form large multimeric complexes with distinct α to β ratios in different brain regions. In contrast, CaM-kinases I and IV appear to be active as monomers. There are three known isoforms of CaM-kinase I; the predominant isoform in brain has an M_r of 41 kDa. The major form of CaM-kinase IV in brain has an M_r of 52 kDa.

Recent investigation has revealed that some of the CaM-kinases engage in quite complex modes of regulation. CaM-kinase II, for example, can autophosphorylate itself and in turn create a form of the enzyme that remains active even after Ca^{2+} levels have returned to normal. Such a sustained period of kinase activation may represent a molecular mechanism that contributes to learning and memory (see Chapter 20). In addition, CaM-kinases I and IV can be activated by a newly identified kinase known as CaM-kinase kinase, which in turn is activated by Ca^{2+}/calmodulin and inhibited by PKA phosphorylation.

Numerous subtypes of PKC are known (Table 5–3), each of which exists as a single polypeptide of approximately 70–80 kDa. Although all of the subtypes exhibit a broad substrate specificity and most likely regulate many aspects of cell function, they differ dramatically in their ability to be regulated by cellular levels of Ca^{2+} and various phospholipids. Some subtypes, for example, are highly sensitive to Ca^{2+}, whereas others are relatively insensitive. A major goal of current research is to identify the signaling role subserved by each of these various PKC subtypes. The **phorbol esters,** which activate all known PKC isoforms, have been a valuable tool in PKC research. The highly carcinogenic nature of phorbol esters supports the critical role played by PKC in the control of cell growth and differentiation.

Several regulatory domains have been identified within the PKC molecule (see Figure 5–11). One critical domain, termed *C2*, appears to mediate the Ca^{2+}-binding property of PKC and is homologous to similar domains in other Ca^{2+}-binding proteins, such as phospholipase C (see Figure 5–9) and the synaptic vesicle protein synaptotagmin (see Chapter 4). Also critical is the phospholipid-binding domain, termed *C1*, which mediates the effect of DAG and phorbol esters on the enzyme. This domain is homologous to similar regions in other proteins that interact with phospholipids, such as the synaptic vesicle-associated proteins discussed in Chapter 4.

Protein kinase-anchoring proteins   An interesting regulatory feature of protein kinases has been uncovered in recent years: their localization in distinct subcellular regions in neurons is controlled by specific anchoring proteins. Such proteins are believed to sequester each type of kinase to the region of a neuron, such as the postsynaptic specialization or cell nucleus, that requires its function.

Table 5–3 Protein Kinase C Family

Subtype	Localization
Regulated by Ca^{2+} and DAG	
α	Ubiquitous
$\beta I/\beta II$	Occurs in many tissues; moderately concentrated in brain
γ	Highly concentrated in brain tissue
Ca^{2+}-independent; but regulated by DAG	
δ	Occurs in many tissues; may occur in brain
ϵ	May be highly concentrated in brain tissue
η	Unknown
θ	Unknown
Ca^{2+}- and DAG-independent, but enzymes are homologous to PKC	
ι	Unknown
ζ	Occurs in some tissues; moderately concentrated in brain
PRKs	Unknown

Note: Cloning studies have revealed an increasing number of PKC-homologous enzymes, with very different regulatory properties. Three classic forms of PKCs require Ca^{2+} and DAG for their activation. Several other forms are Ca^{2+}-independent, yet are activated by DAG; these forms are missing a portion of the C2 domain (see Figure 5–11). Some forms are not regulated by Ca^{2+} or DAG; these are missing portions of their C1 and C2 domains. PRKs, PKC-related kinases.

The A kinase-anchoring proteins (AKAPs) are some of the best characterized examples of these proteins. AKAPs, each approximately 75 kDa, bind to specific microtubule-associated proteins as well as to the regulatory subunits of PKA, and thereby tether PKA to neuronal regions that are rich in microtubules, such as distal dendrites. In this way, AKAPs keep inactive PKA holoenzyme close to synaptic regions. In response to increased cAMP levels, free catalytic subunits are released from the microtubule-AKAP-regulatory subunit complex in proximity to their physiologic substrates, for example, channels and receptors. Some AKAPs, in addition to anchoring PKA, also may anchor isoforms of PKC and certain protein phosphatases, such as calcineurin, and thereby build even larger and more complex multifunctional enzyme complexes that subserve important aspects of synaptic transmission.

Several types of PKC-anchoring proteins also exist and are believed to target PKC to specific subcellular sites. Receptors for activated C kinase (RACKs) bind to PKC at domains that are distinct from the active site of the enzyme; thus activated PKC may remain bound to these receptors. In contrast, substrate-binding proteins (SBPs) bind to PKC near the active site of the enzyme and are phosphorylated by PKC in response to activation of the enzyme by Ca^{2+} and phospholipids. Accordingly, SBPs may perform a function analogous to that of AKAPs; they may target PKC to a subcellular site and subsequently release enzyme at that site as it is activated.

Many more anchoring proteins for protein kinases, as well as for other intracellular signaling proteins, are likely to be identified. One exciting possibility is that some of these proteins will represent targets for the development of novel pharmacotherapeutic agents for neuropsychiatric disorders.

Protein kinase inhibitors   There has been intense interest in the development of protein kinase inhibitors for use as research tools and as potential therapeutic agents. The most specific of these are peptide inhibitors, which are directed at the active site of a particular enzyme. The prototype, a naturally occurring 17-kDa protein known as protein kinase inhibitor (PKI), is a highly specific inhibitor of PKA that is expressed in many tissues. It inhibits PKA by binding to the catalytic site of the enzyme. The physiologic role of PKI is unknown. Synthetic peptide inhibitors are also available for most second messenger-regulated protein kinases; however, their utility is limited because they do not penetrate cells. Consequently, investigators have focused on discovering small-molecule kinase inhibitors. Although their clinical use may be limited because of the ubiquity of many kinases, small-molecule kinase inhibitors have been extremely important tools in deter-

mining the roles of protein kinases in neural phenomena. The primary experimental limitation associated with most of these inhibitors is their lack of specificity: most affect a range of kinases and other proteins. Thus caution must be used in interpreting the results of experiments involving these agents. The best rule of thumb is to compare the effects of several types of inhibitors of distinct chemical classes and to characterize such effects over a wide range of doses. Some examples of protein kinase inhibitors used experimentally are listed in Table 5–4.

Protein phosphatases   The brain contains four major types of protein phosphatases that undo the actions of the second messenger-dependent protein kinases. These protein phosphatases, termed *protein serine–threonine phosphatases*, differ in their regional distribution in the brain and in their regulatory properties. These enzymes, which are summarized in Table 5–5, are termed *protein phosphatases 1, 2A, 2B, and 2C*. This terminology is based on the biochemical properties of these enzymes as they were first identified.

Neurotransmitters can regulate protein phosphatases, and in turn influence protein phosphorylation, by means of two known mechanisms. Phosphatase 2B, also referred to as calcineurin, is activated directly when it is bound to Ca^{2+}/calmodulin. Thus neurotransmitters that alter cellular Ca^{2+} levels can influence the phosphorylation of cellular proteins by influencing

Table 5–4 Examples of Protein Kinase Inhibitors

Inhibitor	Target(s)[1]
Rp-cAMPS[2]	PKA
H7[3]	PKC, PKA, PKG, and others
H89[3]	PKA, PKG
Bisindolylmaleimide I	PKC
Calphostin	PKC
R59949[4]	PKC
Chelerythrine	PKC
KN-62	CaM-Ks
Roscovitine	cdk-5
Staurosporine	PKC, PTKs
Genistein	PTKs
Tyrphostins	PTKs
PP1	Src family PTKs

[1]Most of these inhibitors show relative specificity at the stated target but are not perfectly selective.
[2]Although this compound is an inhibitor of the type-I regulatory subunit, it is a partial agonist at the type-II subunit. The stereoisomer of the compound, Sp-cAMPS, is an activator of PKA.
[3]Examples of a large series of isoquinolone inhibitors that show varying specificity at different protein kinases.
[4]One of a series of DAG site inhibitors.
PKA, protein kinase A; PKG, protein kinase G; PKC, protein kinase C; CaM-K, Ca^{2+}/calmodulin-dependent protein kinase; cdk-5, cyclin-dependent kinase type 5; PTK, protein tyrosine kinase; PP1, 4-amino-5-(4-methylphenyl)-7-(t-butyl) pyrazole[3,4-D]pyrimidine.

Table 5-5 Protein Serine-Threonine Phosphatases

Class	Inhibitor Proteins
PP1	
α; β; γ1; γ2	Inhibitor 1; inhibitor 2; DARPP-32; and NIPP-1
PP2A	Inhibitor 1^{2A}; inhibitor 2^{2A}
PP2B (calcineurin)	Immunophilins: cyclosporin A-cyclophilin FK506-FK506 binding protein
PP2C	
PP4	
PP5	
Dual-function phosphatases (VH1 family) MKP (MAP-kinase phosphatases); cdc25	

PP1, protein phosphatase; DARPP-32, dopamine and cAMP-regulated phosphoprotein of 32 kDa; NIPP-1, nuclear inhibitor of PP1; VH, vaccinia virus; cdc25, cell division cycle protein 25.

calcineurin activity. Calcineurin activity is also regulated by immunophilins. This class of proteins, including cyclophilin and FKBP–FK506 binding protein, was originally discovered in lymphocytes and are the targets of several important immunosuppressive agents, such as **cyclosporin** and **FK506.** Immunophilins are also expressed in the brain, although little is known about their physiologic regulation in this area. However, when they are bound to FK506 and related drugs, the immunophilins inhibit calcineurin activity.

The other mechanism of protein phosphatase regulation is indirect and involves a class of proteins referred to as protein phosphatase inhibitors. Among these, the best known are termed *phosphatase inhibitors 1* and *2* and *dopamine- and cAMP-regulated phosphoprotein of 32 kDa* (DARPP-32). DARPP-32 is especially concentrated in neurons in the brain that receive dopaminergic innervation. Another phosphatase inhibitor, which is localized in the nucleus, is termed the *nuclear inhibitor of protein phosphatase* (NIPP). These proteins are highly potent inhibitors of protein phosphatase 1, one of the major protein serine–threonine phosphatases in mammalian cells. Phosphorylation of most of these inhibitor proteins by PKA or by other protein kinases greatly enhances their inhibitory activity. In neurons that contain these inhibitors, neurotransmitters that alter cellular cAMP levels can influence the phosphorylation of cellular proteins by altering protein phosphatase 1 activity as well as by activating PKA. This process, as it applies to DARPP-32, is illustrated in Figure 5–12.

Studies of the physiologic functions of phosphatases have been facilitated by the identification of natural small molecules that are relatively specific phosphatase inhibitors. Among these, the best known is **okadaic acid,** which inhibits protein phosphatases 1 and 2A.

The anchoring of protein phosphatases to specific cellular domains by a series of regulatory subunits, which can be tissue-specific, represents another level of regulation. The GL and GM subunits, which target protein phosphatase 1 to liver and skeletal muscle, respectively, are the best established examples of these subunits. Research also suggests that a recently described protein, termed *spinophilin,* may function as a protein phosphatase 1-anchoring protein that selectively tethers the enzyme to dendritic spines. In contrast, the protein phosphatase 1 nuclear targeting subunit (PNUTS) may target the same phosphatase to the cell nucleus.

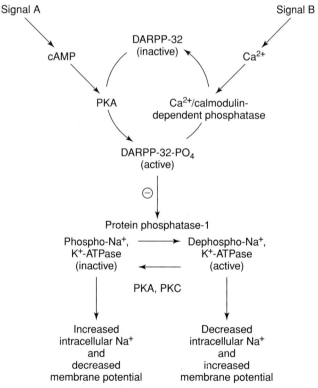

Figure 5-12. Proposed physiologic role of DARPP-32. The figure illustrates how DARPP-32 might integrate cellular cAMP and Ca^{2+} signals. DARPP-32 might be converted by cAMP into an active phosphatase inhibitor by activation of PKA, which phosphorylates DARPP-32, whereas Ca^{2+} might have the opposite effect by activating a phosphatase that dephosphorylates DARPP-32. Phosphorylated (active) DARPP-32, by inhibiting protein phosphatase 1, may increase the phosphorylation state of numerous phosphoproteins, for example, the Na^+, K^+-ATPase shown here, to regulate numerous physiologic processes. (Borrowed from P. Greengard, The Rockefeller University, with permission.)

NEUROTROPHIC FACTOR-REGULATED PROTEIN PHOSPHORYLATION CASCADES

Significant progress has been made in the delineation of intracellular signal transduction pathways for neurotrophic factors, which are discussed in detail in Chapter 11. As mentioned previously, most of these pathways involve the activation of protein tyrosine kinases, which occurs by different mechanisms, depending on the neurotrophic factor involved. These pathways illustrate the extraordinary complexity of intracellular regulation, and keeping track of them can be daunting, even for scientists who study them. Although neurotrophic factors and their signaling pathways typically have been studied because of their central role in neural development and differentiation, research has confirmed that they are critical for mediating responses to a wide array of external stimuli throughout the adult life of an organism.

Neurotrophin signaling pathways Neurotrophic factor signal transduction cascades are best established for the neurotrophins, as summarized in Figure 5–13 (see Chapter 11). Neurotrophins bind to a plasma membrane receptor, termed *Trk*, and in turn trigger the dimerization of Trk and the activation of a protein tyrosine kinase that is intrinsic to the Trk protein. Thus Trk is considered a receptor tyrosine kinase. The Trk receptor subsequently undergoes autophosphorylation whereby one activated Trk of the dimer phosphorylates the other. Such phosphorylation enables other intracellular signaling proteins to recognize the receptor by interacting with its src homology-2 (SH2) domain. Slight variations in SH domains allow intricate interactions among numerous types of proteins in neural and non-neural cells. Indeed, major discoveries in recent years have revealed that many protein–protein interaction domains (e.g., SH, PDZ, and leucine zipper domains) are integral to protein signaling (Box 5–3).

After phosphorylation, the Trk complex interacts with additional linker proteins (see Figure 5–13) and, through an unknown mechanism, activates Ras, a small-molecular-weight G protein (see Box 5–1). Such activation in turn activates a cascade of protein serine–threonine kinases: Ras activates Raf, which phosphorylates and activates MAP-kinase/ERK kinase (MEK), which phosphorylates and activates extracellular signal-regulated kinases (ERKs). ERKs are one of the three major types of MAP-kinases; the others, JNK and p38, are described later in this chapter. Interestingly, MEK phosphorylates ERK on both threonine and tyrosine residues, both of which are required for ERK activation; for this reason, MEK is sometimes referred to as a

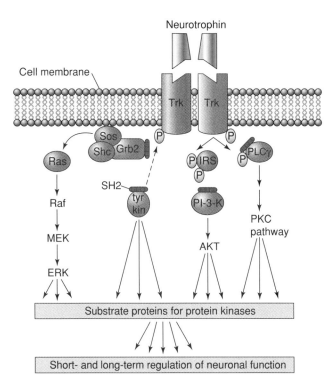

Figure 5–13. Intracellular pathways of neurotrophins in the brain. The activation of a neurotrophin receptor (Trk) stimulates protein tyrosine kinase activity and results in the autophosphorylation of the receptor. The phosphorylated receptor subsequently associates with other proteins, such as Grb2, Shc, and Sos, to activate the small G protein Ras, which in turn leads to the activation of Raf, a protein serine–threonine kinase. Raf phosphorylates and activates a MAP-kinase kinase (MEK), which subsequently activates a MAP-kinase (ERK) by phosphorylating it on threonine and tyrosine residues. In alternative pathways, Trks: (1) attract by means of SH2 domains, phosphorylate, and activate phospholipase C (PLCγ); (2) activate phosphatidylinositol-3-kinase (PI-3-K) by means of insulin receptor substrate (IRS) proteins, which contain SH2 domains and act as linker proteins; or (3) activate other cytoplasmic protein tyrosine kinases that lack a receptor domain. P represents phosphorylation of the indicated proteins on tyrosine residues.

dual-function kinase. Finally, ERK phosphorylates and activates protein kinases such as ribosomal S6-kinase (RSK) and MAP-kinase-activating protein kinase (MAP-KAP-kinase), which in turn join ERK in phosphorylating an array of effector proteins.

Although the activation of ERK represents the best characterized effector pathway through which neurotrophins produce their varied effects on neuronal function, other pathways have been implicated. Trk can, for example, phosphorylate and activate certain subtypes of phospholipase C (PLCγ), which in turn can trigger the activation of the phosphatidylinositol and cellular Ca^{2+}

Box 5–3 Protein–Protein Interactions as Novel Drug Targets

Noncatalytic protein–protein interactions are important for the regulation of enzyme activity, in the transport and subcellular localization of proteins, and in the formation of specialized multiprotein complexes. These protein interactions mediate or regulate diverse neuronal functions, including signal transduction, control of gene expression, cytoskeletal organization, synaptic connectivity, and neurotransmission. During the past decade, researchers have identified protein subregions, or domains, that are responsible for recognizing and binding to other proteins with high affinity and specificity (see table). Many of these sites of protein–protein interaction are modular and contain distinct three-dimensional structures that retain their binding capacity even when they are separated from the rest of the protein. Domains with similar amino acid sequences, structures, and binding activities have been found in proteins that are otherwise unrelated, and these domain families have been given special names.

Selected Protein-Protein Interaction Domains

Domain	Interaction	Domain-Containing Proteins	Binding-Target Proteins	Functions
Leucine zipper	Hydrophobically binds other leucine zipper domains	Fos Jun CREB	Jun Fos CREB	Homodimers or heterodimers of transcription factors
Pleckstrin homology	Binds to inositol lipids, $G_{\beta\gamma}$ subunits, and PKC	Pleckstrin IRSs PLCs GRKs AKT/PKB Sos Dynamin	$G_{\beta\gamma}$ PKC	Targets proteins to membrane; permits regulation of enzyme activity by inositol lipids, and perhaps by $G_{\beta\gamma}$, PKC.
PDZ	Binds to C-terminal in consensus S/TXV, or to other PDZ domains	PSD95 GRIP Homer nNos	Shaker K^+ channels, NMDARs, AMPARs, mGluRs	Allows ion channel clustering; forms signal transduction complexes
Phosphotyrosine binding domain interacting	Binds phosphotyrosines in NPXpY consensus	IRSs Shc	RTKs, JAKs	Forms signal transduction complexes
Regulator of G protein signaling	Binds to specific G protein α subunits	RGS family	$G_{\alpha i}/G_{\alpha o}$ $G_{\alpha q}$ $G_{\alpha t}$ (transducin)	Down-regulates signaling through G proteins by increasing their GTPase activity
Src homology 2	Binds phosphotyrosines in YXXphi consensus, both intermolecular and intramolecular interactions occur	Src family PTKs PLCγ PI-3-K RasGAP PTP1C Shc Grb2 STATs	IRSs RTKs	Forms signal transduction complexes; allows regulation of enzyme activity by tyrosine kinases
Src homology 3	Binds polyproline sequences, with PXXP consensus	Src family PTKs PLCγ PI-3-K RasGAP Grb2 Amphiphysin	Sos Shc Dynamin	Forms signal transduction complexes
WW	Binds polyproline sequences, with XPPXY consensus	FE65 YAP	WBPs	Unknown

RGS, regulator of G protein signaling; SH, src homology; PTB, phosphotyrosine binding; YAP, Yes-associated protein (Yes is a PTK); Grb2, growth factor receptor binding protein 2; PLC, phospholipase C; PI-3-K, phosphoinositol-3-kinase; STAT, signal transducer and activator of transcription; JAK, janus kinase; RTK, receptor tyrosine kinase; PTK, protein tyrosine kinase; Shc, src homology containing protein; NMDAR, NMDA glutamate receptor; AMPAR, AMPA glutamate receptor; mGluR, metabotropic glutamate receptor; PSD, post-synaptic density; nNOS, neuronal nitric oxide synthase; IRS, insulin receptor substrate; WBP, WW domain binding protein; GRK, G protein-coupled receptor kinase; GAP, GTPase activating protein; PTP, protein tyrosine phosphatase.

The Src homology 2 (SH2) domain, roughly 100 amino acids long, was among the first domains discovered and initially was found in the oncogenic protein tyrosine kinase known as Src. SH2 domains bind short amino acid sequences that contain a phosphorylated tyrosine residue. A highly conserved core amino acid sequence common to all members of the SH2 domain family is responsible for binding the phosphotyrosine residue. In addition, less conserved flanking sequences impart specificity to particular SH2-target interactions. SH2 domains allow tyrosine kinases to act as molecular on–off switches for a distinct subset of protein–protein interactions. Neurotrophin receptors (Trks), for example, have a tyrosine kinase activity that is activated in response to the binding of neurotrophin to the extracellular domain, causing receptor autophosphorylation on intracellular tyrosine residues (see Figure 5–13; also see Chapter 11). Multiple proteins can then bind to these phosphotyrosines by means of their SH2 domains, and are in turn phosphorylated by the kinase. This phosphorylation causes the enzymatic activation of some substrates (PLCγ), and also recruits more SH2-containing proteins, such as Shc and Grb2. The resulting cascade produces a large activated signaling complex; its many downstream effects mediate the neuronal growth, survival, and differentiation of the neurotrophins.

Many other families of protein–protein interaction domains have been identified in recent years through the analysis of protein sequence databases, and some of their mechanisms of interaction, their target proteins, and their roles in cellular processes have been determined (see table).

A particularly important type of protein–protein interaction involves scaffolding or anchoring proteins. The Drosophila eye provides perhaps the most striking example of the role played by scaffolding proteins in the organization of intracellular signaling. In Drosophila photoreceptors, the InaD protein, which contains five PDZ domains, functions as a multivalent adapter that brings together multiple components of the phototransduction signaling cascade. Phototransduction in Drosophila photoreceptors proceeds from the activation of rhodopsin by a single photon to the generation of an electrical potential in just a few tens of milliseconds. Scientists have long believed that signaling cascades permit the amplification of input signals; for example, a single activated G protein in a signaling cascade might be permitted to stimulate many molecules of a second messenger-generating enzyme. However, evidence that supports this theory has been drawn from the observation of reconstituted systems that lack scaffolding proteins. If scaffolding proteins in vivo were to assemble signaling molecules into macromolecular complexes, such assembly would severely interfere with the molecules' ability to diffuse and interact with multiple targets, and in turn would hinder amplification. Genetic manipulations that alter the availability of different components of the Drosophila phototransduction signaling cascade indicate that such assembly of signaling molecules improves the speed and reliability of signaling, and may improve feedback regulation, even though it limits amplification. Whether this model from Drosophila is typical of other signaling cascades is currently under investigation.

Because of their functional importance, their specificity, and their variety, protein–protein domains are extremely attractive targets for experimental and therapeutic drugs. Cell-permeable peptides and synthetic nonpeptide agents that block protein–protein interactions are currently being developed, as are agents that facilitate these interactions. This exciting and rapidly expanding field should become an increasingly integral part of basic and clinical neuropharmacology.

pathways as previously outlined. PLCγ is drawn by means of its SH2 domains to the proximity of activated Trk. Phosphorylated Trk also can phosphorylate linker proteins termed insulin receptor substrate (IRS) proteins, which were initially found for the insulin receptor (another receptor tyrosine kinase). Phosphorylated IRS proteins bind to the SH2 domains of phosphatidylinositol-3-kinase (PI-3-kinase), causing the activation of this enzyme. PI-3-kinase eventually activates certain protein serine–threonine kinases, such as AKT. Activation of Trk also triggers its binding (through SH2 domains) to and activation of several cytoplasmic protein tyrosine kinases, such as src (see the next section of this chapter), thereby further multiplying the effects of the neurotrophin. A major challenge associated with current research involves determining which of the many effects of neurotrophins are mediated by these various signaling cascades.

The Ras–Raf–MEK–ERK cascade that is activated by neurotrophins is homologous to a key signaling cascade used by yeast; in fact, it was through the application of yeast genetics that the mammalian counterparts of the pathway were first identified. Currently it is known that mammalian cells express several variants of this cascade, each of which follows a general pattern: a small G protein (homologous to Ras) activates a protein kinase termed MAP-kinase kinase kinase (M-KKK), or MEK-kinase, that is homologous to Raf; M-KKK phosphorylates and activates a MAP-kinase kinase (M-KK) homologous to MEK; M-KK phosphorylates and activates a MAP-kinase (M-K) homologous to ERK; and M-K phosphorylates many effector proteins and additional protein kinases (Figure 5–14). Remarkably, yet another kinase (a MAP-kinase kinase kinase kinase or M-KKKK) may be required for G protein activation of the MAP-KKK.

Mammalian signaling		General scheme	Yeast signaling
ERK pathway	SAP-kinase pathway		
RAS	Rac, Cdc-42	Small G protein	Cdc-42
?	PAK	MAP-kinase kinase kinase kinases	Ste20
Raf	MEKK	MAP-kinase kinase kinases	Ste11
MEK	SEK	MAP-kinase kinases	Ste7
ERK	SAP-kinase (JNK)	MAP-kinases	Fus3,Kss1
RSK	MAPKAP kinase	MAP-kinase activated kinases	

Figure 5–14. MAP-kinase pathways. Pathways originally delineated in yeast (*right*) are compared with homologous pathways more recently identified in mammalian cells (*left*). MEK, MAP-kinase and ERK kinase; ERK, extracellular signal-regulated kinase; RSK, ribosomal S6 kinase; SEK, SAP-kinase kinase; SAP-kinase, stress-activated protein kinase; JNK, Jun kinase; MAPKAP-kinase, MAP-kinase activated protein kinase.

A parallel pathway is activated by certain cytokines and noxious stimuli. Tumor necrosis factor-α or UV light, for example, leads to the activation of the small G protein Rac. In response, Rac activates a protein kinase termed MEK-kinase, which phosphorylates and activates a distinct form of MEK, which in turn phosphorylates and activates the Jun N-terminal kinase (JNK). JNK phosphorylates the transcription factors Jun and activating transcription factor-2 (ATF2) and thereby enables them to regulate gene expression (see Chapter 6). Because this pathway is involved in responses to cellular stress, JNK is often referred to as a stress-activated protein kinase, or SAP-kinase (see Chapter 11). Another SAP-kinase is a 38-kDa protein known as p38.

JAK–STAT pathway   Another prominent family of cytokines employs a very different mechanism of signal transduction. This family includes ciliary neurotrophic factor (CNTF), leptin, prolactin, leukemia inhibitory factor (LIF), interleukin 6 (IL-6), and oncostatin-M (see Chapter 11). Although these cytokines were first studied because of their actions on the immune system, they are known to exert potent effects on the brain. Each cytokine interacts with a specific plasma membrane α receptor named for the associated cytokine (e.g., CNTF α receptor). The α subunits of these receptors subsequently form heterotrimeric complexes with other pro-

teins (see Chapter 11). After these complexes are formed, the tripartite receptor associates with a protein tyrosine kinase called Janus kinase (JAK), which normally exists in the cytoplasm in its inactive form. The association of JAK with the receptor complex leads to JAK's activation and to the phosphorylation and activation of a family of transcription factors called *signal transducers and activators of transcription* (STATs). The activation of STATs in turn leads to many of the long-term effects of the cytokine on cell function. JAK most likely also phosphorylates other effector proteins that mediate further effects of the cytokine on cell function.

GDNF signaling pathway   A similar pattern characterizes signaling by glial cell line-derived neurotrophic factor (GDNF) and the related neurotrophic factors known as neurturin and persephin. These factors are distant relatives of the transforming growth factor-β family and are of particular interest because of their potent neurotrophic effects on dopaminergic neurons. GDNF, neurturin, and persephin each bind to a unique receptor that dimerizes and interacts with the protein tyrosine kinase Ret (see Chapter 11). Activation of Ret is believed to mediate all of the actions of these neurotrophic factors on cell function, although the signaling mechanisms underlying such effects remain poorly understood.

Cytoplasmic protein tyrosine kinases   The first protein tyrosine kinase discovered was Src, which we now know is a prototype of a large family of such kinases that exist in the cell cytoplasm and in general are not physically part of a plasma membrane receptor complex. Src family members that are expressed at high levels in neurons include Fyn, Yes, Lck, and Lyn, in addition to Src, itself.

The activity of these enzymes can be regulated in response to a wide range of extracellular and intracellular signals. The enzymes are phosphorylated and thereby activated or inhibited by several other kinases. In addition, Src family kinases contain SH2 or related domains, which enable them to bind to particular tyrosine-phosphorylated proteins and form large multimeric signaling complexes. By phosphorylating many types of substrates, such as ion channels, glutamate receptor subunits, synaptic vesicle proteins, and transcription factors, Src family kinases have been implicated in the regulation of numerous neuronal processes, including synaptic transmission, neurotransmitter release, cell survival, and gene expression.

Protooncogenes   Many of the proteins involved in neurotrophic factor signaling cascades are normal cellular homologues of genes responsible for the transforming, or cancer-causing, potential of oncogenic viruses; thus these proteins were originally described as protooncogenes. A viral form of Ras, for example, has been implicated in human colon and other cancers. In most cases, the difference between a protooncogene and an oncogene is a relatively minor mutation that alters the regulatory properties of the protein. The effects of such minor mutations underscore the critical role these proteins play in cell function and attest to the exquisite control of intracellular messenger pathways required for the normal regulation of physiologic processes.

Protein tyrosine kinase inhibitors   Given the role of tyrosine phosphorylation in carcinogenesis, it is not surprising that researchers are attempting to develop small-molecule inhibitors of protein tyrosine kinases that might function as anticancer agents. Such agents are not yet in clinical use, but one such compound, **genistein,** is a naturally occurring isoflavone in legumes. Although interest in the compound as a dietary supplement exists, there are as yet no data concerning its efficacy in cancer prevention. Several protein tyrosine kinase inhibitors (see Table 5–4) have been used experimentally to study the role of tyrosine phosphorylation in neural phenomena. Development of inhibitors that are selective for the many distinct protein tyrosine kinases is a major goal of future research.

Protein tyrosine phosphatases   Interestingly, many more types of protein tyrosine phosphatases occur in the brain than do types of protein serine–threonine phosphatases. Some protein tyrosine phosphatases are selective for ERK and related MAP-kinases because they can dephosphorylate these proteins at both threonine and tyrosine residues. Other enzymes are membrane-associated and contain extracellular domains that may represent recognition sites for as yet unknown intercellular signals. Still other forms of protein tyrosine phosphatases are soluble and are present throughout the neuronal cytoplasm. Certain membrane- and cytosol-associated forms, which exhibit highly restricted distributions in the nervous system, may subserve specialized functions. For example, the striatal-enriched phosphatases (STEPs) are expressed at high levels in striatal medium spiny neurons and presumably contribute to the unique features of these cells. Although inhibitors of protein tyrosine phosphatases might be expected to promote the survival of neurons, this remains an unproven hypothesis. **Vanadate,** which inhibits most if not all protein tyrosine phosphatases, has been used as an experimental tool to study these enzymes in neural phenomena.

OTHER PROTEIN PHOSPHORYLATION CASCADES

Second messenger-dependent protein kinases and the protein kinases that function in neurotrophic factor

signaling cascades represent a relatively small fraction of the more than 70 forms of protein kinases that have been identified in mammalian cells (Table 5–6). We are not sure how most of these other kinases affect neural functioning, but research has yielded some clues. G protein receptor kinases (GRKs), for example, have been proven to phosphorylate G protein-coupled receptors and to influence the regulation of receptor desensitization (Box 5–4). Many protein kinases were first characterized according to their role in basic cellular functions, such as cell division or intermediary metabolism (e.g., glycogen synthase kinases, casein kinases, and cyclin-dependent kinases); however, recent evidence indicates that several of these enzymes operate in particular signal transduction cascades in the brain. Cyclin-dependent kinase-5 (cdk-5), for example, is believed to be one of the protein kinases responsible for the hyperphosphorylation of a microtubule-associated protein in the brain known as tau; such hyperphosphorylation contributes to several types of dementia, including **Alzheimer disease** and **Pick disease** (see Chapter 20).

Table 5–6 Major Classes of Protein Serine–Threonine Kinases[1]

Second messenger-dependent protein kinases
cAMP kinase
cGMP kinase
Ca^{2+}/calmodulin kinases
Protein kinase C
MAP kinases
ERKs
JNKs or SAP-kinases
MAP kinase-regulating kinases
MEKs
SEKs
Raf
MEKK
Cyclin-dependent protein kinases (Cdks)
cdk-2
cdk-5
Cdk regulating kinases
Cdk-activating kinase (CAK)
CAK-kinase
G protein receptor kinases (GRKs)
Others
Ribosomal S6 kinases (RSKs)
Casein kinases

[1]This list is not intended to be comprehensive. These protein kinases, are present in many cell types and are included here because their multiple functions in the nervous system include the regulation of neuron-specific phenomena. Not included are other protein kinases present in diverse tissues (including brain) that play a role in generalized cellular processes, such as intermediary metabolism, but that may not play a role in neuron-specific phenomena.

ERK, extracellular signal-regulated kinase; JNK, jun kinase; SAP-kinase stress-activated kinase; MEK, MAP-kinase or ERK kinase; SEK, SAP, kinase, or ERK kinase; MEKK, MEK kinase; cdc-2, cell division cycle-protein 2; cdk-5, cyclin-dependent kinase type 5; CAK, cdk-activating kinase.

Box 5–4 Desensitization of the β-Adrenergic Receptor

One of the dramatic features of G protein-coupled receptors is their rapid desensitization in response to agonist stimulation. An important mechanism underlying this desensitization is phosphorylation of the receptor by a second messenger-activated kinase such as PKA and by a β-adrenergic receptor kinase (β-ARK) that has been renamed G protein receptor kinase (GRK; see figure).

threonine kinase that is constitutively active and not regulated by second messengers (see part B of figure). This kinase can phosphorylate the receptor only when the receptor is bound to agonist because such binding alters the receptor's conformation in such a way that it becomes a good substrate for the kinase. After it undergoes phosphorylation by β-ARK, the receptor is able to bind a protein

A   β-receptor

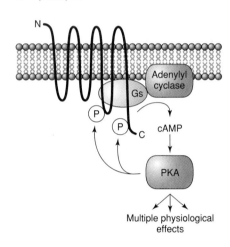

B   β-receptor

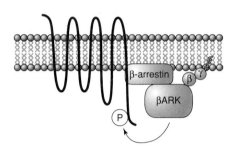

The details of GRK action are best established for the β-adrenergic receptor. Agonist binding to the receptor stimulates G_s, which leads to the activation of adenylyl cyclase, increased levels of cAMP, and the activation of PKA. The activation of PKA subsequently triggers many of the physiologic effects of β-adrenergic receptor stimulation through the phosphorylation of numerous substrate proteins. However, among the proteins phosphorylated by the kinase is the receptor itself, which is phosphorylated on several serine residues in its cytoplasmic domains. This process reduces the subsequent ability of agonists to activate the receptor. For example, phosphorylation of the receptor may trigger its endocytosis or internalization from the plasma membrane, sequestering it from further agonist binding. An internalized receptor may be returned to the plasma membrane after its dephosphorylation or may undergo proteolysis during periods of prolonged agonist exposure.

Phosphorylation of the β-adrenergic receptor by PKA can be viewed as an example of negative feedback: activation of the receptor stimulates intracellular cascades that reduce further receptor activation. Phosphorylation of the receptor by PKA also can mediate heterologous desensitization of the receptor; any neurotransmitter–receptor system that works through cAMP stimulates β-adrenergic receptor phosphorylation by means of PKA and leads to receptor desensitization. Thus this process enables one neurotransmitter–receptor system to affect another.

The β-adrenergic receptor is also phosphorylated on several distinct serine residues by β-ARK, a protein serine–

known as β-arrestin, which effectively sequesters the receptor and prevents its further interaction with the ligand or the G protein. Recent studies indicate that the βγ subunits of G proteins are required to bring β-ARK, a predominantly cytosolic enzyme, into close association with the plasma membrane-associated receptors occupied by ligand. This process represents an elegant mechanism by which β-ARK is specifically recruited to receptors that have been recently activated, as evidenced by nearby free βγ complexes.

Phosphorylation of the β-adrenergic receptor by β-ARK, like its phosphorylation by the cAMP-dependent enzyme, occurs through a process involving negative feedback. However, unlike phosphorylation by PKA, phosphorylation by β-ARK represents an example of homologous desensitization: only the β adrenergic receptor molecules occupied by the agonist are affected in this process.

This model of receptor desensitization may explain why many G protein-coupled receptors are desensitized after persistent ligand binding. Accordingly, at least six forms of β-ARK-like GRKs have been cloned to date. These enzymes are differentially expressed in the nervous system, and each GRK appears to phosphorylate a distinct subset of G protein-coupled receptors. Moreover, GRKs have been proven to phosphorylate and desensitize several G protein-coupled receptors in addition to the β-adrenergic receptor and may be prominent mediators of homologous desensitization in the brain. Investigators also have identified several forms of arrestins that are believed to contribute to the specific desensitization of G protein-coupled receptor function by the various GRKs.

Another substrate for cdk-5 in the brain is DARPP-32. As previously discussed, phosphorylation of DARPP-32 by PKA converts it into an inhibitor of protein phosphatase 1. Recent research has shown that phosphorylation of DARPP-32 by cdk-5 on a different amino acid residue converts DARPP-32 into an inhibitor of PKA. Thus DARPP-32 can serve as a switch, alternately inhibiting the phosphorylation or dephosphorylation of various phosphoproteins, depending on the level of activity of PKA versus cdk-5 in the neuron.

CENTRALITY OF PROTEIN PHOSPHORYLATION

The final step of most signal transduction pathways is the regulation of phosphoproteins, or third-messenger proteins, which include an array of substrate proteins for each protein kinase and protein phosphatase involved in phosphorylation. Because an increasing number of neuronal proteins are included among known phosphoproteins (Table 5-7), it is now well established that protein phosphorylation underlies the regulation of diverse aspects of neuronal function, a possibility first proposed by Greengard and colleagues in the 1970s. The phosphorylation of neuronal proteins influences the regulation of ion channel activity; neurotransmitter receptor sensitivity; neurotransmitter synthesis, release, and reuptake; axoplasmic transport; the elaboration of dendritic and axonal processes; and the differentiation of neurons. Many forms of neural plasticity, including learning and memory, are similarly governed by the phosphorylation of neuronal proteins.

Table 5-7 Neuronal Proteins Regulated by Phosphorylation

Regulated Protein	Protein Kinase	Effect
Enzymes involved in neurotransmitter biosynthesis and degradation		
Tyrosine hydroxylase	PKA, PKC, CaM-KII	Increase in enzyme activity
Tryptophan hydroxylase	CaM-KII	Increase in enzyme activity
G protein-coupled receptors		
β-adrenergic receptor	PKA, GRKII	Receptor desensitization
Opioid receptors	GRKII	Receptor desensitization
Neurotransmitter-gated ion channels		
GluR1 (AMPA subunit)	PKA	Increase in response
NMDAR1 (NMDA subunit)	PKC, tyrosine kinase	Increase in response
Ion channels		
Voltage-gated Na^+ channel	PKA, PKC	Decrease in channel conductance
Voltage-gated Ca^{2+} channel	PKA	Increase in channel conductance
Enzymes and other proteins involved in the regulation of second messengers		
Phospholipase Cγ	Tyrosine kinase	Increase in enzyme activity
IP_3 receptor	PKA	Increase in Ca^{2+} release
Protein kinases		
PKA	PKA	Increase in dissociation and activity
CaM-KI and IV	CaM-KK	Increase in enzyme activity
Trk	Trk	Increase in signaling
Protein phosphatase inhibitors		
DARPP-32	PKA, PKG	Increase in inhibitory activity
Inhibitor 1	PKA	Increase in inhibitory activity
Inhibitor 2	GSK3	Decrease in inhibitory activity
Cytoskeletal proteins		
MAP-2	PKA	Promotion of microtubule assembly
Tau	cdk-5 and others	Increase in aggregation
Myosin light chain	MLC-K	Increase in binding to actin
Synaptic vesicle proteins		
Synapsin	PKA, CaM-KII	Increase in neurotransmitter release
Transcription factors		
CREB	PKA, CaM-KIV, RSK	Increase in transactivation
STAT proteins	JAK	Increase in transactivation

This list is not intended to be comprehensive but instead indicates the diverse types of neuronal proteins that are regulated by phosorylation.
PKA, protein kinase A; PKC, protein kinase C; CaM-K, Ca^{2+}/calmodulin-dependent protein kinases; GRK, G protein-coupled receptor kinase; CaM-KK, CaM-K kinase; Trk, Trk receptor; PKG, protein kinase G; GSK3, glycogen synthase kinase 3; MAP-2, microtubule-associated protein-2; MLC-K, myosin light chain kinase; RSK, ribosomal S6 kinase; STAT, signal transducers and activators of transcription; JAK, Janus kinase.

Although proteins are covalently modified in many ways—for example, by ADP-ribosylation, acylation, carboxymethylation, tyrosine sulfation, and glycosylation—none of these mechanisms is as widespread or as readily subject to regulation by synaptic and hormonal stimuli as phosphorylation.

NEUROMODULATORS

As mentioned in Chapter 4, a distinction is sometimes made between neurotransmitters and neuromodulators. Accordingly, a neurotransmitter may be considered a substance that acts through ligand-gated ion channels, whereas a neuromodulator acts through intracellular second messengers. Yet our knowledge of the brain's signal transduction pathways indicates that such a distinction is arbitrary for several reasons. First, some neurotransmitters elicit postsynaptic potentials by enabling direct G protein coupling between a receptor and an ion channel in addition to activating a receptor ionophore or causing second messenger-dependent phosphorylation of ion channels (see Figure 5–1).

Second, many neurotransmitters produce effects through all three of these mechanisms; for example, glutamate, GABA, serotonin, and acetylcholine produce some of their postsynaptic potentials in target neurons by means of ligand-gated channels and produce others by means of G protein-coupled receptors and intracellular messengers.

Third, the activation of ligand-gated channels does not always have a more pronounced effect on the electrical properties of postsynaptic neurons, as implied by the distinction between neurotransmitter and neuromodulator. Indeed a postsynaptic potential mediated by cAMP- or Ca^{2+}-dependent protein phosphorylation can have a pronounced impact on the activity of target neurons or other target cells. An example of the latter are the robust effects of the sympathetic nervous system on peripheral smooth muscle.

Fourth, although neurotransmitters that activate ligand-gated channels produce their initial postsynaptic potentials without the involvement of G proteins or intracellular messengers, the activation of such channels leads to multiple effects that are mediated by intracellular messenger pathways. Many of these effects may be crucial to the overall functioning of the brain. Thus a single substance can be both a neurotransmitter and neuromodulator, and sometimes a combination of these, depending on the cell types, receptor subtypes, and specific physiologic responses involved.

The distinction between neurotransmitters and neurotrophic factors also is becoming increasingly arbitrary. Current evidence suggests that traditional neurotransmitters (e.g., glutamate, monoamines, and opioid peptides) can regulate the phenotype, growth, and survival of neurons in addition to their synaptic activity. Likewise, neurotrophic factors most likely regulate synaptic activity in addition to neural phenotype, growth, and survival. Moreover, the intracellular signaling pathways influenced by neurotransmitters and by neurotrophic factors exhibit extensive similarities and overlap. Indeed, a substance such as dopamine or an opioid peptide may be viewed as entirely analogous to brain-derived neurotrophic factor (BDNF) in terms of the host of physiologic functions subserved by these substances.

HETEROGENEITY IN BRAIN SIGNAL TRANSDUCTION PATHWAYS

Molecular biologic research has revealed a degree of heterogeneity in intracellular messenger pathways not suspected by classic biochemical, pharmacologic, or physiologic studies. Molecular cloning studies currently confirm the existence of at least 22 distinct G protein α subunits, 7 distinct subunits of PKA, 9 subtypes of adenylyl cyclase, and 7 subtypes of PKC, whereas biochemical and pharmacologic research led to the identification of only 4 types of G_α proteins (G_s, G_i, G_o, and G_t), 2 types of PKA, 2 forms of adenylyl cyclase, and 1 type of PKC. Moreover, individual subtypes of these proteins possess unique regulatory properties and exhibit varying levels of expression in different neuronal cell types. These discoveries hint at even greater functional specificity within and between neuronal cell types in the brain. In addition, such heterogeneity may enable the development of drugs that interfere with a particular subtype of intracellular messenger. This point can be illustrated by consideration of RGS proteins. With more than 20 RGS subtypes known, many of which show highly restricted patterns of expression within the brain, it is conceivable that drugs aimed at antagonizing one particular subtype could exert a potent, and clinically useful, effect on the signaling of G protein-coupled receptors within brain regions of interest.

In a similar vein, our knowledge of the intracellular signaling cascades for neurotrophic factors may lead to the discovery of novel targets for pharmacotherapeutic agents. However, because neurotrophic factors are relatively large proteins (e.g., BDNF has a molecular mass of approximately 10,000 kDa), it may prove particularly difficult to generate small molecules that can cross the blood–brain barrier and activate neurotrophic factor receptors. An alternative approach might involve activating these pathways at a step distal to ligand binding, perhaps by facilitating dimerization of the receptor subunits or by activating some of their intracellular signaling proteins.

SELECTED READING

Berman DM, Gilman AG. 1998. Mammalian RGS proteins: Barbarians at the gate. *J Biol Chem* 273:1269–1272.

Bernards A. 1995. Neurofibromatosis type I and Ras-mediated signaling: Filling in the GAPs. *Biochim Biophys Acta* 1242:43–59.

Berridge MJ. 1997. Elementary and global aspects of calcium signaling. *J Physiol* 499:291–306.

Catterall WA. 1997. Modulation of sodium and calcium channels by protein phosphorylation and G proteins. *Advances Second Messenger Phosphoprotein Research* 31:159–181.

Clapham DE, Neer EJ. 1997. G protein beta gamma subunits. *Annu Rev Pharmacol Toxicol* 37:167–203.

Conti M, Jin SL. 1999. The molecular biology of cyclic nucleotide phosphodiesterases. *Prog Nucleic Acid Res Mol Biol* 63:1–38.

Cooper DM, Karpen JW, Fagan KA, Mons NE. 1998. Ca(2+)-sensitive adenylyl cyclases. *Advances Second Messenger Phosphoprotein Research* 32:23–51.

Dohlman HG, Thorner J. 1997. RGS proteins and signaling by heterotrimeric G proteins. *J Biol Chem* 272:3871–3874.

Duman RS, Nestler EJ. 1999. Cyclic nucleotides. In: Siegel GJ, Agranoff BW, Alberts RW, et al (eds): *Basic Neurochemistry*, 6th ed, pp. 433–452. Philadelphia: Lippincott-Raven Publishers.

Edwards AS, Scott JD. 2000. A-kinase anchoring proteins: protein kinase A and beyond. *Curr Opin Cell Biol* 12:217–221.

Foord SM, Marshall FH. 1999. RAMPs: Accessory proteins for seven transmembrane domain receptors. *Trends Pharmacol Sci* 20:184–187.

Fukunaga K, Miyamoto E. 1998. Role of MAP kinase in neurons. *Mol Neurobiol* 16:79–95.

Greengard P, Allen PB, Nairn AC. 1999. Beyond the dopamine receptor: the DARPP-32/protein phosphatase-1 cascade. *Neuron* 23:435–447.

Hamm HE. 1998. The many faces of G protein signaling. *J Biol Chem* 273:669–672.

Holler C, Freissmuth M, Nanoff C. 1999. G proteins as drug targets. *Cell Mol Life Sci* 55:257–270.

Houslay MD, Sullivan M, Bolger GB. 1998. The multienzyme PDE4 cyclic adenosine monophosphate-specific phosphodiesterase family: intracellular targeting, regulation, and selective inhibition by compounds exerting antiinflammatory and antidepressant actions. *Adv Pharmacol* 44:225–342.

Hunter T. 2000. Signaling—2000 and beyond. *Cell* 100:113–127.

Klee CB, Ren H, Wang X. 1998. Regulation of the calmodulin-stimulated protein phosphatase calcineurin. *J Biol Chem* 273:13367–13370.

Lefkowitz RJ. 1998. G protein-coupled receptors: III. New roles for receptor kinases and beta-arrestins in receptor signaling and desensitization. *J Biol Chem* 273:18677–18680.

Lewis TS, Shapiro PS, Ahn NG. 1998. Signal transduction through MAP kinase cascades. *Adv Cancer Res* 74:49–139.

Marshall CJ. 1996. Ras effectors. *Curr Opin Cell Biol* 8:197–204.

McDonald LJ, Murad F. 1996. Nitric oxide and cyclic GMP signaling. *Proc Soc Exp Biol Med* 211:1–6.

Mielke K, Herdegen T. 2000. JNK and p38 stress kinases—degenerative effectors of signal-transduction-cascades in the nervous system. *Prog Neurobiol* 61:45–60.

Nakanc M, Murad F. 1994. Cloning of guanylyl cyclase isoforms. *Adv Pharmacol* 26:7–18.

Nestler EJ, Greengard P. 1984. *Protein Phosphorylation in the Nervous System.* New York: Wiley.

Nestler EJ, Duman RS. 1999. G proteins. In: Siegel GJ, Agranoff BW, Alberts RW, et al (eds): *Basic Neurochemistry*, 6th ed, pp. 401–414. Philadelphia: Lippincott-Raven Publishers.

Nestler EJ, Greengard P. 1999. Serine and threonine phosphorylation, In: Siegel GJ, Agranoff BW, Alberts RW, et al (eds), pp. 471–496. *Basic Neurochemistry*, 6th ed. Philadelphia: Lippincott-Raven Publishers.

Nishizuka Y. 1995. Protein kinase C and lipid signaling for sustained cellular responses. *FASEB J* 9:484–496.

Rodbell M. 1997. The complex regulation of receptor-coupled G-proteins. *Adv Enz Reg* 37:427–435.

Sabatini DM, Lai MM, Snyder SH. 1997. Neural roles of immunophilins and their ligands. *Mol Neurobiol* 15:223–239.

Sala A, Zarini S, Bolla M. 1998. Leukotrienes: Lipid bioeffectors of inflammatory reactions. *Biochemistry* 63:84–92.

Schnabel P, Bohm M. 1995. Mutations of signal-transducing G proteins in human disease. *J Mol Med* 73:221–228.

Schneider T, Igelmund P, Hescheler J. 1997. G protein interaction with K+ and Ca2+ channels. *Trends Pharmacol Sci* 18:8–11.

Scott K, Zuker CS. 1998. Assembly of the *Drosophila* phototransduction cascade into a signaling complex shapes elementary responses. *Nature* 395:805–808.

Segal RA, Greenberg ME. 1996. Intracellular signaling pathways activated by neurotrophic factors. *Annu Rev Neurosci* 19:463–489.

Shenolikar S. 1995. Protein phosphatase regulation by endogenous inhibitors. *Cancer Biol* 6:219–227.

Soderling SH, Beavo JA. 2000. Regulation of cAMP and cGMP signaling: new phosphodiesterases and new functions. *Curr Opin Cell Biol* 12:174–179.

Sunahara RK, Dessauer CW, Gilman AG. 1996. Complexity and diversity of mammalian adenylyl cyclases. *Annu Rev Pharmacol Toxicol* 36:461–480.

Vane JR, Bakhle YS, Botting RM. 1998. Cyclooxygenases 1 and 2. *Annu Rev Pharmacol Toxicol* 38:97–120.

Winston LA, Hunter T. 1996. Intracellular signalling: Putting JAKs on the kinase MAP. *Curr Biol* 6:668–671.

Zhang X, Majerus PW. 1998. Phosphatidylinositol signaling reactions. *Semin Cell Dev Biol* 9:153–160.

Chapter 6
Signaling to the Nucleus

KEY CONCEPTS

- Many intracellular signaling pathways ultimately regulate gene expression.

- Chromatin plays a critical role in eukaryotic gene regulation by blocking the access of transcription factors to DNA; thus, the activation of gene expression often requires a modification in chromatin structure.

- The initiation of transcription is a critical biologic control point gating the flow of information out of the genome.

- Transcription typically occurs when an activator protein displaces nucleosomes, the major component of chromatin, permitting a complex of proteins, called general transcription factors, to bind DNA at a core promoter and recruit RNA polymerase.

- RNA polymerase II transcribes genes that yield messenger RNA and hence proteins.

- DNA binding sites for regulatory proteins are called *cis*-regulatory elements, and the proteins that bind them are called *trans*-acting factors, which are directly involved in the regulation of transcription.

- Each gene has a unique pattern of cellular expression and response to physiologic signals based on the combinatorial interaction of *cis*-regulatory elements found within its regulatory region and on the *trans*-acting factors available within a cell to bind those *cis* elements.

- Transcription factors typically contain physically distinct domains, including a DNA binding domain, a transcription activation domain, and most often an interaction domain that permits the formation of dimers and higher order complexes of proteins.

- Response elements, *cis*-regulatory sequences that confer responsiveness to physiologic signals, work by binding transcription factors that are modified, for example, via phosphorylation, by specific signaling pathways.

- Eukaryotic cells increase the diversity of proteins that can be produced from a single gene by alternatively splicing the exons within the primary transcript; alternative splicing is utilized to a great degree by neurons in the brain.

- Mature (spliced) messenger RNAs are transported from the nucleus into the cytoplasm, where they are translated to proteins on organelles called ribosomes.

- During and after translation, proteins are processed by cleavage into smaller proteins and by a variety of covalent modifications such as glycosylation.

All living cells depend on the regulation of gene expression by extracellular signals for their development, homeostasis, and adaptation to the environment. Indeed, many signal transduction pathways function primarily to modify transcription factors that alter the expression of specific genes. Thus, neurotransmitters, growth factors, and drugs change patterns of gene expression in cells and in turn affect many aspects of nervous system functioning, including the formation of long-term memories. Many drugs that require prolonged administration, such as antidepressants and antipsychotics, trigger changes in gene expression that are in fact therapeutic adaptations to the initial action of the drug.

The mechanisms underlying the control of gene expression are becoming increasingly well understood. These are subject to various forms of dynamic regulation in the cell, including structural changes in chromatin, transcription of DNA into RNA, splicing of RNA into mRNA, editing and other covalent modifications of mRNA, translation of mRNA into protein, and post-translational modification of a protein into its mature, functional form. Although we have learned the molecular details of some these regulatory processes, such information has not yet been exploited for the medical treatment of CNS disorders. This chapter provides a detailed overview of the regulation of gene expression in cells, underscoring its profound impact on neural and behavioral plasticity. Central to this chapter is the belief that the therapeutic effects of drugs that influence the CNS often depend on alterations in gene expression, as well as the expectation that novel therapeutic agents for neuropsychiatric disorders will one day target some of the mechanisms that govern the transcription and translation of genes into mature proteins.

CONTROL OF GENE EXPRESSION

DNA REPLICATION AND TRANSCRIPTION

Gene expression is governed by the regulated transcription of deoxyribonucleic acid (DNA), which contains the genetic blueprint for all living organisms. DNA transmits information from generation to generation and is the repository of information required to guide an organism's development and interaction with the environment. This information is stored in a double helix composed of deoxyribose–phosphate backbones bridged by paired purine–pyrimidine nucleotide bases. The purine bases in DNA are adenine (A) and guanine (G), and the pyrimidines are cytosine (C) and thymine (T); within the double

helix, A is complementary to T, and G is complementary to C.

Because DNA is a linear polymer, it is an ideal template for the synthesis of other macromolecules and thus an ideal vehicle for the transfer of information. The fundamental process by which information is transferred with high fidelity from a template strand of DNA to a new molecule of DNA (as occurs in DNA replication), or to a new molecule of RNA (as occurs in transcription), is known as complementary base pairing. In accordance with this process, the directionality of a DNA or RNA strand is designated by the free phosphate group of its terminal nucleotide, which is either 5′ or 3′. During DNA replication, which is required before cell division can occur, the double helix unwinds, and each existing strand of DNA serves as a template for the synthesis of a new complementary strand in the 5′ to 3′ direction. Because every new double helix contains one old strand and one that is newly synthesized but complementary, this process is described as semiconservative. During transcription, the first step in gene expression, the DNA unwinds in a local region of the chromosome and only one of the two DNA strands is used as a template to synthesize a complementary single-stranded molecule of RNA. The RNA subsequently dissociates from the DNA, thus permitting the original double helix to reanneal (Figure 6–1).

Although it is ideal for stable information storage and transfer, the chemical simplicity and rigid helical structure of DNA prohibit it from assuming other functions in the cell. Consequently, the information

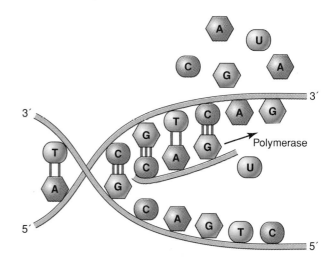

Figure 6–1. Complementary base pairing of DNA. A DNA double helix unwinds, allowing the transcription of a new, complementary strand of RNA catalyzed by an RNA polymerase in the 5′ to 3′ direction.

contained in DNA must be expressed through RNA and proteins. RNA, like DNA, is a linear polymer that comprises four nucleotide building blocks; however, in RNA the nucleotide uracil (U) takes the place of T. Unlike DNA, RNA is a flexible single strand, which is free to fold into a variety of conformations; thus its functional versatility greatly exceeds that of DNA. For example, some types of RNA, such as ribosomal RNA (rRNA), transfer RNA (tRNA), and small nuclear RNA (snRNA), perform functions other than information transfer. In contrast, messenger RNA (mRNA) is an intermediate for the synthesis of proteins.

REGULATION OF GENE EXPRESSION BY CHROMATIN

In eukaryotic cells, DNA is contained within a discrete organelle called the nucleus, which is the site of DNA replication and transcription. Transcriptionally quiescent regions of DNA are tightly packed into a coiled coil, whereas regions characterized by active transcription may be more than a 1000-fold more extended. Chromosomes are extremely long molecules of DNA, which are wrapped around histone proteins to form nucleosomes, the major subunits of chromatin. Although chromatin serves a structural function, in eukaryotes it also plays a critical role in transcriptional regulation because it can repress gene expression by inhibiting the ability of transcription factors to access DNA. In fact, chromatin ensures that genes are inactive unless their expression is required (Figure 6–2). To activate gene expression, cells must attenuate nucleosome-mediated repression of an appropriate subset of genes by means of activator proteins that modify chromatin structure. This activation process, which involves transcription factors, histones, and cofactors, displaces or remodels chromatin and opens up regions of DNA to permit the binding of regulatory proteins. Recent work has demonstrated that genetic defects in the remodeling of chromatin cause **Rett syndrome,** an **autism**-like disorder (Box 6–1).

GENES AND THE GENOME

Only a small percentage of chromosomal DNA in the human genome (approximately 4%) is responsible for encoding the roughly 40,000 genes that encode RNA strands. Among RNA strands, only a minority—for example, rRNA, tRNA, and snRNA—have cellular functions themselves; most RNA is mRNA that serves as an intermediate between DNA and protein. Chromosomal DNA comprises both genes and more extensive intergenic regions. The spacing of genes on chromo-somes is far from uniform: some chromosomal regions, and indeed whole chromosomes, are gene-rich or gene-poor. Intergenic regions alternately consist of unique sequences and long stretches of tandemly repeated sequences referred to as satellite DNA. Whether this extragenic DNA performs a structural or regulatory role, or simply represents parasitic DNA that is replicated in conjunction with functional regions of DNA, is currently a matter of debate.

DNA sequences in genes either code for RNA or assume control functions. Some interact with regulatory proteins and thereby determine the boundaries of segments of DNA that can be transcribed into RNA. Other closely linked DNA sequences determine whether a segment of DNA can be transcribed in a given cell type and, if it can, under what circumstances. Regulation of gene expression conferred by the nucleotide sequence of a DNA molecule is referred to as *cis*-regulation because the regulatory and transcribed regions occur on the same DNA molecule. The sequences involved in *cis*-regulation serve as binding sites for regulatory proteins. Because these proteins may be encoded anywhere in the genome and are not coded by the stretches of DNA to which they bind, they are sometimes described as *trans*-acting factors. *Trans*-acting factors that regulate the transcription of DNA are called transcription factors.

REGULATED STEPS OF TRANSCRIPTION

Transcription occurs in regions of open chromatin, and thus may require an activator protein that displaces nucleosomes (see Figure 6–2). Such displacement permits a complex of proteins, called general transcription factors, to bind DNA at a core promoter and to recruit RNA polymerase. The construction of this protein complex at the transcription start site and the synthesis of the first phosphodiester bond between nucleotides is referred to as transcription initiation. In the elongation step, the RNA polymerase must successfully transcribe an appropriate length of RNA without undergoing premature termination; regulated termination appears to be a mechanism that controls the expression of a small number of genes. The final step in the transcription of RNA is appropriate termination.

The resulting nuclear RNA engages in a posttranscriptional process called *splicing*, which removes internal sequences that will not be translated into protein in that particular cell (Figure 6–3). Subsequently the RNA is exported from the nucleus into the cytoplasm. Within the cytoplasm, mRNA may be regulated by processes that increase its rate of degradation or, alternatively, stabilize it; this regulation is important experi-

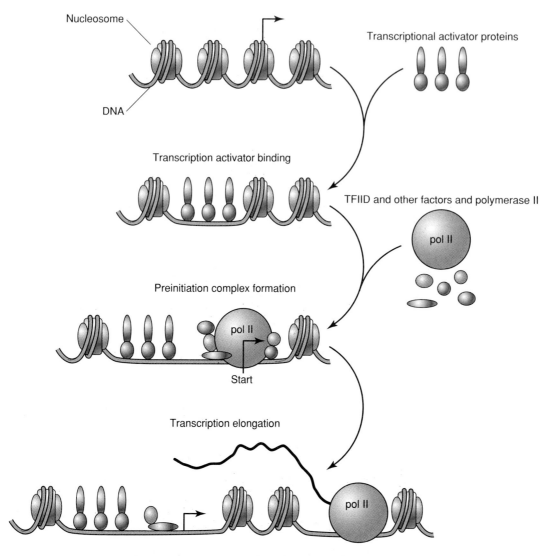

Figure 6–2. Inhibition of gene expression by the nucleosomal structure of chromatin. To activate the transcription of DNA, activator proteins such as histone acetylases must displace nucleosomes. The acetylation of histones appears to be a critical step in the chromatin remodeling that permits transcription. Additional nucleosomes must be displaced to permit general transcription factors (collectively called TFIID) and RNA polymerase (pol) II to bind to the transcription initiation site in a gene (*start arrow*). Still more nucleosomes must be displaced to permit transcription elongation.

mentally because many compounds that inhibit protein synthesis in cells also stabilize subsets of mRNA. Coincident with or subsequent to translation, the newly synthesized protein may undergo a variety of chemical modifications and cleavages and must be targeted to the appropriate cellular compartment.

ALTERNATIVE SPLICING OF PRIMARY RNA TRANSCRIPTS

Stretches of noncoding DNA are found not only between genes but also within them. Although mRNA in prokaryotes is almost invariably encoded by a single uninterrupted stretch of DNA, the sequences that code for mRNA in eukaryotes are frequently interrupted by intervening DNA sequences. DNA sequences that code for a segment of mRNA are called *exons* because the information they contain is exported from the nucleus; the intervening sequences, which remain in the nucleus, are called *introns*. When a protein-coding gene is first transcribed, the product RNA is termed the *primary transcript* and is colinear with the DNA; thus it contains both exons and introns (see Figure 6–3). RNA that contains both introns and exons is called

Box 6–1 Rett Syndrome

Rett syndrome is a pervasive developmental disorder that occurs predominantly in females and shares certain clinical features with **autism-spectrum disorders.** Infants appear normal at birth and show normal developmental milestones until approximately 6 months of age, when severe developmental arrest occurs. Thereafter, patients are afflicted by gross deterioration in mental, social, and motor functioning.

Most cases of Rett syndrome are caused by loss-of-function mutations in the gene that encodes methyl-CpG-binding protein 2 (MECP2), which is located on the X chromosome. MECP2, through interactions with mSin3A (a transcriptional repressor) and certain histone acetylases, binds to methylated CpG dinucleotides in the genome and represses gene transcription. Thus MECP2 is part of the normal mechanisms

by which methylation of DNA causes repression of gene expression. Such mechanisms are implicated in the phenomenon of genetic imprinting, which explains why certain traits are preferentially inherited from the mother or the father independent of the dominance or recessiveness of the trait. For example, if a paternal gene is highly methylated, it remains inactive in the offspring, regardless of whether it is dominant or recessive.

A major goal of future research is to determine how loss of MECP2 leads to the pervasive developmental arrest that is characteristic of patients with Rett syndrome. Research also is needed to determine which genes are overexpressed in the absence of MECP2, and why developmental arrest occurs during mid-infancy.

heteronuclear RNA (hnRNA). Before the transcript exits the nucleus, its introns are removed and its exons are spliced together to form mature mRNA. Such splicing is catalyzed by RNA–protein complexes called *spliceosomes.* Spliced mRNA subsequently leaves the nucleus and binds to a ribosome in the cytoplasm, where it can direct the synthesis of a protein. However, some parts of the mature mRNA molecule are not translated. All mRNA molecules contain untranslated regions (UTRs)

at their 5′ and 3′ ends in which *cis*-regulatory elements may affect mRNA stability and translatability.

Many genes expressed in the brain contain multiple introns and exons that may not be spliced identically in every cell type, at every stage of development, or under every condition in a given cell type. Current estimates suggest an average of five splice variants per gene. Alternative splicing may be accomplished by a number of different mechanisms. A particular exon–intron

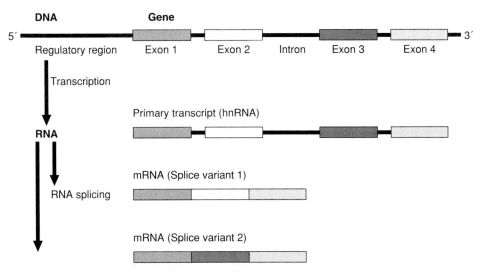

Figure 6–3. Transcription and RNA splicing. Horizontal black lines represent DNA regulatory regions and introns. Blue, gray, and white rectangles represent exons. The region to the left of the first exon is the 5′ regulatory region of the gene, but *cis*-regulatory elements are also found in introns and sometimes even downstream of the last exon. The primary transcript, also known as heterogeneous RNA (hnRNA), contains both exons and introns and gives rise to two alternatively spliced mRNA: one containing exons 1, 2, and 4, and one containing exons 1, 3, and 4. If these splice variants were exported from the nucleus and translated in the cytoplasm, they would give rise to distinct proteins.

boundary may, for example, be utilized or ignored by the splicing machinery in some cells but not in others. Some genes undergo extensive alternative splicing; for example, the gene that encodes the NR1 subunit of the NMDA glutamate receptor gives rise to at least eight different proteins by means of alternative splicing (see Chapter 7). Moreover, each of these proteins exhibits distinct variations in tissue distribution and function. Thus the true molecular diversity of mammalian cells is significantly underrepresented by the approximately 40,000 genes contained in the genome.

Calcitonin and calcitonin gene-related peptide (CGRP), two peptides derived from the same primary transcript, were among the first proteins to be identified as products of alternative splicing. The production of one rather than the other peptide depends on use of alternative 3′ splice acceptor sites in particular cell types. Many cell types in the nervous system, including primary afferent nociceptive neurons, express the neuropeptide CGRP, which is translated from mRNA containing exons 1, 2, 3, 5, and 6. Medullary cells of the thyroid gland express the hormone calcitonin, which is involved in Ca^{2+} homeostasis, from mRNA containing exons 1, 2, 3, and 4. Exons 1, 2, and 3 contain the 5′ untranslated region of both types of mRNA; exon 3 also contains shared protein coding sequences. Exon 4 encodes the calcitonin-specific peptide sequence and a 3′ polyadenylation site. Exons 5 and 6 encode the CGRP-specific peptide sequence and a second polyadenylation site utilized by the CGRP mRNA. The mechanisms by which alternative splice sites are selected in particular cell types are not well understood but probably involve the tissue-specific expression of proteins that regulate the splicing machinery. Examples of brain-specific regulators of alternative splicing include a group of recently discovered proteins termed *Nova*. In addition, a single gene might give rise to several different types of mRNA and proteins by use of alternative promoters present with the gene.

REGULATION OF mRNA STABILITY AND TRANSLATABILITY

A poly(A) tail is coupled to mRNA by means of an endonucleolytic cleavage step that produces the 3′ end of a mature mRNA molecule. In higher eukaryotes, but not in yeast, essentially all mRNA contains *cis*-regulatory information for cleavage and polyadenylation in the form of the sequence AAUAAA just 5′ to the cleavage site. In some genes, alternative polyadenylation sites may be used in different cells to give rise to different mRNA molecules. Both the stability and translata-

bility of an mRNA molecule are regulated by its polyadenylation. Stability refers to the half-life of the mRNA, or the amount of time it remains in the cytoplasm and is available for translation. Translatability refers to the rate at which it can be translated into protein. The mechanism by which polyadenylation regulates mRNA stability and translatability is not known.

The untranslated 3′ regions of some mRNA molecules also contain sequences, such as AUUUA, or secondary structures—for example, stem-loops in the mRNA—that bind proteins that in turn regulate the stability and translatability of the mRNA. Such regulation may prove to be quite important for neural and behavioral plasticity, given that particular perturbations can alter the levels of some proteins in the brain without an associated change in gene transcription.

Eukaryotic mRNA molecules not only undergo polyadenylation but are modified at their 5′ ends with the addition of a cap referred to as 7mGpppN. The 7mG refers to a 7-methylguanosine residue linked to a triphosphate (ppp) at the 5′ end of the RNA transcript, and N refers to the first nucleotide in the RNA sequence. This cap not only increases the stability of mRNA, it is also essential for efficient protein synthesis because it binds to protein factors that are required to initiate the assembly of a translation-competent ribosome.

TRANSLATION OF MATURE mRNA IN THE CYTOPLASM

The genetic code comprises the rules that govern the translation of mRNA into protein. The sequence of nucleotides in a molecule of mRNA is read on ribosomes in serial order and in groups of three. Each triplet of nucleotides, called a codon, specifies a single amino acid. Because there are more triplet codons than amino acids, some amino acids are specified by more than one codon. The codons in mRNA do not interact directly with the amino acids they specify; rather, the translation of mRNA into protein depends on the presence of adaptor RNA molecules, called tRNA, that recognize the three bases in a codon and carry a corresponding amino acid. A specific tRNA exists for each codon. Ribosomes, which are themselves composed of proteins and specific rRNA, provide the structure on which tRNA can interact with the codons of mRNA in sequential order. After the ribosome finds a specific start site on the mRNA, which is always the codon AUG (specifying methionine), it moves along the mRNA molecule and translates the nucleotide sequence one codon at a time, using tRNA to add amino acids to the growing end of the polypeptide chain. When the ribosome reaches a stop codon in the message, both the mRNA and the newly synthesized protein are released from the ribosome, which subsequently dissociates into individual subunits.

POSTTRANSLATIONAL PROCESSING OF PROTEINS

During and after translation, proteins are further processed by cleavages that produce smaller proteins by the covalent modification—for example, glycosylation—of constituent amino acid residues and by folding mechanisms. Such processing is determined by the protein's amino acid sequence and by the presence of enzymes that catalyze these modifications. Amino acid sequences also specify the locations to which proteins are targeted within the cell. Details regarding posttranslational alterations and the associated sorting of proteins to different cellular locations are addressed in subsequent chapters in this book.

The stability of a protein, like that of an mRNA molecule, is highly regulated. This is necessary because the level of a protein in a cell is determined by its rate of synthesis and by its rate of degradation, or proteolysis. Some proteins, such as those in the Fos family of transcription factors, are highly unstable because they contain specific amino acid sequences, such as PEST sequences, that serve as substrates for proteolytic enzymes, or proteases. The stability of certain proteins depends on their association with other proteins; for example, when the catalytic subunit of protein kinase A binds to its regulatory subunit (see Chapter 5), the stability of the kinase is dramatically enhanced. Moreover, when protein kinase A is activated by cAMP, the catalytic and regulatory subunits dissociate, thereby producing a free, active catalytic subunit that is vulnerable to proteolysis and that regulates the amount of the kinase by means of negative feedback.

Many cellular proteins, including protein kinase A, undergo proteolysis by means of the ubiquitin–proteasome pathway, whereby specific enzymes add ubiquitin groups to the targeted protein. This addition tags the protein for proteolysis by proteasomes, which are large multiprotein complexes. Specific inhibitors of proteasomes, such as **leu-leu-leu** and **lactacystin**, are used experimentally to study the role of proteasomes in cell regulation. The processes that control protein stability require further elucidation. However, because the protein levels in neurons are often altered without corresponding changes in their mRNA, it is likely that these processes are important contributors to neural and behavioral plasticity.

REGULATION OF TRANSCRIPTION

TRANSCRIPTION INITIATION: A CRITICAL BIOLOGIC CONTROL POINT

As the preceding sections have indicated, transcription can be divided into three discrete steps: initiation, mRNA chain elongation, and chain termination. Although biologically significant regulation may occur at any step in this process, transcription initiation appears to be one of the most significant control points because it gates the flow of information out of the genome. Indeed this is the step in gene expression that is most highly regulated by extracellular signals.

Transcription initiation involves two critical processes: positioning of the appropriate RNA polymerase at the correct transcription start site, and efficient control of the rate of transcription. To ensure that these control functions operate smoothly, *cis*-regulatory elements must recruit appropriate transcription factors to the DNA. Many of these factors bind to DNA directly; others interact with DNA indirectly by means of protein–protein interactions. *Cis*-regulatory elements that determine a gene's transcription start site are called basal, or core, promoters; other *cis*-elements are responsible for tethering different activator and repressor proteins to the DNA.

CORE PROMOTERS

In eukaryotes, transcription is carried out by three distinct RNA polymerases. Each of these acts on a distinct type of core promoter whose characteristics are exploited by a distinct class of genes. Polymerase I (pol I) promoters are utilized by genes that encode large rRNA molecules. Polymerase II (pol II) promoters are utilized by genes that are transcribed to yield mRNA and hence proteins; these promoters are also used by a subset of genes that encode snRNA involved in RNA splicing. Polymerase III (pol III) promoters interact with genes that encode other small RNA molecules, including snRNA that is not involved in RNA splicing, small rRNA molecules, and tRNA.

RNA polymerases do not bind to DNA directly; rather, they are recruited to DNA by other proteins that bind to core promoters. Core promoters for the three different polymerases contain distinct elements on which different types of basal transcription complexes are assembled. Because this chapter focuses on the regulated expression of protein-encoding genes, only the core promoters used by pol II are described here.

Pol II promoters are surprisingly diverse but share certain key features. The most common of these is the TATA box, a sequence rich in nucleotides A and T and

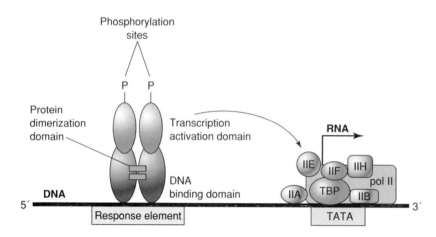

Figure 6–4. A generalized polymerase II promoter. Two *cis*-regulatory elements, including a hypothetical activator, or response element, and the TATA box are located on a stretch of DNA (*black line*). The TATA element binds the TATA binding protein (TBP), which associates with multiple general transcription factors (TFIIA, B, E, F, and H). This basal transcription apparatus recruits RNA polymerase (pol) II and also forms the substrate for interactions with various activator proteins, which typically contain DNA-binding domains, dimerization domains, and transcription activation domains. Several of these proteins may be modified by phosphorylation.

located between 25 and 30 bases upstream of the transcription start site (Figure 6–4). The TATA box determines the start site of transcription and orients the basal transcription complex; thus it establishes the 5' to 3' direction in which pol II synthesizes RNA. A mutation of this sequence can inhibit or interfere with the accuracy of transcription initiation. Many pol II promoters, including those for many genes expressed in neurons, lack a TATA box and possess instead a poorly conserved core promoter element called an initiator.

A TATA-binding protein (TBP) initiates the formation of the basal transcription complex by binding the core promoter together with multiple TBP-associated factors (or TAFs) and other general transcription factors. Each of the transcription factors in Figure 6–4 is a mixture of proteins, the terminology of which is based on their original identification as chromatographic fractions derived from cell nuclei. TBP, together with its TAFs, was first identified as a fraction called TFIID, whereby TFII identifies general transcription factors associated with pol II, and the final letter designates the fraction. TFIID is also required to build a basal transcription complex from TATA-less promoters.

TRANSCRIPTION FACTORS: KEY REGULATORS OF GENE EXPRESSION

The basal transcription apparatus alone is not adequate to initiate more than low levels of transcription. To achieve higher levels, this multiprotein assembly requires help from transcriptional activators that recognize and bind to *cis*-regulatory elements found elsewhere in the gene. Because they are tethered to specific recognition sequences in the DNA, such *trans*-acting factors can be described as sequence-specific transcription factors.

The functional *cis*-regulatory elements for a particular gene typically are located within several hundred

bases of its start site but occasionally can be found many thousands of base pairs away, either upstream (i.e., in the 5' direction) or downstream (i.e., in the 3' direction) of the start site. Regulatory elements that exert control near the core promoter are referred to as *promoter elements* and those that act at a distance are called *enhancer elements*, but the distinction between these elements is artificial from a mechanistic point of view. Both represent short spans of DNA that are 7 to 15 base pairs in length, each of which is a specific binding site for one or more transcription factors. Each gene has a particular combination of *cis*-regulatory elements, the nature, number, and spatial arrangement of which determine the gene's unique pattern of expression; thus transcriptional regulation in eukaryotes may be described as combinatorial. Promoter or enhancer elements control the cell types in which the gene is expressed, when the gene is expressed, and the level at which it is expressed both basally and in response to physiologic and environmental signals.

Sequence-specific transcription factors typically contain physically distinct functional domains (Figure 6–5). The *DNA-binding domain* recognizes and binds to a specific nucleotide sequence; the *transcription activation domain* interacts with co-activators or with general transcription factors (i.e., components of the pol II complex) to form a mature or fully active transcription complex; and the *multimerization domain* permits the formation of homomultimers or heteromultimers in conjunction with other transcription factors. The presence of distinct types of domains contributes to the categorization of transcription factors into various families. Domains from different activators can be swapped experimentally to produce novel hybrid proteins that are functionally active.

Many transcription factors are active only when they form dimers or higher-order complexes. Multimerization domains are diverse and include so-called leucine zippers, Src homology (SH2) domains, and certain helical moieties (see Chapter 5). Whether transcription factor dimers are homodimers or heterodimers, both partners commonly contribute to the DNA binding domain and to the activation domain. Interestingly, dimerization sometimes can be a mechanism for the negative control of transcription, as illustrated by interactions among members of the helix-loop-helix (HLH) family of transcription factors, which are so named because they contain two conserved amphipathic α-helices connected by an unconserved loop of variable length. These proteins must dimerize through their α-helical domains so that they can bind to DNA and activate transcription; for example, when the muscle-specific

A

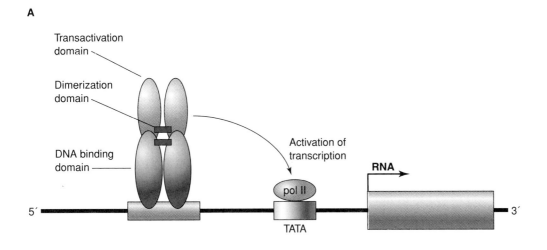

B

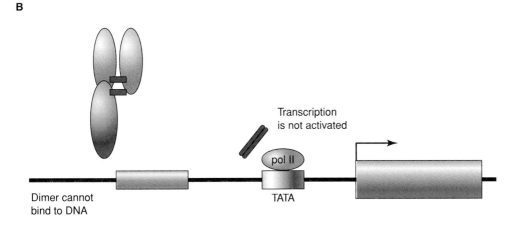

C

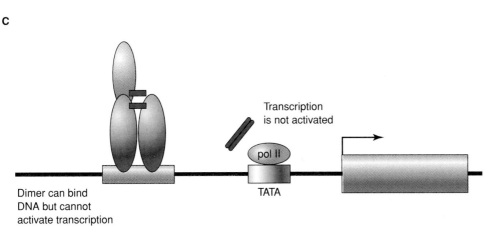

Figure 6–5. **A.** A normal or wildtype transcription factor, which contains a DNA-binding domain, a dimerization domain, and a transactivation domain. The transactivation domain interacts with a RNA polymerase (pol) II complex to induce transcription. **B.** A dominant negative inhibitor that dimerizes with a wildtype protein but lacks a DNA-binding domain and thus cannot activate transcription. **C.** A dominant negative inhibitor that dimerizes with a wildtype protein but lacks a transactivation domain and thus cannot activate transcription.

HLH protein known as MyoD is dimerized with the ubiquitous HLH protein E12/E47, it activates a variety of genes in muscle cells that contribute to the differentiated state of the tissue. In contrast, these muscle genes are not transcribed in proliferating myoblasts because, despite their high levels of MyoD and E12/E47, myoblasts express a negative partner of MyoD called Id. Id lacks the basic DNA-binding domain that is found just N terminal to the first α helix in HLH proteins that are transcriptional activators. Thus MyoD-Id dimers cannot bind DNA and cannot activate transcription.

The negative regulation of MyoD by Id involves an activator that is titrated out, or sequestered, by an inactive dimerization partner. In other cases of negative regulation, the dimer formed by an activator and its negative regulator can bind DNA, but the negative regulator lacks an activation domain and thereby disrupts the formation of the mature transcription complex. Such inhibitory mechanisms, which occur naturally in cells, have also been exploited experimentally for the purpose of designing *dominant negative inhibitors* of protein function. Such inhibitors have proved to be powerful tools in the functional analysis of transcription factors (see Figure 6–5).

Regulation by heterodimers is not an all-or-none proposition. Some members of the Fos family of transcription factors, such as c-Fos, are strong activators when dimerized with a partner from the Jun family, such as c-Jun. Other Fos-related proteins, such as Fos-related antigen-1 (FRA-1), form heterodimers with c-Jun that bind DNA but provide weaker activation than c-Fos, or perhaps slightly different preferences for a particular region of DNA containing an AP-1 site. The formation of heterodimers and other multimers increases the diversity of transcription factor complexes in cells and in turn increases the complexity of regulatory information that can be exerted on gene expression.

Although sequence-specific transcription factors may directly contact several proteins in the basal transcription complex, they sometimes interact with this apparatus through the mediation of coactivator or adapter proteins (Figure 6–6). In either scenario, transcription factors that bind at a distance from the core promoter can interact with the basal transcription apparatus because the DNA forms loops that bring distant regions in contact with each other.

Many activator proteins become involved in the assembly of the mature transcription apparatus only after modification, such as phosphorylation, has occurred in response to extracellular signals (see Chapter 5). Phosphorylation alters the ability of the phosphoprotein to interact with other proteins, as illustrated by the activity of the transcription factor *cAMP response element-binding protein* (CREB). CREB can activate transcription only when it is phosphorylated on a particular serine residue (ser133) because phosphorylation of this residue permits CREB to interact with an adapter protein known as CREB-binding protein (CBP), which in turn contacts and activates the basal transcription apparatus. Interestingly, mutations in CBP have been shown recently to cause abnormalities in mice that resemble **Rubinstein-Taybi** syndrome, an autosomal dominant disorder characterized by mental retardation, bone and palatal abnormalities, and cardiac dysfunction.

REGULATION OF GENE EXPRESSION BY EXTRACELLULAR SIGNALS

The precise control of transcription by extracellular signals such as neurotransmitters, growth factors, and cytokines permits the regulation of processes such as cell proliferation and differentiation and assists cells in adapting to their environments. Each cell in an organism contains a complete copy of that organism's genome. However, selective expression of this common genome is required for the formation of distinct cell types during development, including the formation of thousands of types of neurons in the brain. Further investigation will be required to determine the precise mechanisms by which genes are transiently or permanently activated in any given cell type, and also the circumstances under which the repressive effects of chromatin must be supplemented by specific repressor proteins.

Studies of invertebrate models suggest that the sequential and hierarchical expression of activator and repressor proteins during development initially depends

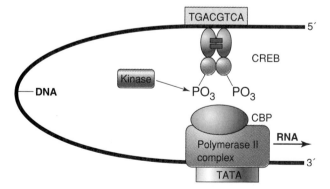

Figure 6–6. Looping of DNA permits activator or repressor proteins binding at a distance to interact with the basal transcription apparatus, or polymerase II complex, which appears as a single box bound at the TATA element. Because the activator protein CREB has been phosphorylated, it is able to interact with a CREB-binding protein (CBP), which in turn mediates CREB's effects on the basal transcription apparatus.

on the asymmetric distribution of critical signaling molecules in the embryo, and in turn the differential expression of genes in embryonic cells. As cells gain individual identities during development, cell–cell interactions mediated by contact, or by the elaboration of autocrine, paracrine, or longer-range signaling molecules, continue the process of specifying the complement of genes they will express. Genes that are silent during particular phases of development may become unavailable for subsequent activation. Extracellular signals also remain critical to the appropriate regulation of gene expression in mature cells. Indeed, from a mechanistic point of view, adult plasticity has much in common with developmental processes.

TRANSCRIPTION FACTORS: TARGETS OF SIGNALING PATHWAYS

Most genes contain *cis*-regulatory sequences that confer responsiveness to physiologic signals. These sequences, known as *response elements*, work by binding transcription factors that are activated or inhibited by specific physiologic signals such as phosphorylation. Two major mechanisms of transcriptional regulation by

extracellular signals are illustrated in Figure 6–7. One of these mechanisms involves transcription factors that are present at significant levels under basal conditions and are rapidly stimulated by signaling cascades to activate or repress the transcription of responsive target genes. By means of the other major mechanism, transcription factors that are expressed at very low levels under basal conditions are induced by a physiologic signal that enables them to regulate the expression of a series of genes.

A critical step in the extracellular regulation of gene expression is the transduction of signals from the cell membrane to the nucleus, which can be accomplished by several mechanisms. Some transcription factors translocate to the nucleus in response to their activation. These include steroid hormone receptors, whose translocation is triggered by the binding of their ligand, and NF-κB, a transcription factor retained in the cytoplasm by a binding protein (IκB) that masks its nuclear localization signal. Signal-regulated phosphorylation of IκB by protein kinase C leads to the dissociation of NF-κB, which in turn is permitted to enter the nucleus to bind DNA; IκB subsequently undergoes proteolysis in the cytoplasm. Other transcription factors

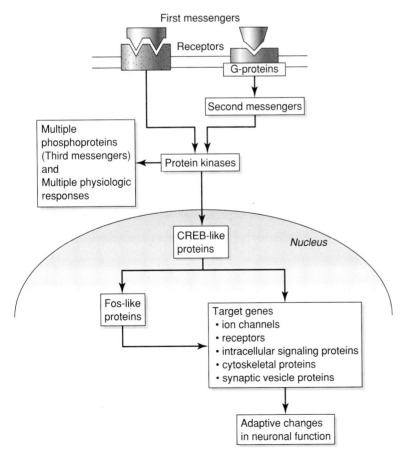

Figure 6–7. Intracellular pathways underlying the regulation of gene expression. The stimulation of neurotransmitter, hormone, or neurotrophic factor receptors activates specific second messenger and protein phosphorylation pathways, which produce effects on neuronal function through the phosphorylation of numerous proteins (see Chapter 5). Changes in gene expression occur by means of two basic mechanisms. When constitutively expressed transcription factors, such as CREB, are phosphorylated by protein kinases, their transcriptional activity is altered and this causes changes in the expression of specific target genes. Among the target genes are those that encode other transcription factors, such as Fos family proteins. Once induced, these transcription factors alter the expression of still other target genes.

must be phosphorylated or dephosphorylated directly before they can bind to DNA; for example, the phosphorylation of *signal transducers and activators of transcription* (STATs) by protein tyrosine kinases in the cytoplasm permits their multimerization, which in turn permits nuclear translocation and the construction of an effective DNA binding site in the multimer.

Some transcription factors are already bound to their cognate *cis*-regulatory elements in the nucleus under basal conditions and are converted into transcriptional activators by phosphorylation. CREB, for example, is bound to DNA elements termed *cyclic AMP response elements* (CREs) before cell stimulation (Figure 6–8). The critical nuclear translocation step for CREB involves the activation of protein kinases such as protein kinase A, which, after entering the nucleus, phosphorylates CREB. Alternatively, CREB activation can involve the nuclear translocation of second messengers, such as Ca^{2+} bound to calmodulin. After entering the nucleus, these second messengers activate Ca^{2+}/calmodulin-dependent protein kinase type IV that in turn phosphorylates CREB (Figure 6–9). As previously mentioned, phosphorylation converts CREB into a transcriptional activator by permitting it to recruit CBP into the transcription complex.

Cyclic AMP response element

$\longrightarrow$

5′ TGACGTCA 3′
3′ ACTGCAGT 5′

$\longleftarrow$

AP-1 element

5′ TGACTCA 3′
3′ ACTGAGT 5′

Figure 6–8. The palindromic structure of consensus cAMP response elements (CREs) and AP-1 elements. Palindromes or near palindromes are common features of *cis*-regulatory elements that bind transcription factors as dimers. In general, perfect palindromes are the strongest binding sites for these factors. An intact CGTCA sequence (*arrows*) may be an absolute requirement for CREs.

The remainder of this chapter focuses on several transcription factor families that have received a great deal of attention as mediators of neural and behavioral plasticity in the adult.

CREB FAMILY OF TRANSCRIPTION FACTORS

CREB regulates transcription by binding to CREs present in a subset of genes. As their name suggests, CREs enable cAMP to activate genes. It has been deter-

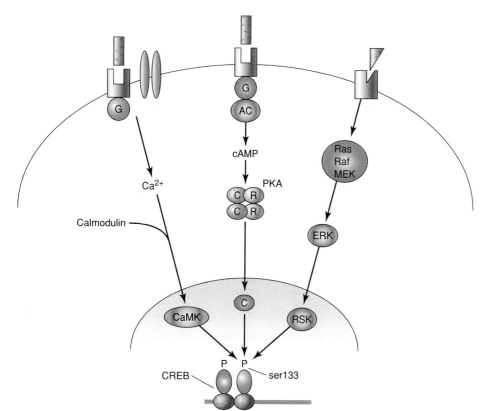

Figure 6–9. Regulation of CREB phosphorylation. Several signaling pathways converge on the phosphorylation of CREB at a single serine residue (ser133). Neurotransmitters that stimulate adenylyl cyclase (AC) increase CREB phosphorylation by activating protein kinase A (PKA). Activated PKA catalytic subunits translocate to the nucleus, where they phosphorylate (P) ser133. Neurotransmitters that inhibit adenylyl cyclase cause the opposite cascade and inhibit CREB phosphorylation. Increased Ca^{2+} permeates the nucleus, where it activates Ca^{2+}/calmodulin-dependent protein kinases (CaMK), particularly CaMK IV, which phosphorylate ser133. Growth factor regulated pathways also lead to CREB phosphorylation by means of the Ras–Raf–MEK pathway that leads to the activation of extracellular signal-regulated kinases (ERKs). ERKs translocate to the nucleus and phosphorylate and activate ribosomal S6 kinase (RSK), which in turn phosphorylates ser133 (see Chapter 5).

mined that CREs also confer responsiveness of genes to Ca^{2+} and to the MAP-kinase pathway. CREs have been identified in many genes expressed in the nervous system, including those that encode neuropeptides (e.g., somatostatin, proenkephalin, and vasoactive intestinal polypeptide), neurotransmitter synthetic enzymes (e.g., tyrosine hydroxylase), signaling proteins (e.g., adenylyl cyclase type VIII), and transcription factors (e.g., c-Fos and CREB).

The characterization of CREs and other *cis*-regulatory elements required that they be deleted or mutated and subsequently reintroduced into eukaryotic cells in culture by transfection (Box 6–2). Mutations in one or more critical nucleotide bases in a *cis*-regulatory element typically destroy the binding site for the relevant transcription factor. When signal-regulated transcription factors can no longer bind their cognate DNA sequences, the corresponding genes cannot be activated by the physiologic stimulus under investigation (e.g., cAMP). By comparing response element sequences from many genes that have been investigated by mutagenesis, an idealized consensus sequence can be derived. For CREs the consensus nucleotide sequence is TGACGTCA, with the nucleotides CGTCA being absolutely required.

The consensus CRE sequence illustrates the palindromic nature of many transcription factor binding sites. Examination of the TGACGTCA sequence reveals that the two complementary DNA strands, which run in opposite directions, are identical (see Figure 6–8). Many *cis*-regulatory elements are perfect or approximate palindromes because many transcription factors bind to DNA as dimers, whereby each member is responsible for recognizing half of the binding site. As mentioned previously, CREB is the major protein that binds to CREs; CREB binds as a homodimer and has a higher affinity for palindromic than for asymmetric CREs.

Regulation of CREB by cAMP, Ca^{2+}, and growth factors cAMP, Ca^{2+}, and growth factors activate CREB by causing its phosphorylation at ser133. cAMP activates protein kinase A, whereas Ca^{2+} activates Ca^{2+}/calmodulin-dependent protein kinase IV, both of which phosphorylate ser133 (see Figure 6–9). CREB is also phosphorylated on ser133 by a growth factor-activated kinase, known as ribosomal S6 kinase (specifically RSK-90), which is phosphorylated and activated by MAP-kinases (see Chapter 5). The activation of CREB thereby illustrates a striking convergence of several signaling pathways on the phosphorylation of a single amino acid residue in the protein. Such phosphorylation is the penultimate step in CREB activation, because only when CREB is phosphorylated on this residue can it bind to the adapter protein CBP, which

interacts with the basal transcription factor complex, to regulate gene expression.

Thus, diverse signaling pathways converge where CREB is phosphorylated and activated. Such convergence may be a critical mechanism for achieving gene regulation when the signal generated by each pathway is relatively weak; in fact some genes may be activated only when multiple pathways are stimulated. Moreover, genes that contain CREs are induced in more than an additive fashion by the interaction of cAMP and Ca^{2+} signaling pathways, although the mechanism by which convergent phosphorylation on the same serine produces synergy is not yet known. Synergy is more readily understood when a particular protein is modified on two different sites, which can result in positively interacting conformational changes. It is important to mention that CREB contains sites other than ser133 that can be phosphorylated, and these sites may assist in fine-tuning the regulation of CREB-mediated transcription. CaM-kinase II, for example, phosphorylates a serine residue in CREB that restricts the ability of other kinases to phosphorylate ser133; thus the activation of CaM-kinase II most likely mediates a dampening of the CREB signal.

CREB mediation of neural plasticity The activation of a single transcription factor by convergent signaling pathways is particularly important in the nervous system because it may represent a mechanism for long-term neural adaptations, such as those underlying long-term memory, drug addiction, and fear conditioning. That some forms of long-term memory require new gene expression is reasonably well established and is discussed in later chapters. Associative memory also depends on the temporally coordinated arrival of two different signals that subsequently must be integrated in target neurons and their circuits. Thus the activation of CREB is likely to mediate aspects of long-term memory and related phenomena (see Chapter 20).

Several experimental findings support CREB's role in learning and memory. *Drosophila* in which CREB is inactivated by a dominant negative transgene, and knockout mice in which CREB is partly inactivated by homologous recombination, both exhibit deficits in long-term memory. Although these findings are intriguing, they must be considered preliminary until alternative explanations for such memory deficits are ruled out. The inactivation in mouse brain of an important transcription factor such as CREB may produce developmental abnormalities not readily detected by light microscopic examination or other routine methodologies, and these may interfere with long-term memory in a number of indirect ways. Moreover, the CREB knockout mouse that has been

Box 6–2 Assaying Promoter Activity

The functional activity of gene promoters is studied in vitro. Before such activity can be observed, a fragment of a promoter must be linked to any gene whose product is easily detectable and quantifiable. Such genes are known as reporter genes and include those that encode β-galactosidase, chloramphenicol acetyltransferase (CAT), luciferase, or green fluorescent protein (GFP). The promoter–reporter construct is transfected into cultured cells, where the reporter gene's rate of expression is controlled by the activity of the gene promoter. Subsequently the cells are challenged with various pharmacologic agents, or transfected with plasmids that encode a specific transcription factor, so that the cellular signaling pathways that control promoter activity may be identified.

Mutants of the promoter often are studied for the purpose of identifying the promoter's regulatory region. Several mutants typically are produced by a series of 5′ deletions, such that less and less of the promoter region is included in the promoter–reporter construct. This process can indicate the general region of a promoter required for some regulation. Subsequently specific nucleotide sequences in the region, such as those comprising a CRE or AP-1 site, are selected to undergo deletion or mutation.

An investigation of response elements required for the regulation of the CREB gene produced the data shown in the figure. For this promoter assay, approximately 1.2 kb of the 5′ promoter of the CREB gene was coupled to a CAT reporter and transfected into C6 glioma cells. Mutants derived from a series of 5′ deletions and also coupled to CAT were studied in parallel (see part A). CREB promoter activity was stimulated in cells treated with **isoproterenol,** a β-adrenergic receptor agonist that increases cellular cAMP levels (see Chapter 8). Because similar activity was observed in a CREB–CAT construct containing only the first 278 bases of the promoter sequence, this effect of isoproterenol is most likely mediated by a response element close to the transcription start site. The 278-base sequence shown in the figure comprises two consensus CRE sites and one consensus SP-1 site. Mutation of either CRE site reduced isoproterenol's effect on the promoter, and the mutation or deletion of both sites completely obliterated it. In contrast, mutation of the SP-1 sites produced no effect. These data indicate that isoproterenol activates CREB promoter activity by means of two CRE sites in the promoter. This autoregulatory mechanism controls CREB gene transcription: activity of CREB regulates its own expression.

Promoters are powerful tools that are widely used in the high throughput screening of new drugs (see Chapter 1). Through this process cultured cells are engineered to express a particular receptor and a promoter–reporter construct sensitive to intracellular signaling. A promoter containing CREs typically is used because it is responsive to the perturbation of cAMP, Ca^{2+}, and MAP-kinase pathways. These cells are exposed to large numbers of compounds, which are determined to be agonists or antagonists based on a decrease or increase in reporter activity. These assays have many advantages over more traditional ligand-binding assays. First, they are more sensitive because the amplification of intracellular signaling pathways allows the detection of compounds whose actions at the receptor may be quite weak. Second, they provide functional information and thereby measure efficacy in addition to affinity. Moreover, if they are appropriately designed, these assays can detect both agonists and antagonists. Third, they do not require knowledge of the receptor's signaling mechanisms because the reporter responds to the perturbation of several signaling pathways.

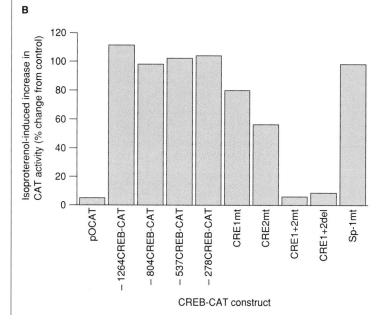

Adapted with permission from Coven E, Widnell KL, Chen JS, et al. 1998 *J Neurochem* 71:1865.

used to investigate hippocampal long-term potentiation and long-term memory exhibits a hypomorphic phenotype that possesses residual CREB activity; it also appears that other CREB-like proteins may compensate, at least partially, for the knockout. As knockout technologies improve, the role of CREB in different types of long-term memory and in the mediation of many types of plasticity is likely to be clarified.

CREB-like proteins   CREB, like many transcription factors, is a member of a large family of related proteins. Other members of this family may compensate for CREB when it is inactivated, and also provide subtle forms of positive and negative regulation analogous to that described for HLH proteins. Among the proteins that are closely related to CREB are *activating transcription factors* (ATFs) and *CRE modulators* (CREMs), which are generated by distinct genes. In addition, several alternative splice forms of CREB, ATFs, and CREMs have been identified.

All of these proteins bind CREs as dimers, and many can heterodimerize with CREB itself. The similarities between ATF-1 and CREB are especially striking because both are activated by cAMP and Ca^{2+} signaling pathways. Many ATF proteins and CREM isoforms also appear to activate transcription; however, some CREMs, such as inducible cAMP element repressor (ICER), act to repress it. CREM isoforms that repress transcription lack the glutamine-rich transcriptional activation domains found in CREBs and ATFs that serve as transcriptional activators. Thus, CREB-ICER heterodimers are able to occupy CREs but may fail to activate transcription. Like CREB, many ATF proteins are produced constitutively, but ATF-3 and some CREM isoforms (such as ICER) are inducible.

The leucine zipper   The dimerization domain used by CREB proteins, and several other families of transcription factors, is called a leucine zipper. This domain, which was first identified in the transcription factor known as *CAATT-enhancer binding protein* (C/EBP), actually forms a coiled coil rather than a zipper. It is composed of an α helix in which every seventh residue is a leucine; the leucines line up along one face of the α helix two turns apart. The aligned leucines of the two dimerization partners interact hydrophobically to stabilize the dimer. The leucine zipper for CREB is located at the carboxy terminus of the protein, and a region of highly basic amino acid residues just upstream of the leucine zipper serves as a DNA binding domain. Dimerization by a leucine zipper juxtaposes the adjacent basic regions of each of the partners so that these regions undergo a conformational change when they bind DNA,

producing what has been described as a scissors grip. The many proteins, in addition to CREB, that utilize these mechanisms of dimerization belong to a superfamily known as basic-leucine zipper, or bZIP, proteins.

AP-1 FAMILY OF TRANSCRIPTION FACTORS

Activator proteins known as AP-1 proteins are among the transcription factors that are indispensable in the regulation of neural gene expression by extracellular signals. The name given to these proteins was derived from their ability to mediate some transcriptional responses to protein kinase C activation. AP-1 proteins bind as heterodimers, and occasionally as homodimers, to the DNA sequence TGACTCA, which is called the activator protein-1 (AP-1) sequence. The consensus AP-1 sequence is a heptamer that forms a palindrome flanking a central C or G base (see Figure 6–8). Although it differs from the CRE sequence by only a single base, AP-1 sites strongly prefer AP-1 proteins as opposed to CREB, which requires an intact CGTCA sequence. As a result, this single base difference between CRE and AP-1 sites significantly influences which transcription factors, and hence which intracellular signaling pathways, can regulate a particular gene.

Many genes expressed in the nervous system contain AP-1 sites in their regulatory regions. Among these are genes that encode neuropeptides (e.g., neurotensin and substance P), neurotransmitter receptors (e.g., D_1 dopamine, NR1 NMDA, and GluR2 AMPA glutamate receptor subunits), neurotransmitter synthetic enzymes (e.g., tyrosine hydroxylase), and cytoskeletal proteins (e.g., neurofilament proteins). Although these sites have been proven to regulate gene promoter activity in vitro, it has been difficult to identify with certainty genes that are regulated by AP-1 transcription factors in the adult brain.

Because the **phorbol ester** known as 12-*O*-tetradecanoyl-phorbol-13-acetate (**TPA**) can induce gene expression by means of AP-1 proteins, the AP-1 sequence initially was described as a TPA-response element (TRE). TPA presumably activates AP-1 by stimulating protein kinase C, which in turn phosphorylates AP-1 proteins; however, the details of this mechanism remain incompletely understood. As discussed later in this chapter, AP-1 proteins are also known to be phosphorylated by certain MAP-kinases, which confers responsiveness of this transcription factor to growth factor-regulated pathways.

AP-1 transcription factors bind to DNA as dimers that comprise two families of proteins, Fos and Jun, both of which are bZIP proteins. The known members of the Fos family are c-Fos, FRA-1, FRA-2, and FosB and its alternative spliced variant ΔFosB. The known members of the Jun family are c-Jun, JunB, and JunD. Most AP-1 complexes are formed by one Fos family member and one Jun family member. Unlike Fos proteins, c-Jun and JunD (but not JunB) also can form homodimers that bind to AP-1 sites, albeit with far lower affinity than Fos-Jun heterodimers. Transcriptional regulation is further complicated by the fact that some AP-1 proteins can heterodimerize, by means of the leucine zipper, with members of the CREB–ATF family.

AP-1 proteins also can form higher order complexes with apparently unrelated families of transcription factors. They can, for example, complex with and apparently inhibit the transcriptional activity of steroid hormone receptors. AP-1 proteins also complex with transcription factors that contain the Rel DNA binding and dimerization domain to form *nuclear factor of activated T cells* (NF-AT). NF-AT, which is also found in the nervous system, was discovered based on its ability to transduce T-cell receptor activation into activation of the interleukin-2 gene.

Among Fos and Jun proteins, only JunD is expressed constitutively at high levels in many cell types. The other AP-1 proteins tend to be expressed at low or even undetectable levels under basal conditions, but with stimulation may be induced to high levels of expression. Thus, unlike regulation by constitutively expressed transcription factors such as CREB, regulation by most Fos/Jun heterodimers requires new transcription and translation of the transcription factors themselves.

Activation of cellular genes by AP-1   The genes that encode most AP-1 transcription factors are termed immediate early genes (IEGs). IEGs, a prototype of which is the c-Fos gene, are activated rapidly (within minutes) and transiently and do not require new protein synthesis. Late response genes, in contrast, are induced or repressed more slowly (over hours) and depend on the synthesis of new proteins. The term IEG initially applied to viral genes in eukaryotic cells that are activated immediately after infection by commandeering host cell transcription factors. Viral IEGs generally encode transcription factors that activate the late expression of viral genes.

The application of IEG terminology to nonviral genes has created some confusion. Many cellular genes are induced independently of protein synthesis but within a time course whose duration is between that of classic IEGs and late response genes. In fact, some of these genes may be regulated differently in response to different extracellular signals. Moreover, many cellular genes that are regulated as IEGs encode proteins that are not transcription factors; for example, any gene induced by CREB could potentially show temporal features of

induction of an IEG. Despite these complications, the concept of IEG-encoded transcription factors has assisted our understanding of gene regulation in the nervous system. In addition, several IEGs have been used as cellular markers of neural activation because of their rapid induction from low basal levels in response to neuronal depolarization and various second messenger and growth factor pathways. Such experimental use of IEGs has permitted novel approaches to functional neuroanatomy (Box 6–3).

Because c-Fos and related AP-1 proteins mediate some of the effects of physiologic stimuli on the expression of late-response genes, they have been designated third messengers in signal transduction cascades whose intercellular first messengers are neurotransmitters and whose second messengers are small intracellular molecules such as cAMP and Ca^{2+} (see Chapter 5). However, some neurobiologists have wrongly assumed that IEGs are a necessary step in the signal-induced expression of most genes involved in the regulation of neural function. In fact, most of these genes, including many that encode neuropeptides and neurotrophic factors, are activated in response to neuronal depolarization or increases in cellular cAMP levels by means of phosphorylation of CREB rather than through IEG third messengers.

Activation by multiple signaling pathways   The most studied cellular IEG is that for c-Fos. Because this gene contains three binding sites for CREB, the strongest of which is shown in Figure 6–10, it is not surprising that it can be activated rapidly by neurotransmitters or drugs that stimulate the cAMP or Ca^{2+} pathways. Yet the c-Fos gene also can be induced by the Ras/MAP-kinase pathway. As discussed in Chapter 5, neurotrophins, such as nerve growth factor, bind a family of receptor tyrosine kinases (Trks) that activate Ras. Ras subsequently triggers a cascade of protein kinases, which results in the phosphorylation and activation of extracellular signal-regulated kinases (ERKs) (types of MAP-kinases). These kinases can phosphorylate and activate other protein kinases, such as RSK, which in turn can phosphorylate CREB's ser133 residue. However, in many cell types ERKs also can induce the c-Fos gene by translocating into the nucleus of the cell, where they phosphorylate the transcription factor Elk-1 (also called the ternary complex factor, or TCF). Elk-1 subsequently complexes with the serum response factor (SRF) to bind to and activate the serum response element (SRE) in the c-Fos gene (see Figure 6–10). SREs are also present in many other growth factor-inducible genes. Compared with cAMP or Ca^{2+} pathways, the Ras/MAP-kinase pathway depends on a complex chain of phosphorylation events, yet these events can occur very rapidly to induce gene expression.

Box 6–3 Anatomic Markers of Neuronal Activation

Because c-Fos and several other cellular IEG products, including c-Jun, JunB, and Zif268 (Egr-1), are strongly and rapidly induced in response to diverse stimuli, they are commonly used as markers in functional neuroanatomy studies. Unstimulated, c-Fos mRNA and c-Fos protein are nearly undetectable in many cell types. However, neural stimuli that activate the cAMP, Ca^{2+}, protein kinase C, Ras-MAP-kinase, or JAK-STAT pathways can produce a rapid and powerful induction of c-Fos gene expression (see Figure 6–10). The lack of background expression and high levels of induction of the c-Fos gene contribute to the sensitivity of this type of marker. Immunohistochemical detection of c-Fos and other IEG-encoded proteins, or alternatively, the in situ hybridization of their mRNA, have become standard tools for mapping neurons and circuits that are activated by diverse in vivo manipulations.

However, there are several drawbacks to mapping cellular activation in the nervous system with these genes. First, most IEGs fail to respond to inhibitory neurotransmission.

Second, some IEGs are not expressed in every cell type; for example, dorsal root ganglia do not appear to express c-Fos. Third, the sensitivity of c-Fos and other IEGs increases their vulnerability to induction by nonspecific stimuli. Despite these disadvantages, the sensitivity, cellular resolution, and versatility of c-Fos immunohistochemistry and other IEG mapping techniques has led to their use in many investigations related to neuropsychiatric disorders.

Among other applications, IEGs have been used to characterize various cellular responses to dopaminergic drugs in the striatum (see figure). Research has indicated that these drugs produce different patterns of Fos induction. Antipsychotic agents that are D_2 antagonists, such as **haloperidol** (5mg/kg ip), induce Fos in striatopallidal neurons that express D_2 dopamine receptors; however, indirect dopamine agonists, such as **amphetamine** (12mg/kg ip) and **cocaine,** induce Fos in striatonigral neurons that express D_1 dopamine receptors (see Chapter 14). IEG mapping also has revealed differences between typical antipsychotic drugs such as haloperidol, which induce Fos in the caudate-putamen and nucleus accumbens, and atypical antipsychotic drugs such as **clozapine,** which induce Fos only in the nucleus accumbens. Such findings may explain the lack of extrapyramidal side effects produced by clozapine, and they may assist in the development of a screen for other antipsychotic agents without these side effects (Chapter 14).

Control   Haloperidol   Amphetamine

Adapted with permission from Nguyen TV, Kosofsky BE, Birnbaum R, et al. 1992 *Proc Natl Acad Sci USA* 89:4270.

Another mechanism of c-Fos induction involves cytokine-activated signaling pathways that trigger the activation of STATs. As previously mentioned, STATs are activated in response to their phosphorylation by protein tyrosine kinases. After they are activated, they form multimeric complexes, translocate to the nucleus, and bind to their specific DNA response elements, called STAT sites. The STAT site in c-Fos was previously named the SIE or SIF-inducible element (SIF itself is an acronym for sis-inducible factor, a factor induced by the oncogene v-sis that activates c-Fos at this site). As discussed in Chapter 11, the cytoplasmic protein tyrosine kinases called Janus kinases (JAKs) that phosphorylate STATs are themselves activated by the class of cytokines that interact with gp130-linked receptors, including ciliary neurotrophic factor (CNTF), leukemia inhibitory factor (LIF), interleukin-6 (IL-6), leptin, and prolactin. There is considerable specificity with respect to the subtypes of JAK and STAT proteins that associate with each of these cytokine receptors. The c-Fos gene (see Figure 6-10) contains an SIE that binds STAT proteins and mediates the induction of the gene by cytokines. Indeed, STAT sites are found in many genes expressed in the nervous system, including the gene that encodes vasoactive intestinal polypeptide (VIP).

Regulation by phosphorylation Several AP-1 proteins are regulated at the posttranslational level by phosphorylation. A well-established example of such regulation involves c-Fos, which is heavily phosphorylated on several closely spaced serine residues in its C-terminal region by protein kinase A, CaM-kinases, and protein kinase C. Phosphorylation appears to be a critical regulatory mechanism for this protein because the

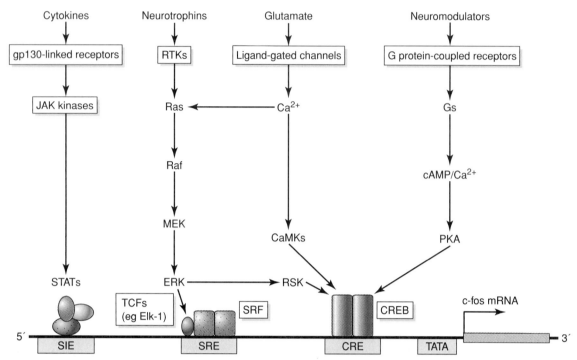

Figure 6–10. Regulatory region of the c-Fos gene. A CRE site binds CREB, a serum response element (SRE) binds serum response factor (SRF) and ternary complex factor (TCF or Elk-1), and a SIF-inducible element (SIE) binds STAT proteins; these three elements represent a small number of all known transcription factor-binding sites. Proteins that bind at these sites are constitutively present in cells and are activated by phosphorylation. CREB can be activated by protein kinase A, Ca^{2+}/calmodulin-dependent protein kinases (CaMKs), or ribosomal S6 kinases (RSKs); Elk-1 can be activated by the MAP-kinases ERK1 and ERK 2; and the STAT proteins can be activated by the JAK protein tyrosine kinases. Because the activation of c-Fos by any of multiple signaling pathways requires only signal-induced phosphorylation rather than new protein synthesis, it can be triggered rapidly by a wide array of stimuli (see Chapter 5). RTKs, receptor tyrosine kinases; STATs, signal transducers and activators of transcription; JAK, Janus kinase.

difference between cellular c-Fos and its viral counterpart v-Fos, which is oncogenic, involves a frame-shift mutation that deletes the serine residues from the viral protein. It has been suggested that phosphorylation of c-Fos allows the protein to suppress its own transcription, thereby providing negative feedback control of its expression.

The phosphorylation of c-Jun also is a critical regulatory mechanism for AP-1-mediated signaling. c-Jun phosphorylation occurs in response to the activation of a MAP-kinase signaling pathway by some form of cellular stress. As described in Chapter 5, a Ras-like G protein can be activated by several types of insult, including ultraviolet radiation, osmotic stress, and the effects of certain toxins and cytokines. Such activation triggers a cascade of protein kinases analogous to that triggered by Ras and culminates in the phosphorylation and activation of MAP-kinases called stress-activated protein kinases (SAP-kinases) or, alternatively,

Jun N-terminal kinases (JNKs). JNKs phosphorylate c-Jun in its transcriptional activation domain, on serine residues 63 and 73, thereby increasing its ability to activate transcription. This process has been implicated in the modulation of synaptic transmission and may, under unique circumstances, trigger the activation of apoptosis (programmed cell death) pathways (see Chapter 11).

Generation of unique AP-1 complexes Stimulation of a cell causes the activation of different members of the Fos family within varying time courses, and thus leads to the generation of distinct AP-1 complexes over time. These unique complexes can be revealed with electrophoretic mobility shift, or gel shift, assays, a common technique for analyzing protein–DNA interactions (Box 6–4).

Under resting conditions, c-Fos mRNA and protein are barely detectable in most neurons; however, a variety of stimuli can induce dramatic expression of the c-Fos

Box 6–4 Gel Shift Assays

The gel shift assay is used to study the interaction between transcription factors and their DNA response elements. It requires a small piece of double-stranded DNA (typically 20 nucleotides long) that contains a particular response element, such as a CRE or AP-1 site, and is labeled with a radioisotope. The radiolabeled probe is incubated in the presence of a tissue extract, and the mixture is separated on a nondenaturing polyacrylamide gel (see figure); a nondenaturing gel must be used because the DNA–protein interaction must be maintained during electrophoresis. In the absence of tissue extract, the radiolabeled probe migrates near the front (*bottom*) of the gel. In the presence of tissue extract, a minute amount of the radiolabeled probe binds to its specific transcription factor and migrates higher on the gel bound to the protein; the protein–oligonucleotide complex migrates much higher on the gel because it is much bigger than the free oligonucleotide. Such migration explains why this procedure is referred to as a gel shift, or electromobility shift, assay. The transcription factor responsible for binding the probe can be determined if antibodies directed against particular transcription factors are added to the incubation mixture before gel electrophoresis. After the probe binds to the transcription factor and the antibody, it migrates higher on the gel, producing what is called a supershift assay. In some cases, the antibody does not produce this shift but instead disrupts the band by preventing DNA–protein interactions. Another way to demonstrate specificity of a band is to incubate the mixture with increasing concentrations of non-radiolabeled oligonucleotide probe. Specific bands will be successfully completed by low concentrations of non-radiolabeled probe, whereas non-specific bands will require much higher concentrations.

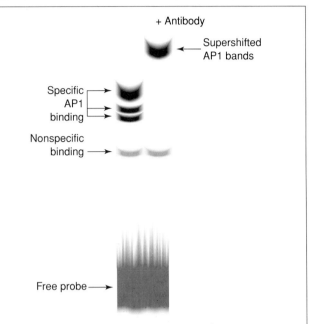

Borrowed with permission from E.J. Nestler, 1997.

In the gel shift assay illustrated in the figure, an aliquot of rat striatal extract was incubated with a ^{32}P-labeled oligonucleotide (19 bases long) that contained an AP-1 site. Another aliquot was incubated with an antibody directed against Fos family proteins and subsequently incubated with the oligonucleotide. The mixtures were separated by polyacrylamide gel electrophoresis and analyzed by autoradiography. Several of the resulting radiolabeled bands represent specific AP-1 binding and contain Fos-like proteins based on their ability to be supershifted by the antibody. Another band is nonspecific and is not supershifted.

---

gene. The experimental induction of a generalized **seizure,** for example, causes marked increases in c-Fos mRNA in the brain within 30 minutes, and similar increases in c-Fos protein within 2 hours; however, because c-Fos is highly unstable it returns to low, basal levels within 4 to 6 hours. The administration of **cocaine** or **amphetamine** causes a similar pattern of c-Fos expression in the striatum. In response to any of these stimuli, other Fos-like proteins are also induced but with a longer temporal latency than that of c-Fos; their peak levels of expression lag behind c-Fos by approximately 1 hour. Moreover, their expression persists slightly longer than that of c-Fos, returning to basal levels within 8 to 12 hours.

If the c-Fos gene is repeatedly stimulated it becomes resistant to further activation. However, the expression of certain other Fos-like proteins is not halted by repeated stimulation. These proteins, originally termed chronic FRAs, are biochemically modified isoforms of ΔFosB that have long half-lives in the brain. Thus these proteins accumulate in neurons in response to repeated perturbations and persist long after such perturbations cease (Figure 6–11). As discussed in subsequent chapters, it has been proposed that ΔFosB may mediate some of the long-term effects on the nervous system produced by drugs of abuse and other pharmacologic agents.

Although the precise biologic significance of these changes in AP-1 complexes is not yet known, it is believed that they can produce varying patterns in the expression of AP-1 regulated genes. This presumably permits neurons to adapt to the pattern of stimulation to which they are being subjected in exact and meaningful ways.

A

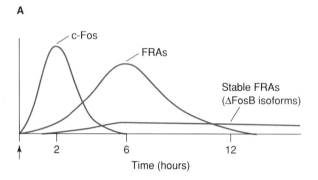

B

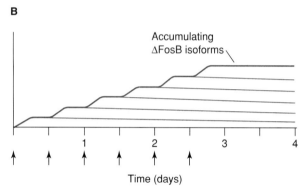

Figure 6–11. Changes in the composition of AP-1 complexes over time. **A.** Several waves of Fos-like proteins (also called Fos-related antigens or FRAs) are induced by acute stimuli in neurons. c-Fos, which is induced most rapidly, degrades within several hours; several FRAs, such as FosB, ΔFosB, FRA-1, and FRA-2, are induced somewhat later and persist somewhat longer than c-Fos. The stable FRAs, which are biochemically modified isoforms of ΔFosB, are also induced by a single stimulus but only at low levels; their enhanced stability allows them to persist in the brain. **B.** With repeated stimulation, each stimulus induces a low level of ΔFosB isoforms, as indicated by the horizontal lines. The result is a gradual increase in total ΔFosB, as indicated by the stepped line; such an increase gradually induces significant levels of a long-lasting AP-1 complex, which may underlie long-lasting forms of neural plasticity in the brain.

STEROID HORMONE RECEPTOR SUPERFAMILY

Steroid hormones (e.g., **glucocorticoids, estrogen, testosterone,** and **mineralocorticoids**), **retinoids, thyroid hormones,** and **vitamin D₃** are small, lipid-soluble ligands that diffuse readily across cell membranes. Unlike the receptors for peptide hormones, which are located in the cell membrane, the receptors for these ligands are localized in the cytoplasm. However, in response to ligand binding, steroid hormone receptors translocate to the nucleus, where they regulate the expression of certain genes by binding to specific hormone response elements (HREs) in their regulatory

regions. Thus these receptors are sometimes collectively referred to as the nuclear receptor superfamily.

The mechanisms by which the glucocorticoid receptor (GR) operates are representative of those utilized by most receptors in this superfamily. Under basal conditions, the GR is retained in the cytoplasm by a large multiprotein complex of chaperone proteins, including the heat shock protein Hsp90 and the immunophilin Hsp56. After it is bound by glucocorticoid, the GR dissociates from its chaperones, translocates to the nucleus, and subsequently functions as a ligand-regulated transcription factor by binding to glucocorticoid response elements (GREs). GREs typically are 15 bases in length and consist of two palindromic half sites, each of which comprises six bases separated by a three-base pair spacer. This palindromic organization of the GRE suggests that the GR, like other transcription factors, binds as a dimer. The receptors in this superfamily also have a modular structure similar to that of other transcription factors. The GR has 3 domains: an N-terminal transcriptional activation domain, a C-terminal ligand binding domain, and an intervening DNA binding domain (Figure 6–12). The DNA-binding domain of the GR is characterized by multiple cysteines organized around a central zinc ion, an arrangement often referred to as a zinc finger. Many other transcription factors, including the IEG product Zif268/Egr1, possess this type of domain, which binds DNA. Experiments involving mutagenesis have demonstrated that dimerization of GR monomers is critical for transcriptional regulation by GREs.

GREs can confer either positive or negative regulation on the genes to which they are linked (see Figure 6–12). Among the first to be characterized as positive was the GRE located in the metallothioneine IIA gene, which encodes a protein that chelates heavy metals. A well-characterized negative GRE is located in the proopiomelanocortin (POMC) gene (see Chapters 10 and 13); it permits glucocorticoids to repress the POMC gene, which encodes adrenocorticotropic hormone (ACTH), and thus acts as an important feedback mechanism by inhibiting further glucocorticoid synthesis.

GRs are responsible for many important physiologic actions that do not appear to be mediated by DNA binding. Moreover, they can interfere with transcriptional activity mediated by other transcription factors—particularly those mediated by AP-1 and NF-κB proteins. Through mechanisms that are not fully understood, GRs appear to interact directly with these proteins to block their ability to activate transcription (see Figure 6–12). Alternatively, glucocorticoids may interfere with NF-κB activity by inducing expression of IκB, the protein that holds NF-κB in the cytoplasm.

Because the lipophilic steroid, thyroid, and retinoid hormones and their nuclear receptors are critical to the development, differentiation, and homeostasis of cells, they are extremely important in CNS pharmacology. Their interactions with various drugs are discussed in Chapters 13 and 15.

Additional members of the nuclear hormone receptor superfamily have been identified in recent years, although the endogenous ligands for many of these receptors are not yet known. Yet there is indirect evidence for their involvement in neural functioning. Nerve growth factor inducible factor B (NGFI-B) and Nurr1, for example, are regulated in the brain by exposure to certain psychotropic drugs, including **cocaine** and **antipsychotic** agents. In addition, retinoid X receptor γ (RXRγ) and retinoic acid receptor α (RARα) are highly concentrated in striatal regions, and mice

lacking these proteins show abnormal behavioral responses to cocaine.

OTHER TRANSCRIPTION FACTORS

The CREB, AP-1, STAT, and steroid hormone receptor families represent just a small portion of the transcription factors that are expressed in neurons and glia. However, other transcription factors are undoubtedly involved in neural signaling. NF-κB is activated by protein kinase C and immunologic signals and most likely assists in regulating neural gene expression. C/EBP and its family members are known to mediate some of the effects of the cAMP pathway on gene expression. Specific protein-1 (SP-1), which binds to the GC-rich regions of many promoters, is often grouped with transcription factors that regulate the basal rate of tran-

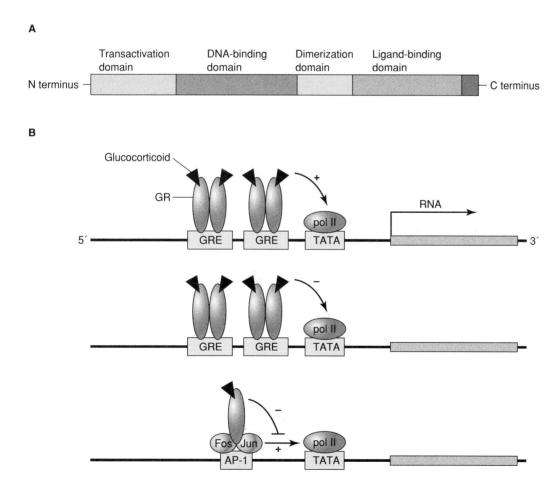

Figure 6–12. The glucocorticoid receptor (GR). **A.** GR domains. **B.** Transcriptional regulation by glucocorticoids and the GR. The idealized promoters represented here contain two glucocorticoid response elements (GREs) or one AP-1 site. GRs act on GREs to activate (*top*) or inhibit (*center*) transcription, and also inhibit AP-1-mediated transcription by binding directly to a Fos-Jun dimer (*bottom*). The TATA box binds the general transcription factors required for activation.

Box 6–5 Transcription Factors as Drug Targets

Most medications used in neurology and psychiatry act directly on neurotransmitter receptors or on proteins that influence levels of neurotransmitters, such as transporters and synthetic enzymes. Collectively, these proteins represent a minute fraction of all proteins expressed in neurons. As discussed in Chapter 5, this diversity currently is being exploited for the development of pharmaceutical agents.

Transcription factors and other proteins involved in the regulation of gene expression may represent viable targets for drugs, particularly if they are expressed in a limited number of cell types or if they exhibit unique temporal patterns (see ΔFosB in Figure 6–11). Conversely, transcription factors such as CREB or c-Fos may not be useful for this purpose because they are ubiquitous. However, efforts to exploit any of these proteins should not be hampered by their location in the nucleus; most drugs that penetrate the blood–brain barrier also cross cell and nuclear membranes.

Although it remains unclear whether protein–DNA binding sites represent suitable targets for drugs, we know that protein–protein interaction domains can be targeted by small molecules. Because most transcription factors bind DNA as dimers or multimeric complexes, these interaction domains may possess the diversity and specificity characteristic of successful pharmaceutical targets. An example is provided by the **thiazolidinedione** drugs, which are used to treat adult-onset (insulin-resistant) **diabetes.** These drugs bind to and activate peroxisome proliferator-activated receptor-γ (PPARγ), a member of the steroid hormone superfamily of nuclear receptors. The PPARγ–thiazolidinedione complex dimerizes with retinoid X receptor (RXR)—another member of the nuclear receptor family—and the dimer binds to target response elements in DNA. Among the genes that contain such response elements are those that encode for proteins that enhance sensitivity to insulin.

scription; however, recent research indicates that some SP-1 family members are subject to dynamic regulation and may mediate transcriptional changes induced by extracellular signals. Activator protein-2 (AP-2) binding sites are present in many genes expressed in the nervous system and have been shown to act synergistically with CREs. Egr family members, including Egr-1 (also known as Zif268), are zinc finger transcription factors that, like c-Fos, are induced rapidly and transiently in the brain by stimuli whose temporal features resemble those of IEGs. The induction of Egr family proteins has been correlated with induction of hippocampal long-term potentiation (see Chapter 20); however, the target genes of these proteins remain poorly characterized.

The functional mechanisms addressed in this chapter are far more intricate than their descriptions suggest. Regulatory regions of genes are often far longer than the coding regions of genes, and regulatory information is contained not only in the 5′ promoter regions of genes but also in intronic and exonic sequences and in 3′ untranscribed regions. Moreover, within the 5′ regions, this chapter focuses on a relatively small number of response elements. Any given gene likely contains many regulatory sites, and these sites do not function in isolation but influence one another. Consequently the temporal and spatial synthesis of multiple signaling pathways affects the expression of most genes. Unraveling this complexity is a daunting task, particularly in vivo, but is likely to yield important clues for understanding neural and behavioral plasticity. One goal of future research, outlined in Box 6–5, is to take advantage of the enormous complexity and

specificity of these mechanisms to generate agents that act more rapidly and more effectively in the treatment of neuropsychiatric disorders.

SELECTED READING

Ahn S, Olive M, Aggarwal S, et al. 1998. A dominant-negative inhibitor of CREB reveals that it is a general mediator of stimulus-dependent transcription of c-Fos. *Mol Cell Biol* 18:967–977.

Amir RE, Van den Veyver IB, Wan M, et al. (1999) Rett syndrome is caused by mutations in X-linked MECP2, encoding methyl-CpG-binding protein 2. *Nature Gen.* 23: 185–188.

Belvin MP, Yin JC. 1997. *Drosophila* learning and memory: Recent progress and new approaches. *Bioessays* 19: 1083–1089.

Berke JD, Paletzki RF, Aronson GJ, et al. 1998. A complex program of striatal gene expression induced by dopaminergic stimulation. *J Neurosci* 18:5301–5310.

Bito H, Deisseroth K, Tsien RW. 1996. CREB phosphorylation and dephosphorylation: A Ca^{2+}- and stimulus duration-dependent switch for hippocampal gene expression. *Cell* 87:1203–1214.

Carey M. Smale ST. 2000. *Transcriptional Regulation in Eukaryotes.* Cold Spring Harbor: Cold Spring Harbor Laboratory Press.

Chong JA, Tapia-Ramirez J, Kim S, et al. 1995. REST: A mammalian silencer protein that restricts sodium channel gene expression to neurons. *Cell* 80:949–957.

De Cesare D, Fimia GM, Sassone-Corsi P. 1999. Signaling routes to CREM and CREB: Plasticity in transcriptional activation. *Trends Biochem Sci* 24:281–285.

Hardingham GE, Chawla S, Cruzalegui SH, Bading H. 1999. Control of recruitment and transcription-activating function of CBP determines gene regulation by NMDA receptors and L-type calcium channels. *Neuron* 22:789–798.

Hill CS, Treisman R. 1995. Transcriptional regulation by extracellular signals: Mechanisms and specificity. *Cell* 80: 199–211.

Jensen KB, Dredge BK, Stefani, et al. 2000. Nova-1 regulates neuron-specific alternative splicing and is essential for neuronal viability. *Neuron* 25:359–371.

Kaplan DR, Miller FD. 2000. Neurotrophin signal transduction in the nervous system. *Curr Opin Neurobiol* 10:381–391.

Karin M. 1995. The regulation of AP-1 activity by mitogen-activated protein kinases. *J Biol Chem* 270:16483–16486.

Karin M. 1998. New twists in gene regulation by glucocorticoid receptor: Is DNA binding dispensable? *Cell* 90: 487–490.

Karin M, Ben-Neriah Y. 2000. Phosphorylation meets ubiquitination: the control of NF-κB activity. *Annu Rev Immunol* 18:621–663.

Kelz MB, Chen JS, Carlezon WA, et al. 1999. Expression of the transcription factor ΔFosB in the brain controls sensitivity to cocaine. *Nature* 401:272–276.

Kornberg RD (1999) Eukaryotic transcriptional control. *Trends Biochem Sci* 24:M46–M49.

Lefstin JA, Yamamoto KR. 1998. Allosteric effects of DNA on transcriptional regulators. *Nature* 392:885–888.

Lin RJ, Kao HY, Ordentlich P, Evans RM. 1998. The transcriptional basis of steroid physiology. *Cold Spring Harb Symp Quant Biol* 63:577–585.

Oike Y, Hata A, Mamiya T, et al. 1999. Truncated CBP protein leads to classic Rubinstein-Taybi syndrome phenotypes in mice: implications for a dominant-negative mechanism. *Human Mol Gen* 8:387–396.

Robertson GS, Matsumura H, Fibiger HC. 1994. Induction patterns of Fos-like immunoreactivity in the forebrain as predictors of atypical antipsychotic activity. *J Pharmacol Exp Ther* 271:1058–1066.

Seeburg PH. 2000. RNA helicase participates in the editing game. *Neuron* 25:261–263.

Struhl K. 1999. Fundamentally different logic of gene regulation in eukaryotes and prokaryotes. *Cell* 98:1–4.

Workman JL, Kingston RE. 1998. Alteration of nucleosome structure as a mechanism of transcriptional regulation. *Annu Rev Biochem* 67:545–579.

PART 2

Neural Substrates of Drug Action

Chapter 7

Excitatory and Inhibitory Amino Acids

KEY CONCEPTS

- The major excitatory neurotransmitter in the brain is glutamate; the major inhibitory neurotransmitter is GABA.

- Glutamate receptors comprise two large families, ligand-gated ion channels called *ionotropic receptors* and G protein-coupled receptors called *metabotropic receptors*.

- Ionotropic glutamate receptors are divided into three classes, AMPA receptors, kainate receptors, and NMDA receptors, which are named after synthetic ligands that activate them.

- In contrast to AMPA receptors and kainate receptors, the NMDA receptor has two important biophysical properties. Because it is highly permeable to calcium and is voltage dependent, it only allows calcium entry if the cell is depolarized.

- AMPA receptors mediate the vast majority of excitatory synaptic transmission in the brain, whereas NMDA receptors play an important role in triggering synaptic plasticity and, when over-activated, in triggering excitotoxicity.

- The eight different subtypes of metabotropic glutamate receptors, when localized to the presynaptic terminal, inhibit neurotransmitter

release, and when localized to the postsynaptic membrane, exert complex modulatory effects through specific signal transduction cascades.

- The $GABA_A$ receptor, a ligand-gated chloride channel, and the $GABA_B$ receptor, a G protein-coupled receptor, are the two major classes of GABA receptors.

- $GABA_A$ receptors, which are highly heterogeneous, mediate the bulk of inhibitory synaptic transmission in the brain. A number of drugs, most notably benzodiazepines and barbiturates, bind to $GABA_A$ receptors and enhance their function.

- $GABA_B$ receptors are localized both presynaptically, where they inhibit neurotransmitter release, and postsynaptically, where they mediate a slow, inhibitory synaptic response.

- Individual excitatory synapses typically express several different subtypes of ionotropic glutamate receptors, such as AMPA and NMDA receptors, as well as metabotropic receptors.

- Glycine, like GABA, is an inhibitory neurotransmitter that activates receptors that are ligand-gated chloride channels. It is critical in inhibitory neurotransmission in the spinal cord and brain stem.

Amino acids, the building blocks of proteins involved in normal intermediary metabolism, are highly concentrated within cells. It is therefore difficult to demonstrate with certainty that amino acids also function as neurotransmitters. However, it has been determined that the amino acids glutamate and, to a lesser extent, aspartate mediate most of the fast excitatory synaptic transmission in the brain; likewise, the amino acids γ-aminobutyric acid (GABA) and, to a lesser extent, glycine mediate most fast inhibitory synaptic transmission. Excitatory amino acids are utilized by nearly every information-bearing circuit in the brain and have been implicated in such diverse pathologic processes as **epilepsy, ischemic brain damage, anxiety,** and **addiction**. In addition, they are necessary for the development of normal synaptic connections. Consequently, amino acid neurotransmitters have been the subject of intensive research during the past two decades. A major advance in the field has been the identification, by molecular cloning techniques, of heterogeneous families of receptors for these neurotransmitters.

GLUTAMATE

THE MAJOR EXCITATORY NEUROTRANSMITTER

Long before glutamate's role in neurotransmission was established, investigators observed that glutamate excites virtually every neuron in the CNS, even at low concentrations. In fact, it is responsible for most neurotransmitter action at excitatory amino acid receptors. Glutamate is present in high concentrations in the adult CNS and can be released in a Ca^{2+}-dependent manner by electrical stimulation in vitro. Autoradiographic, immunohistochemical, and pharmacologic techniques have enabled researchers to identify highly selective receptor binding sites for glutamate. Furthermore, enzymes responsible for glutamate synthesis and degradation are located in both neurons and glial cells, as are high-affinity excitatory amino acid reuptake transporters (EAATs), which terminate the synaptic actions of glutamate. Many of these reuptake and receptor proteins also respond to aspartate, which is believed to mediate transmission at a small number of central excitatory synapses.

SYNTHETIC AND DEGRADATIVE PATHWAYS

Glutamate and aspartate are nonessential amino acids that do not cross the blood–brain barrier and thus are not supplied to the brain by the circulatory system. Instead, they are synthesized in the brain from glucose and a variety of other precursors. Glutamate, which is the reduced form of glutamic acid, is in a metabolic pool with α-oxoglutaric acid and glutamine. Glutamate that is destined to be used for neurotransmission is packaged into synaptic vesicles and released from nerve terminals in response to nerve impulses (Figure 7–1). After it is released, glutamate is primarily taken up by glial cells, where it is converted into glutamine by glutamine synthetase. The resulting glutamine is transported out of glia by system N-1 (SN1), a Na^+- and H^+-dependent pump that is homologous to the vesicular GABA transporter (VGAT). Glutamine is subsequently taken up by glutamatergic nerve cells, by means of a transport process that remains poorly described, and is converted back into glutamate by glutaminase. As discussed later in this chapter, glutamine also replenishes the transmitter pool of GABA.

RELEASE AND REUPTAKE

Synaptic vesicles actively accumulate glutamate through a Mg^{2+}- and adenosine triphosphate (ATP)-dependent uptake process that is driven by an electrical gradient across their membranes. During uptake, concentrations of glutamate in these vesicles are likely to exceed 20 mM. Substances that destroy the electrochemical gradient across vesicles, such as *Evans blue* and related dyes, prevent the concentration of this amino acid. Glutamate's vesicular transporter, extensively characterized biochemically, is highly specific with a low affinity for aspartate; one such trasporter (VGluT1) has been cloned recently. When an action potential arrives in the presynaptic terminal of a neuron, it initiates a complex cascade that results in the fusion of synaptic vesicles with the presynaptic membrane and the liberation of glutamate, which enters the synaptic cleft (see Chapter 4). Glutamate freely diffuses across this narrow cleft to interact with its corresponding receptors on the postsynaptic face of an adjacent cell.

As discussed in Chapter 4, the reuptake of glutamate and aspartate serves to control the extracellular concentrations of these amino acids in the CNS. At least two families of glutamate transporters are located in the plasma membrane. Only the Na^+-dependent transporter is coupled to electrochemical gradients for Na^+, K^+, and H^+. Because such coupling permits the transport of glutamate and aspartate against their concentration gradients, Na^+-dependent glutamate transporters are capable of lowering extracellular glutamate concentrations to submicromolar levels. These transporters take up L-glutamate and L-aspartate with similar affinity and maximum velocity (V_{max}). Unlike many stereoselective transporters in the CNS, they also transport the D isomer of aspartate; however, they do not trans-

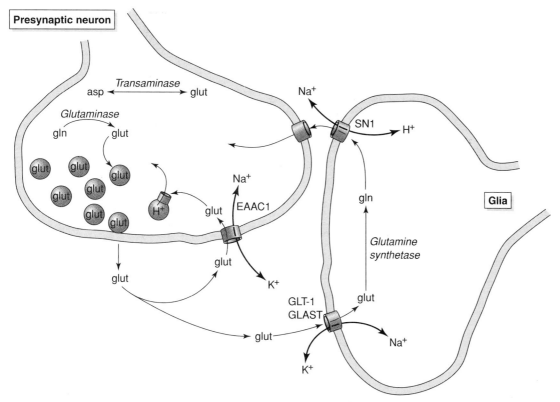

Figure 7–1. Synthesis and degradation of the neurotransmitter pool of glutamate. In the mitochondrial compartment of glutamatergic nerve terminals, glutamine (gln) is converted to glutamate (glut) by the enzyme glutaminase. Alternatively, glutamate is synthesized by the transamination of aspartate (asp) by transaminase. Newly synthesized glutamate is packaged into synaptic vesicles by means of a Mg^{2+}- and ATP-dependent proton gradient-coupled uptake process. After it is released from nerve terminals, most of it is taken up into glial cells, where it is converted into glutamine by glutamine synthetase. Glutamine is then pumped out of the glia by SN1 and taken up by nerve terminals, where it is converted back to glutamate to replenish the transmitter pool. Uptake of glutamate into glial (and to a lesser extent, neural) compartments is achieved by the Na^+-dependent glutamate transporters GLT-1, GLAST, and EAAC1.

port D-glutamate. Glutamate transport is electrogenic: three Na^+ ions and one H^+ ion are translocated with every molecule of glutamate transported in exchange for the outward movement of one K^+ ion. Such exchange results in the net inward movement of positive charge during each transport cycle.

Four principal members of the high-affinity Na^+-dependent family of glutamate transporters have been cloned from rat and salamander: GLAST (glutamate-aspartate transporter), GLT-1 (glutamate transporter-1), EAAC1 (excitatory amino acid carrier-1), and sEAAT5 (salamander excitatory amino acid transporter-5). The human homologs of these transporters are EAAT1, EAAT2, EAAT3, and EAAT5, respectively; in addition, EAAT4 has been cloned from human motor cortex. Each of these transporters belongs to a large superfamily whose members transport a wide range of neurotransmitters and related substances (see Chapters 4, 8,

and 9). Considerable evidence suggests that the cloned transporters GLAST and GLT-1, which are expressed by glial cells, are responsible for the majority of glutamate uptake in the CNS (see Figure 7–1).

Several pathologic conditions, such as **ischemia**, can lead to the accumulation of glutamate or aspartate in extracellular spaces, which results in the excessive activation of glutamate receptors (see Chapter 21). Such activation can in turn cause a variety of pathologic changes and can in its extreme form result in cell death. Glutamate transporters limit the concentrations of free glutamate and aspartate in extracellular spaces, and thereby prevent the excessive stimulation of glutamate receptors. Consequently, agents capable of facilitating transporter function might limit the damage caused by ischemia and other neurologic insults that produce an increase in extracellular glutamate. Currently, however, only inhibitors of glutamate transporters are available. Two such inhibitors are D,L-threo-3-hydroxyaspartate (**THA**), a broad-spectrum antagonist of glutamate and aspartate transport, and dihydrokainate (**DHK**), an inhibitor selective for the glial GLT-1 transporter. Although these drugs are useful experimental tools, they have no apparent clinical use.

GLUTAMATE RECEPTORS

Glutamate receptors comprise two large families: the ionotropic and the metabotropic receptors. The glutamate binding site and associated ion channel for ionotropic glutamate receptors are incorporated into the same macromolecular complex. Agonists at these receptors act to increase a channel's tendency to open. Three classes of ionotropic glutamate receptors, *N*-methyl-D-aspartate (**NMDA**), α-amino-3-hydroxy-5-methyl-4-isoxazole propionic acid (**AMPA**), and **kainate,** were originally named based on the ability of these drugs to serve as selective agonists (Table 7–1).

Table 7–1 Glutamate Receptors

Ionotropic

Functional Classes	Gene Families	Agonists	Antagonists
AMPA	GluR1	Glutamate	CNQX
	GluR2	AMPA	NBQX
	GluR3	Kainate	GYK153655
	GluR4	(S)-5-flurowillardine	
Kainate	GluR5	Glutamate	CNQX
	GluR6	Kainate	LY294486
	GluR7	ATPA	
	KA1		
	KA2		
NMDA	NR1	Glutamate	D-AP5, D-APV
	NR2A	Aspartate	2R-CPPene
	NR2B	NMDA	MK-801
	NR2C		Ketamine
	NR2D		Phencyclidine

Metabotropic

Group I	mGluR1	1S, 3R-ACPD	AIDA
	mGluR5	DHPG	CBPG
Group II	mGluR2	1S, 3R-ACPD	EGLU
	mGluR3	DCG-IV	PCCG-4
		APDC	
Group III	mGluR4	L-AP4	MAP4
	mGluR6	1S, 3R-ACPD	MPPG
	mGluR7		
	mGluR8		

It has since been determined that these classifications are represented by distinct families of receptor genes.

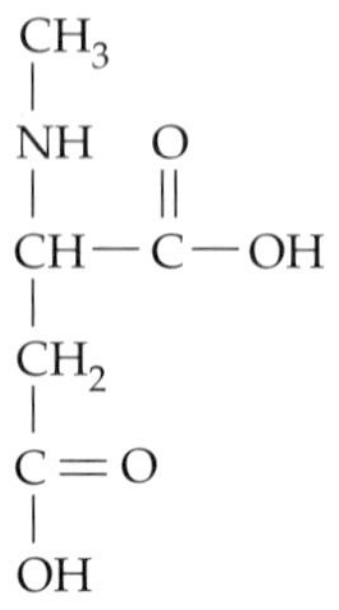

NMDA

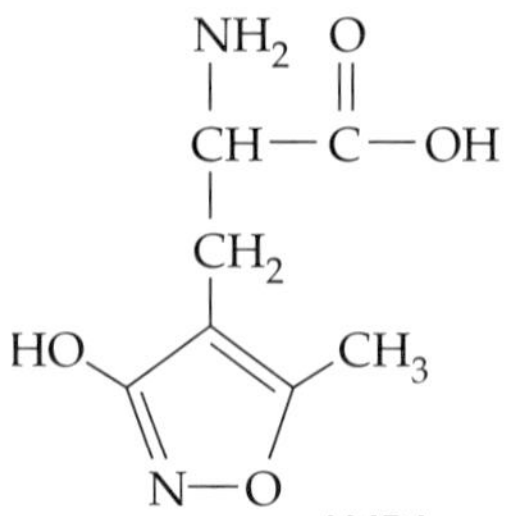

AMPA

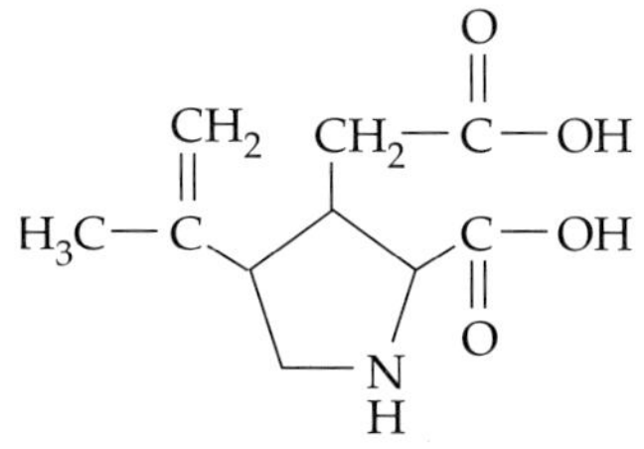

Kainic acid

Metabotropic glutamate receptors belong to the large superfamily of G protein-coupled receptors. These receptors, which are characterized by seven transmembrane domains, couple to G proteins and in turn mediate the biologic effects of receptor activation (see Chapters 4 and 5). The term *metabotropic* was used to indicate that these receptors affect cellular metabolic processes, unlike the ionotropic receptors, which form ion channels. However, this nomenclature is highly misleading because metabotropic glutamate receptors, like other G protein-coupled receptors, can exert profound effects on neuronal function through the regulation of ion channels, second messenger cascades, and protein phosphorylation.

Mediation of fast excitatory transmission Synaptically released glutamate interacts with postsynaptic receptors located on immediately adjacent cells or on the nerve terminals from which glutamate is released (see Chapter 4). The binding of glutamate to AMPA and NMDA receptors opens postsynaptic cation channels and initiates a two-component excitatory postsynaptic current (EPSC) at most central synapses (Figure 7–2). Considerable evidence suggests that AMPA and NMDA receptors co-localize at many functional excitatory synapses. However, the ratio of AMPA to NMDA receptors at individual synapses can vary greatly; indeed, some synapses may contain only NMDA or AMPA receptors. In contrast, only a small number of kainate receptors are present in most CNS regions.

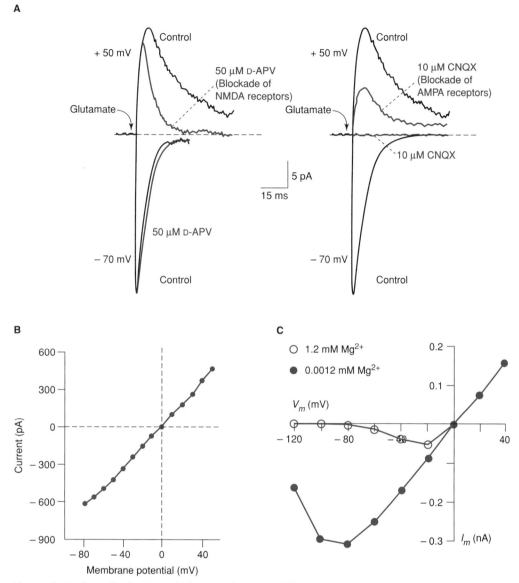

Figure 7–2. Synaptically released glutamate interacts with postsynaptic AMPA and NMDA receptors. **A.** Excitatory postsynaptic currents (EPSCs) caused by glutamate in a hippocampal neuron. When glutamate binds to NMDA and AMPA receptors, postsynaptic cation channels open, initiating a two-component EPSC. These components can be pharmacologically separated. Blockade of NMDA receptors by the antagonist D-APV (*left*) reveals a rapid AMPA receptor-mediated component of the EPSC. Conversely, blockade of AMPA receptors by CNQX (*right*) reveals a slowly rising and decaying NMDA receptor-mediated component of the EPSC at positive voltages. In contrast, application of D-APV at negative voltages (*lower left*) reveals little NMDA receptor contribution to the EPSC due to the profound block of these channels by Mg^{2+} ions. **B.** The current–voltage relationship for AMPA receptors. This relationship is roughly linear and reverses at approximately 0 mV, indicating that the channels do not discriminate well between Na^+ and K^+ ions. **C.** The current–voltage relationship for NMDA receptors. The concentration of Mg^{2+} in the extracellular fluid of the brain (approximately 1 mM) is sufficient to virtually abolish ion flux through NMDA receptor channels at membrane potentials close to resting potential (approximately -70 mV). As the membrane potential becomes less negative or even positive, the affinity of Mg^{2+} for its binding site decreases, permitting the passage of ionic current. Removal of extracellular Mg^{2+} linearizes the current–voltage relationship and permits significant current flow at negative voltages.

The activation of an AMPA receptor mediates a synaptic current that has a rapid onset and decay, whereas the current mediated by a NMDA receptor has a slower onset and a decay that lasts as long as several milliseconds (see Figure 7–2). The decay time of the NMDA receptor-mediated current is approximately 100 times longer than the mean open time of its channel. Such prolonged activation is believed to be caused by glutamate's high affinity (K_d = 3–8 nM) for and consequent slow dissociation from these receptors. In contrast, glutamate has a much lower affinity for AMPA receptors (K_d = 200 nM), from which it rapidly dissociates.

The slower time course of NMDA receptor activation may provide a mechanism by which temporal or spatial summation of synaptic transmission can occur. The depolarization caused by one input may allow other synaptic inputs or nonsynaptic membrane channels to initiate action potential firing. Thus their slow activation, in conjunction with their special voltage dependence (described later in this chapter), allow NMDA receptors to act as coincidence detectors that can sense the activity of many independent synaptic inputs converging on the same cell (Figure 7–3; see Chapter 20).

AMPA receptors: physiology and pharmacology

Current is carried through AMPA receptors primarily by the movement of Na^+ from the extracellular space into the intracellular compartment. However, because the reversal potential of current (the membrane potential at which net current flow is zero; see Chapter 3) through AMPA channels is close to 0 mV, an outward current carried by K^+ must counterbalance the inward flow of Na^+ ions. The resulting current–voltage relationship for these AMPA receptors is roughly linear (see Figure 7–2). Experimentally, Cs^+ can be substituted for K^+ to maintain the reversal potential at a value close to zero; thus AMPA channels most likely do not discriminate well among Na^+, K^+, and Cs^+ ions.

Some AMPA receptors, on neurons and astrocytes in structures as diverse as the striatum, hippocampus, and cerebellum, are also permeable to Ca^{2+}. The translocation of Ca^{2+} from the extracellular space to the intracellular compartment plays a key role in the regulation of several second messenger systems (see Chapters 5, 20, and 21). Thus the permeability of some AMPA receptors to Ca^{2+} may have great functional importance, particularly in cells that do not contain NMDA receptors, which always flux Ca^{2+}. Some AMPA receptor channels that are permeable to Ca^{2+} exhibit a rectifying type of current–voltage relationship (see Chapter 3). This relationship results when intracellular **polyamines** such as **spermine** and **spermidine** prohibit current from passing through these ion channels.

AMPA receptors also can be blocked selectively by certain quinoxaline diones, the most notable of which is 6-nitro-7-sulphamobenzo-quinoxaline 2,3-dione (**NBQX;** see Table 7–1). NBQX is a potent and selective competitive antagonist of AMPA receptors; its effect on other receptors is weak or nonexistent. Drugs in the 2,3-benzodiazepine class, such as **GYKI 53655,** are noncompetitive antagonists of AMPA receptors and show promise as neuroprotective drugs for the treatment of **stroke**. Because it has minimal effects on kainate or NMDA receptors, this class of drug permits unequivocal separation of the AMPA receptors from other categories of glutamate receptors.

AMPA receptors desensitize within milliseconds of exposure to AMPA, and kainate receptors desensitize just as swiftly after exposure to kainate. Currently, AMPA and kainate receptors can be reliably distinguished from one another only by their response to two drugs, **cyclothiazide** and the lectin **concanavalin A**. Cyclothiazide relieves AMPA receptor desensitization but does not affect kainate receptors. Concanavalin A relieves the desensitization of kainate receptors, most likely by interacting with surface sugar chains, but has insignificant effects on AMPA receptors. Until selective

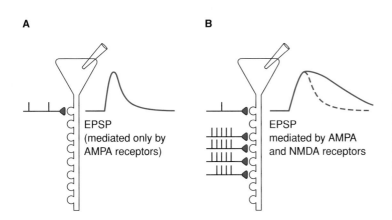

Figure 7–3. The NMDA glutamate receptor as a coincidence detector. **A.** A single synaptic input results in the generation of a short-lasting excitatory postsynaptic potential (EPSP) that is mediated entirely by AMPA receptors. **B.** When multiple inputs occur simultaneously, the same single synaptic input generates a longer-lasting EPSP that is mediated by both AMPA and NMDA receptors. Thus the NMDA receptor can "sense" the activity in adjacent inputs.

kainate receptor antagonists are developed, these two drugs, together with GYKI 53655, are the most valuable agents for determining whether a given synaptic current is mediated by AMPA or kainate receptors.

Molecular composition of AMPA and kainate receptors

Three families of ionotropic glutamate receptor subunits, encoded by at least 16 genes, assemble to form functional AMPA, kainate, or NMDA receptors (see Table 7–1). Within each family there is greater than 80% identity at the amino acid level over membrane spanning domains. Between families, a lower degree of identity exists (~50%). Ionotropic glutamate receptors are believed to exist as pentamers. Different subunit combinations produce functionally different glutamate receptors. Moreover, in situ hybridization and immunohistochemistry have revealed striking regional differences in the expression of genes that encode these subunits. Such differences illustrate the rich diversity of glutamate receptors throughout the CNS.

Four subunits, termed GluR1 through GluR4 (or GluRA through GluRD), coassemble with one another to form proteins whose pharmacologic profiles are identical to those of AMPA receptors. Each of these subunits is encoded by a distinct gene, and each exists in two forms, termed *flip* and *flop*. The flip and flop forms are generated by alternative splicing, exhibit region-specific patterns of expression in the brain, and give rise to receptors that differ in desensitization rates. The best characterized AMPA receptor subunit is GluR1, which is predicted to be 889 amino acids long; other ionotropic receptor subunits, such as those of nicotinic, GABA$_A$, or glycine receptors, are approximately 420 amino acids long (Table 7–2). The extra length of GluR1 results from an unusually large N-terminal extracellular domain.

Table 7–2 Molecular Masses of Representative Ionotropic Receptor Subunits

Subunit	Molecular Mass, (kDa)	No. of Amino Acid Residues
NMDAR1	103.4	920
NR2A	162.8	1442
NR2B	163.2	1456
NR2C	133.3	1218
NR2D-1	143.7	1333
NR2D-2	140.7	1300
GluR1	99.6	889
GluR5-1	100.8	890
KA1	104.9	936
ACh α	50.1	437
GABA$_A$ α$_1$	48.7	429
Gly α$_1$	48.4	422
5-HT$_2$	58.6	465

Based on heterologous expression systems in vitro, subunits GluR5 through GluR7 appear to coassemble with KA1 or KA2 subunits to form functional kainate receptors. Experiments with radioligands have revealed that homomeric GluR5, GluR6, and GluR7 receptors expressed in mammalian cell lines bind [^{3}H]-kainate with an affinity of approximately 80–100 nM. These homomeric receptors may correspond to low-affinity kainate binding sites previously identified in membrane fractions of the brain. In contrast, homomeric KA1 receptors bind kainate with an affinity of 4 nM and may correspond to high-affinity kainate binding sites in the brain. However, when they are expressed alone, KA1 and KA2 are virtually inactive because they lack functional channels. Consequently, it is believed that they serve as modulatory subunits that confer high-affinity kainate binding on channels formed by GluR5 through GluR7.

As previously indicated, the AMPA and kainate glutamate receptor families have a topology that differs from that of certain other ligand-gated ion channels, such as GABA$_A$ and glycine receptors (Figure 7–4). Glutamate receptor subunits possess only three transmembrane spanning domains. What appears to be an abridged transmembrane domain, located between M2 and M3 in glutamate subunits, is a reentrant loop whose ends both face the cytoplasm. Homology mapping of glutamate receptors onto the crystal structure of bacterial amino acid-binding proteins suggests that agonist binding requires portions of both the large N terminus and the short region between M2 and M3 (see Figure 7–4).

AMPA receptors lacking the GluR2 subunit are highly permeable to Ca^{2+} ions. This Ca^{2+} permeability has been traced to a single amino acid in the reentrant loop of GluR2, which is known as the Q/R site (see Figure 7–4). In GluR1, GluR3, and GluR4, a glutamine (Q) resides at this position, but in GluR2 an arginine (R) is present. When heteromeric receptors contain GluR2 they are relatively impermeable to calcium, most likely because the positive charge of the arginine residue repels Ca^{2+} from the channel pore. The replacement of glutamine with arginine in GluR2 occurs because of a special form of *RNA editing*: the gene for GluR2 encodes a glutamine, and the resulting form of GluR2 is expressed in various regions of the brain during development. However, virtually all of the GluR2 mRNA present in adult mammalian brain is edited to a codon that encodes arginine at this site. This editing changes a single base within GluR2 transcripts by RNA editing enzymes. Inhibition of such RNA editing in mice by molecular genetic means can be lethal, presumably because many AMPA receptors that normally are Ca^{2+} impermeable become Ca^{2+} permeable,

A AMPA receptors (GluR1-4)

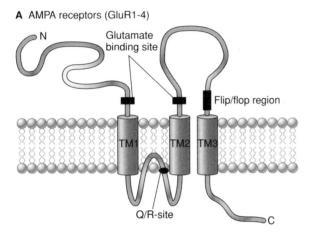

B GABA and glycine receptors

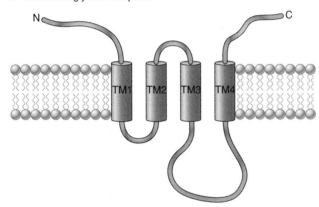

Figure 7–4. Membrane topology of AMPA glutamate, GABA$_A$, and glycine receptors. **A.** AMPA glutamate receptor subunits (GluR1-4) possess only three transmembrane spanning domains. The channel lining domain between TM1 and TM2 is a reentrant loop with both ends facing the cytoplasm. The Q/R site, which controls the Ca^{2+} permeability of AMPA receptor subunits, is located in this loop. The flip-flop site, located extracellularly between TM2 and TM3, yields two splice variants of each subunit. The glutamate binding site of AMPA receptors is formed by several amino acids in the N-terminal and extracellular loop. **B.** In contrast to AMPA receptors, GABA$_A$ and glycine receptors possess four putative membrane-spanning domains.

making cells vulnerable to the neurotoxic effects of excessive intracellular Ca^{2+}.

In addition to Ca^{2+} permeability, the Q/R site of GluR2 influences the single channel conductance properties of associated AMPA receptors and the sensitivity of the receptor complex to blockage by **polyamine spider toxins** and endogenous **polyamines**. AMPA receptors that do not contain edited GluR2 show greater overall conductance. In addition, they show voltage-dependent inhibition at positive membrane potentials by endogenous, intracellular polyamines, which gives rise to inward rectification.

The flip and flop splice variants of receptor subunits GluR1 through GluR4, together with the products of Q/R editing, represent a wide range of proteins yielded by genes that encode these subunits. This diversity provides neurons with an extraordinary degree of flexibility in the construction of a large number of AMPA receptors. The degree of AMPA receptor heterogeneity employed by neurons in vivo remains unknown. Although Ca^{2+}-permeable AMPA receptors are consistently found at excitatory synapses on GABAergic interneurons—whereas most principal cells (i.e., projection neurons) express Ca^{2+}-impermeable AMPA receptors that contain the edited form of GluR2—the physiologic significance of these findings remains to be determined.

Although AMPA receptors function primarily as ion channels, there are recent reports that they also may produce physiologic effects by other mechanisms. Activation of AMPA receptors by glutamate has been shown to stimulate the protein tyrosine kinase Lyn, which leads to the activation of MAP-kinase signaling pathways (see Chapter 11). Stimulation of Lyn is independent of AMPA receptor-mediated Na^{+} and Ca^{2+} influx. The physiologic importance of this mechanism is still being investigated, but this finding underscores the notion that neurotransmitter receptors may act through several distinct signaling mechanisms to produce their myriad effects on target neurons.

NMDA receptors: physiology and pharmacology NMDA receptors have several properties that set them apart from other ligand-gated receptors. At membrane potentials more negative than approximately −50 mV, the concentration of Mg^{2+} in the extracellular fluid of the brain is sufficient to virtually abolish ion flux through NMDA receptor channels, even in the presence of glutamate. Thus at resting membrane potentials of approximately −70 mV, the activation of these receptors results in little current flow, even when glutamate or aspartate is bound to the receptor, because the entry of Mg^{2+} into the channel pore blocks the movement of monovalent ions across the channel.

In the presence of Mg^{2+} ions, this receptor's current–voltage relationship has a region of slope-negativity that produces a characteristic J shape when plotted (see Figure 7–2). As the receptor's membrane potential becomes less negative, the affinity of Mg^{2+} for its binding site decreases, and the blocking action of Mg^{2+} becomes ineffective; consequently, ionic current can pass through the channel. As it enters the ion channel, Mg^{2+} undergoes slow dehydration so that its own passage through the channel is impeded; accordingly, Mg^{2+} rapidly moves in and out of the open channel, giving rise to a flickery channel block in single-channel recordings. This blocking action is mimicked by a variety of divalent cations, including Co^{2+}, Mn^{2+}, and Ni^{2+}, but is not produced by Zn^{2+}.

As previously mentioned, NMDA receptors are often thought of as coincidence detectors that are capable of sensing simultaneous, repetitive activity at a number of adjacent synapses (see Figure 7–3). They have this capability because at individual synapses they are believed to function only when they are activated by synaptically released glutamate and when adjacent synaptic inputs occur repetitively. Repetitive stimulation is required because the depolarization produced by single inputs is not sufficient to relieve the blockage of the NMDA receptor channel by Mg^{2+}.

The activation of NMDA receptors, like that of AMPA receptors, produces a nonspecific increase in permeability to the monovalent cations Na^+ and K^+. However, unlike most AMPA and kainate receptors in the adult CNS, NMDA receptors are highly permeable to Ca^{2+}; in fact, their permeability to Ca^{2+} is approximately 10-fold greater than their permeability to Na^+. Several other divalent cations can also permeate these receptors, with the following relative permeability: $Ca^{2+} > Ba^{2+} > Sr^{2+} \gg Mn^{2+}$. Thus, although their activation results in appreciable current and tends to depolarize the cell membrane toward the threshold for action potential firing, such activity is unlikely to represent the primary function of these receptors when activated at resting membrane potentials. Instead, researchers believe that NMDA receptors provide one of the most significant mechanisms by which synaptic activity can increase the level of intracellular Ca^{2+} at individual synapses.

NMDA receptor agonists, such as glutamate, aspartate, and NMDA, typically are short-chain dicarboxylic amino acids. Glutamate, which acts at the conventional binding site, is the most potent agonist endogenous to the mammalian brain. NMDA, although a very selective agonist at these receptors, is 30-fold less potent than glutamate in electrophysiologic assays.

Competitive antagonists of the glutamate recognition site are formed from corresponding agonists whose carbon chains have been extended, often in a ring structure; in addition, the agonist's ω-carboxyl group is typically replaced in the antagonist by a phosphonic acid group. Numerous competitive antagonists of this recognition site are available, notably D-2-amino-5-phosphonopentanoic acid (**AP-5**) and 3-(2-carboxypiperazin-4-yl)1-propenyl-1-phosphonic acid (**2R-CPPene**); however, these compounds are polar and penetrate the blood–brain barrier poorly. Several competitive NMDA receptor blockers developed recently have better access to the brain.

The NMDA receptor is unique among all neurotransmitter receptors in that its activation requires the simultaneous binding of two different agonists. In addition to the binding of glutamate at the conventional agonist-binding site, the binding of glycine appears to be required for receptor activation (Figure 7–5). Because neither of these agonists alone can open this ion channel, glutamate and glycine are referred to as coagonists of the NMDA receptor. The physiologic significance of the glycine binding site is unclear because the normal extracellular concentration of glycine is believed to be saturating; however, some contradictory evidence suggest that extracellular glycine concentrations may be physiologically regulated. Nevertheless, the glycine site on the NMDA receptor may prove to be an important drug target. **Cycloserine,** originally developed as an antitubercular drug, is a weak partial agonist at this site and thus can modulate NMDA receptor function in vitro and in vivo. Cycloserine is reported to enhance the effects of **antipsychotic** drugs in patients with **schizophrenia.** More specific agonists, such as **HA966,** have been used in laboratory animals but are not yet available for clinical investigation. Derivatives of **kynurenic acid,** such as 5,7-dichlorokynurenic acid (**5,7-DCK**) and **quinolinecarboxylic acid,** are also competitive antagonists at the glycine site. It is important to note that the glycine site on NMDA receptors is distinct from the **strychnine**-sensitive glycine receptor, which mediates the neurotransmitter functions of glycine.

Another important binding site on the NMDA glutamate receptor exists for **phencyclidine (PCP or "angel dust")** and related drugs such as **MK801** and **ketamine** (see Figure 7–5). These drugs, which bind at or near the Mg^{2+}-binding site, occlude the NMDA receptor channel. Thus they act as noncompetitive receptor antagonists, and their actions, like those of Mg^{2+}, are somewhat voltage dependent. These drugs exert potent effects on the brain. At lower concentrations they are **psychotomimetic** and produce effects, such as cognitive defects, hallucinations, and delusions, that are similar to some of the symptoms of **schizophrenia** (see Chapter

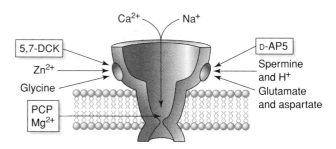

Figure 7–5. Pharmacologic binding sites of the NMDA receptor. Sites for drugs that promote receptor function (Na^+ and Ca^{2+} influx) appear in normal type, and sites for drugs that inhibit receptor function appear in boxes.

17). At higher doses, these drugs are **dissociative anesthetics**. Many are used predominantly in veterinary practice; however, **ketamine** has been used successfully as a pediatric anesthetic because children are less likely than adults to exhibit psychotic-like side effects. Interestingly, doses of **ethanol** associated with the upper range of intoxication in humans exert effects on NMDA receptors that are similar to those produced by phencyclidine and related drugs.

An important endogenous allosteric modulator of NMDA receptor activation is pH. Protons limit the frequency with which NMDA receptor channels open, such that at a pH of 6.0, receptor activation is almost completely suppressed. The effect of pH on these receptors suggests that an ionizable histidine or cysteine residue may play a key role in their activation. In addition, NMDA receptors have one or more modulatory sites that bind polyamines. The occupancy of one of these sites relieves tonic proton block and thereby potentiates NMDA receptor activation in a pH-dependent manner. At higher concentrations, however, polyamines act on an extracellular site to produce a voltage-dependent block of the ion channel and consequently inhibit receptor activation.

Because they mediate a large number of important physiologic functions, and also contribute to cell damage and death when they are overactivated (see Chapter 21), NMDA receptors are a compelling target for therapeutic drugs. Many drugs that target these receptors have been developed and are being tested in clinical trials for conditions, such as stroke or head trauma, in which excitotoxicity may play a significant role. However, compounds with clear efficacy and tolerable side effects have yet to be identified. The large number of modulatory sites on the NMDA receptor increase the likelihood that clinically useful compounds will be discovered.

Molecular composition of NMDA receptors

Two families of NMDA receptor subunits have been identified. One family is represented by a single gene (NR1) that encodes proteins composed of approximately 900 amino acids; the other is represented by four genes (NR2A–NR2D; see Tables 7–1 and 7–2) that encode proteins composed of approximately 1450 amino acids. Although homomeric NR1 receptors appear to possess all of the pharmacologic features characteristic of bona fide NMDA receptors, recent evidence suggests that the physiologically relevant glutamate-binding site is located on the NR2 subunit. Moreover, the very small currents supported by homomeric NR1 receptors increase by more than 100-fold when such receptors are coexpressed with NR2 subunits. Thus it is believed that NMDA receptors in the brain exist as NR1–NR2 heteromeric complexes.

More than nine splice variants of NR1 have been cloned. These variants differ with regard to their regional patterns of expression in the CNS, their regulation (e.g., by phosphorylation, polyamines, Zn^{2+}, and protons), the electrophysiologic properties of channels they form, and their affinity for elements of the neuronal cytoskeleton. Such distinguishing features suggest that these variants may be involved in different components of the synapse.

The subtype of NR2 subunit that combines with NR1 subunits can influence the biophysical and pharmacologic properties of endogenous NMDA receptors. A well-documented example of this phenomenon occurs during early postnatal development, when many synaptic NMDA receptors are composed of NR1 and NR2B. This subunit combination yields a receptor that produces very long-lasting synaptic responses and one that is strongly inhibited by the NMDA receptor antagonist **ifenprodil**. Gradually during the first few weeks of development, the NR2B subunit is replaced by NR2A (and perhaps NR2C), yielding a receptor that produces shorter synaptic currents and that is no longer sensitive to ifenprodil. The mechanism of action of ifenprodil is unknown.

In addition to the many regulatory mechanisms that have been described for NMDA receptors (see Figure 7–5), an interesting form of Ca^{2+}-dependent inactivation of these receptors is brought about by the Ca^{2+}-binding protein calmodulin. In response to Ca^{2+} entry, calmodulin interacts with the C-terminal domain of the NR1 subunit, reducing the frequency with which the receptor channel opens and also the length of time that it remains open. In addition, calcineurin, a $Ca^{2+}/$calmodulin-dependent protein phosphatase, inactivates NMDA receptors by dephosphorylating them. Thus one form of NMDA receptor modulation may occur through a two-step process, whereby the receptor undergoes dephosphorylation and subsequent binding to Ca^{2+}-calmodulin.

Metabotropic glutamate receptors

Eight metabotropic glutamate receptors, termed mGluR1 through mGluR8, have been cloned (see Table 7–1). mGluRs are considerably larger than other G protein-coupled receptors, and a comparison of their amino acid sequences with those of other receptors reveals little homology or common features. Thus mGluRs constitute a new family of receptors. Like other G protein-coupled receptors, mGluRs contain seven membrane-spanning domains; however, like the ionotropic receptors, they also possess an unusually large N-terminal extracellular domain that precedes the membrane-spanning segments (Figure 7–6).

mGluRs comprise three functional groups based on amino acid sequence homology, agonist pharmacology,

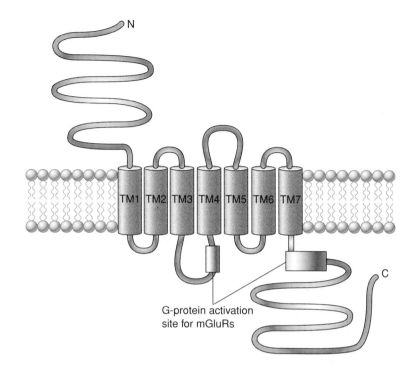

Figure 7–6. Proposed membrane topology of mGluRs and GABA$_B$ receptors. mGluRs and GABA$_B$ receptors contain seven transmembrane domains and are members of the G protein-coupled receptor superfamily. These receptors can be distinguished from most other G protein-coupled receptors by their unusually large extracellular N-terminal domains. In mGluRs, the second intracellular loop and the intracellular C-terminal domain determine the specificity of G protein coupling. The G protein-interaction domains of GABA$_B$ receptors have not yet been identified.

and the signal transduction pathways to which they are coupled. Group I comprises mGluR1 and mGluR5; group II, mGluR2 and mGluR3; and group III, mGluR4, mGluR6, MGluR7, and mGluR8. Members of each group share approximately 70% sequence homology, with approximately 45% homology exhibited between groups. Alternatively spliced variants also have been described for mGluR1, mGluR4, mGluR5, and mGluR7.

The classification of mGluRs into three groups is supported by their signal transduction mechanisms. Group I mGluRs stimulate phospholipase C activity by means of the G protein G$_q$, and thereby release Ca^{2+} from cytoplasmic stores through IP$_3$. Yet group I mGluRs vary in their ability to increase intracellular Ca^{2+} levels, most likely because each receptor has a different affinity for G$_q$ (see Chapter 5). Activation of phospholipase C leads to the formation of not only IP$_3$ but also diacylglycerol, which, in conjunction with increases in intracellular Ca^{2+}, activates protein kinase C. In contrast to group I mGluRs, group II and group III mGluRs inhibit adenylyl cyclase and regulate specific K$^+$ and Ca^{2+} ion channels, actions believed to be mediated by G proteins of the G$_i$ family.

Glutamate itself activates all of the recombinant mGluRs, with potencies that range from 2 nM for mGluR8 to 1 μM for mGluR7. Highly selective agonists for each of the three groups also have been identified. 3,5-dihydroxyphenylglycine (**DHPG**) appears to be a selective group I agonist; 2*R*,4*R*-4-aminopyrrolidine-2-4-dicarboxylate (**APDC**) is a highly selective and moder-

ately potent (400 nM) agonist for group II mGluRs; and L-amino-4-phosphonobutyrate (**L-AP4**) is a selective agonist of the group III mGluRs. A recently developed group II-selective mGluR agonist, termed **LY354740,** is currently in clinical development as an **anti-anxiety** (and possibly **antipsychotic**) agent, as discussed later in this chapter. mGluR antagonists include some phenylglycine derivatives, but most of these do not distinguish among the various groups of receptors.

Modulation of ion channel activity mGluRs located on the postsynaptic membrane modulate a variety of ligand- and voltage-gated ion channels expressed on central neurons (Figure 7–7). An unexpected related finding is that glutamate or **L-AP4** can act on group III mGluRs in retinal bipolar neurons to close Na$^+$-selective ion channels, thereby causing membrane hyperpolarization. This discovery is surprising because glutamate usually depolarizes central neurons. The hyperpolarization is brought about by the activation of a G protein that in turn appears to activate a phosphodiesterase. The latter hydrolyzes a cyclic nucleotide that normally maintains the Na$^+$ channel in an open state.

The activation of each of the three groups of mGluRs has been found to inhibit L-type voltage-gated Ca^{2+} channels, and groups I and II are capable of inhibiting N-type Ca^{2+} channels. mGluRs also decrease high-threshold Ca^{2+} currents in spiking neurons of *Xenopus* retina. Moreover, mGluR activation closes voltage-gated K$^+$ channels in hippocampal neurons, in neurons of the nucleus tractus solitarius, and in cholinergic interneurons of the caudate putamen. Such closure of voltage-gated K^+ channels produces a slow depolarization and results in neuronal excitation. The exact mechanism by which mGluRs modulate K^+ currents is not yet clear. In cerebellar granule cells, mGluRs increase the activity of Ca^{2+}-dependent K^+ channels, termed *BK channels*, and thereby reduce cell excitability. mGluRs also activate G protein-coupled, inwardly rectifying K^+ channels. Thus postsynaptic mGluRs can have a wide range of effects, depending on the cell type involved and the mGluR subtype that is activated.

Mediation of presynaptic inhibition at excitatory synapses   Immunohistochemical studies at both light and electron microscopic levels have firmly established that several types of mGluRs are located on the presynaptic terminals of central neurons. The activation of presynaptic mGluRs blocks both excitatory glutamatergic and inhibitory GABAergic synaptic transmission in many CNS regions (see Figure 7–7). Experiments designed to identify the locus of mGluR action have suggested that mGluR agonists exert a direct effect on receptors located on presynaptic terminals. In the hippocampus, mossy fiber-evoked EPSPs on CA3 pyramidal neurons are blocked by **DCG-IV,** which acts on presynaptic group II mGluRs located on granule cell terminals. Similar effects have been observed throughout the cerebral neocortex. In contrast, synaptic transmission between Schaeffer collaterals and CA1 pyramidal cells is resistant to DCG-IV but is reduced by **L-AP4,** suggesting that group III mGluRs modulate presynaptic function. One mechanism by which activation of mGluRs decreases neurotransmitter release may involve the inhibition of voltage-gated Ca^{2+} channels on

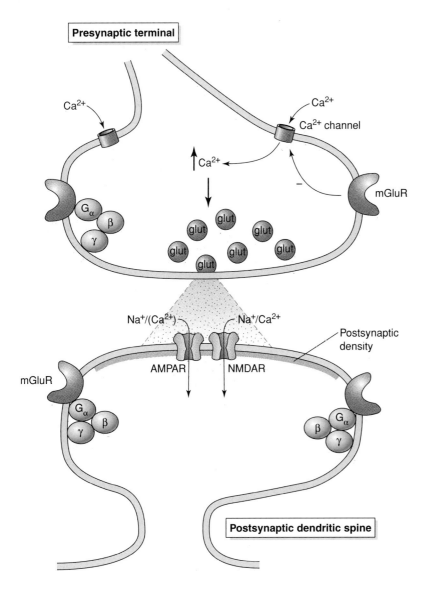

Figure 7–7. Typical excitatory synapse. AMPA and NMDA receptors (AMPAR, NMDAR), which are ionotropic, and mGluRs, which are G protein-coupled, are all localized in the postsynaptic spine but have different subcellular locations. mGluRs are also located on the presynaptic terminal, where they act as inhibitory autoreceptors, in part by reducing Ca^{2+} influx. Not shown are kainate receptors, which can have either postsynaptic or presynaptic locations, depending on the synapse.

the presynaptic nerve terminal membrane. Such activity has been observed directly at certain glutamatergic synapses, where mGluR agonists suppress voltage-gated P/Q-type Ca^{2+} channels and thereby inhibit transmitter release. Accordingly, mGluRs most likely function as inhibitory autoreceptors at many glutamatergic nerve terminals.

The numerous effects that mGluRs can have on both postsynaptic cells and presynaptic terminals is confusing, especially because the conditions under which these receptors are physiologically activated are not always clear. Yet the diversity that characterizes mGluRs and their actions promises to further the development of subtype-specific drugs for the treatment of neuropsychiatric disorders. **LY354740,** for example, is a group II mGluR agonist under evaluation for the treatment of **anxiety disorders** and **schizophrenia** whose inhibitory effects on presynaptic glutamate nerve terminals may repress central glutamatergic function. A reduction in glutamatergic function also may be useful in the treatment of **epilepsy**.

Synaptic clustering of glutamate receptors
Effective synaptic communication requires the precise localization of high concentrations of appropriate presynaptic and postsynaptic proteins at the synapse. On the postsynaptic side of the synapse, neurons must be able to target glutamate receptors to excitatory but not inhibitory synapses and must ensure that the receptors are appropriately clustered opposite presynaptic terminals that release glutamate. Research during the past 5 years has isolated a family of proteins that appear to be involved in these important tasks. Several of these proteins contain single or multiple copies of an amino acid sequence termed the *PDZ domain*, which is important for mediating many specific protein–protein interactions (Box 7–1).

Evidence supports the evolving premise that each subtype of glutamate receptor interacts with distinct proteins at the synapse. Accordingly, the subcellular localization of these receptors may be independently regulated under physiologic conditions. Although these mechanisms remain poorly understood, they may underlie certain forms of neural plasticity.

ROLE OF GLUTAMATE IN NEURAL PLASTICITY

The high permeability of NMDA receptor channels to divalent cations, especially to Ca^{2+}, has many implications for cell function. The concentration of Ca^{2+} in the cell interior typically is heavily buffered to approximately 100 nM and is tightly regulated by several mechanisms, including storage in intracellular organelles.

Ca^{2+} entry through NMDA receptor channels can lead to a transient increase in intracellular Ca^{2+} concentrations to the micromolar range. Such an increase can in turn result in the activation of many Ca^{2+}-dependent enzymes, including Ca^{2+}/calmodulin-dependent protein kinases, calcineurin (protein phosphatase 2B), protein kinase C, phospholipase A_2, phospholipase C, nitric oxide synthase, and several proteases (see Chapter 5).

One of the most important consequences of NMDA receptor activation is the generation of often long-lasting changes in synaptic function termed *synaptic plasticity*. Many forms of synaptic plasticity have been discovered in the mammalian CNS, but long-term potentiation (*LTP*) and long-term depression (*LTD*) of excitatory synaptic responses in CA1 pyramidal cells in the hippocampus have been the most extensively characterized. LTP and LTD are activity-dependent alterations in synaptic efficacy that can last as long as several weeks in vivo. The bidirectional control of synaptic strength by LTP and LTD is believed to underlie some forms of learning and memory in the mammalian brain (see Chapter 20).

Some of the principal mechanisms involved in the induction of LTP and LTD in the hippocampus have been elucidated (see Chapter 20). Much of this research has focused on synapses between Schaeffer collateral axons and CA1 pyramidal neurons. Both LTP and LTD require the activation of postsynaptic NMDA receptors and the elevation of intracellular Ca^{2+} levels; depending on the characteristics of the Ca^{2+} signal, these activities may in turn lead to the activation of protein kinases or protein phosphatases. Specific Ca^{2+}-dependent enzymes that have been implicated in LTP include Ca^{2+}/calmodulin-dependent protein kinase II and protein kinase C, whereas LTD may involve the preferential activation of calcineurin. It is likely that AMPA receptors, whose functioning is modified by phosphorylation, are among the most important targets of these protein kinases and protein phosphatases (Box 7–2).

ROLE OF GLUTAMATE IN NEURONAL TOXICITY

A large body of literature has placed glutamatergic neurotransmission at the center of a wide array of mechanisms that underlie neuronal toxicity (see Chapter 21). Moreover, animal models of ischemic cell injury have highlighted the potential benefits of neuroprotectant drugs aimed at blocking glutamatergic function. In animal models of **stroke,** for example, the administration of an NMDA receptor antagonist within several hours after the initial insult results in appreciable protection of CNS tissue. Likewise, these receptor antagonists have been effective at reducing both the intensity and duration of

Box 7–1 PDZ Proteins and Synaptic Clustering of Glutamate Receptors

Immunocytochemical and ultrastructural studies have revealed that individual excitatory synapses can contain profoundly different densities of AMPA, NMDA, and metabotropic glutamate receptors. Furthermore, even at synapses that contain all three subtypes, their localization in dendritic spines usually differs (see Figure 7–7). The ionotropic receptors (AMPA and NMDA) are located in the central part of the postsynaptic density opposite presynaptic release sites. In contrast, mGluRs are located at the periphery of synapses. This anatomic subsynaptic segregation of ionotropic and metabotropic receptors may permit the differential activation of these receptors based on patterns of presynaptic activity and may contribute significantly to certain forms of neural plasticity. A series of proteins have been identified in recent years that assist in clustering glutamate receptors at synapses. Most of these contain several PDZ domains, structures known to mediate many intracellular protein–protein interactions (see Chapter 5).

The first of these proteins to be isolated was the *postsynaptic density protein of 95 kDa* (PSD-95); as its name implies, this protein occurs in high concentrations in the postsynaptic density, the most prominent structural specialization of the postsynaptic membrane of excitatory synapses (Chapter 4). PSD-95 contains three PDZ domains, two of which interact with the C terminus of NMDA receptor NR2 subunits. These two domains also permit the binding of PSD-95 to Shaker K$^+$ channels. PSD-95 is believed to be a critical component of the molecular mechanism responsible for the clustering of NMDA receptors at synapses (see figure), and of Shaker K$^+$ channels in axons and other cellular compartments. Because NMDA receptors and Shaker K$^+$ channels are located in different regions of the neuron, other molecules must be involved in targeting these proteins to their appropriate subcellular locations.

AMPA receptors and mGluRs do not bind to PSD-95 but instead bind to their cognate PDZ-containing proteins.

AMPA receptors bind to a protein known alternately as the *glutamate receptor interacting protein* (GRIP) or AMPA receptor binding protein (ABP). This protein contains seven PDZ domains, the fourth and fifth of which bind to the C-terminal tail of AMPA receptor subunits. AMPA receptors also bind to PICK1 (protein interacting with C-kinase 1). Homer, a protein that binds to the C terminus of group I mGluRs, contains a single PDZ-like domain. Interestingly, expression of some splice variants of Homer can be regulated by neuronal activity; thus nerve impulses may influence the efficacy of mGluR synaptic transmission by regulating receptor clustering at physiologic sites.

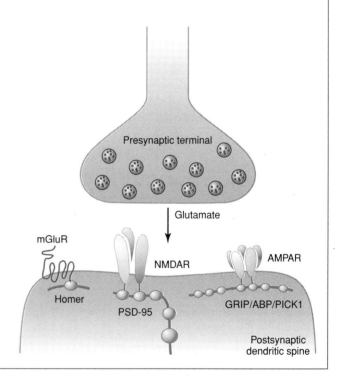

seizure activity in several animal models of **epilepsy**. NMDA receptor antagonists work by counteracting the excessive stimulation of glutamatergic pathways that precipitates seizures in these animal models, caused for example, by the blockade of glutamate reuptake transporters or other pharmacologic manipulations.

GABA

MAJOR INHIBITORY NEUROTRANSMITTER IN THE BRAIN

GABA is present in highly diverse inhibitory interneurons and projection neurons throughout the brain. In the past, the action of GABA on its receptors was considered to be solely inhibitory, based on the observation that GABA receptor activation moves the membrane potential of a cell away from action potential threshold. However, recent evidence suggests that the role of GABA is more complex. During development, GABA also may function as an excitatory transmitter because in certain circumstances GABA transmission can depolarize neurons. In addition, GABA released from local-circuit inhibitory interneurons assists in generating membrane oscillations such as the theta rhythm.

The wide-ranging and ubiquitous role of GABA as an inhibitory transmitter is supported by evidence that links numerous neuropsychiatric disorders with altered GABA function and, in some cases, the degeneration of GABAergic neurons. These disorders include **epilepsy,**

Box 7–2 Modulation of Glutamate and GABA Receptors by Phosphorylation

Among all synapses in the brain, the most ubiquitous are excitatory synapses that require glutamate and inhibitory synapses that require GABA. Thus the modulation of glutamate and GABA receptors by intracellular second messenger cascades is believed to be of paramount importance for a host of normal brain functions (see Chapter 5).

The functioning of all subtypes of ionotropic glutamate receptors, including that of kainate, AMPA, and NMDA receptors, can be dramatically altered by phosphorylation. The AMPA receptor subunit GluR1 is phosphorylated by three major protein serine–threonine kinases: protein kinase A, protein kinase C, and Ca^{2+}/calmodulin-dependent protein kinase II (CaM-kinase II). All three kinases increase the current elicited by agonist activation of a GluR1-containing AMPA receptor by phosphorylating distinct residues in its intracellular C terminus. Specifically, protein kinase A phosphorylates serine 845, whereas protein kinase C and CaM-kinase II both appear to phosphorylate serine 831. Similarly, when the kainate receptor subunit GluR6 is phosphorylated by protein kinase A at serine 684, receptors that contain GluR6 become more responsive. Such modulation most likely underlies activity-dependent forms of synaptic plasticity believed to be involved in learning and memory (see Chapter 20).

The modulation of NMDA receptor function, in contrast to that of AMPA and kainate receptors, appears to involve protein tyrosine kinases in addition to serine–threonine kinases. Activation of the tyrosine kinase src, for example, causes an increase in NMDA-induced currents in both native and recombinant NMDA receptors. The biochemical mechanism responsible for this process is unclear but may involve phosphorylation of the intracellular C terminus of NR2A (and perhaps NR2B). Protein kinase C also has been found to enhance NMDA receptor function, and to disrupt the clustering of NMDA receptors, perhaps by interfering with the interaction between cytoskeletal elements and the C terminus of NR1. Whether CaM-kinase II modifies NMDA receptors is unclear, but calmodulin itself binds directly to NR1 and reduces the frequency with which channels open in heteromeric NMDA receptors containing NR1.

$GABA_A$ receptors are phosphorylated by at least two different protein serine–threonine kinases: protein kinase C and protein kinase A. In most studies, protein kinase C appears to inhibit $GABA_A$ receptor function, in part by phosphorylating serine residues 409 and 343 on β_1 and γ_2 subunits, respectively. The effects of protein kinase A on $GABA_A$ receptors are more variable. Protein kinase A, like protein kinase C, can phosphorylate serine 409 on the β_1 subunit and thereby attenuate $GABA_A$ receptor-mediated currents; however, the biophysical consequences of protein kinase A phosphorylation depend on the exact subunit composition of the $GABA_A$ receptor. In certain cell types, such as cerebellar Purkinje and retinal bipolar cells, the activation of protein kinase A potentiates GABA-mediated responses, although the molecular mechanisms responsible for these effects remain to be determined.

Because G protein-coupled receptors are linked to the activation or inhibition of protein kinases, many types of neurotransmitters, such as the monoamines, acetylcholine, and several neuropeptides (see Chapters 8–10), probably modulate glutamate or GABA receptor function; indeed examples of such modulation have been identified in several neuronal preparations. Similarly, changes in the amount of intracellular Ca^{2+} can regulate protein phosphorylation cascades and thereby modify receptor function. Furthermore, the phosphorylation states of these receptors are controlled by protein phosphatases, the inhibition of which often mimics the effects of increased protein kinase activity. An important goal of current research is to determine how phosphorylation of glutamate and GABA receptor subunits regulates the functioning of neural circuits and in turn the complex behaviors they underlie.

Huntington disease, tardive dyskinesia, alcoholism, and **sleep disorders**. In addition, animal models of epilepsy have been generated with the use of agents that compromise GABAergic transmission; such interference results in an imbalance of excitation and inhibition and leads to hyperexcitability and various forms of epileptiform activity. Enhancement of GABAergic function is a highly effective approach for the treatment of some forms of anxiety (see Chapter 15) and epilepsy (see Chapter 21).

SYNTHETIC AND DEGRADATIVE PATHWAYS

The portion of cellular GABA that functions as a neurotransmitter is formed by a metabolic pathway commonly referred to as the GABA shunt (Figure 7–8). As with glutamate synthesis, the most common precursor for GABA formation is glucose; pyruvate also can act as a precursor. The first step in the GABA shunt is the conversion of α-ketoglutarate into glutamate by the action of α-oxoglutarate transaminase (GABA transaminase or GABA-T). Glutamic acid decarboxylase (GAD) catalyzes the decarboxylation of glutamic acid to produce GABA.

Like most neurotransmitters, GABA is packaged into vesicles in the presynaptic terminals for its ultimate release into the synaptic cleft. The vesicular transporter for GABA has been cloned; its primary sequence predicts a protein with 10 transmembrane domains and a very large cytoplasmic N terminus of approximately 130 amino acids. Like the vesicular glutamate transporter, the vesicular GABA transporter is highly dependent on the electrical potential across the vesicle membrane.

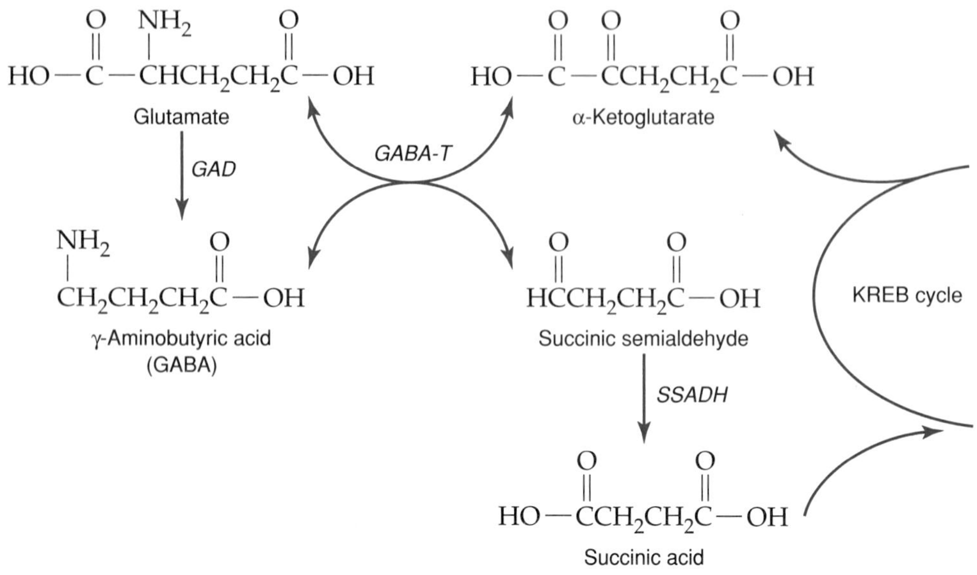

Figure 7–8. The GABA shunt. This metabolic pathway traces the synthesis and degradation of the neurotransmitter pool of GABA. GAD, glutamic acid decarboxylase; GABA-T, GABA transaminase; SSADH, succinic semialdehyde dehydrogenase.

The vesicular GABA and glutamate transporters differ from the vesicular transporters for monoamines and acetylcholine in terms of this bioenergetic dependence. Specific inhibitors of vesicular GABA transport have not yet been identified.

After it is released, GABA is removed from the synaptic cleft by the actions of several types of plasma membrane GABA transporters (see Chapter 4). Through this action GABA can be returned to GABAergic nerve terminals where it is repackaged for release; it can also be taken up by glial cells. In glia, GABA is metabolized into succinic semialdehyde by the action of GABA-T. To conserve the available supply of GABA, this transamination step occurs only when the precursor α-ketoglutarate is also present to accept the amino group removed from GABA. GABA is then reconverted to glutamic acid, which is transferred back to the neuron. Because GAD is not present in glia, glutamic acid is returned to neurons, where it can be converted by GAD to regenerate GABA. GABA-T inhibitors are being developed for use as **anticonvulsant** agents. One such drug, **vigabatrin,** has shown promise in clinical trials.

RELEASE AND REUPTAKE

The arrival of a depolarizing stimulus such as an action potential in a presynaptic terminal initiates a sequence of events that ultimately results in vesicular fusion and the liberation of GABA into the synaptic cleft. The **anticonvulsant** drug **gabapentin** inhibits GABA release, although its underlying mechanism of action remains unclear. Once released, GABA freely diffuses across the cleft to interact with its appropriate receptors on the postsynaptic membrane. Free synaptic GABA, including GABA that has dissociated from its receptors, is taken back into the presynaptic terminal or into glial cells by plasma membrane GABA transporters. This is the major mechanism for terminating the synaptic actions of GABA. Such transport requires extracellular Na^+ and Cl^-; two Na^+ ions and one Cl^- ion are transported for each GABA molecule. Molecular cloning techniques have revealed the genes for four distinct GABA transporters (GAT-1, GAT-2, GAT-3, and BGT-1), disclosing a greater heterogeneity than previously suspected. GABA transporters are expressed on nerve terminals and glial cell membranes throughout the nervous system.

Hydroxynipecotic acid, a rigid GABA analogue, has been used as an inhibitor of GABA transport. Its selectivity for glial transporters is approximately 20-fold greater than its selectivity for GABA transporters on nerve terminals. Related inhibitors **nipecotic acid** and **guvacine** block nerve terminal and glial transporters with similar potency. The cloning of GABA transporters led to a clearer understanding of their pharmacology, which was established with the use of recombinant expression techniques. With these techniques, researchers determined that guvacine, nipecotic acid, and hydroxynipecotic acid are equipotent blockers of the GAT-1 transporter, with IC_{50}s between 20 and 40 μM. **L-DABA** (2,4-diaminobutyric acid) and **ACHC** are approximately four times less potent, and **β-alanine, hypo-**

taurine, and **taurine** all have a low potency at GAT-1. One of the most potent compounds at this transporter is **NNC-711,** a lipophilic derivative of guvacine with an IC_{50} of less than 400 nM. NNC-711 is 40,000 times more selective for GAT-1 than for GAT-3. The **anticonvulsant** drug **tiagabine** and the lipophilic inhibitors **Cl-966** and **SKF89976** also act at the GAT-1 transporter. By inhibiting GABA transport, these drugs act to potentiate the inhibitory effects of GABA on CNS function.

The pharmacologic profiles of GAT-2 and GAT-3 are quite distinct from those of GAT-1. GAT-2 and GAT-3 have a lower affinity for guvacine, nipecotic acid, and hydroxynipecotic acid. GAT-2 and GAT-3 also can be distinguished pharmacologically by their sensitivity to β-alanine, taurine, and hypotaurine. BGT-1, which is not expressed to an appreciable extent in the CNS but is located primarily in the kidney, also has a distinct pharmacology. Its transport, for example, is inhibited by **phloretin** and **quinidine,** known inhibitors of the so-called betaine transporter. Moreover, β-alanine, L-DABA, and nipecotic acid are weak inhibitors of BGT-1.

Interestingly, several tricyclic and related tetracyclic **antidepressants** have been shown to affect particular GABA transporters. **Desipramine** and **maprotiline** inhibit all subtypes of GABA transporters with similar potencies; however, the affinity of these drugs for GABA transporters is considerably lower than their affinity for the norepinephrine transporter (see Chapter 8). In contrast, **amitriptyline** blocks transport through both GAT-1 and GAT-3 with an affinity only 10 times lower than that for the serotonin transporter (see Chapters 9 and 15). Whether such inhibition of GABA transport contributes to the clinical effects of these drugs remains to be determined.

GABA RECEPTORS

Like glutamate receptors, GABA receptors are divided into two main functional groups. The ionotropic $GABA_A$ receptor is a heterooligomeric protein complex that consists of a GABA binding site coupled to an integral Cl^- channel (Figure 7–9). This receptor is remarkable because it is the site of action for **anxiolytic** benzodiazepines and other **sedative hypnotics,** which are among the most widely prescribed medications in the world. $GABA_A$ receptors are blocked by the convulsant **bicuculline,** a competitive antagonist at the GABA binding site.

$GABA_B$ receptors belong to the superfamily of G protein-coupled receptors. Thus they are considered to be metabotropic: their ligand-binding domain is not directly associated with their ion channel effector. These receptors, which are resistant to bicuculline, are activated by **baclofen,** a competitive agonist, and inhibited by **phaclofen,** a competitive antagonist.

Recent evidence supports the existence of GABA receptors that are distinct from $GABA_A$ and $GABA_B$ receptors and are resistant to the actions of both bicuculline and baclofen. These novel receptors have been given a variety of names including $GABA_C$; GABA-non-A, non-B (GABA-NANB); and GABA receptor cloned from retina ($GABA_R$). These receptors are found in many CNS locations, including the retina, cerebellum, hippocampus, optic tectum, and spinal cord. It has been hypothesized that the more complex $GABA_A$ receptor evolved from the simpler, possibly homomeric, $GABA_C$ receptor. However, because little is known about the function of the $GABA_C$ receptor, and because it is not known to be the specific target of any drug, it is not discussed further in this chapter.

Molecular composition of $GABA_A$ receptors   The cloning of the first $GABA_A$ receptor subunits occurred in 1987. Since then, 15 different subunits have been identified and placed into seven functionally distinct families. The α subfamily comprises six known subunits, the β subfamily four, the ρ subfamily three, and the γ subfamily two; the δ, ε, and π subfamilies each have one member (Table 7–3). $GABA_A$ subunits are approximately 50 kDa in size. All possess a similar putative membrane topology, comprising a long N-terminal extracellular domain, four α-helical transmembrane spanning segments (M1–M4),

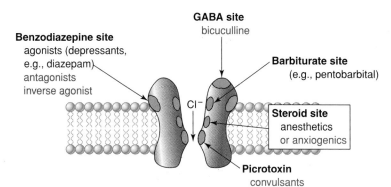

GABA site
bicuculline

Benzodiazepine site
agonists (depressants,
e.g., diazepam)
antagonists
inverse agonist

Barbiturate site
(e.g., pentobarbital)

Cl^-

Steroid site
anesthetics
or anxiogenics

Picrotoxin
convulsants

Figure 7–9. Pharmacologic binding sites of the $GABA_A$ receptor. Drugs that promote receptor function appear in black, and drugs that inhibit receptor function appear in blue. Only drugs that interact with the GABA binding site are considered competitive agonists or antagonists; all other drugs are considered noncompetitive agonists or antagonists.

Table 7–3 γ-Aminobutyric Acid (GABA) Receptors

Ionotropic GABA$_A$ Receptor	Metabotropic GABA$_B$ Receptor
Gene Families	
α1-α6	GABA$_B$R$_{1a}$
β1-β4	GABA$_B$R$_{1b}$
γ1-γ2	
δ	GABA$_B$R$_2$
ρ1-ρ3	
ε	
π	
Agents That Bind to the GABA Site	
Agonists	Agonists
GABA	L-Baclofen
Isoguvacine	CGP27492
Muscimol	
THIP	
Piperidine 4-sulphonic acid	
Antagonists	Antagonists
Bicuculline	2-OH-*s*-saclofen
	CGP35348
	CGP55845
	CGP64213
Agents That Bind to the Benzodiazepine Site	
Agonists	
Flunitrazepam	
Zolpidem	
Abecarnil	
Inverse agonists	
DMCM	
Rol94603	
Antagonists	
Flumazenil	
ZK93426	
Antagonists That Bind to Other Sites	
Picrotoxin	
Zn^{2+}	

a long intracellular sequence between M3 and M4, and a short extracellular C-terminal loop (see Figure 7–4). In the rat, a high degree of conservation exists among members of a subfamily, with 70–80% sequence homology at the amino acid level. Although GABA$_A$ subunits exhibit a low sequence homology (approximately 10–25%) with glycine, 5-HT$_3$, and nicotinic acetylcholine receptors, they are distantly related and are placed within the same superfamily of ionotropic receptors. Thus the genes for these receptor subunits most likely evolved from a common ancestral sequence by means of gene duplication and mutation.

The heterogeneity of GABA$_A$ receptors is partly due to the existence of multiple splice variants. Alternative exon splicing generates, for example, two versions of the γ$_2$ and of the β$_2$ subunits. These isoforms differ in

terms of the presence of a short peptide sequence between transmembrane domains M3 and M4, which carries a protein kinase C phosphorylation site (see Box 7–2). Alternative splicing of the α$_6$, α$_5$, and β$_3$ subunits also has been described.

Heteromeric subunit assembly can occur among members of the α, β, γ, and δ subfamilies; members of the ρ subfamily, which are present only in the retina, are believed to form homomeric receptors. The π subfamily is expressed primarily in reproductive tissues and also is believed to exist only in homomeric form.

Like most ionotropic receptors, GABA$_A$ receptors probably exist as a pentameric complex positioned around a water-filled ion-conducting pore. The size of a GABA$_A$ receptor complex (approximately 275 kDa) is estimated to be five times that of its individual subunits. The individual subunits that comprise native receptors remain largely unknown. It is generally assumed that GABA$_A$ receptors in the CNS are composed of nα, nβ, and nγ subunits, where the value of n is between 1 and 3. Based on available evidence, the most likely subunit combination is 2α-2β-1γ. Within most receptor complexes, members of α, β, and γ subunit families are believed to be identical; that is, a given receptor is not expected to contain two different forms of an α (or β or γ) subunit. However, a minority of receptors may contain more than one form. Based on the large number of receptor subunits and their potential combinations, calculations indicate that more than 2000 distinct GABA$_A$ receptors may be formed. It is highly unlikely that so many receptor types exist in the mammalian CNS; indeed, a major challenge in current research involves the identification of combinations that actually occur in vivo. That several combinations do exist in vivo is supported by binding, immunohistochemistry, immunoprecipitation, and electrophysiologic experiments that have revealed considerable heterogeneity among native GABA$_A$ receptors.

The composition of GABA$_A$ receptors in vivo is ultimately influenced by the relative levels of expression of subunits in a given cell type. Immunohistochemical and immunoprecipitation studies have determined that the major GABA$_A$ receptor subtype in brain is α$_1$, β$_2$, γ$_2$. The most prevalent subunit in the brain is α$_1$. Receptors containing the α$_2$ subunit are most abundant in regions where the α$_1$ subunit is absent or expressed at low levels, such as the hippocampus, striatum, and olfactory bulb. Similarly, the α$_3$ subunit is expressed in regions complementary to the α$_1$ subunit, including the lateral septum, reticular nucleus of the thalamus, and brain stem nuclei. Notably, the α$_6$ subunit is expressed almost exclusively in cerebellum.

The difficulty associated with ascertaining the exact subunit combinations of native GABA$_A$ receptors is best illustrated by a consideration of cerebellar granule cells. Inhibitory input to these cells is provided solely by Golgi cells. In adult rats, six GABA subunits (α_1, α_6, β_2, β_3, γ_2, and δ) are expressed abundantly in granule cells, and these are coassembled into at least four distinct receptor types. Yet recent evidence suggests that specific subunit combinations are targeted to synaptic and extrasynaptic sites in individual granule cells. Receptors containing the δ subunit are almost exclusively restricted to extrasynaptic sites and are believed to assist in tonic inhibitory activity. In contrast, three possible receptor types containing α_1, α_6, β_2, β_3, and γ_2 are concentrated in synapses made with Golgi cells and are believed to underlie phasic inhibitory synaptic transmission. Thus, even within a single neuron, cells are able to compartmentalize subunits to particular synaptic and nonsynaptic targets. The mechanisms responsible for this targeting remain unknown but likely involve anchoring proteins, based on analogy with mechanisms responsible for glutamate receptor clustering at synapses (see Box 7–1). Indeed a recently discovered protein, termed *GABARAP* (GABA$_A$ receptor-associated protein), is reported to anchor the γ_2 subunit of the receptor to tubulin and may contribute to GABA$_A$ receptor clustering in neurons.

Characteristics of subunit expression during development contribute to the complexity of subunit composition in native GABA$_A$ receptors. Embryonic GABA$_A$ receptors contain both α_2 and α_5 subunits but not α_1 subunits. Shortly after birth these receptors begin to adopt an adult pattern of expression: the α_1 subunit predominates and only minor populations of receptors contain the embryonic α_2 and α_5 subunits. The developmental switch in subunit expression is controlled by a variety of factors, including the innervation pattern of the developing tissue. It is likely that such plasticity of subunit expression is maintained throughout adult life: many experimental models indicate that the expression of one subunit can be up- or down-regulated or even replaced by the expression of another subunit. Studies of the mechanisms of GABA$_A$ subunit expression should shed light not only on the physiology of receptor adaptation but also on the pathophysiology of diseases such as **Huntington disease, epilepsy,** and **alcoholism** in which GABA$_A$ receptor expression is known to be altered.

GABA$_A$ receptor pharmacology GABA$_A$ receptor pharmacology originated in the 1970s, when researchers discovered that the convulsant alkaloid **bicuculline** antagonizes certain inhibitory actions of GABA. This observation paved the way for the discovery of GABA's role as a principal inhibitory neurotransmitter in the brain. Other antagonists of GABA$_A$ receptors include **pitrazepin,** the convulsant **securinine,** the aminidine steroid analogue **RU5135,** and the pyridazinyl derivative **SR95531 (gabazine).** In addition to GABA, selective agonists at this site include **muscimol, isoguvacine, THIP** (4,5,6,7-tetrahydroisoxazolo[5,4-*c*]-pyridone), and **piperidine-4-sulphonic acid** (see Table 7–3). Competitive agonists and competitive antagonists of GABA$_A$ receptors interact with the GABA binding site (see Figure 7–9), which for most receptor complexes is located on the β subunit. However, the affinity of GABA for the receptor can be modulated by other subunits in the heteromeric complex. In *Xenopus* oocytes, for example, GABA receptors whose subunit composition is α_1, β_1, γ_2 have an EC$_{50}$ for GABA of 41 μM, whereas α_3, β_1, γ_2 receptors have an EC$_{50}$ of approximately 100 μM.

In addition to the previously mentioned competitive GABA$_A$ receptor antagonists are antagonists that do not bind to the GABA binding site. The best known are the potent convulsants **pentylenetetrazol** and **picrotoxin** (and the related **picrotoxinin**), which appear to bind at or near the Cl$^-$ channel and occlude ion flow.

In the early 1970s, when GABA receptors were not yet cloned or biochemically isolated, **benzodiazepines** were proven to potentiate the effects of GABA at its receptors. Shortly thereafter, investigators discovered that benzodiazepines potentiate GABAergic inhibitory synaptic transmission by binding directly to the GABA$_A$ receptor. The benzodiazepine site, which is clearly distinct from the GABA-binding site, is an allosteric modulatory site on the GABA$_A$ receptor pentamer (see Figure 7–9). Recent evidence indicates that the site is formed by the apposition of α and β subunits but also requires the presence of a γ subunit, which itself is not part of the benzodiazepine binding site.

Drugs targeted at the benzodiazepine site exist on a continuum that ranges from full agonist to full inverse agonist. Indeed, GABA$_A$ receptor pharmacology played an important role in the development of the concept of inverse agonists (see Chapter 1). Agonists at the benzodiazepine site, including anxiolytic benzodiazepines such as **diazepam, chlordiazepoxide, lorazepam,** and **alprazolam,** act to increase the receptor's affinity for GABA at its own binding site and consequently increase the frequency of channel openings. Such drugs, in addition to being anxiolytic, are anticonvulsant and sedative and sometimes function as muscle relaxants. Partial agonists increase the frequency with which channels open but exert a milder effect on GABA$_A$ receptor functioning. Conversely, inverse agonists such as β-**carboline,** or β-**CCE,** whether partial or full, decrease both the frequency of channel openings and the efficacy of GABA binding, and thereby antagonize GABA$_A$ receptor function. Such inverse agonists tend to be **convulsant** and

anxiogenic, although a weak partial inverse agonist may exert less of an activational effect (a possibility not yet tested in humans). Antagonists such as **flumazenil** typically bind to and occlude the benzodiazepine-binding site, but do not affect channel function; they can be used to reverse the actions of an agonist or inverse agonist, as in the treatment of an overdose with a benzodiazepine agonist.

The responsiveness of $GABA_A$ receptors to drugs targeted at the benzodiazepine site varies considerably. Although the γ_2 subunit appears necessary for benzodiazepine binding, the presence of a γ_1 subunit may exert the opposite effect. Of particular interest are the findings that numerous benzodiazepine site agonists and inverse agonists exert α subunit-selective effects on $GABA_A$ receptors. These discoveries have important clinical ramifications, as discussed later in this chapter.

$GABA_A$ receptors also are the site of action for a large number of sedative–hypnotic and anesthetic agents, including **barbiturates** and related drugs, **ethanol** and other alcohols, and **volatile anesthetics.** Barbiturates and other sedative-hypnotics, such as **methaqualone** and **chloral hydrate,** exert a modulatory effect on the $GABA_A$ receptor similar to the effect produced by benzodiazepine agonists, but do so by binding to a distinctly separate location, most likely near the Cl^- channel pore (see Figure 7–9). Barbiturates increase the duration of channel openings and decrease the likelihood of short-lived openings without affecting the frequency with which channels open; thus they maximize the opportunity for Cl^- to flow down its concentration gradient. **Pentobarbital** and **phenobarbital** are the most commonly used barbiturates; phenobarbital has been in use as an anticonvulsant since the early part of the 20th century. Variation in the subunit composition of $GABA_A$ receptors does not seem to alter their sensitivity to barbiturates. A similar mechanism of action may operate with neuroactive steroids, some of which may be synthesized endogenously in the brain. These agents can allosterically regulate $GABA_A$ receptor function to enhance or attenuate Cl^- conductance (see Chapter 13).

The effects that **ethanol** exerts on the $GABA_A$ receptor complex are similar to those produced by benzodiazepines and barbiturates: it facilitates GABA's ability to activate the receptor and prolongs the time that the Cl^- channel remains open. Interestingly, the alternatively spliced forms of the γ_2 subunit include a short form (γ_{2S}) and a long form (γ_{2L}), and ethanol potentiates $GABA_A$ responses only in receptors containing γ_{2L}. This splice variant also contains a consensus sequence for protein kinase C phosphorylation; when this sequence is mutated, the receptor's sensitivity to ethanol is lost.

Volatile anesthetics such as **enflurane** represent another class of drugs that prolong channel opening of $GABA_A$ receptors. Molecular mutagenesis has been used to identify sites in most $GABA_A$ receptor subunits that are responsible for the potentiating effects of both ethanol and volatile anesthetics. Given their location, typically near the extracellular regions of transmembrane domains M2 and M3, these sites may be part of the protein pocket that binds both ethanol and the volatile anesthetics, although this hypothesis remains unproved.

Because barbiturates, benzodiazepines, and ethanol have related actions on a shared receptor substrate, the use of these agents can result in clinical complications. Their pharmacologic synergy increases the dangers associated with overdose and can lead to the development of cross-dependence. In fact, such cross-dependence often is exploited in **alcohol detoxification: benzodiazepines** are the treatment of choice and are used to prevent the emergence of alcohol withdrawal symptoms such as hallucinosis, delirium tremens, and seizures.

Prolonged exposure to benzodiazepines results in tolerance to some of their pharmacologic actions, particularly to their sedative and anticonvulsant effects. Thus their effectiveness in the prolonged treatment of chronic insomnia is limited, and they are used infrequently in the long-term treatment of epilepsy. Surprisingly, tolerance to the anxiolytic effects of benzodiazepines may not develop; patients often benefit from these effects for many years. In addition to tolerance, benzodiazepines and related sedative–hypnotics can produce profound dependence, which is manifested by rebound withdrawal symptoms that appear when drug administration ceases. Both tolerance and dependence are characterized by a down-regulation of GABAergic transmission and by a reduction in the benzodiazepine modulation of $GABA_A$ currents. Despite considerable research, little consensus exists as to the mechanisms that underlie tolerance caused by prolonged exposure to benzodiazepines. Several reports have suggested that tolerance is caused by the down-regulation of the benzodiazepine recognition site on $GABA_A$ receptor complexes, indicating that distinct receptor subunits that lack such sites may be expressed in response to continued exposure to benzodiazepines.

The extensive heterogeneity of $GABA_A$ receptors, and the broad array of pharmacologic agents that are currently known to modulate these receptors, offer hope that more specific therapeutic agents can be engineered in the future. Such optimism has been bolstered by the hypothesis that $GABA_A$ receptors responsible for mediating the effects of benzodiazepine agonists are located in distinct brain regions and are composed of distinct α subunits. A striking endorsement of this hypothesis emerged several years ago with the development of **RO 15-4513**, a benzodiazepine site antagonist that acts selectively on $GABA_A$ receptors that contain the α_6 subunit, which is concentrated in the cerebellum. This drug reduces the ataxia produced by ethanol without altering ethanol's other actions. Thus researchers have been encouraged in their attempts to develop drugs that selectively inhibit the anxiolytic, sedative, or anticonvulsant actions of nonselective agents such as diazepam. Early progress along these lines occurred with the development of **zolpidem**, a nonbenzodiazepine sedative hypnotic that binds at the benzodiazepine site of the $GABA_A$ receptor. Zolpidem is somewhat selective for $GABA_A$ receptors that possess the α_1 subunit, which is believed to mediate the sedative actions of this drug.

Drug research is also aimed at developing agents that target $GABA_A$ receptors without producing tolerance or dependence, or triggering abuse. One strategy may involve the development of partial agonists that are sufficiently efficacious but less likely than full agonists to elicit compensatory adaptations. A related approach may involve the development of partial inverse agonists that are selective for $GABA_A$ receptors associated with cognitive function and attentional states. Although a full inverse agonist is convulsant and anxiogenic, a weak partial inverse agonist with the right α subunit selectivity may effectively enhance cognition. Indeed, it is conceivable that a single agent might reduce anxiety and enhance cognitive function simultaneously by acting as a partial agonist at anxiolytic $GABA_A$ receptors, and as a weak inverse partial agonist at cognitive $GABA_A$ receptors. However, it is important to note that drugs with these various mechanisms of action have not yet been developed.

$GABA_B$ receptors $GABA_B$ receptors were initially recognized because of their insensitivity to bicuculline and other $GABA_A$ ligands. Subsequently, the GABA analog and **muscle relaxant** known as **baclofen** proved to be a potent agonist at $GABA_B$ receptors. The physiologic roles of $GABA_B$ receptors were further elucidated after the development and analysis of specific antagonists such as **phaclofen, CGP 35348**, and **2-OH-s-(−)-saclofen**.

In addition, molecular cloning techniques revealed that $GABA_B$ receptors are members of the G protein-coupled receptor superfamily and contain seven transmembrane domains (see Figure 7–6). Two major $GABA_B$ subunits have been cloned: $GABA_BR_{1a}$ and R_{1b}, both of which couple to G_i. $GABA_B$ receptors, which are larger than most G protein-coupled receptors, are composed of 850–960 amino acids and are structurally similar to mGluRs. A novel $GABA_B$ receptor subunit, termed $GABA_BR_2$, has been identified and has been shown to heterodimerize with $GABA_BR_{1a}$ or R_{1b} to form a functional receptor. Thus these are the first G protein-coupled receptors known to function as multimeric complexes.

$GABA_B$ receptors are expressed on both presynaptic and postsynaptic membranes and, like other G_i-linked receptors, have been proven to open K^+ channels, decrease Ca^{2+} conductances, and inhibit adenylyl cyclase. Compared with $GABA_A$ receptors, postsynaptic $GABA_B$ receptors produce a slower but longer-lasting form of inhibition, an effect largely ascribed to the opening of inwardly rectifying K^+ channels. The physiologic role of $GABA_B$ receptors has not been determined with certainty because the precise population of neurons that exhibit $GABA_B$ responses has yet to be identified. In structures such as the hippocampus, thalamus, and cortex, low-intensity stimulation of inhibitory interneurons evokes inhibitory postsynaptic potentials (IPSPs) mediated entirely by $GABA_A$ receptors; IPSPs mediated by $GABA_B$ receptors require much stronger stimulation or stimuli of longer duration and higher frequency. These findings have led to the conclusion that the synaptic location of these receptor subtypes may differ. $GABA_A$ receptors are believed to localize at the synapse proper, directly opposite the site of GABA release; thus they can be activated by the release of a single quantum of neurotransmitter. In contrast, $GABA_B$ receptors may be extrasynaptic. An extrasynaptic location would explain their need for high-intensity stimulation or for prolonged, high-frequency stimuli, either of which would increase GABA release and make it possible for GABA to diffuse out of the synaptic cleft.

On the presynaptic side, $GABA_B$ receptors can function as so-called autoreceptors and inhibit further GABA release from GABAergic nerve terminals. Other $GABA_B$ receptors are located on excitatory terminals, where their activation inhibits the release of glutamate. Receptors at this location are activated by synaptically released GABA that has, in a paracrine fashion, spilled out from an inhibitory synapse and diffused to adjacent excitatory synapses (Figure 7–10). $GABA_B$ autoreceptors and heteroreceptors appear to regulate GABA and glutamate release, respectively, during repetitive activity. The activation of presynaptic $GABA_B$ receptors can

Baclofen

Phaclofen

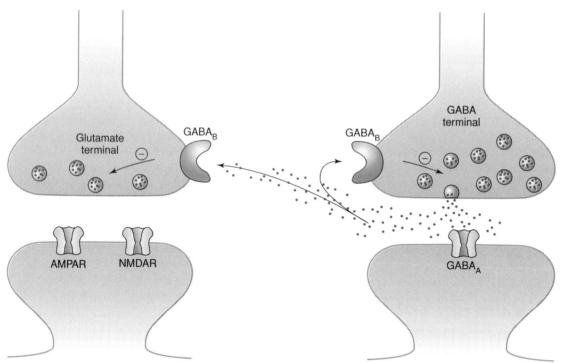

Figure 7-10. Presynaptic actions of GABA$_B$ receptors. An excitatory, glutamatergic synapse (*left*) is compared with an inhibitory, GABAergic synapse (*right*). In the latter, synaptically released GABA activates presynaptic GABA$_B$ autoreceptors located on the same inhibitory nerve terminal. Under certain conditions, GABA can also diffuse out of the synaptic cleft and activate GABA$_B$ receptors on adjacent excitatory nerve terminals. At both types of nerve terminals, GABA$_B$ receptors inhibit transmitter release.

also inhibit the release of several other neurotransmitters, including norepinephrine, dopamine, serotonin, and substance P. In each of these situations, GABA$_B$-mediated inhibition of transmitter release occurs, at least in part, through the inhibition of Ca^{2+} channels and the consequent decreases in Ca^{2+} influx that occur in a terminal invaded by an action potential. Such inhibition also may involve K$^+$ conductances, or direct modulation of the release machinery in the terminal through the regulation of cAMP and protein kinase A, and the phosphorylation of synaptic vesicle proteins (see Chapters 4 and 5).

The only major drug in clinical use that interacts with GABA$_B$ receptors is **baclofen,** which acts as a **muscle relaxant** and is used to decrease spasticity in a variety of neurologic disorders. It is used less frequently for the treatment of **trigeminal neuralgia**. Inhibition of glutamate release is believed to underlie its clinical efficacy. Other applications for GABA$_B$ receptor agonists are currently under investigation and may include their use in the treatment of **seizure disorders, anxiety,** and **depression**. GABA$_B$ antagonists may be used in the future to enhance cognition.

GLYCINE

SYNTHETIC AND DEGRADATIVE PATHWAYS

Most of the glycine in the mammalian CNS is synthesized de novo from glucose through serine. Serine is converted to glycine by serine hydroxymethyltransferase (SMHT), a pyridoxal phosphate-dependent enzyme. Pyridoxal phosphate is a derivative of **vitamin B$_6$**. It is believed that this conversion occurs in the mitochondrial compartment because the distribution of mitochondrial SMHT mirrors the distribution of glycine (Figure 7–11).

Glycine is an amino acid that is used primarily in the synthesis of proteins in all tissues of the body. Only a small fraction of the cellular pool of glycine in a small subset of neurons is packaged into synaptic vesicles for release as neurotransmitter. This packaging is mediated by a vesicular transport system identical to that previously described for GABA. Glycine acts as a neurotransmitter predominantly in the brain stem and spinal cord, where, like GABA, it is a principal mediator of inhibitory neurotransmission.

The degradation of glycine occurs mainly by means of the glycine cleavage system (GCS), which has four protein components (see Figure 7–11). A defect in the GCS, which is located in the inner mitochondrial membrane, causes a group of metabolic disorders termed **nonketotic hyperglycinemias,** which are characterized by high concentrations of glycine in the cerebrospinal fluid (Box 7–3).

GLYCINE RELEASE AND REUPTAKE

As with the release of other neurotransmitters, the arrival of an action potential in the presynaptic terminal of a glycinergic neuron initiates a cascade involving vesicular fusion with the presynaptic membrane and the release of glycine into the synaptic cleft. Glycine thus released is free to diffuse and bind with its receptors clustered on the postsynaptic face of adjacent cells.

Glycine is removed from the synaptic cleft by uptake transporters located on glial cells and on the presynap-

tic terminals of neurons (see Figure 7–11). The electrochemical gradients of Na^+ and Cl^- assist in transporting glycine against its concentration gradient. This uptake mechanism is electrogenic and results in a net movement of positive charge. Two glycine transporters have been cloned thus far: GLYT1 and GLYT2. However, GLYT1 exists in three isoforms, which most likely are generated by alternative splicing; these exhibit no known variation in their uptake properties but possess distinct patterns of expression in the CNS.

Because only GLYT1 isoforms are sensitive to **sarcosine** (*N*-methylglycine), GLYT1 and GLYT2 can be differentiated pharmacologically. Both GLYT1 and GLYT2 are expressed in caudal regions of the CNS, a location consistent with their role in terminating glycinergic neurotransmission. In addition, GLYT1 is expressed in several forebrain regions that are devoid of glycinergic transmission. This forebrain GLYT1 might regulate NMDA glutamate receptor function in these areas by controlling levels of glycine in the

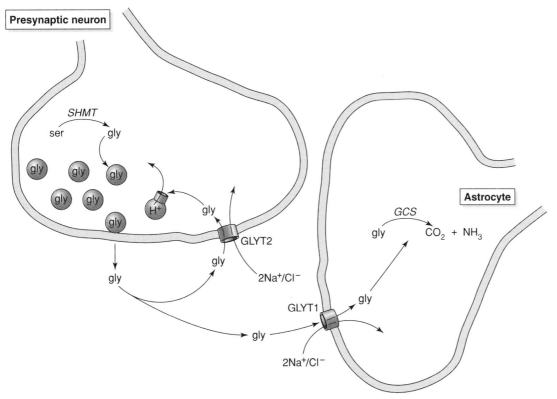

Figure 7–11. Synthesis and metabolism of the neurotransmitter pool of glycine. Serine (ser) is converted to glycine (gly) by the enzyme serine hydroxymethyltransferase (SHMT) in the mitochondrial compartment of a presynaptic neuron. Glycine is packaged into vesicles for release as neurotransmitter by a vesicular transport system identical to that used for GABA. Subsequently, glycine is removed from the synaptic cleft by uptake transporters located on glial cells (GLYT1) and on presynaptic nerve terminals (GLYT2). The transport of glycine against its concentration gradient and along the electrochemical gradients of Na^+ and Cl^- produces a net movement of positive charge. The degradation of glycine occurs mainly by means of the glycine cleavage system (GCS) in the inner mitochondrial membrane.

Box 7–3 Inherited Disorders Related to Abnormal Functioning of Amino Acid Neurotransmitters

The critical roles played by glutamate and GABA in controlling normal brain function suggest that naturally occurring mutations in any of the receptors for these neurotransmitters may be important causes of inherited human disorders. Yet, surprisingly, no such disorder has been connected definitively with a mutation in the genes for these receptors. In contrast, inactivation of the GABA$_A$ β_3 subunit in mice causes developmental abnormalities that include **cleft palate.** Moreover, the ataxia characteristic of the mutant mouse known as *lurcher* results from a loss of cerebellar Purkinje cells during development, recently attributed to a missense mutation in the *GRID2* homolog. This gene encodes the orphan glutamate receptor subunit δ_2, the normal function of which is unknown. Whether similar mutations occur in humans also remains unknown.

One disease clearly associated with glutamate receptor dysfunction is **Rasmussen's encephalitis,** a childhood autoimmune disorder characterized by epileptic seizures and associated with progressive destruction of a single cerebral hemisphere. One of the targeted autoantigens is the glutamate receptor subunit GluR3. Presumably, the disease is caused by antiGluR3 antibodies entering the brain, where they precipitate an immune response that destroys nervous tissue. Indeed, some affected children benefit from plasma exchange that removes circulating antiGluR3 antibodies.

Mutations in the protein components of the glycine

cleavage system (GCS), which is responsible for the degradation of glycine, cause metabolic disorders known as **nonketotic hyperglycinemias.** These diseases, which are characterized by high concentrations of glycine in the cerebrospinal fluid, develop early in infancy and are associated with severe neurologic defects such as lethargy, hypotonia, myoclonus, and generalized seizures.

Mutations in glycine receptor subunits contribute to abnormalities in two mouse mutants and also underlie a hereditary disease in humans. The mouse mutant known as *spasmodic* contains a recessive missense mutation in the α_1 subunit that causes a twofold to threefold decrease in its affinity for glycine. A similar mutation is responsible for **hyperekplexia,** a relatively rare dominant heredity disorder that affects humans. This disease is characterized by increased muscle tone and an exaggerated startle reflex, and is caused by point mutations at position 271 of the α subunit. These mutations result in more than a 100-fold decrease in glycine affinity. Hyperekplexia shows a dominant mode of inheritance. The mouse mutant known as *spastic* also displays a complex motor disorder that is caused by reduced expression of the adult form of glycine receptor. This phenomenon results from the insertion of a transposable element into intron 5 of the β subunit gene, which produces aberrations in the splicing of β transcripts and leads to a reduction in correctly spliced β subunit mRNA.

---

extracellular fluid available to allosterically modulate these receptors. This would suggest the **GLYT1 inhibitors** may be useful clinically in promoting NMDA receptor function. GLYT1 is expressed in both astrocytes and neurons, whereas GLYT2 is localized on axons and terminal boutons of neurons that contain vesicular glycine.

GLYCINE RECEPTORS

Glycine receptors are primarily restricted to the brain stem and spinal cord. Like GABA$_A$ receptors, the glycine receptor is a receptor ionophore that contains a Cl$^-$ channel. It is also similar in size to the GABA$_A$ receptor (approximately 250 kDa) and is believed to possess a quasisymmetrical pentameric structure that surrounds a water-filled ion conduction pore. Glycine receptors, which are unrelated to the glycine binding sites present on NMDA glutamate receptors, are

defined pharmacologically by **strychnine,** a selective antagonist and a potent convulsant. Agonists at these receptors, which are competitive and limited to a few ligands, are ranked according to potency as follows: glycine > β-alanine > taurine > L- and D-alanine > L-serine $\gg$ D-serine. The potent convulsants **picrotoxin** and **picrotoxinin** are noncompetitive inhibitors of some of these receptors and are believed to interact directly with the receptor's ion channel to block Cl$^-$ permeation.

Glycine receptors are composed of two types of glycosylated integral transmembrane proteins: 48-kDa α subunits and 58-kDa β subunits. Both of these are closely associated with gephyrin, a large (approximately 93 kDa) cytoplasmic protein in native receptors. The α and β subunits possess similar sequence homologies (see Figure 7–4), which in turn are similar to those of other receptor ionophores; thus glycine receptors belong to the same superfamily as nicotinic cholinergic, GABA$_A$, and 5-HT$_3$ receptors. Like other members of this superfamily, glycine receptors are believed to possess a large N-terminal extracellular domain and four transmembrane spanning regions. The glycine receptor pentamer is formed by α subunits either alone or in association with a β subunit; only the α subunit contains the functional glycine binding site. Three α subunits and a single β subunit have been cloned, and each of these is known to have several splice variants. Gephyrin associates with the intracellular region of the β subunit and links the receptor to cytoplasmic tubulin; thus it functions as an anchoring protein for glycine receptors.

The composition of the glycine receptor is developmentally regulated. In rat embryonic tissue, these receptors are exclusively composed of α_2 subunits; however, in the adult they typically are composed of $3\alpha_1$ and 2β subunits (Figure 7–12). The transient expression of α_2 subunits during development occurs in most regions of the CNS, including the telencephalon, diencephalon, midbrain, and spinal cord. In mature animals, only a few neurons in the spinal cord exhibit persistent expres-

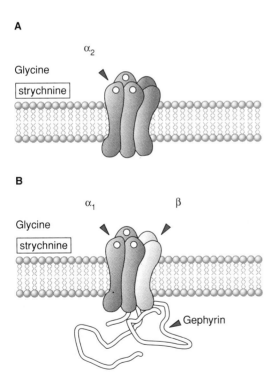

Figure 7–12. Developmental differences in the molecular composition of glycine receptors. **A.** In embryonic tissue, glycine receptors comprise only α_2 subunits. **B.** Adult receptors typically comprise $3\alpha_1$ and 2β subunits. The β subunit allows the glycine receptor to interact with gephyrin, which links it to cytoplasmic tubulin. Strychnine antagonizes both forms of glycine receptors.

sion of α_2. In adults, the distribution of α_1 corresponds closely to the distribution of strychnine binding sites throughout the spinal cord, in brain stem nuclei associated with general motor and somatosensory systems, and in the reticular, auditory, and vestibular systems. An increase in α_3 transcription during development is restricted to the infralimbic system; in the adult such transcription is restricted to the hippocampal complex and cerebellar granule cell layer. Interestingly, β mRNA transcripts are found throughout the mammalian adult CNS, although β subunits alone are incapable of forming functional glycine receptors.

Homomeric α_1 receptors exhibit channel properties that are strikingly similar to those of glycine receptors assembled from rat brain poly(A)$^+$ mRNA or cultured spinal cord neurons. They also have an agonist profile identical to that previously described for native glycine receptors. This is consistent with α_1 predominating in the adult CNS. In contrast, homomeric α_2 channels are selective for glycine. Single-channel recordings reveal a higher main conductance state for homomeric α_2 and α_3 than for α_1 receptors. Homomeric α_1 receptor channels have a short life span compared with those of homomeric α_2 receptors; this difference is consistent with the observation that the mean open time of the glycine receptor decreases during development. Although the β subunit does not form functional channels when expressed alone, its presence can alter the single-channel conductance of heteromeric receptors. Indeed, when β and α subunits are coexpressed, channel conductance values diminish and approach those observed in adult tissue.

The pharmacology of glycine receptors remains limited. Among the known antagonists of these receptors, **strychnine** is the most commonly used experimentally because it blocks receptors composed of all α subunits. The binding pocket of the glycine receptor binds both strychnine and glycine agonists and is composed of several discontinuous domains of the α subunit. Interestingly, the residues important for ligand binding are homologous to amino acid positions that determine the ligand-binding affinities of nicotinic cholinergic and GABA$_A$ receptors; thus it appears that the ligand-binding pockets of all members of this receptor superfamily may share a common architecture. Other glycine receptor antagonists include **cyanotriphenylborate** (CTB), which preferentially binds to receptors containing the α_1 subunit; **picrotoxin,** which most effectively blocks recombinant α_2 homomeric receptors; and **picrotoxinin,** which most effectively blocks α_1 homomeric receptors. The presence of the β subunit enables glycine receptors to resist antagonism by picrotoxinin.

SELECTED READING

Alexander SPH, Peters JA. 2000. 2000 Receptor and ion channel nomenclature supplement. *Trends Pharmacol Sci* (suppl).

Bellocchio EE, Reimer RJ, Fremeau RT, Edwards RH. 2000. Uptake of glutamate into synaptic vesicles by an inorganic phosphate transporter. *Science* 289:957–960

Bennett JA, Dingledine R. 1995. Topology profile for a glutamate receptor: Three transmembrane domains and a channel-lining reentrant membrane loop. *Neuron* 14: 373–384.

Borden LA. 1996. GABA transporter heterogeneity: Pharmacology and cellular localization. *Neurochem Int* 29: 335–356.

Bowery NG. 1993. GABA$_B$ receptor pharmacology. *Annu Rev Pharmacol Toxicol* 33:109–147.

Chaudhry FA, Reimer RJ, Krizaj D, et al. 1999. Molecular analysis of system N suggests novel physiological roles in nitrogen metabolism and synaptic transmission. *Cell* 99: 769–780.

Conn PJ, Pin J-P. 1997. Pharmacology and functions of metabotropic glutamate receptors. *Annu Rev Pharmacol Toxicol* 37:205–237.

Hayashi T, Umemori H, Mishina M, Yamamoto T. 1999. The AMPA receptor interacts with and signals through the protein tyrosine kinase Lyn. *Nature* 397:720–726.

Hollmann M, Heinemann S. 1994. Cloned glutamate receptors. *Annu Rev Neurosci* 17:31–108.

Hsueh YP, Sheng M. 1998. Anchoring of glutamate receptors at the synapse. *Prog Brain Res* 116:123–131.

Johnston GAR. 1996. GABA$_A$ receptor pharmacology. *Pharmacol Ther* 69:173–198.

Kaupmann K, Malitschek B, Schuler V, et al. 1998. GABA$_B$-receptor subtypes assemble into functional heteromeric complexes. *Nature* 396:683–687.

Knuessel M, Betz H. 2000. Clustering of inhibitory neurotransmitter receptors at developing postsynaptic sites: the membrane activation model. *Trends Neurosci* 23:429–435.

Kornau HC, Seeburg PH, Kennedy MB. 1997. Interaction of ion channels and receptors with PDZ domain proteins. *Curr Opin Neurobiol* 7:368–373.

Kuhse J, Betz H, Kirsch J. 1995. The inhibitory glycine receptor: Architecture, synaptic localization and molecular pathology of a postsynaptic ion-channel complex. *Curr Opin Neurobiol* 5:318–323.

MacDonald RL, Olsen RW. 1994. GABA$_A$ receptor channels. *Annu Rev Neurosci* 17:569–602.

McBain CJ, Mayer ML. 1994. NMDA receptor structure and function. *Physiol Rev* 74:723–760.

Mihic SJ, Ye Q, Wick MJ, et al. 1997. Sites of alcohol and volatile anaesthetic action on GABA$_A$ and glycine receptors. *Nature* 389:385–389.

Pin JP, De Colle C, Bessis AS, Acher F. 1999. New perspectives for the development of selective metabotropic glutamate receptor ligands. *Eur J Pharmacol* 375:277–294.

Robinson MB, Dowd LA. 1997. Heterogeneity and functional properties of subtypes of sodium-dependent transporters in the mammalian nervous system. *Adv Pharmacol* 37:69–115.

Schoepp DD, Jane DE, Monn JA. 1999. Pharmacological agents acting at subtypes of metabotropic glutamate receptors. *Neuropharmacology* 38:1431–1476.

Seeburg PH. 1996. The role of RNA editing in controlling glutamate receptor channel properties. *J Neurochem* 66:1–5.

Seeburg PH. 1993. The TiPS/TINS lecture: The molecular biology of mammalian glutamate receptor channels. *Trends Pharmacol Sci* 14:297–303.

Sheng M, Pak DT. 2000. Ligand-gated ion channel interactions with cytoskeletal and signaling proteins. *Annu Rev Physiol* 62:755–778.

Takamori S, Rhee JS, Rosenmund C, Jahn R. 2000. Indentification of a vesicular glutamate transporter that defines a glutamatergic phenotype in neurons. *Nature* 407: 189–194.

Vannier C, Triller A. 1997. Biology of the postsynaptic glycine receptor. *Int Rev Cytol* 176:201–244.

Wang H, Bedford FK, Brandon NJ, et al. 1999. GABA$_A$-receptor-associated protein links GABA$_A$ receptors and the cytoskeleton. *Nature* 397:69–72.

Zafra F, Aragon C, Giminez C. 1997. Molecular biology of glycinergic neurotransmission. *Mol Neurobiol* 14: 117–142.

Chapter 8

Catecholamines

KEY CONCEPTS

- The monoamines and acetylcholine have a striking organization in the brain: their cell bodies are restricted to a small number of nuclei but their axons project widely throughout the nervous system.

- All receptors for catecholamine neurotransmitters are G protein-coupled receptors; norepinephrine interacts with α- and β-adrenergic receptors and dopamine with D_1 through D_5 dopamine receptors.

- Norepinephrine is synthesized in a small number of brain stem nuclei, the most prominent of which is the nucleus locus ceruleus found in the dorsal pons.

- Norepinephrine is believed to play important roles in sleep and arousal, attention and vigilance, and learning and memory.

- The norepinephrine system is an important target of drugs that treat depression, anxiety, hypertension, and other disorders.

- Dopamine neurons have cell bodies in the midbrain within the substantia nigra pars compacta and the ventral tegmental area and in the hypothalamus; dopamine is also produced by local circuit neurons in the retina.

- Midbrain dopamine neurons projecting to the forebrain influence motor control, emotion and motivation, and cognitive processes, including multiple forms of memory.

- Hypothalamic dopamine neurons regulate neuroendocrine function, most notably inhibiting the synthesis and release of prolactin.

- Dopamine plays a critical role in human disease; for example, substantia nigra dopamine neurons degenerate in Parkinson disease and ventral tegmental area dopamine neurons are important in the pathogenesis of drug addiction.

- In neuropharmacology, the psychostimulants cocaine and amphetamine are indirect dopamine agonists; the dopamine precursor L-dopa is used to treat Parkinson disease; and D_2 receptor antagonists have antipsychotic properties.

- Tyrosine hydroxylase, the rate-limiting enzyme in catecholamine biosynthesis, is regulated by phosphorylation of at least four distinct serine residues by at least nine distinct protein kinases.

- The action of catecholamines in synapses is terminated by specific transporters, the norepinephrine transporter and dopamine transporter.

- Many commonly used antidepressants inhibit the norepinephrine transporter; cocaine and related psychostimulants act on the dopamine and norepinephrine transporters to increase catecholaminergic function.

- The uptake of catecholamines into synaptic vesicles for release is accomplished by distinct vesicular monoamine transporter proteins.

- Catecholamines are metabolized by monoamine oxidase (MAO), which exists in two forms, MAO-A and MAO-B, and by catechol-*O*-methyl transferase.

Of the approximately 100 billion neurons in the human brain, only about 500,000, or 0.0005%, are estimated to use catecholamines as neurotransmitters. Yet, more research has been devoted to catecholaminergic processes than to the workings of any other neurotransmitter system. Why do these neurotransmitters warrant such attention? Why is normal brain function so dependent on the activity of such a small number of neurons, and what relevance do catecholamines have to modern clinical neuropharmacology?

This chapter addresses these questions as they relate to the catecholamine neurotransmitters **dopamine, norepinephrine,** and **epinephrine.** Together with serotonin and histamine, which are discussed in the next chapter, these substances often are collectively referred to as monoamine neurotransmitters because each contains a single amine group. Monoamine transmitters exert modulatory effects on virtually every circuit in the brain, acting to dampen or facilitate communication among neurons and to regulate the plasticity of these circuits.

Neural systems involved in higher brain functions such as voluntary movement, emotion, and cognition are subserved by parallel, distributed circuits that process information by means of fast excitatory transmission at well-defined synapses. Superimposed on this precise information-processing scheme are modulatory systems that involve not only the monoamine transmitters but also neurotransmitters such as acetylcholine, neuropeptides, and purines. The most remarkable of these modulatory systems are those that utilize the monoamines or acetylcholine because, in contrast to glutamate and γ-aminobutyric acid (GABA), these substances are synthesized in a highly restricted number of nuclei in the brain stem and basal forebrain, whose neurons project widely to targets in cortical and subcortical regions in the brain and in the spinal cord. The anatomic organization of these neurotransmitter systems is such that a relatively small number of neurons innervate wide areas of the CNS, and this is consistent with the belief that these systems perform a unique set of intrinsic regulatory functions. Unlike neurotransmitters that are involved in communication of precise individual bits of data about the external world, catecholamines and other monoamines operate through G protein-coupled receptors and second messenger systems to regulate the responsiveness of large areas of brain circuitry.

Norepinephrine (NE), also known as noradrenaline, is synthesized in a small number of brain stem nuclei, the most prominent of which is the locus ceruleus (LC). NE is also used by sympathetic neurons of the autonomic nervous system (see Chapter 12). It targets both α- and β-adrenergic receptors and plays a role in multiple brain functions, including sleep, arousal, attention, learning, and memory. Because the NE system is also involved in the actions of many antidepressant and anti-anxiolytic medications, it has been implicated in the pathogenesis of depression and anxiety disorders. Uncovering how the NE system might be altered in these states, either as a primary or downstream aspect of pathophysiology, remains an important avenue of research (see Chapter 15).

Dopamine (DA) is the biochemical precursor to NE. Like NE, it is produced by a small number of nuclei in the brain, whose projections are less diffuse. DA targets five distinct receptor subtypes (D_1 through D_5) to influence motor activity, cognitive processes, emotion, motivation, and neuroendocrine functions. Moreover, DA systems are involved in **Parkinson disease, schizophrenia,** and **drug addiction,** among other neuropsychiatric disorders.

Epinephrine, or adrenaline, is the major hormone of the adrenal medulla; hence its names in Greek (epinephron) and in Latin (ad-renal), which mean "by the kidney." It is produced by a very small population of neurons in the brain stem, whose precise functions have yet to be determined.

SYNTHETIC PATHWAYS

Catecholamines are molecules with a catechol nucleus and an ethylamine group attached at its 1 position (Figure 8–1). Catecholaminergic neurotransmitters such as NE, DA, and epinephrine are synthesized by means of a shared biosynthetic pathway that begins with the amino acid precursor tyrosine (Figure 8–2). Dietary tyrosine is actively transported into the brain and concentrated in neurons; in catecholaminergic neurons it is hydroxylated at the 3 position by the enzyme tyrosine hydroxylase (TH) to form dihydroxyphenylalanine

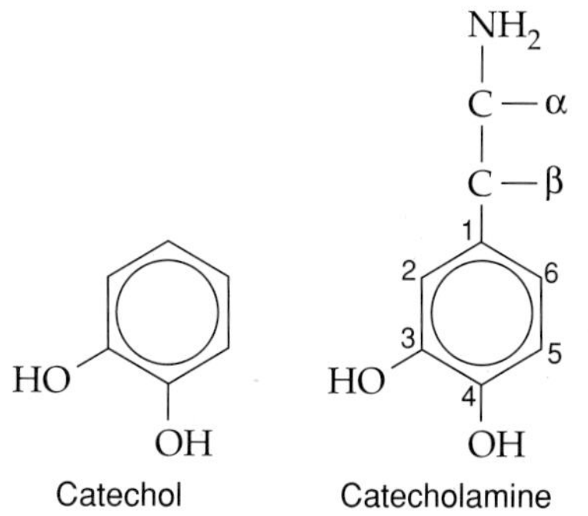

Figure 8–1. Catecholamine structure. An ethylamine group is attached to a catechol nucleus at the 1 position.

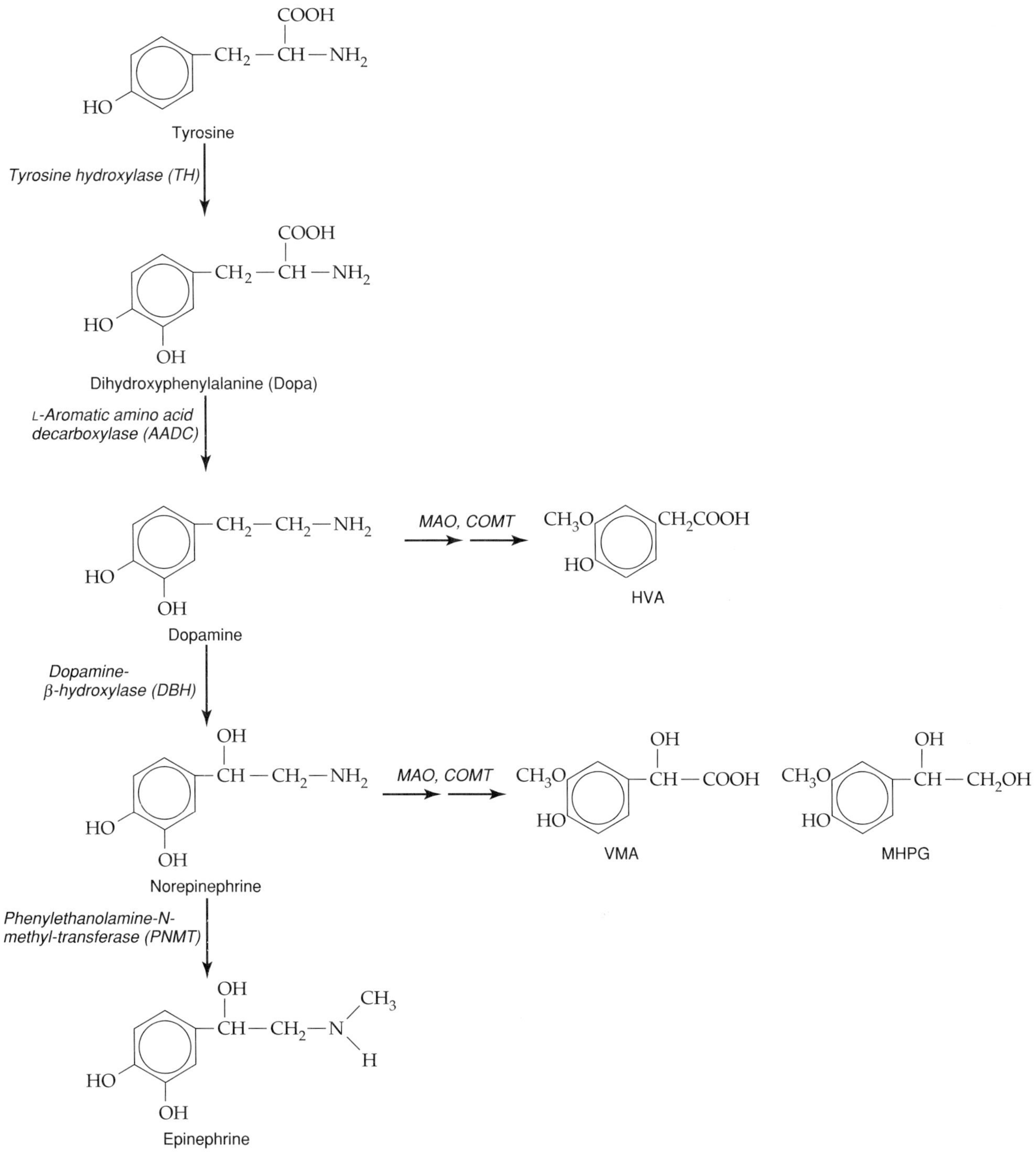

Figure 8-2. Biosynthetic pathway of catecholamines. Dopamine, norepinephrine, and epinephrine are derived from the multistep processing of tyrosine, a dietary amino acid that is actively transported across the blood–brain barrier and concentrated in catecholaminergic neurons. Region-specific expression of the enzymes shown here determine which neurotransmitters are expressed in a given cell; for example, both dopaminergic and noradrenergic cells express tyrosine hydroxylase (TH) and amino acid decarboxylase (AADC), but only noradrenergic cells express dopamine-β-hydroxylase (DBH). The principal metabolites of dopamine and norepinephrine are HVA, VMA, and MHPG. MAO, monoamine oxidase; COMT, catechol-O-methyl transferase; HVA, homovanillic acid; VMA, 3-methoxy-4-hydroxy-mandelic acid (also known as vanillylmandelic acid); MHPG, 3-methoxy-4-hydroxy-phenylglycol.

(dopa). This enzyme exists as a homotetramer; it requires Fe^{2+} as a cofactor, as well as molecular oxygen and tetrahydrobiopterin (a hydrogen donor). An inhibitor of TH known as **α-methylparatyrosine (AMPT)** is used in laboratory animals and in humans as an experimental tool to study catecholamine function. In dopaminergic neurons, only one additional enzyme is expressed in this synthetic pathway, L-aromatic amino acid decarboxylase (AADC), which converts dopa to DA. AADC is a cytoplasmic enzyme that requires pyridoxal phosphate, a substance derived from **vitamin B₆**, for its activity. It was originally known as dopa decarboxylase until molecular cloning revealed that AADC is responsible for the decarboxylation of many substances in the brain, including that of 5-hydroxytryptophan, a precursor of serotonin (see Chapter 9).

In noradrenergic neurons, the synthetic pathway continues with the conversion of DA to NE by the enzyme dopamine-β-hydroxylase (DBH). To form NE, DBH requires Cu^{2+} and ascorbic acid, or **vitamin C,** as cofactors. Based on studies of sympathetic neurons and the adrenal medulla, it is believed that DBH is associated with synaptic vesicles that store NE; indeed, some vesicles release DBH together with NE. Whether this occurs in the CNS remains unknown. In epinephrinergic neurons and in the adrenal medulla, the pathway contains an additional enzyme known as phenylethanolamine-*N*-methyl-transferase (PNMT), which converts NE to epinephrine. *S*-adenosyl-L-methionine, a methyl donor in cells, is a required cofactor for this step. Table 8–1 summarizes the functional properties of the enzymes involved in the biosynthesis of catecholamines. The most highly regulated of these is TH.

TYROSINE HYDROXYLASE

Because TH is the rate-limiting enzyme in catecholamine synthesis, it controls the neuronal concentrations of all catecholamines. Consequently, the regulation of TH and the gene that encodes this enzyme have been the focus of intensive research. In general, when a catecholaminergic neuron or adrenal medullary cell is activated, the activity of TH is increased so that the cell can keep pace with the demands of neurotransmission. Such regulation of TH occurs at the transcriptional, translational, and posttranslational levels.

Very rapid, short-term regulation of TH activity occurs through the posttranslational phosphorylation and dephosphorylation of at least four distinct serine residues in the N terminus of the protein (Figure 8–3). These sites can be phosphorylated by at least nine distinct protein kinases, including protein kinase A, Ca^{2+}/calmodulin-dependent protein kinase II, and protein kinase C. It is believed that phosphorylation by most of these kinases induces a conformational change in the protein that results in a higher affinity for its tetrahydrobiopterin cofactor and a lower affinity for catecholamines that trigger end-product inhibition of TH. The end result is an increase in the catalytic activity of TH, which subsequently leads to an increase in cellular concentrations of DA, NE, or epinephrine. Thus extracellular signals or pharmacologic agents that

Table 8-1 Enzymes Involved in the Synthesis of Catecholamines

Enzyme	Substrate	Product	Requirements	Inhibitors
Amino acid residues (aa)				
Tyrosine hydroxylase (TH) (4 splice variants) TH-1 497 aa TH-2 501 aa TH-3 524 aa TH-4 528 aa	Tyrosine	Dihydroxyphenylalanine (Dopa)	O_2; Fe^{2+}; Tetrahydropteridine cofactor	Amino acid analogs (e.g., α-methyl-*p*-tyrosine); catechol derivatives; tropolones; iron chelators
L-Aromatic amino acid decarboxylase (AADC) (2 splice variants) 442 aa 480 aa	Dopa	Dopamine	Vitamin B₆	Carbidopa; benserazide
Dopamine-β-hydroxylase (DBH) 578 aa	Dopamine	Norepinephrine	Cu^{2+}	Copper chelators; coenzyme A
Phenylethanolamine-*N*-methyl-transferase (PNMT) 282 aa	Norepinephrine	Epinephrine	*S*-adenosyl methionine	

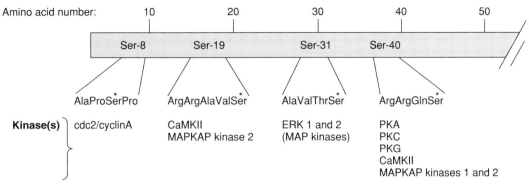

Figure 8–3. Regulatory domains in the N terminus of tyrosine hydroxylase (TH). Short-term regulation of TH enzyme activity occurs through the phosphorylation of at least four serine residues (indicated with an asterisk) in the first forty amino acids of the enzyme. Listed below each residue are the types of kinases that catalyze this phosphorylation. The activities of the kinases themselves are tightly regulated by cellular processes, which means that the phosphorylation state and catalytic activity of TH are regulated by numerous stimuli. Cdc2, cyclin-dependent kinase-2; CaMKII, Ca²⁺/calmodulin-dependent protein kinase II; MAPKAP, MAP-kinase activated kinase; ERK, extracellular signal-regulated kinase; PKA, protein kinase A; PKC, protein kinase C; PKG, protein kinase G. (Adapted with permission from Kumer SC, Vrana KE. 1996. *J Neurochem* 67:446.)

activate protein kinases or phosphatases can control the amount of catecholamine synthesized in a given neuron. Recent efforts to determine the crystal structure of TH have been successful and have paved the way for further advances in our understanding of TH and its catalytic activity.

Longer-term changes in TH activity can occur through transcriptional regulation of the TH gene by numerous extracellular stimuli including neurotransmitters, hormones, and drugs. Stimuli that up-regulate TH expression include chronic environmental stress and drugs such as **caffeine, nicotine,** and **morphine;** among those that down-regulate TH expression are **antidepressants.** These disparate stimuli elicit their effects by activating or repressing transcriptional regulatory elements in the TH gene promoter. The TH promoter (Figure 8–4) contains several DNA regulatory elements, including CRE, GRE, AP-1, and NF-kB sites (see Chapter 6). Among these, the cAMP response element (CRE) appears to play a particularly important role in inducing TH expression in response to physiologic and pharmacologic signals. Increased levels of TH subsequently result in increases in catecholamine biosynthesis. Overall, regulation of TH gene expression by environmental stress or psychotropic drugs represents one of the best established means by which external stimuli produce adaptive changes in target neurons at the transcriptional level.

Under normal conditions, for example, during normal dietary intake of amino acids, tyrosine hydroxylase is fully saturated by levels of circulating tyrosine. Although the ability of peripherally administered tyrosine to penetrate the brain depends on an active transport process at the blood–brain barrier, the transporter involved is saturated under normal circumstances. Consequently, the administration of supplemental tyrosine cannot produce significant increases in catecholamine synthesis in the CNS. However, increased catecholamine synthesis can be achieved by peripheral administration of **levodopa** (L-dopa), which bypasses this rate-limiting enzymatic step and readily penetrates the blood–brain barrier. For this reason, L-dopa is used in the treatment of **Parkinson disease** (see Chapter 14).

Four different splice variants of the TH gene have been detected in humans, although the functional significance of these isoforms is not yet known (see Table 8–1). Rodents express only a single variant of the protein. The stability of TH mRNA and its rate of translation are reported to be regulated as well, although the biologic significance of such regulation has yet to be determined.

TH is only one member of a family of amino acid hydroxylases. Another member is tryptophan hydroxylase, the rate-limiting enzyme involved in the synthesis of serotonin (see Chapter 9). Yet another member of this family, phenylalanine hydroxylase, is the enzyme responsible for converting phenylalanine to tyrosine; mutations in this enzyme are associated with reduced enzyme activity and result in **phenylalaninemias** (e.g., **phenylketonuria**) that, if untreated, can cause severe mental retardation after birth. Interference with the degradation of phenylalanine causes the buildup of oxidized derivatives such as phenylketones, which in turn directly exert toxic effects on nerve cells. An affected individual can nevertheless avoid such complications by eliminating phenylalanine from his or her diet.

A

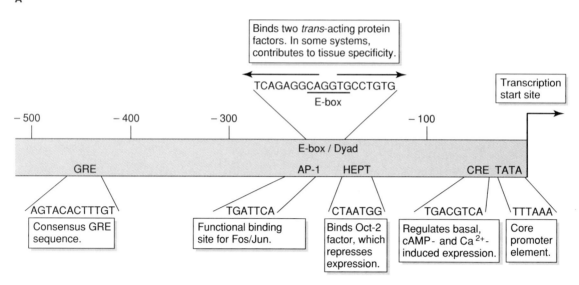

Binds two *trans*-acting protein factors. In some systems, contributes to tissue specificity.

TCAGAGGCAGGTGCCTGTG
E-box

Transcription start site

−500   −400   −300   −100

E-box / Dyad

GRE   AP-1   HEPT   CRE TATA

AGTACACTTTGT
Consensus GRE sequence.

TGATTCA
Functional binding site for Fos/Jun.

CTAATGG
Binds Oct-2 factor, which represses expression.

TGACGTCA
Regulates basal, cAMP- and Ca^{2+}-induced expression.

TTTAAA
Core promoter element.

B

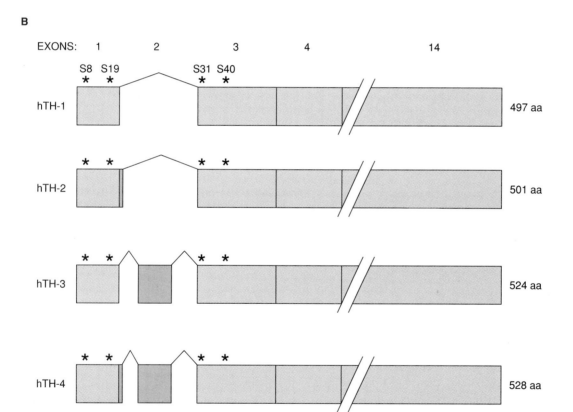

EXONS: 1   2   3   4   14

hTH-1   S8 S19   S31 S40   497 aa

hTH-2   501 aa

hTH-3   524 aa

hTH-4   528 aa

Figure 8–4. Regulation of tyrosine hydroxylase (TH) gene expression. **A.** The TH promoter contains numerous DNA regulatory sequences that participate in gene regulation. Transcription factors that bind to these sites modulate activation and repression of the TH gene (see Chapter 6). **B.** Alternative processing of the tyrosine hydroxylase gene. The human TH gene contains 14 exons; alternative splicing of the first and second of these leads to the production of four different RNA transcripts. All four of the serine phosphorylation sites (indicated with an asterisk and described in Figure 8–3) are conserved in each of the subsequent proteins; the sizes of these proteins are indicated to the right of each transcript. aa, amino acids. (Adapted with permission from Kumer SC, Vrana KE. 1996. *J Neurochem* 67:451.)

DEGRADATIVE PATHWAYS

Catecholamines can be catabolized enzymatically; however, it is important to emphasize that the functional activity of synaptically released catecholamines is primarily terminated through their reuptake into the nerve terminal. The major products that emerge from the enzymatic breakdown of catecholamines include homovanillic acid (HVA), 3-methoxy-4-hydroxy-phenylglycol (VMA), and 3-methoxy-4-hydroxy-phenylglycoaldehyde (MHPG) (see Figure 8–2). Historically, these metabolites have been measured in cerebrospinal fluid, blood plasma, and urine as putative markers of catecholaminergic function in the CNS in disorders such as depression and schizophrenia (see Chapters 15 and 17). However, levels of these metabolites are confounded by activity of the sympathetic nervous system and adrenal medulla and many other factors. Thus their usefulness as markers of CNS catecholamine function is limited. Indeed, despite decades of research, analysis of these markers has not revealed information about the pathophysiology of neuropsychiatric disorders.

MONOAMINE OXIDASE

Catecholamines are converted to their aldehyde derivatives by monoamine oxidase (MAO), a major degradative enzyme that requires flavin adenine dinucleotide (FAD) as a cofactor. Because MAO exists both intracellularly and extracellularly, its inhibition increases presynaptic intracellular transmitter concentrations and prolongs the availability of synaptically released transmitter. **MAO inhibitors (MAOIs)**, such as **tranylcypromine** and **deprenyl,** are used clinically to treat **depression** and **Parkinson disease** (see Chapters 14 and 15). However, the clinical use of MAOIs as antidepressants has been limited because of their potentially serious side effects, which can be traced to the presence of MAO in both the brain and peripheral tissues (Box 8–1).

Two major forms of MAO have been described: MAO_A and MAO_B. These forms are derived from distinct genes and differ with regard to several biochemical properties, including their substrate specificity, cellular localization, and regulation by pharmacologic agents (Table 8–2). The significant clinical ramifications of these differences are discussed in Box 8–1.

CATECHOL-O-METHYL TRANSFERASE

Catecholamines also can be catabolized by catechol-*O*-methyl transferase (COMT), which is found in the synaptic cleft. This enzyme acts to methylate catecholamines and requires *S*-adenosyl-methionine as a methyl donor. COMT inhibitors, such as **entacapone** and **tolcapone,** increase levels of catecholaminergic neurotransmitter in the synaptic cleft and prolong receptor activation. In rare cases, COMT inhibitors are coadministered with L-dopa to enhance dopaminergic function in individuals with Parkinson disease. The crystal structure of COMT has been determined and may be used to guide the development of more specific inhibitors.

FUNCTIONAL ANATOMY

NOREPINEPHRINE

The locus ceruleus, which is located on the floor of the fourth ventricle in the rostral pons, contains more than 50% of all noradrenergic neurons in the brain. This region of the brain is also known in the rat as area A6, based on the Falck–Hillarp method of mapping monoamine systems in the rat brain. This method involves the autofluorescence of monoaminergic neurons after exposure of brain sections to formaldehyde. The locus ceruleus on each side of the brain stem contains only about 12,500 neurons in humans, and even fewer neurons in rodents, yet this exceedingly small number is misleading in terms of the importance of NE to overall brain function. Indeed, mutant mice that are deficient in NE cannot survive. Although they are few in number, the cells of the locus ceruleus have widely distributed axons that project to virtually every area of the brain and spinal cord (Figure 8–5). Thus changes in neuronal activity in the locus ceruleus can alter NE release to postsynaptic sites throughout the neuroaxis. The other noradrenergic neurons in the brain occur in loose collections of cells in the brain stem, such as the lateral tegmental regions, which have been designated areas A1, A2, A5, and A7 in the rat. The axons of these neurons also project to the spinal cord and brain but are not as widely distributed as those of neurons in the locus ceruleus.

As previously mentioned, epinephrine occurs in only a small number of neurons in the CNS, whose functioning remains poorly understood. These cells also are located in lateral tegmental regions (designated area C1), as well as in the dorsal medulla (area C2) and medial longitudinal fascicle (area C3).

The noradrenergic system is implicated in several critical brain functions (see Chapters 17 and 18). It is believed, for example, that this system is involved in regulating the stages of the sleep–wake cycle. The firing of neurons in the locus ceruleus increases during waking and dramatically decreases during slow-wave and paradoxical sleep. (Paradoxical sleep in rats is equivalent to REM sleep in humans.) Moreover, drowsi-

Box 8–1 Monoamine Oxidases and Their Inhibitors

Although MAO_A and MAO_B share structural similarities, and although 70% of their constituent amino acids are identical, they are quite different enzymes. They arise from distinct genes on the X chromosome and are expressed in different regions of the nervous system. MAO_A mRNA is expressed almost exclusively in noradrenergic neurons, such as those in sympathetic ganglia and in the locus ceruleus. MAO_B mRNA is detected predominantly in serotonergic neurons, such as those that comprise the raphe nuclei, and in histaminergic neurons of the hypothalamus. Neither of the genes for these enzymes appears to be expressed in dopaminergic neurons, although this remains a matter of controversy.

Both enzymes oxidize monoamines but differ somewhat in their affinity for substrates. MAO_A displays a strong affinity for norepinephrine and serotonin. In contrast, MAO_B exhibits the highest affinity for β-phenylethylamine, an endogenous brain amine. However, because β-phenylethylamine is expressed in very small amounts in the brain, it is unclear whether a true substrate for MAO_B has been determined. MAO_A and MAO_B have similar affinities for dopamine.

Most MAO inhibitors that are used clinically are nonselective; that is, they block both MAO_A and MAO_B. Examples include **phenelzine, tranylcypromine, and isocarboxazid.** The first available MAO inhibitor, a congener of isoniazid known as **iproniazid,** was tested in the mid-1900s as an antimicrobial agent for the treatment of tuberculosis. Although it was ineffective against mycobacteria, it relieved the depression that was common among patients hospitalized with TB. Iproniazid is no longer used clinically because it causes hepatitis, but the other MAO inhibitors continue to be highly effective in the treatment of depression and panic disorder. They may even be more effective than tricyclic antidepressants in the treatment of so-called **atypical depression,** which is characterized by a reversal of the usual neurovegetative symptoms of depression (e.g., hypersomnia instead of insomnia, and hyperphagia instead of anorexia).

MAOs are localized not only in the brain but also in peripheral tissues. MAO_A is expressed in both gut and liver, where it catabolizes biogenic amines present in foods. Some aged or fermented foods, including many wines and cheeses, have particularly high levels of biogenic amines such as tyramine. When MAO_A is inhibited, as in response

to the therapeutic use of nonselective MAO inhibitors, biogenic amines in foods can enter the general circulation and can be taken up into sympathetic nerve terminals by norepinephrine reuptake transporters. This process can lead to the massive displacement and release of norepinephrine from sympathetic nerve terminals, and also can cause the release of epinephrine from the adrenal medulla. Such release typically results in a hyperadrenergic crisis, which is characterized by headache, hypertension that can be severe, and chest pain. Alternatively, tyramine and related substances may serve as false transmitters that, after displacing norepinephrine from nerve terminals, are themselves released from the terminals to act on adrenergic receptors; however, this hypothesis remains unproven. To prevent a potentially dangerous hyperadrenergic syndrome, individuals who take nonselective MAO inhibitors must eliminate tyramine-containing foods from their diet.

Because the inhibition of MAO_A appears to be required for antidepressant action and also necessitates dietary restrictions, there has been considerable interest in the development of reversible inhibitors of MAO_A (so-called **RIMAs** such as **meclobemide**). Such medications currently are used in Europe, but they are less efficacious than other antidepressants and ultimately may not be used in the United States.

MAO inhibitors also have been used to treat **Parkinson disease.** They were initially tested for this purpose after investigators discovered that the dopamine neurotoxin **MPTP,** which was known to cause Parkinson disease in drug abusers, must be converted to MPP^+ by MAO_B before it can exert toxic effects on dopaminergic neurons (see Box 8–2). Consequently the MAO_B-selective inhibitor **deprenyl** (also known as **selegiline**) was administered in clinical trials as a putative neuroprotective agent. Although it has been used to treat the early stages of Parkinson disease, its mechanism of action remains unclear; for example, it is not known whether the modest but real benefits of this drug are related to its neuroprotective effect or to its ability to increase levels of synaptic dopamine. More investigation is needed to evaluate these possibilities. At low doses deprenyl does not affect MAO_A and thus does not require alterations in diet. However, at the high doses required for antidepressant effects, the drug becomes a nonselective MAO inhibitor and its use requires dietary precautions.

ness has been associated with a reduction in cell firing in this region of the brain, and alertness typically is accompanied by an increase in neuronal discharge. In rodents and nonhuman primates who are awake, the locus ceruleus acts principally to control vigilance and perhaps contribute to working memory. Firing in the locus ceruleus is correlated with the onset of new sensory stimuli; when an animal is awake yet inattentive to external stimuli, firing rates are lower.

Cells in the locus ceruleus are most responsive to stimuli that are noxious or stressful. Phasic, fear-associated stimuli produce the greatest increases in firing among cells in this region and, in turn, an increase in NE release in the brain. Drugs such as the α_2-adrenergic receptor antagonist **yohimbine,** which increase firing in the locus ceruleus by blocking inhibitory autoreceptors, induce fear and anxiety in laboratory animals and in humans. Agents such as **opiates,** which act on μ opi-

Table 8-2 Properties of Catecholaminergic Metabolic Enzymes

Metabolic Enzyme	Neurotransmitter Substrates	Selective Inhibitors	Clinical Uses of Inhibitors
Amino acid residues (aa)			
Monoamine oxidase B (MAO$_A$) 528 aa	Norepinephrine; serotonin; dopamine	Clorgyline; tranylcypromine	Depression; anxiety
Monoamine oxidase B (MAO$_B$) 528 aa	β-phenylethylamine; dopamine	Deprenyl	Parkinson disease; possibly Alzheimer disease; stroke; ALS; and epilepsy
Catechol-O-methyl transferase (COMT) 221 aa (soluble) 271 aa (membrane-bound)	Norepinephrine; dopamine	Tolcapone; entacapone	Parkinson disease

oid receptors (see Chapter 10), and **benzodiazepines,** which act on GABA$_A$ receptors (see Chapter 7), decrease firing and thereby decrease anxiety behaviors. Although these agents affect many brain regions, it is believed that the locus ceruleus and other noradrenergic systems contribute to normal fear and stress responses and may play a role in neuropsychiatric conditions associated with fear and stress, such as **panic disorder** and **posttraumatic stress disorder** (**PTSD**).

It is important to note that the cell physiology of the locus ceruleus can be altered by several classes of abused drugs, including **opiates, nicotine, stimulants** (e.g., **amphetamine** and **cocaine**), **alcohol,** and **halluci-** **nogens**. The role of the locus ceruleus in addictive behaviors is discussed in greater detail in Chapter 16.

DOPAMINE

The total number of dopaminergic neurons in the human brain (excluding those in the retina and olfactory bulb) is estimated to be between 300,000 and 400,000. The three primary dopaminergic nuclei in the rat brain are the substantia nigra pars compacta (designated area A9), the ventral tegmental area (area A10), and the arcuate nucleus (Figure 8–6). Similar clusters of neurons exist in the primate brain, although they

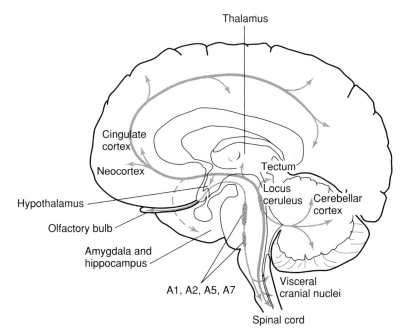

Figure 8-5. Noradrenergic systems of the brain. The locus ceruleus of the rostral pons is the principal noradrenergic nucleus of the brain. It projects to almost all areas of the CNS, as indicated by thick arrows. Other sources of norepinephrine are found in loose clusters of cells designated areas A1, A2, A5, and A7. The projections from these cells are much more limited than those from cells of the locus ceruleus.

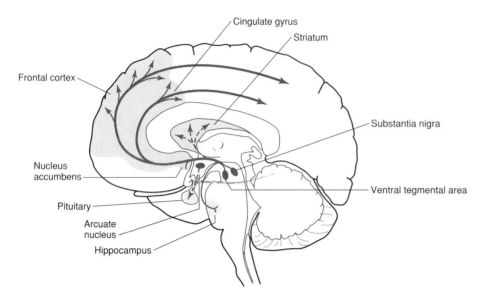

Figure 8–6. Dopaminergic systems of the brain. Three main dopaminergic nuclei occur in the brain. The substantia nigra pars compacta projects to the striatum (*upward dashed arrows*); the ventral tegmental area projects to the nucleus accumbens and some regions of cerebral cortex (*solid arrows*); and the arcuate nucleus of the hypothalamus projects to the tuberoinfundibular area of the hypothalamus, which is in close proximity to the pituitary stalk. (*downward dashed arrow*).

are generally less compact. Cells of the substantia nigra pars compacta reside in the ventral midbrain and project primarily to the caudate and putamen, which are referred to collectively as the neostriatum, to form the nigrostriatal DA system. Cells of the ventral tegmental area, also found in the ventral midbrain just medial and posterior to the substantia nigra, project to limbic structures including the nucleus accumbens, prefrontal cortex, and cingulate cortex (cortical innervation by DA neurons is particularly dense in primates). Together, these structures and the connections between them form the mesolimbocortical DA system. Dopaminergic cells of the hypothalamic arcuate nucleus release DA that affects the pituitary gland and constitute the tuberoinfundibular DA system. Several other cell types in the CNS also utilize DA, including periglomerular cells of the olfactory bulb and amacrine cells of the retina.

The three major dopaminergic systems in the brain serve distinct functions and elicit very different behavioral effects when disrupted. The tuberoinfundibular DA system controls prolactin release from the anterior pituitary; thus disruption of its function can lead to neuroendocrine effects. **Antipsychotic** drugs, which antagonize DA D_2 receptors and thereby disrupt this regulatory control, can precipitate **hyperprolactinemia** and even lactation. Conversely, **bromocriptine**, a DA D_2 receptor agonist, is used to treat hyperprolactemia, which is most commonly caused by prolactin-secreting **pituitary adenomas** (see Chapter 13).

The neostriatum, which is a component of the basal ganglia, regulates motor control and the learning of motor programs and habits. DA release in the nigrostriatal system plays an integral part in the complex circuitry of the basal ganglia and is required for voluntary movement. If dopaminergic neurons of the substantia

nigra pars compacta die, as occurs in **Parkinson disease,** DA levels in the striatum decrease, and voluntary motor control is severely compromised. **L-Dopa** is still the mainstay in the treatment of Parkinson disease. When L-dopa is administered to a patient with Parkinson disease, it is absorbed into the bloodstream and transported across the blood–brain barrier to dopaminergic nerve terminals, where it is converted by aromatic amino acid decarboxylase (AADC) to dopamine. However, because AADC also resides in peripheral tissues, a significant fraction of L-dopa is decarboxylated into dopamine before it can be transported into the brain. Thus the clinical benefits of a dose of L-dopa often are severely compromised because dopamine cannot penetrate the blood–brain barrier. Moreover, the peripheral conversion of L-dopa to dopamine produces nausea and other side effects. Consequently, L-dopa typically is coadministered with an AADC inhibitor such as **carbidopa** that cannot penetrate the brain. When delivered in this manner, the peripheral side effects of L-dopa are significantly diminished, and the fraction of administered drug that enters the brain is greatly enhanced. Because antipsychotic drugs antagonize DA D_2 receptors, as previously mentioned, they can produce serious motor disturbances, or extrapyramidal side effects, which are similar to the symptoms of Parkinson disease. The circuitry of the basal ganglia, and the role of dopaminergic transmission in Parkinson disease and other motor disorders, are described in greater detail in Chapter 14.

The mesolimbocortical dopamine system has both cognitive and emotive functions. One of the best characterized attributes of this system is its role as a reward pathway. Specifically, dopaminergic connections between the ventral tegmental area and the nucleus accumbens appear to mediate the reinforcing, or rewarding, properties of drugs of abuse (see Chapter 16). In addition, this system is believed to be the anatomic target for the therapeutic actions of antipsychotic drugs, which antagonize DA function and in turn ameliorate psychotic symptoms in patients with schizophrenia or other psychotic disorders (see Chapter 17).

STORAGE, RELEASE, AND REUPTAKE

Most catecholamine synthesis does not occur in the cell bodies of noradrenergic and dopaminergic neurons; rather, enzymes involved in the formation of these transmitters are transported from cell bodies to nerve terminals, where the bulk of transmitter synthesis takes place. DA is synthesized in the nerve terminal cytoplasm and is packaged in storage vesicles by means of vesicular monoamine transporter proteins (VMATs); thus the synapse maintains a reservoir of neurotransmitter that is protected from rapid metabolism by MAO. In noradrenergic terminals, DA is converted to NE by DBH, which also is located in storage vesicles. Two human VMATs have been cloned: VMAT1, a 526-amino acid protein expressed in the adrenal medulla and other neuroendocrine tissues but not in the brain, and VMAT2, a 515-amino acid protein that is expressed in brain. The predicted structural features of both VMATs are very similar to those described for the

plasma membrane transporters discussed in the next section of this chapter.

Reserpine and related compounds (e.g., **tetrabenazine**) inhibit catecholamine uptake into storage vesicles through the blockade of VMATs, and thereby deplete available stores of transmitter. Such depletion manifests itself physiologically in dramatic fashion; for example, it may result in a rapid and profound decrease in blood pressure. Reserpine is best known as an antihypertensive agent, but it also was the first antipsychotic drug available. Its clinical use today is rare because of its side effects; for example, approximately 15% of individuals who use this medication experience serious depression. These side effects may result from the profound depletion of both catecholamines and serotonin.

Catecholamines released into the synaptic cleft may undergo one or more of the following: 1) degradation by COMT or MAO, as previously discussed; 2) diffusion from the synaptic cleft; 3) presynaptic receptor activation; 4) postsynaptic receptor activation; or 5) transporter-mediated reuptake into the presynaptic terminal (Figure 8–7). The latter three events are discussed in greater detail in the sections that follow.

PLASMA MEMBRANE TRANSPORTERS

As explained in Chapter 4, both DA and NE transporters (DAT and NET, respectively) are transmembrane proteins that function to remove transmitter

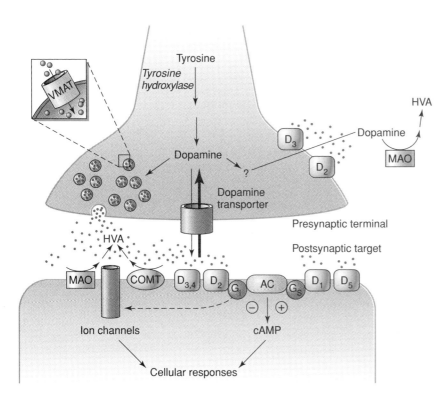

Figure 8–7. Model of a dopaminergic synapse. Presynaptic and postsynaptic molecular entities associated with the synthesis, release, signaling, and reuptake of dopamine are shown. Note that tyrosine hydroxylase (TH) is transported to the synaptic terminal so that dopamine may be synthesized on site. Also note that the D_2 receptor resides in both presynaptic and postsynaptic locations; in the former it functions as an autoreceptor and in the latter it assists in intercellular signaling. The D_3 receptor is also present on the presynaptic terminal, but its function is unclear. The question mark in the dopamine nerve terminal refers to persisting controversy as to whether MAO is expressed in dopaminergic neurons or whether most dopamine metabolism occurs in other cells, particularly glia. VMAT, vesicular monoamine transporter; G_i and G_s, inhibitory and stimulatory guanine nucleotide-binding proteins; MAO, monoamine oxidase; COMT, catechol-O-methyltransferase; AC, adenylyl cyclase.

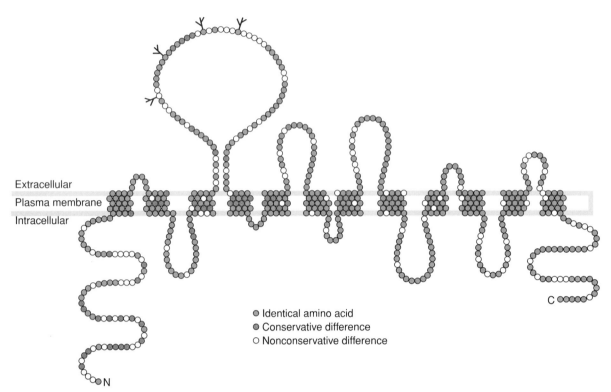

Figure 8–8. Two-dimensional model of a catecholamine transporter. This beads-on-a-string model illustrates several features of these proteins. First, both the N terminus (N) and C terminus (C) are believed to reside intracellularly. Second, the protein possesses 12 hydrophobic, membrane-spanning domains with intervening extracellular and intracellular loops. The second extracellular loop is the largest and contains several potential glycosylation sites (indicated with tree-like symbols). Third, the color coding of the beads reveals the similarity between norepinephrine and dopamine transporters in terms of constituent amino acids. The most highly conserved regions of these transporters are located in transmembrane domains; the most divergent areas occur in N and C termini. (Adapted with permission from Buck KJ, Amara S. 1995. *Mol Pharmacol* 48:1035.)

from the synapse and return it to the presynaptic terminal (Figure 8–8). The rapid reuptake of released transmitter by these transporters has several consequences that are vitally important to signaling among neurons. First, reuptake limits the duration of presynaptic and postsynaptic receptor activation. Second, it limits the diffusion of transmitter molecules to other synapses. Third, it allows for the recycling and reuse of unmetabolized transmitter. Accordingly, NET and DAT are targets for two major classes of psychotropic drugs. Various **tricyclic** and related **antidepressants** act initially by antagonizing NE and serotonin transporters (see Chapter 15). Some **psychostimulants** such as **cocaine** block DA, NE, and serotonin transporters. Other psychostimulants, such as **amphetamine** and related drugs, serve as substrates for these transporters; after they enter the nerve terminal, they cause the transporters to actively pump neurotransmitter out of the terminal (see Chapter 16). Table 8–3 lists some drugs that are known to inhibit or reverse reuptake by catecholamine transporters.

Table 8–3 Binding Properties of Catecholamine Transporters

Norepinephrine (NET)		Dopamine (DAT)	
Drug	K_i or K_m (nM)	Drug	K_i or K_m (nM)
Mazindol	1.4	Mazindol	11
Desipramine	4.0	Nomifensine	17
Imipramine	65	Benztropine	55
Amitriptyline	100	GBR 12783	13
Nortriptyline	16.5	GBR 12209	17
Cocaine	140	Cocaine	58
D-amphetamine	55	D-amphetamine	2260

NOREPINEPHRINE TRANSPORTER

The human NET is a 617-amino acid with 12 hydrophobic transmembrane domains, three extracellular *N*-linked glycosylation sites, and one cytoplasmic serine–threonine phosphorylation site. Among the members of the neurotransmitter transporter superfamily, NET is most similar to DAT in terms of constituent amino

Substrate (protein abbreviation)

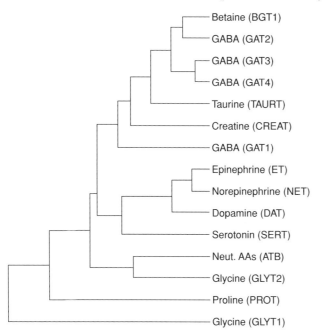

Betaine (BGT1)

GABA (GAT2)

GABA (GAT3)

GABA (GAT4)

Taurine (TAURT)

Creatine (CREAT)

GABA (GAT1)

Epinephrine (ET)

Norepinephrine (NET)

Dopamine (DAT)

Serotonin (SERT)

Neut. AAs (ATB)

Glycine (GLYT2)

Proline (PROT)

Glycine (GLYT1)

Figure 8–9. Neurotransmitter transporter gene tree. The alignment of the amino acid sequences of cloned neurotransmitter transporters has revealed the relatedness of their corresponding genes. The lengths of the branches in this tree are proportional to the degree of similarity among sequences. The colored lines indicate that NET and DAT genes are most homologous to one another and are more closely related to the serotonin transporter than to other members of the transporter family. (Borrowed with permission from E. Adkins and R. D. Blakely, Vanderbilt University.)

acids (Figure 8–9). NET mRNA is expressed predominantly in the locus ceruleus; it also has been detected in other noradrenergic regions, including areas A4, A5, and A7, the lateral tegmentum, and the nucleus tractus solitarius. After the NET protein is translated, it is transported from noradrenergic cell bodies to the vast terminal fields projecting from the locus ceruleus and other noradrenergic nuclei.

Although antibodies to DAT have enabled researchers to determine the cellular and subcellular distribution of the protein, antibodies suitable for NET immunocytochemistry have yet to be developed. Consequently, localization of NET must rely on binding studies involving the use of a highly selective NET radioligand, such as [³H]**nisoxetine**. In situ binding autoradiography reveals [³H]nisoxetine sites throughout the brain; most binding at these sites occurs in the locus ceruleus and anteroventral thalamic nucleus, and the least occurs in the striatum. Interestingly, fairly high levels of binding are detected in the dorsal raphe nucleus, which is the

primary source of serotonin in brain (see Chapter 9). Because the dorsal raphe contains few noradrenergic cells, the dense [³H]nisoxetine binding in this location is believed to involve NETs on noradrenergic terminals that heavily innervate raphe neurons. This hypothesis is consistent with studies indicating that the noradrenergic system strongly influences serotonergic cell physiology in the dorsal raphe.

Many commonly used antidepressant drugs exhibit high affinity for NET, including the tricyclic antidepressants **desipramine, imipramine, amitriptyline,** and **nortriptyline** (see Table 8–3). More recently developed inhibitors, which also are used as antidepressants, include **venlafaxine** and **reboxetine**. Some of these, including desipramine, nortriptyline, and reboxetine, are highly selective for NET. The clinical efficacy of these various compounds is believed to be related to their interference with noradrenergic reuptake. However, because antagonism of NET occurs very soon after drug administration, and the clinical benefits of these drugs are not evident until several weeks after continued administration, the exact role of NET blockade in antidepressant action remains unknown. Understanding the long-term adaptive mechanisms that result from NET blockade is a goal of current research in the field of depression (see Chapter 15).

DOPAMINE TRANSPORTER

The human DAT is a 620-amino acid protein believed to have 12 hydrophobic membrane-spanning domains, two to four extracellular *N*-linked glycosylation sites, and as many as five cytoplasmic serine–threonine phosphorylation sites. As previously mentioned, human DAT and NET exhibit 66% homology at the amino acid level but are considerably less homologous to other members of the neurotransmitter transporter superfamily (see Figure 8–9). The critical role played by DAT in maintaining homeostasis of the brain's DA systems is highlighted by the extraordinary abnormalities that occur in mice that lack this one protein. DAT knockout mice display multiple compensatory adaptations in numerous synthetic enzymes and receptors that appear to counter the elevated synaptic levels of DA caused by the absence of DAT. However, despite such adaptations, these mice exhibit an extreme level of hyperactivity, which is indicative of a hyperdopaminergic state.

Northern blot and in situ hybridization studies reveal that DAT gene expression occurs exclusively in brain regions in which DA is synthesized. DAT mRNA is most abundant in the substantia nigra and ventral tegmental area, and is less prevalent in the arcuate nucleus, olfactory bulb, and inner nuclear layer of the retina. It is most commonly translated in cell bodies, and transported to dendrites and axon fibers. Antibodies raised against DAT have been used to determine the specific cellular and subcellular localization of the protein. Dense immunoreactivity in perikarya is limited to the substantia nigra and ventral tegmental areas; only faint staining occurs in other dopaminergic regions, including the arcuate nucleus and olfactory bulb. Fibers and terminal regions most immunoreactive for DAT are found throughout the striatum and nucleus accumbens, the primary projection areas of neurons from the substantia nigra and ventral tegmental area, respectively. Other regions that exhibit immunoreactivity in fibers or terminal fields include the amygdala, hippocampus, zona incerta, olfactory bulb, islets of Calleja, and medial prefrontal and cingulate cortices.

Ultrastructurally, DAT immunoreactivity in terminal fields throughout the CNS has proven to be plasma membrane-associated, in accordance with the view that synaptic DATs reside in the presynaptic membrane. In addition, dendritic plasma membranes in both the substantia nigra and ventral tegmental area are immunoreactive for DAT and thus are also sites for the presynaptic reuptake of DA. This finding is consistent with the results of earlier neurochemical studies that implicated dendritic release of DA in ventral midbrain function. Interestingly, DAT immunoreactivity also has been detected in axonal plasma membranes, where Ca^{2+}-mediated DA release would not be expected. DAT may act as a reverse transporter that conveys DA out of the axon; although it remains controversial, such DAT-mediated transmitter release has been demonstrated experimentally. DAT staining in cell bodies is confined to cytoplasmic membranous structures and therefore is indicative of DAT localization in endoplasmic reticulum and Golgi saccules. Such localization is consistent with the synthesis of DAT in cell bodies and its subsequent transport to neuronal processes.

DAT function has been studied in several neuropsychiatric disorders—particularly those related to drug addiction and Parkinson disease. **Cocaine**, for example, binds to DAT and blocks the reuptake of synaptically released DA. Such antagonism of DAT function in the mesolimbic DA system is believed to mediate the reinforcing properties of this drug (see Chapter 16). Study of chimeric DAT and NET proteins has revealed that the cocaine binding site in DAT is distinct from the substrate recognition site. This finding suggests the exciting possibility that one or more compounds may be developed to antagonize cocaine's affinity for DAT without hindering DA transport. Such compounds, or "cocaine antagonists," might be useful clinical tools in the treatment of cocaine addiction.

DAT has been implicated in experimental models of **Parkinson disease**, although the relevance of these models to common forms of the disease is not clear. As previously indicated, this progressive disease of motor control is characterized by the degeneration of dopaminergic cells of the substantia nigra, which leads to the depletion of DA in the striatum. One model of Parkinson disease suggests that it may be traced to a DAT-mediated accumulation of neurotoxins in the DA neurons of the substantia nigra. This model, together with DAT's possible role in certain other neuropsychiatric disorders, is discussed in Box 8–2.

RECEPTORS

Synaptically released NE or DA that is not degraded enzymatically or transported back into the presynaptic cell may activate receptors. All catecholaminergic receptors belong to the G protein-coupled receptor superfamily. The binding of a catecholamine to a membrane-bound receptor initiates a conformational change in the receptor such that it activates a G protein, which in turn is coupled to an ion channel or second messenger system (see Chapter 5). Although only one transporter has been identified for each transmitter, numerous adrenergic and dopaminergic receptors have been cloned. Each type of receptor is unique with regard to its pharmacologic properties, its localization in brain and peripheral tissues, its effector coupling, and its role in both normal brain function and pathophysiology.

The nomenclature associated with adrenergic and dopaminergic receptors is complicated because most of the names were assigned when receptors were identified according to their unique pharmacologic profiles, before the advent of modern molecular cloning techniques. Cloning led to the definitive identification of distinct receptor subtypes and generated a different classification scheme for many of these receptors. Thus modern receptor nomenclature is a hybrid of two types of classification.

Cloned adrenergic receptors are divided into α and β categories, both of which comprise multiple receptor subtypes (Table 8–4). Each subtype responds in varying degrees to both NE and epinephrine. All β receptors are G_s-coupled, and most α_1 receptors are G_q-coupled; α_2 receptors, which are generally G_i-coupled, function not only as heteroreceptors but also as autoreceptors for catecholaminergic neurons. Drugs that act on adrenergic receptors and some of their common clinical uses are discussed in Box 8–3.

Cloned dopaminergic receptors are classified as D_1-like or D_2-like (Table 8–5). The D_1-like receptors, which include D_1 and D_5 receptors, are G_s-coupled. The D_2-like receptors, which comprise D_2, D_3, and D_4 receptors, are G_i-coupled. The D_2 receptor, which appears to be the major autoreceptor for dopaminergic neurons, has two splice variants, D_{2short} and D_{2long}; however,

Box 8-2 DAT in Neuropsychiatric Disorders

One of the most common animal models of Parkinson disease involves the use of the synthetic toxin 1-methyl-4-phenyl-1,2,3,6-tetrahydropyridine (**MPTP**). MPTP initially was determined to be a contaminant in a preparation of the opiate **meperidine,** and was responsible for inducing a severe Parkinson disease-like syndrome in a group of individuals who were addicted to opiates. Subsequently MPTP proved to be a selective toxin for dopamine neurons in animal studies.

MPTP is believed to exert its selective toxic effect according to the following scheme. Because it is relatively lipophilic, MPTP can pass through the blood–brain barrier. In the brain, it is converted into 1-methyl-4-phenylpyrdinium (MPP$^+$) by MAO$_B$. MAO$_B$ currently is believed to be a glial enzyme and may not be expressed in dopamine neurons themselves, although this hypothesis remains controversial. MPP$^+$ subsequently is tranported into dopaminergic nerve terminals by the dopamine transporter (DAT); its ability to serve as a substrate only for DAT, and not for other transporters, explains MPP$^+$'s selective effect on dopamine neurons. From inside nerve terminals MPP$^+$ is believed to exert a direct toxic effect on neurons, either by acting on nerve terminal mitochondria to generate oxygen-reactive species or by inhibiting complex I of the respiratory chain of the inner mitochondrial membrane (see Chapter 11). Both actions lead to the degeneration of dopaminergic neurons. Consistent with this scheme is

the observation that knockout mice that lack DAT are resistant to MPTP toxicity. Moreover, the high level of DAT expression in terminal fields and dendrites of dopaminergic neurons in the substantia nigra make this region especially vulnerable to toxins such as MPTP and may account for the relatively selective destruction of nigral cells in Parkinson disease. However, whether this disease is caused by environmental exposure to as yet unidentified toxins remains a matter of considerable debate (see Chapter 14).

Several other disorders may involve DAT dysfunction. Elevated levels of DAT binding have been detected in positron emission tomography and single-photon emission computed tomography (SPECT) studies of patients with **Tourette syndrome,** a condition marked by motor tics (Chapter 14). SPECT studies also reveal that **Lesch-Nyhan disease,** an X-linked disorder characterized by dystonia, choreoathetosis, and compulsive self-injury, is associated with a dramatic 50–75% reduction in DAT binding levels in the striatum. A significant reduction in DAT binding is also seen in the striatum of patients with **Rett syndrome,** a neurodevelopmental disorder caused by a defect in chromatin remodeling (see Chapter 6), which is characterized by mental retardation, autistic behavior, and motor dysfunction. Although all of these findings are largely preliminary, they point to DAT as a possible target for new therapies for these disorders.

Table 8-4 The Adrenergic Receptor Family

Receptor	Agonists[1]	Antagonists[1]	G Protein Coupling	Areas of Localization
Amino acid residues (aa)				
α_{1A} 466 aa	A61603* Phenylephrine Methoxamine	Nigulpidine* Prazosin Indoramin	$G_{q/11}$	Cortex Hippocampus
α_{1B} 519 aa	Phenylephrine Methoxamine	Spiperone* Prazosin Indoramin	$G_{q/11}$	Cortex Brain stem
α_{1D} 572 aa	Phenylephrine Methoxamine	Prazosin Indoramin	$G_{q/11}$	
α_{2A} 450 aa	Oxymetazoline*; clonidine	Yohimbine; rauwolscine; prazosin	$G_{i/o}$	Cortex; brain stem; midbrain; spinal cord
α_{2B} 450 aa	Clonidine	Yohimbine; rauwolscine; prazosin	$G_{i/o}$	Diencephalon
α_{2C} 461 aa	Clonidine	Yohimbine; rauwolscine; prazosin	$G_{i/o}$	Basal ganglia; cortex; cerebellum; hippocampus
β_1 477 aa	Isoproterenol; terbutaline*	Alprenolol*; betaxolol*; propranold	G_s	Olfactory nucleus; cortex; cerebellar nuclei; brain stem nuclei; spinal cord
β_2 413 aa	Procaterol*; zinterol*	Propranolol	G_s	Olfactory bulb; piriform cortex; hippocampus; cerebellar cortex
β_3 408 aa		Pindolol*; bupranolol*; propranolol	$G_s/G_{i/o}$	

[1]Asterisks indicate selective agonists and antagonists.

Box 8–3 Common Clinical Uses of Adrenergic Receptor Ligands

Drugs that act on adrenergic receptors are among the most widely used medications. Many of their actions are related to the functioning of the autonomic nervous system and are discussed in greater detail in Chapter 12. β-Adrenergic receptor (β-AR) agonists are used in the treatment of asthma and other obstructive pulmonary diseases; their activation, through G_s and activation of the cAMP pathway, promotes the relaxation of the smooth muscle that lines the bronchial tree and thereby relieves obstruction of lower airways. Selective β_2 agonists, such as **terbutaline** and **salbutamol,** are used for this purpose because of the concentration of their corresponding receptors in bronchial smooth muscle. In contrast, β-AR antagonists, which are used in the treatment of **hypertension, angina,** and **tachyarrhythmias,** act by reducing the tonic influence of catecholamines on cardiac contraction; selective β_1 antagonists such as **alprenolol** are used for these purposes because of the concentration of their receptors in cardiac myocytes. Related β-AR antagonists, such as **timolol,** are also used to reduce ocular pressure in patients with certain types of **glaucoma. Propranolol,** a β-AR antagonist that does not distinguish among β receptor subtypes, crosses the blood–brain barrier and is used not only for cardiovascular disorders but also for the treatment of stimulus-bound forms of **social phobia,** most notably stage fright. By means of a central action that is not yet well understood, it reduces the excessive activation of the sympathetic nervous system that occurs in some people with anxiety disorders.

Agonists at α_1 receptors are the principal components of many commonly used decongestant drugs, including **ephedrine, pseudephedrine,** and **phenylephrine.** Although these agents are not highly selective α_1 agonists in vitro, their clinical effectiveness appears to be related to their actions on this receptor subtype. In contrast, antagonists at α_1 receptors, such as **prazosin,** are potent antihypertensive agents because they block the tonic effect of catecholamines on vascular smooth muscle contraction.

Agonists at α_2 receptors, such as **clonidine** and **guanfacine,** potently inhibit the sympathetic nervous system and are used in the treatment of **hypertension.** Their effects are mediated by noradrenergic neurons of the locus ceruleus and other brain stem regions; the activation of inhibitory α_2 autoreceptors on these cells reduces their drive of the sympathetic system. **α-Methyl-dopa,** another antihypertensive agent, acts by a similar central mechanism but is less specific and is associated with a greater incidence of side effects. α_2 agonists are also used to treat physical withdrawal from opiates, an effect mediated in part by inhibition of the locus ceruleus (see Chapter 16). In addition, they have been used in the treatment of **Tourette syndrome** and **attention deficit disorder,** although the mechanism of action that underlies these applications remains unknown. Antagonists at α_2 receptors, such as **yohimbine,** are anxiogenic. Used clinically to treat certain forms of male erectile dysfunction, they are only modestly efficacious.

Table 8–5 The Dopaminergic Receptor Family

Receptor	Agonists[1]	Antagonists[1]	G Protein Coupling	Areas of Localization[2]
Amino acid residues (aa)				
D_1 466 aa	SKF82958*; SKF81297*	SCH23390;* SKF83566; haloperidol	G_s	Neostriatum; cerebral cortex; olfactory tubercle; nucleus accumbens
D_2 443 aa	Bromocriptine*	Raclopride; sulpiride; haloperidol	$G_{i/o}$	Neostriatum; olfactory tubercle; nucleus accumbens
D_3 400 aa	Quinpirole*; 7-OH-DPAT	Raclopride	$G_{i/o}$	Nucleus accumbens; islands of Calleja
D_4 387 aa		Clozapine	$G_{i/o}$	Midbrain; amygdala
D_5 477 aa	SKF38393	SCH23390	G_s	Hippocampus; hypothalamus

[1]Asterisks indicate selective agonists and antagonists.
[2]mRNA expression has been determined predominantly in rat brain and may differ from the expression patterns found in human brain.
[3]D_2 long and D_2 short forms, which differ in the length of the third cytoplasmic loop, have been cloned. Although they are expressed in different brain regions, the funtional significance of these splice variants is not known.

functional differences between these D_2 receptor isoforms have not been identified. As previously discussed, DA receptor ligands currently have numerous clinical applications. First-generation **antipsychotic** drugs are D_2-like antagonists. D_2-like agonists, such as **bromocriptine**, are used in the treatment of Parkinson disease and hyperprolactemia. **Amantadine,** an anti-influenza drug that can stimulate DA release—perhaps through weak antagonism of NMDA glutamate receptors—also is used as an adjunct treatment for Parkinson disease. Because D_1 agonists are associated with nausea and vomiting, their clinical application is limited. These side effects are not surprising given DA's action as an emetic in the chemoreceptor trigger zone within the area postrema of the brain stem, where both D_1 and D_2 receptors are located. Indeed, D_2 antagonists such as **compazine** are highly effective **antiemetic** medications.

Because of the great number of catecholamine receptors, only one or two for each transmitter are described here to illustrate general differences among receptor families. The adrenergic α_2 receptor and the dopaminergic D_2 receptor are discussed briefly to introduce the concept of the autoreceptor. Discussion of the adrenergic β_2 receptor addresses the important structural features and intracellular trafficking of catecholamine receptors, and discussion of the dopaminergic D_1 and D_2 receptors demonstrates that even receptors for the same neurotransmitter can have unique and widely divergent patterns of expression in the brain. The pharmaceutical industry aims to exploit this diversity to develop drugs that target catecholamine receptors with greater selectivity.

PHYSIOLOGY OF CATECHOLAMINE RECEPTORS

The physiologic responses elicited by the activation of catecholamine receptors are quite varied. Responses vary not only among receptors but also for any given receptor, depending on the neuronal cell type involved. The latter phenomenon occurs because the regulation of ion channels by G protein-coupled receptors is indirect (as described in Chapter 5) and different signaling molecules and ion channels are found in different types of cells. For example, an ion channel inhibited by protein kinase A phosphorylation may predominate in one cell type, but a distinct ion channel that is activated by protein kinase A phosphorylation may predominate in another, leading to very different responses of the two cell types to receptor activation. (See Chapter 3 for a more detailed discussion of the regulation of ion channels.) Because the physiologic responses elicited by catecholamine receptor activation are numerous and complex, only general themes related to these responses are presented here.

The activation of β-adrenergic receptors (β-ARs) by means of G_s coupling leads to the activation of both adenylyl cyclase and protein kinase A. Such activation in turn leads to excitatory or inhibitory effects in neurons, depending on the cell type. In addition, cAMP can itself, independent of protein kinase A, activate a newly described class of channels that are gated by this cyclic nucleotide. In many pyramidal cells in the cortex and hippocampus, β-AR activation facilitates the excitation of pyramidal cells by blocking the activity of a Ca^{2+}-activated K^+ channel. In the heart, β-AR activation leads to the phosphorylation and activation of voltage-gated Ca^{2+} channels, which in turn mediate the stimulatory effects of norepinephrine and circulating epinephrine on the force and rate of cardiac contraction.

The activation of α_1 receptors by means of G_q coupling triggers the phosphatidylinositol cascade, which can have multiple effects on neuronal excitability. In contrast, the activation of α_2 receptors, typically through G_i coupling, has been determined to cause inhibitory responses in many cells, based on the autoreceptor functions subserved by these receptors.

The electrophysiologic consequences associated with the activation of D_1-like receptors have been extremely difficult to pin down because of conflicting reports. Such inconsistencies most likely reflect the heterogeneity of the cell types that have been studied, and also the complex cascades of protein kinases and protein phosphatases that are influenced by D_1-like receptors and that regulate many types of ion channels. The consequences of D_2 receptor activation appear to be more uniform, and frequently give rise to inhibitory responses caused by the activation of inwardly rectifying K^+ channels and other actions described in the following section. Responses to the activation of dopaminergic D_3 and D_4 receptors appear to be similar to those produced by D_2 receptor activation; however, such findings have yet to be confirmed.

AUTORECEPTORS

The adrenergic α_2 receptor and the dopaminergic D_2 receptor often serve as autoreceptors because their activation can inhibit the cells in which they reside. DA released from a nerve terminal, for example, can activate D_2 receptors residing on the same presynaptic terminal and can in turn curtail the synthesis or release of more DA. By this means, the D_2 receptor acts as a negative feedback mechanism to modulate or terminate DA signaling at a particular synapse. Autoreceptors also may reside on cell bodies. Adrenergic α_2 receptors, for example, are expressed on both the cell bodies and terminals of locus ceruleus neurons; when these receptors are activated, regardless of their location, they dampen the firing rate of the cells and limit the release of NE from noradrenergic terminals. The functional properties of these autoreceptors are illustrated in Figure 8–10. Other examples of receptors that can function as autoreceptors include GABA_B receptors, some metabotropic glutamate receptors, and the 5-HT$_{1a}$ serotonin receptor (see Chapters 7 and 9).

Most, if not all, autoreceptors couple to G_i and thus are believed to inhibit neurotransmitter release by one or more of several possible mechanisms, including: 1) inhibition of voltage-gated Ca^{2+} channels; 2) activation of inwardly-rectifying K^+ channels; and 3) inhibition of adenylyl cyclase, which inhibits protein kinase A and thereby may directly regulate proteins involved in the release process. The mechanism by which an autoreceptor inhibits neurotransmitter release may vary depending on its location in a neuron.

STRUCTURAL FEATURES OF G PROTEIN-COUPLED RECEPTORS

A two-dimensional representation of the β$_2$-AR can be seen in Figure 8–11. As with all G protein-coupled receptors, the β$_2$-AR must be capable of: 1) proper insertion and folding within the plasma membrane; 2) ligand recognition and binding; and 3) G protein coupling.

Through mutational analysis and chimeric receptor construction, the components of the β$_2$-AR that are critical for each of these functions have been elucidated. The asparagine glycosylation sites in the N terminus of the β$_2$-AR are essential for the transport of newly synthesized protein through the cell and for the proper folding of the protein within the plasma membrane. Deletion of any of the seven hydrophobic membrane-spanning domains (M1–M7) also alters protein folding in the membrane. Such folding is not affected by the deletion of the hydrophilic intracellular and extracellular loops; however, the cysteine residues in the first and second extracellular loops, which are conserved by a majority of G protein-coupled receptors, most likely form a disulfide bond that helps to maintain the three-dimensional structure of the protein in the membrane.

In three dimensions, the seven membrane-spanning domains of the G protein-coupled receptor are believed to form a pore-like structure, within which a corresponding ligand is recognized and bound. Deletion of the receptor's conserved cysteine residues alters the conformation of this pore and changes the binding properties of the receptor. Other residues critical for ligand binding in adrenergic receptors include the acidic amino acids in transmembrane domains M2 and M3,

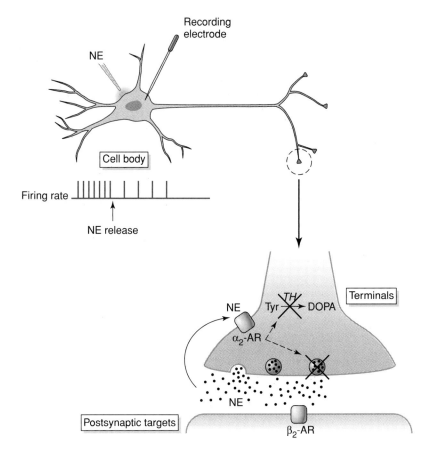

Figure 8–10. Autoreceptors. Autoreceptors typically function to inhibit activity in cell bodies and in synaptic terminals. Activation of α$_2$-adrenergic receptors (α$_2$-ARs) in a noradrenergic cell body, illustrated by the micropipette release of norepinephrine (NE), leads to a decrease in the firing rate of the cell, which can be recorded experimentally with an extracellular electrode. In the synaptic terminal, release of NE into the synaptic cleft allows for the diffusion of transmitter and the activation of presynaptic α$_2$-ARs. Such activation can inhibit further synthesis of norepinephrine and block the release of more transmitter. Thus autoreceptors function in negative feedback loops to modulate signaling between neurons. Tyr, tyrosine; TH, tyrosine hydroxylase.

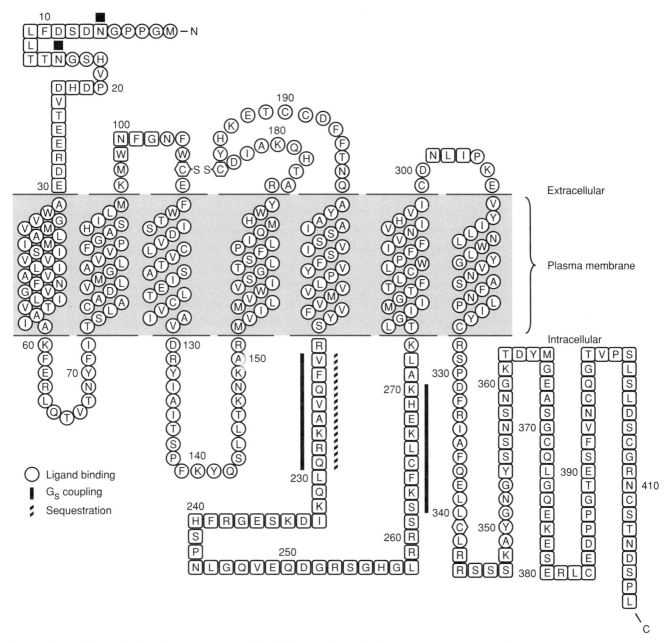

Figure 8–11. Model of a β-adrenergic receptor (β-AR). This two-dimensional beads-on-a-string model illustrates features common to most catecholamine receptors. The N terminus (N) is extracellular and the C terminus (C) is intracellular; in between are seven hydrophobic membrane-spanning domains and alternating intracellular and extracellular loops. Glycosylation sites (*black boxes*) reside near the N terminus; consensus phosphorylation sites (not shown) reside intracellularly. Amino acid residues that can be deleted from the protein without disrupting ligand binding or receptor insertion into the membrane are indicated with open boxes. Residues that alter ligand binding or protein folding when deleted appear in circles. The residues in bolded circles in transmembrane domains M3, M5, and M6 have been shown to be important for ligand binding specificity. The amino acids adjacent to the black bars are critical for G protein-coupling, and those adjacent to the striped bar are necessary for ligand-mediated internalization. (Reproduced with permission from Strader CD, Sigal IS, Dixon RIF. 1989. *FASEB J* 3:1826.)

most likely because they interact with the amine group of NE or epinephrine. In addition, residues conserved by various receptors in transmembrane domains M5 through M7 are believed to interact with the catechol ring of these transmitters.

After a ligand is recognized by a receptor and bound in its pore, the conformational change in the pore triggers a conformational change in the G protein α subunit to which it is bound, or coupled. Because inverse agonists have been proven to reduce receptor–G protein coupling, a certain low level of coupling most likely

occurs under basal conditions (see Chapter 1). Deletion analysis has revealed that two regions in the third intra-cellular loop are essential for such receptor binding to the G protein α subunit. What remains to be determined for adrenergic receptors and for most G protein-coupled receptors are the precise segments of the receptor responsible for the specificity of G protein coupling. The question of why coupling occurs to a given type of G protein, for example, only to G_s, G_i, or G_q, still must be answered. Coupling specificity may be determined not only by particular sequences in a re-

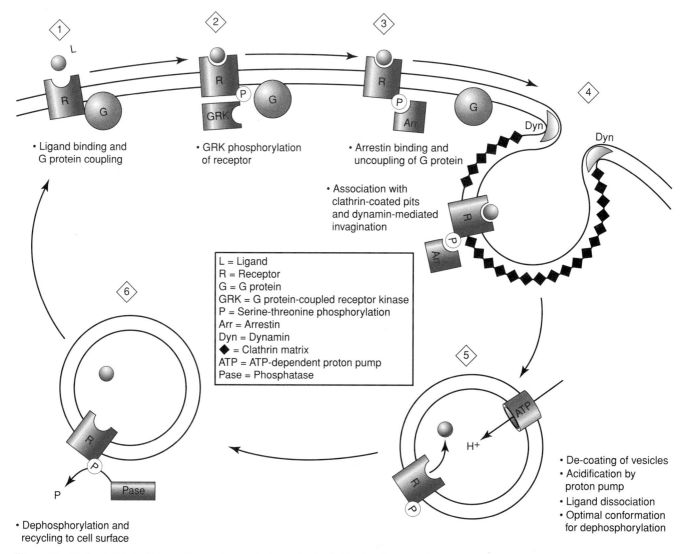

Figure 8–12. Receptor trafficking. G protein-coupled receptor trafficking involves a series of molecular events after ligand binding takes place (step **1**). Phosphorylation of the ligand-bound receptor occurs (step **2**); arrestin then binds to the phosphorylated receptor–ligand complex (step **3**). Bound arrestin complexes with clathrin lattices to bring about receptor sequestration in clathrin-coated pits and internalization by means of a dynamin-mediated process (step **4**). After the receptor is internalized in a vesicle, acidification alters its conformation and triggers the release of the ligand (step **5**). The receptor is dephosphorylated before it is recycled to the cell membrane (step **6**).

ceptor but also by the types of G proteins expressed in a given cell and by the subcellular localization of a G protein in relation to a receptor. Recent research on metabotropic glutamate receptors has indicated that their subcellular localization is determined in part by specific anchoring proteins (see Chapter 7); whether this holds true for adrenergic receptors remains unknown.

RECEPTOR TRAFFICKING

After a neurotransmitter binds to a receptor, several events take place in addition to receptor activation (Figure 8–12). In particular, receptor desensitization may occur, whereby the transmitter no longer causes a cellular response. Several modes of desensitization are known. The most rapid involves receptor phosphorylation by protein kinase A, protein kinase C, or G protein receptor kinases (GRKs). Phosphorylation by protein kinase A or protein kinase C can be stimulated by receptor activation but may not require continued receptor occupation by an agonist. GRKs phosphorylate only agonist-occupied receptors and can act within seconds of ligand binding. The best studied GRK is β_2-AR kinase (β-ARK). β-ARK phosphorylation of β_2-AR does not directly uncouple the receptor from its G protein; rather phosphorylation by β-ARK alters the conformation of the receptor–ligand complex such that it binds to a cytosolic protein called arrestin, which functionally uncouples the receptor (see Chapter 5).

A second means of rapid desensitization, which is believed to be phosphorylation-dependent, involves receptor sequestration and internalization. Receptor internalization is a multistep process that ultimately leads to the receptor's return to the cell membrane (see Figure 8–12). The first step involves arrestin's interaction with a matrix composed of clathrin protein that is located in clathrin-coated pits in the cell membrane (see Chapter 4). When arrestin, already bound to its ligand–receptor complex, subsequently binds to clathrin in these pits, endocytosis of the pit occurs in an adenosine triphosphate (ATP)-dependent fashion. This process requires a dynamin protein that serves to pinch off the clathrin-coated vesicle from the rest of the cell membrane. After they are internalized, the pits are uncoated, and the newly formed vesicles are acidified by ATP-driven H^+ pumps. This acidification serves to dissociate the ligand from its receptor and also alters the conformation of the receptor so that its phosphorylated domain is optimally exposed to cytoplasmic protein phosphatases. The dephosphorylated receptor is subsequently recycled to the cell surface, where it can repeat this cycle of ligand binding, phosphorylation, and internalization. Under certain circumstances, usually in the sustained presence of an agonist, the inter-

nalized receptor can be degraded; however, the cellular signals involved in the shift from reversible internalization to degradation are poorly understood.

RECEPTOR DISTRIBUTION IN THE BRAIN

Each catecholamine receptor has a unique pattern of expression in the brain. Some receptors, such as β_2-AR, may exhibit diffuse expression throughout the brain; others, such as the dopaminergic D_4 receptor, are localized in only a few structures. The regional patterns associated with the dopaminergic D_1 and D_2 receptors are discussed here to illustrate some of the interesting features of receptor gene expression.

D_1 and D_2 receptors are encoded by distinct genes and are only about 29% homologous at the amino acid level. Nevertheless, these receptors exhibit remarkably similar patterns of expression in the CNS. Their mRNA are concentrated in many of the same brain regions, most strikingly in the neostriatum (Figures 8–13 and

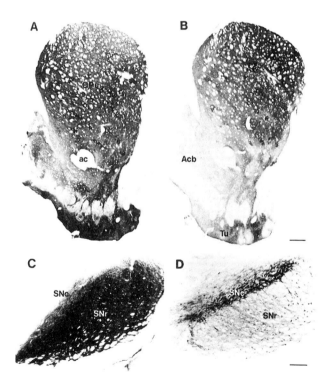

Figure 8–13. Dopamine receptor expression in rat brain. Immunocytochemistry with antibodies directed against the D_1 receptor (**A, C**) and the D_2 receptor (**B, D**) reveals the patterns of expression for these proteins in the nigrostriatal system. High levels of D_1 receptor immunoreactivity are seen throughout the striatal complex (**A**), and in the substantia nigra pars reticulata (SNr, **C**). In contrast, high levels of D_2 receptor immunoreactivity occur in the dorsal striatum (**B**) and in the substantia nigra pars compacta (SNc, **D**). Ac, anterior commissure; Acb, nucleus accumbens; Tu, olfactory tubercle. (Adapted with permission from Levey AI, Hersch SM, Rye DM, et al. 1993. *Proc Natl Acad Sci USA* 90:8863.)

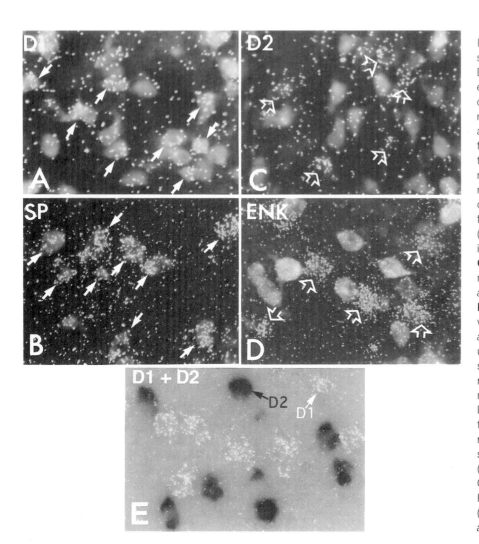

Figure 8–14. Cell type-specific expression of dopamine receptors in striatum. Dopaminergic D$_1$ and D$_2$ receptor mRNA expression tends to colocalize with different neuropeptide mRNA. Striatal neurons that project to the substantia nigra are labeled with the fluorescent dye fluorogold (whitish cell bodies in A–C) and thereby differentiated from striatopallidal neurons. In situ hybridization signals of mRNA appear as white grains on top of cells. **A.** D$_1$ receptor mRNA is localized in fluorogold-labeled striatonigral cells (*arrows*). **B.** The peptide substance P also is expressed in these neurons (*arrows*). **C.** D$_2$ receptor mRNA signals appear over nonfluorescing striatopallidal cells (*open arrows*) but not over striatonigral cells. **D.** The peptide enkephalin is colocalized with expression of the D$_2$ receptor (*open arrows*). **E.** An ^{35}S-labeled riboprobe is used to detect D$_1$ receptor mRNA expression (*white grains*), and a digoxigenin riboprobe is used to detect D$_2$ receptor mRNA (*dark immunoreactivity*). Double labeling of the same sections with these two probes reveals that D$_1$ and D$_2$ receptors are largely segregated into separate populations of striatal neurons. (Reproduced with permission from Gerfen CR, Wilson CJ. 1996. The basal ganglia. In Swanson LW, Björklund A, Hökfelt T (editors): *Handbook of Chemical Neuroanatomy,* vol 12, p 441.)

8–14). At the microscopic level, however, they largely segregate to separate subpopulations of neurons (see Figure 8–14). D$_1$ receptors occur predominantly in striatonigral cells—GABAergic medium spiny neurons that contain substance P and dynorphin and that project to the substantia nigra. In contrast, D$_2$ receptors are expressed predominantly in striatopallidal cells—GABAergic medium spiny neurons that project to the globus pallidus. Striatopallidal cells do not contain substance P or dynorphin but rather contain the neuropeptide enkephalin (see Chapter 14). Hence, the specificity of receptor expression in the striatum, and in other regions of the brain, may be determined by the connections between a particular brain structure and its projection sites.

The location of a receptor protein in a neuron cannot be determined exclusively from information about its mRNA. In situ hybridization can indicate the location of a receptor gene transcript in the brain, but not the location of the receptor protein. Often a receptor's mRNA and its corresponding protein are located in the

same region; for example, antibodies to the dopaminergic D$_1$ receptor protein have indicated that the protein is concentrated throughout the neostriatum (see Figure 8–13), in accordance with the location of its mRNA. However, the same D$_1$ antibodies have detected immunoreactivity in the substantia nigra, which does not express D$_1$ mRNA. If nigral cell bodies do not express the D$_1$ gene, how is the presence of the receptor protein explained? Based on studies of lesions in the striatonigral pathway, and receptor binding assays, it is believed that D$_1$ receptors in the substantia nigra reside not in nigral cells but on GABAergic terminals of nigrostriatal medium spiny neurons that project to the nigra. Hence, D$_1$ receptors in the substantia nigra are not nigral in origin; rather they arise from D$_1$ receptor mRNA transcribed and translated in the striatum and transported axonally to nigral terminals.

Although the foregoing discussion of dopaminergic D$_1$ and D$_2$ receptors relies on studies of the rat, similar findings have been confirmed in primates. Moreover, advances in brain imaging have enabled researchers to

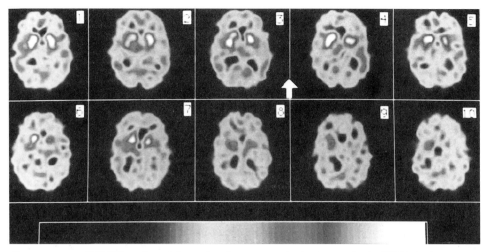

Figure 8–15. SPECT imaging of dopamine D$_2$ receptors in the human brain. [^{123}I]-IBZM administered intravenously to awake human subjects crosses the blood–brain barrier and binds to dopamine D$_2$ receptors. The most intense signals, which represent the greatest density of D$_2$ receptor expression, are found in the striatum. The dopaminergic D$_2$ receptor antagonist haloperidol, administered intravenously 80 minutes after [^{123}I]-IBZM injection (*arrow*), competes with the radioligand for receptor occupancy. In panels **4–10,** the intensity of radiolabeling in the striatum gradually decreases as haloperidol displaces bound [^{123}I]-IBZM. (Reproduced with permission from Seibyl JP et al. 1992. *J Nucl Med* 33:1969.)

visualize receptor binding in the living human brain. The SPECT images in Figure 8–15, which show D$_2$-like receptor labeling in an awake human subject, were created with the use of [^{123}I]-IBZM, a highly specific ligand for D$_2$ and related receptors. The intense labeling discernible in the striatum agrees with the immunocytochemistry data previously described for these receptors. Figure 8–15 also shows the brain's response to the administration of an antipsychotic agent; **haloperidol,** a D$_2$ receptor antagonist, competes with the [^{123}I]-IBZM radioligand and eventually displaces it from the receptor. Studies similar to this one are beginning to provide information about potentially abnormal patterns of receptor expression in neuropsychiatric disorders such as Parkinson disease and schizophrenia. Such studies also may enable researchers to establish dosages of novel therapeutic agents based on measurements of in vivo receptor binding.

SELECTED READING

Abell CW, Kwan SW. 2000. Molecular characterization of monoamine oxidases A and B. *Prog Nucleic Acid Res Mol Biol* 65:129–156.

Alexander SPH, Peters JA. 2000. 2000 Receptor and ion channel nomenclature supplement. *Trends Pharmacol Sci* Supplement.

Amara SG, Sonders MS, Zahniser NR, et al. 1998. Molecular physiology and regulation of catecholamine transporters. *Adv Pharmacol* 42:164–168.

Blakely RD, Bauman AL. 2000. Biogenic amine transporters: regulation in flux. *Curr Opin Neurobiol* 10:328–336.

Bloch B, Dumartin B, Bernard V. 1999. In vivo regulation of intraneuronal trafficking of G protein-coupled receptors for neurotransmitters. *Trends Pharmacol Sci* 20:315–319.

Boulton AA, Eisenhofer G. 1998. Catecholamine metabolism: From molecular understanding to clinical diagnosis and treatment. *Adv Pharmacol* 42:273–292.

Bremner JD, Krystal JH, Southwick SM, Charney DS. 1996. Noradrenergic mechanisms in stress and anxiety: I. Preclinical studies. *Synapse* 23:28–38.

Cooper JR, Bloom FE, Roth RH. 1996. *The Biochemical Basis of Neuropharmacology,* 7th ed. New York: Oxford University Press.

Foote SL, Aston-Jones GS. 1995. Pharmacology and physiology of central noradrenergic systems. In Bloom FE, Kupfer DJ (editors): *Psychopharmacology: The Fourth Generation of Progress,* pp 335–345. New York: Raven Press.

Gainetdinov RR, Jones SR, Caron MG. 1999. Functional hyperdopaminergia in dopamine transporter knock-out mice. *Biol Psychiatry* 46:303-311.

Gerfen CR, Engber TM, Mahan LC, et al. 1990. D$_1$ and D$_2$ dopamine receptor-regulated gene expression of striatonigral and striatopallidal neurons. *Science* 250:1429–1432.

Kim DS, Szczypka MS, Palmiter RD. 2000. Dopamine-deficient mice are hypersensitive to dopamine receptor argonists. *J Neurosci* 20:4405–4413.

Kumer SC, Vrana KE. 1996. Intricate regulation of tyrosine hydroxylase activity and gene expression. *J Neurochem* 67:443–462.

Lefkowitz RJ. 1998. G protein-coupled receptors III: New roles for receptor kinases and beta-arrestins in receptor signaling and desensitization. *J Biol Chem* 273:18677–18680.

Missale C, Nash SR, Robinson SW, et al. 1998. Dopamine receptors: From structure to function. *Physiol Rev* 78:189–225.

Mukherjee S, Ghosh RN, Maxfield FR. 1997. Endocytosis. *Physiol Rev* 77:759–803.

Nagatomo T, Koike K. 2000. Recent advances in structure, binding sites with ligands and pharmacological function of beta-adrenoceptors obtained by molecular biology and molecular modeling. *Life Sci* 66:2419–2426.

Nicola SM, Surmeier DJ, Malenka RC. 2000. Dopaminergic modulation of neuronal excitability in the striatum and nucleus accumbens. *Annu Rev Neurosci* 23:185–215.

Nirenberg MJ, Vaughan RA, Uhl GR, et al. 1996. The dopamine transporter is localized to dendritic and axonal plasma membranes of nigrostriatal dopaminergic neurons. *J Neurosci* 16:436–447.

Nirenberg MJ, Chan J, Vaughan RA, et al. 1997. Immunogold localization of the dopamine transporter: An ultrastructural study of the rat ventral tegmental area. *J Neurosci* 17:4037–4044.

Oakley RH, Laporte SA, Holt JA, et al. 1999. Association of beta-arrestin with G protein-coupled receptors during clathrin-mediated endocytosis dictates the profile of receptor resensitization. *J Biol Chem* 274:32248–32257.

Ordway GA, Stockmeier CA, Cason GW, Klimek V. 1997. Pharmacology and distribution of norepinephrine transporters in the human locus ceruleus and raphe nuclei. *J Neurosci* 17:1710–1719.

Reimer RJ, Fon EA, Edwards RH. 1998. Vesicular neurotransmitter transport and the presynaptic regulation of quantal size. *Curr Opin Neurobiol* 8:405–412.

Rohrer DK, Kobilka BK. 1998. Insights from in vivo modification of adrenergic receptor gene expression. *Annu Rev Pharmacol Toxicol* 38:351–373.

Saura J, Bleuel Z, Ulrich J, et al. 1995. Molecular neuroanatomy of human monamine oxidases A and B revealed by quantitative enzyme radioautography and in situ hybridization histochemistry. *Neurosci* 70:755–774.

Strader CD, Sigal IS, Dixon RAF. 1989. Structural basis of β-adrenergic receptor function. *FASEB J* 3:1825–1832.

Vickery RG, von Zastrow M. 1999. Distinct dynamin-dependent and -independent mechanisms target structurally homologous dopamine receptors to different endocytic membranes. *J Cell Biol* 144:31–43.

Wong DF, Ricaurte G, Gründer G, et al. 1998. Dopamine transporter changes in neuropsychiatric disorders. *Adv Pharmacol* 42:219–223.

Chapter 9

Serotonin, Acetylcholine, and Histamine

KEY CONCEPTS

- Neurons that synthesize and release serotonin (5-HT) are found almost exclusively in the raphe nuclei of the brain stem. Their axon projections are diffuse and reach many different brain regions, including limbic structures and all areas of the cerebral cortex.

- The serotonin transporter, which pumps serotonin back into the nerve terminal after it is released, is inhibited by many different antidepressant medications.

- There are 14 different 5-HT receptors, 13 of which are G protein-coupled receptors and 1 of which is a ligand-gated ion channel.

- 5-HT receptors are found on postsynaptic membranes as well as on 5-HT nerve terminals where they function as autoreceptors to inhibit 5-HT release.

- Several different psychotropic drugs including hallucinogens, such as LSD, and antipsychotic medications, such as clozapine and risperidone, interact with specific subtypes of 5-HT receptors.

- Acetylcholine is the neurotransmitter at nerve-muscle synapses. In the brain it is used both by neurons localized in the brain stem, by neurons in the forebrain that project to the cerebral cortex and hippocampus, and by interneurons in the striatum.

- Two major classes of acetylcholine receptors are nicotinic receptors, which are ligand-gated ion channels, and muscarinic receptors, which are G protein-coupled receptors.

- The five different subtypes of muscarinic receptors, which can be divided into two families based on the subtype of G protein to which they couple, are targets for drugs used in the treatment of Parkinson disease.

- Nicotinic receptors, pentamers composed of a subset of 12 different subunits, trigger muscle contractions at the neuromuscular junction. In the CNS, where these receptors are found both pre- and postsynaptically, they are the critical site of action of nicotine.

- Histamine is produced by neurons in the tuberomammillary nucleus of the posterior hypothalamus that send projections throughout the brain, including the cerebral cortex and limbic structures.

- Histamine receptors, of which there are three subtypes, are members of the G protein-coupled receptor superfamily.

In addition to the amino acids and catecholamines discussed in previous chapters, many small molecules function as neurotransmitters in the brain. Among the most important of these are serotonin, acetylcholine, and histamine, which are discussed in this chapter. Serotonin and histamine, together with the catecholamines, often are referred to as the monoamine neurotransmitters because each contains a single amine group. Indeed, the monoamines share many similarities, the most significant of which is their release from a relatively small number of neurons in the brain that project widely throughout the neuraxis. Monoamines also exhibit important differences, including distinct biosynthetic pathways; for example, all catecholamines are derived from tyrosine, whereas serotonin is derived from tryptophan and histamine from histidine. Although acetylcholine is not a monoamine, it is often grouped with these neurotransmitters because it also is released by a relatively small number of neurons, most of which are components of widely projecting systems in the brain.

SEROTONIN

Serotonin is an enigma. It is at once implicated in virtually everything but responsible for nothing.

B.L. Jacobs and C.A. Fornal

Although serotonin has been studied extensively, its precise role in the brain remains poorly understood, at least in part because selective pharmacologic probes for each subtype of serotonin receptor are not yet available. Under normal conditions serotonin is implicated in numerous processes from mood to sleep, and alterations in its activity are hypothesized to contribute to many neuropsychiatric conditions from migraine headaches to depression. A surprisingly large number of serotonin receptors have been identified; thus teasing out serotonin's influence on normal brain functions and on the pathophysiology of disease has been challenging.

SYNTHETIC AND DEGRADATIVE PATHWAYS

Also known as 5-hydroxytryptamine (5-HT), serotonin is an indolamine that possesses a hydroxy group at the 5 position and a terminal amine group on the carbon chain (Figure 9–1). It is synthesized from the amino acid tryptophan (Figure 9–2), which is actively transported across the blood–brain barrier and hydroxylated by tryptophan hydroxylase (TPH). The resulting 5-hydroxytryptophan molecule is decarboxylated into serotonin by L-aromatic amino acid decarboxylase (AADC)—the same enzyme involved in the

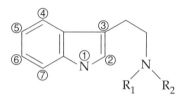

Figure 9–1. Chemical structure of an indolamine. Serotonin is an indolamine where R_1 and R_2 are hydrogen atoms, and a hydroxy group is substituted at the 5 position.

biosynthesis of catecholamines (see Chapter 8). In the pineal gland, additional enzymatic steps convert serotonin to melatonin (Box 9–1).

TPH is a rate-limiting enzyme that requires molecular oxygen and tetrahydrobiopterin as cofactors; some of its biochemical properties are summarized in Table 9–1. This enzyme is subject to short-term and long-term regulatory processes similar to those described for tyrosine hydroxylase (see Chapter 8); indeed, both enzymes belong to the same family of amino acid hydroxylases. TPH can be activated by protein kinase A and also by a calcium/calmodulin-dependent protein kinase, perhaps CaM-kinase II. Studies of the TPH gene indicate that its promoter can be activated by cAMP in vitro, although a consensus cAMP-response element (CRE) has not been identified. Presumably, increased TPH activity and expression, which occurs in response to the activation of serotonergic neurons, enables the neurons to synthesize the greater amount of serotonin required for neurotransmission.

Levels of serotonin in the brain can be manipulated by several means. Drugs such as **_p_-chlorophenylalanine** (PCPA), for example, can irreversibly inhibit TPH to produce a long-lasting depletion of serotonin. Halogenated amphetamines such as **fenfluramine** induce a rapid release of serotonin from neurons, most likely by disrupting vesicular storage of the transmitter; such disruption increases cytoplasmic serotonin, which in turn is transported out of the terminal by the serotonin transporter, working in reverse of its normal direction.

Table 9–1 Properties of Tryptophan Hydroxylase

Amino acid residues	445
Substrate	Tryptophan
Product	5-Hydroxytryptophan
Requirements	Fe^{2+}; tetrahydrobiopterin; O_2
Inhibitors	Desferrioxamine; dopamine[1]; _p_-chlorophenylalanine

[1]Like desferrioxamine, dopamine complexes iron, an element required for the the catalytic activity of tryptophan hydroxylase.

Prolonged exposure to these drugs can cause a lasting depletion of serotonin from neurons, accompanied by a down-regulation of TPH and of the serotonin transporter; however, the mechanism underlying this depletion remains unknown. Fenfluramine, which was prescribed as an appetite suppressant, was removed from the market in the United States because it was associated with cardiac valve disease and, in rare cases, with primary pulmonary hypertension. It was prescribed alone or in combination with **phentermine,** a

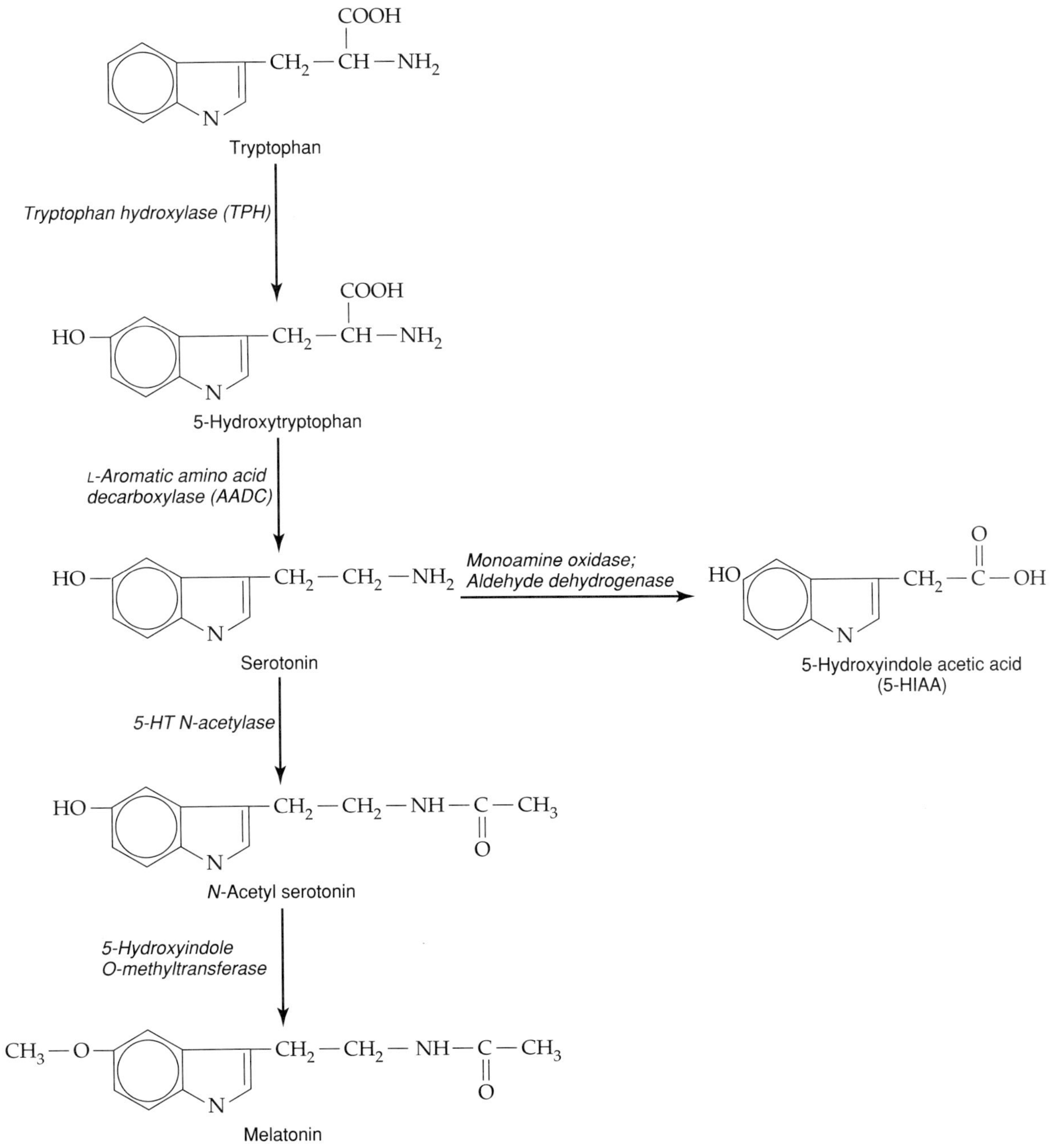

Figure 9-2. Biosynthetic pathways of serotonin and melatonin. Serotonin, also known as 5-hydroxytryptamine or 5-HT, and melatonin are both derived from the multistep processing of the dietary amino acid tryptophan. Serotonin is synthesized neuronally in various brain stem nuclei and is converted by monoamine oxidase and aldehyde dehydrogenase into its primary metabolite, 5-HIAA. Serotonin is also produced in cells of the pineal gland, which contain two enzymes—5-HT N-acetylase and 5-hydroxyindole-O-methyl transferase—not expressed in serotonergic cells. These enzymes rapidly convert serotonin to melatonin.

Box 9–1 Melatonin

Melatonin is synthesized from serotonin in the pineal gland by means of the biochemical pathway shown in Figure 9–2. This pathway is highly regulated by environmental lighting: in humans melatonin synthesis and release is stimulated in the dark and inhibited in the light. This effect is mediated by means of the suprachiasmatic nucleus of the hypothalamus, the major circadian pacemaker in the brain (see Chapter 18). In the dark, neurons of the suprachiasmatic nucleus activate the superior cervical sympathetic ganglion, which innervates the pineal gland. Norepinephrine released from ganglionic nerve terminals activates β-adrenergic receptors on pineal cells, which signal through the cAMP pathway. cAMP, through the activation of protein kinase A, dramatically stimulates the enzymes that catalyze the conversion of serotonin into melatonin and promotes melatonin release into the general circulation.

Although it is not expressed in neurons, melatonin released from the pineal gland binds to receptors in the brain and spinal cord and can influence several neuroendocrine functions and peripheral organs. In lower vertebrates, such as Amphibia, melatonin produces a potent skin-lightening effect; indeed, it was originally isolated based on its ability to stimulate the aggregation of pigment in melanocytes. Melatonin also has been proven to regulate circadian rhythms and reproductive behavior in many animal species.

Despite our knowledge of its function in animals, melatonin's effects in humans remain elusive. It is used clinically in the treatment of certain pigment disorders, although it produces less skin lightening in humans than in lower species. Because it is believed to promote sleep, it also has been proposed as a treatment for jet lag and other sleep disorders.

Three melatonin receptors have been identified; two of these, Mel_{1A} and Mel_{1B}, have been isolated in humans, and a third has been isolated only in nonmammalian species. All three are members of the superfamily of G protein-coupled receptors. Many pharmaceutical companies are attempting to develop agonists that selectively target melatonin receptors in humans for use in the treatment of sleep disorders. Studies suggest that these agonists may induce sleep and that their repeated administration may reset the circadian pacemaker in the suprachiasmatic nucleus (see Chapter 18 for further discussion of circadian rhythms and sleep). Thus melatonin currently is sold as an over-the-counter sleep aid, and its benefits are routinely hailed by the lay press. However, its effectiveness in treating sleep disorders has not been confirmed by well-designed studies. Moreover, the long-term effects of its use, which are unknown, may include the disruption of neuroendocrine function. Further research is necessary to determine whether selective melatonin receptor agonists can be used as safe and effective sleep aids.

---

sympathomimetic drug with amphetamine-like actions (see Chapter 12).

The exclusion of tryptophan from the diet also can reduce levels of serotonin in the brain. Individuals who are asked to follow a low-tryptophan diet and subsequently are challenged with a beverage containing many common amino acids but lacking tryptophan typically experience not only a dramatic reduction in blood tryptophan levels but also a greater than 90% reduction in serotonin in the brain; these findings are based on direct measurements in nonhuman primates and on indirect measurements obtained from humans by means of brain imaging techniques. Such procedures have been used to explore the involvement of serotonin in depression and in the actions of psychotropic drugs; for example, among patients who have recovered from depression, tryptophan depletion induces a return of depressive symptoms in those who were treated with a **selective serotonin reuptake inhibitor** (**SSRI**), but not in those treated with another antidepressant. Tryptophan depletion does not cause relapse in patients with obsessive-compulsive disorder after treatment with the same agents and has no discernible effect on normal subjects given the drugs experimentally. Together these findings suggest that a loss of serotonin per se cannot cause depression in subjects without this disorder and that an

intact serotonin system is required for maintaining clinical improvement in depression induced by a SSRI (see Chapter 15).

Some anecdotal reports suggest that serotonin synthesis increases in response to the oral administration of L-tryptophan, most likely because TPH is not fully saturated by normal circulating levels of tryptophan; however, such synthesis is likely to have a minor impact on overall serotonin function. The infusion of tryptophan has been used as an experimental tool to probe the serotonin system in humans. Rapid intravenous infusion of as much as 7 g can cause a very mild sedative effect that is usually clinically insignificant, and also can cause small changes in plasma levels of pituitary hormones (e.g., prolactin) known to be regulated by serotonin. Although L-tryptophan is a natural substance, the tryptophan preparations sold in health food stores can be dangerous; several years ago, contaminated tryptophan preparations available throughout the world caused a serious form of **eosinophilia–myalgia syndrome**.

Like catecholamine neurotransmitters, serotonin is degraded by monoamine oxidases (see Chapter 8). Paradoxically, serotonergic neurons express MAO_B, which has a much lower affinity for serotonin than does MAO_A. Because these neurons maintain a pool of cytoplasmic serotonin, it is believed that the function of MAO_B may be not to oxidize intracellular stores of serotonin, but rather to metabolize other trace amines that might act as false transmitters. Extracellularly, serotonin appears to be oxidized by MAO_A derived from other sources.

After serotonin is oxidized, aldehyde dehydrogenase converts the metabolite to 5-hydroxyindole-acetic acid (5-HIAA). Many studies have used levels of 5-HIAA in cerebrospinal fluid (CSF), blood, or urine to assess central serotonergic function in neuropsychiatric disorders. During the past two decades, the reduction of 5-HIAA in CSF has been reported to correlate with impulsive violence in some circumstances, most notably among individuals who have attempted suicide by violent means. Yet despite considerable research, the significance of these findings remains unclear. Because measurements of CSF cannot provide information about specific neural circuits or receptor types, they are unlikely to reveal the pathogenic mechanisms that underlie a particular behavior or disorder.

FUNCTIONAL ANATOMY

It has been estimated that several hundred thousand serotonergic neurons reside in the human brain. These neurons are confined almost exclusively to discrete nuclei in the midline, or raphe, of the brain stem (Figure 9–3), termed areas B1–B9 in original histochemical studies of the rat conducted by Dahlstrom and Fuxe. The most caudal clusters innervate the medulla as well as the spinal cord. The dorsal raphe (area B7) and median raphe (area B8) innervate much of the rest of the CNS by means of numerous and sometimes diffuse projection pathways. The dorsal raphe is located in the midbrain and forms the ventralmost portion of the periaqueductal gray matter. The median raphe is located ventral to the dorsal raphe in roughly the same anterior–posterior position of the midbrain. Although these two nuclei have overlapping terminal fields, the dorsal raphe preferentially innervates the cerebral cortex, thalamus, striatal regions (caudate-putamen and nucleus accumbens), and dopaminergic nuclei of the midbrain (e.g., the substantia nigra and ventral tegmental area), and the median raphe innervates the hippocampus, septum, and other limbic structures. Projections from these and other raphe nuclei are so extensive that virtually every neuron in the brain may be contacted by a serotonergic fiber. Interestingly, neurons of the dorsal raphe appear to be more susceptible than other serotonergic neurons to the toxic effects of the drug of abuse known as **MDMA**, or **ecstacy** (Box 9–2).

Partly because of the expansive nature of the serotonergic system, it is difficult to determine with cer-

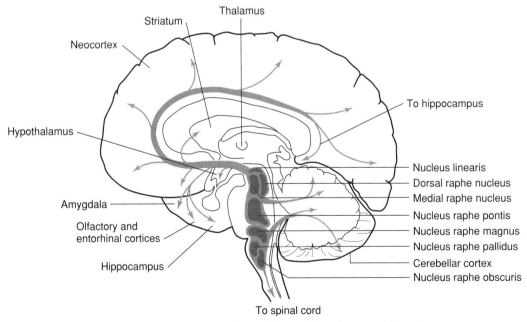

Figure 9–3. Serotonergic systems in the brain. Serotonin is produced by several discrete brain stem nuclei, which appear here in rostral and caudal clusters. The rostral nuclei, which include the nucleus linearis, dorsal raphe, medial raphe, and raphe pontis, innervate most of the brain, including the cerebellum. The caudal nuclei, which comprise the raphe magnus, raphe pallidus, and raphe obscuris, have more limited projections that terminate in the cerebellum, brain stem, and spinal cord. Together the rostral and caudal nuclei innervate most of the CNS.

Box 9–2 Ecstacy

Ecstacy is a popular name that was given to 3,4-methylenedioxymethamphetamine (**MDMA**), a drug of abuse that began circulating on college campuses in the 1980s and that continues to be widely used at so-called rave parties and as a "club" drug.

MDMA is a substrate for the serotonin transporter (SERT) and also has a high affinity for 5-HT$_2$ receptors. These two actions cause a moderate elevation of mood and mild perceptual alterations. Side effects of its use include tachycardia, agitation, hyperthermia, and panic attacks.

Unfortunately, MDMA also has been proven to selectively destroy serotonergic axons and cell bodies in rodents and nonhuman primates. After it is transported into serotonergic neurons by means of SERT, MDMA is believed to produce toxic effects through mechanisms of oxidative stress. Thus the actions of MDMA on serotonergic neurons appear to be analogous to those of MPTP on dopaminergic neurons (see Chapter 8). If the toxic effects of MDMA in humans are similar to those produced in laboratory animals, particularly in nonhuman primates, its use may lead to significant and permanent damage to serotonergic systems in the brain. Indeed, the tolerance to some of MDMA's euphorigenic effects, which occurs with repeated use, may be attributed in part to the loss of serotonergic neurons. However, long-term behavioral sequelae associated with the use of MDMA have not been adequately described.

tainty its function in the brain. At least 14 different serotonin receptors have been identified, each of which is characterized by a unique structure, pharmacology, pattern of expression, and second messenger effector. Selective agonists and antagonists are in great demand, not only for possible clinical use but also as tools to probe serotonin function in the CNS.

STORAGE, RELEASE, AND REUPTAKE

Serotonin is concentrated in presynaptic storage vesicles by the same vesicular monoamine transporter protein (VMAT) responsible for the vesicular concentration of the catecholamines (see Chapter 8). Consequently, the same drugs that disrupt catecholamine storage by inhibiting VMAT (i.e., **reserpine** and **tetrabenazine**) also disrupt serotonin storage and cause profound serotonin depletion after prolonged use.

Serotonin that is released synaptically may undergo one of several molecular processes (Figure 9–4). These include 1) diffusion away from the synapse; 2) metabolism by MAO; 3) presynaptic receptor activation; 4) postsynaptic receptor activation; and 5) reuptake by means of a presynaptic serotonin transporter.

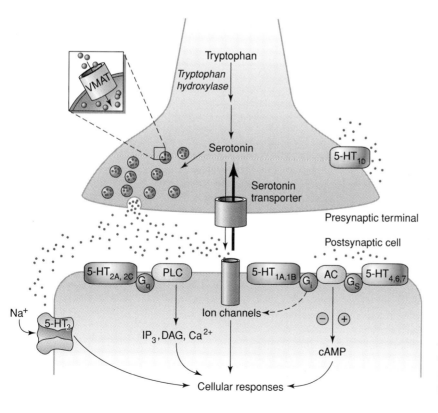

Figure 9–4. Model of a serotonergic synapse. Presynaptic and postsynaptic molecular entities involved in the synthesis, release, signaling, and reuptake of serotonin are shown. Tryptophan hydroxylase is transported to serotonergic synapses, where it initiates the synthesis of serotonin. After serotonin is synthesized and released, 5-HT activates as many as 14 different receptors. The 5-HT$_{1D}$ autoreceptor is located on the presynaptic side of the synapse. Several receptors coupled to their respective G proteins are located postsynaptically. The 5-HT$_3$ receptor, which is not G protein-coupled, functions as a receptor ionophore. VMAT, vesicular monoamine transporter; PLC, phospholipase C; AC, adenylyl cyclase; IP$_3$, inositol triphosphate; DAG, diacylglycerol.

The serotonin transporter The reuptake of synaptic serotonin into serotonergic nerve terminals represents the most important mechanism by which this neurotransmitter's signals are terminated. Serotonin reuptake is mediated by the serotonin transporter (SERT). The human SERT, for which there is only one gene, is a 630-amino acid protein with two putative extracellular *N*-linked glycosylation sites and eight canonical serine–threonine phosphorylation sites. It is roughly 48% homologous to both norepinephrine and dopamine transporters at the amino acid level. Moreover, its proposed structure is similar to that described for NET and DAT (see Chapters 4 and 8): it has 12 membrane-spanning domains joined by alternating intracellular and extracellular loops that have intracellular N and C termini.

DNA and RNA probes derived from the cloned SERT, as well as antibodies raised against it, have enabled researchers to localize its expression in the CNS. SERT mRNA expression occurs almost exclusively in the raphe nuclei, and especially high levels are detected in the dorsal and median raphe. Such expression is absent from other brain stem nuclei, including the locus ceruleus and substantia nigra. In contrast to its mRNA, the SERT protein is ubiquitous in the CNS, consistent with its transport to the extensively projecting nerve terminals of serotonergic neurons. Immunoreactive fibers, which can be detected throughout the brain and spinal cord, are most densely located in the neostriatum, amygdala, cerebral cortex, septum, and substantia nigra. In both the spinal cord and brain, SERT immunoreactivity tends to occur in axonal varicosities and terminals. Because serotonin immunoreactivity is also concentrated in these varicosities, it is believed that they are important sites of transmitter release.

Drugs that inhibit SERT activity prolong serotonergic signaling. Many antidepressants, among other psychoactive drugs, bind with very high affinity to SERT (Table 9–2). In fact, SSRIs, which are among the most widely prescribed antidepressants, were given their name because of their ability to bind relatively selectively to SERT and thereby inhibit the reuptake of serotonin. Some older tricyclic drugs, especially **clomipramine,** have relatively selective affinities for SERT as well. Other antidepressants, including many tricyclic compounds and **venlafaxine,** have similar affinities for NET and SERT and inhibit them with comparable efficacy. Tables 8–3 (see Chapter 8) and 9–2 indicate the relative affinities of several compounds for various monoamine transporters (see also Chapter 15). SSRIs in current use include **fluoxetine, sertraline, fluvoxamine, paroxetine,** and **citalopram**. As discussed in Chapter 15, these agents are effective in the treatment of **depression** and **panic disorder**. Unlike other antidepressants, the SSRIs and clomipramine can be used at higher doses to treat obsessive–compulsive disorder. SSRIs also are somewhat effective in the treatment of **bulimia** (a type of eating disorder), **posttraumatic stress disorder, generalized anxiety disorder,** and several other neuropsychiatric conditions.

Several drugs of abuse interfere with SERT activity. **Cocaine** is roughly equipotent at inhibiting SERT and DAT. Similarly, **amphetamine** is equally effective at serving as a substrate for SERT and DAT and thereby stimulating both serotonin and dopamine release. Cocaine's and amphetamine's actions on DAT and the dopamine

Table 9–2 Binding Properties of the Cloned Serotonin Transporter

Drug	Classification	K_i or K_m value (nM)
Fluoxetine	SSRI antidepressant	3.1
Sertraline	SSRI antidepressant	0.8
Paroxetine	SSRI antidepressant	0.25
Imipramine	Tricyclic antidepressant	2.1
Clomipramine	Tricyclic antidepressant	0.3
Desipramine	Tricyclic antidepressant	40
Amitriptyline	Tricyclic antidepressant	15
Nortriptyline	Tricyclic antidepressant	130
Mazindol	Undetermined	100
Serotonin	Indolamine	460
Cocaine	Psychostimulant	4200
D-amphetamine	Psychostimulant	>10,000
Norepinephrine	Catecholamine	>10,000
Dopamine	Catecholamine	>10,000

K_i and K_m values were determined in cultured cells transfected with the human SERT cDNA. See Table 8–3 in Chapter 8 for a comparison of affinities for the norepinephrine (NET) and dopamine (DAT) transporters.
(Adapted with permission from Barker EL, Blakely RD. 1995. Norepinephrine and serotonin transporters. Molecular targets of antidepressant drugs. In: Bloom FE, Kupfer DJ (eds). *Psychopharmacology: The Fourth Generation of Progress.* New York: Raven Press, p. 323.)

system are believed to be most strongly related to the addicting qualities of these drugs; it is likely that their effects on the serotonin system are also involved but to a lesser extent (see Chapter 16). **MDMA,** a drug of abuse previously mentioned in this chapter, also produces its effects by targeting SERT (see Box 9–2).

A unique feature of SERT is its large number of potential phosphorylation sites; it has eight such sites, whereas the norepinephrine transporter has only one. It is possible that these phosphorylation sites tightly regulate the activity of SERT by producing rapid, short-term changes in the transport of serotonin into neurons. Preliminary studies indicate that SERT is highly phosphorylated by both protein kinase A and protein kinase C; moreover, in vitro SERT phosphorylation by protein kinase C leads to the internalization of the protein and to a reduction in serotonin reuptake.

Although antidepressants, including SSRIs and inhibitors of norepinephrine reuptake, act immediately to inhibit monoamine transport, they require several weeks of repeated administration to produce therapeutic benefits. It is believed that such prolonged treatment causes long-term changes in neuronal gene expression, which in turn must alter the functioning of neural circuits to lead to an improvement in mood and to the amelioration of several symptoms of depression. Because of these findings, a central goal of neuropharmacologic research is to identify the specific genes that are regulated by antidepressant drugs (see Chapter 15).

The promoter of the human SERT gene contains consensus sequences for AP-1, AP-2, SP-1, and CRE sites (see Chapter 6); thus the gene may be transcriptionally regulated by numerous second messenger systems. Moreover, studies of rats have demonstrated that the expression of SERT mRNA in raphe nuclei is regulated by prolonged antidepressant administration. The possibility that antidepressants may have similar effects on humans is suggested by postmortem studies that have revealed altered levels of SERT binding in the brains of patients with mood disorders. In addition, recent brain imaging studies conducted with SERT radioligands have detected elevated levels of SERT binding in the midbrain regions of depressed patients; presumably these regions represent the raphe nuclei. However, it is important to emphasize that these studies are preliminary and, despite decades of research, little direct evidence supports SERT's involvement in the pathophysiology of depression.

SEROTONIN RECEPTORS

The extraordinary size of the serotonin receptor family has many intriguing implications. Fourteen distinct serotonin receptors have been cloned thus far, and the completion of the human genome project should indicate whether there are others. The classification of these receptors is complicated by the fact that many were first categorized by their pharmacologic properties. Subsequent studies of cloned receptors have indicated that early pharmacologic classifications do not correspond to the structural and functional properties of serotonin receptors; current nomenclature, shown in Table 9–3, represents a hybrid of two classification systems. This nomenclature is further complicated by the incomplete characterization of many recently identified receptors.

Thirteen serotonin receptors belong to the superfamily of G protein-coupled receptors. Investigators have determined that each of these receptors is derived from a distinct gene. Although little is known about their splice variants, a novel form of the 5-HT_{2C} receptor is generated by RNA editing. Such editing, which previously had not been attributed to a G protein-coupled receptor, suggests that RNA editing may increase the diversity of other members of this receptor superfamily. Although exceptions to patterns of G protein coupling may exist, 5-HT_1 receptors generally couple to G_i proteins; 5-HT_2 receptors to G_q proteins; and 5-HT_4, 5-HT_6, and 5-HT_7 receptors to G_s proteins; coupling for the 5-HT_5 receptor has not been determined.

The 5-HT_3 receptor is unique among all monoamine receptors in that it does not couple to a G protein; instead it is a ligand-gated ion channel that is homologous to other receptor ionophores, including the AMPA and NMDA glutamate receptors, the γ-aminobutyric acid $(GABA)_A$ receptor, and the nicotinic cholinergic receptor. Activation of the 5-HT_3 receptor by serotonin opens a nonselective cation channel and triggers a rapid, transient depolarizing current that is carried by Na^+ and K^+. The ultrastructure of this receptor has been deduced from electron microscopic examination (Figure 9–5); like other receptor ionophores, the 5-HT_3 receptor appears to be a pentamer whose subunits surround a central pore. However, unlike other ionotropic receptors, for which multiple subunits are known, only a single subunit of the 5-HT_3 receptor has been identified. Moreover, this subunit forms a functional channel when it is expressed in vitro, indicating that additional subunits are not absolutely required for 5-HT_3 receptor activity.

Autoreceptors   Serotonin signaling, like signaling in most neurotransmitter systems, is characterized by the participation of autoreceptors. Serotonergic 5-HT_{1A} receptors, for example, are termed *somatodendritic autoreceptors* because they reside on serotonergic cell bodies and dendrites; their activation reduces cell firing and curtails the synthesis and release of serotonin. The activation of serotonergic autoreceptors in the presynaptic nerve terminal, which are believed to be 5-HT_{1D}

Table 9–3 The Serotonergic Receptor Family

Receptor[1] (amino acid residues)	Agonists	Antagonists	G protein	Localization[2]
5-HT$_{1A}$ (421 aa)	8-OH-DPAT; buspirone, gepirone	WAY 100135	G$_{i/o}$	Hippocampus; septum; amygdala; dorsal raphe; cortex
5-HT$_{1B}$ (390 aa)	Sumatriptan and related triptans		G$_{i/o}$	Substantia nigra; basal ganglia
5-HT$_{1D}$ (377 aa)	Sumatriptan and related triptans	GR 127935	G$_{i/o}$	Substantia nigra; striatum nucleus; accumbens; hippocampus
5-HT$_{1E}$ (365 aa)			G$_{i/o}$	
5-HT$_{1F}$ (366 aa)			G$_{i/o}$	Dorsal raphe; hippocampus; cortex
5-HT$_{2A}$ (471 aa)	DMT and related pscyhedelics[3]	Ketanserin; cinanserin; MDL900239	G$_{q/11}$	Cortex; olfactory tubercle; claustrum
5-HT$_{2B}$ (481 aa)	DMT		G$_{q/11}$	Not located in brain
5-HT$_{2C}$ (458 aa)	DMT; MCPP	Mesulergine; fluoxetine	G$_{q/11}$	Basal ganglia; choroid plexus; substantia nigra
5-HT$_3$ (478aa) (per subunit)		Ondansetron; granisetron	Ligand-gated channel	Spinal cord; cortex; hippocampus; brain stem nuclei
5HT$_4$ (387 aa)	Metoclopramide	GR 113808	G$_s$	Hippocampus; nucleus accumbens; striatum substantia nigra
5HT$_{5A}$ (357 aa)		Methiothepin	G$_s$	Cortex; hippocampus; cerebellum
5-HT$_{5B}$ (aa unknown)		Methiothepin	Unknown	Habenula; hippocampal CA1
5-HT$_6$ (440 aa)		Methiothepin; clozapine; amitriptyline	G$_s$	Striatum; olfactory tubercle; cortex; hippocampus
5-HT$_7$ (445 aa)		Methiothepin; clozapine; amitriptyline	G$_s$	Hypothalamus; thalamus; cortex; suprachiasmatic nucleus

[1]The nomenclature of 5-HT receptors is extremely complicated because so many subtypes have been cloned. Some require further characterization before definitive classifications may be made. Represented in the table is the nomenclature recently approved by the International Union of Pharmacology Classification of Receptors Subcommittee on 5-HT Receptors.
[2]mRNA expression has been determined for some subtypes in rat brain and may differ from patterns of expression in human brain.
[3]Other examples include lysergic acid (LSD), psilocybin, and mescaline.
DMT, *N,N*-dimethylamine; MCPP, metachlorophenylpiperazine

receptors in humans (and 5-HT$_{1B}$ receptors in rodents), decreases the local synthesis and release of transmitter. 5-HT$_{1A}$ and 5-HT$_{1D}$ receptors are highly homologous, and both signal by coupling to G$_i$ proteins. It is believed that their inhibitory effects on serotonergic neurons, like those of other G$_i$-linked receptors, are mediated by the activation of inwardly rectifying K$^+$ channels, the inhibition of voltage-gated Ca^{2+} channels, and perhaps the inhibition of adenylyl cyclase. The actions of both types of autoreceptor are represented in Figure 9–6.

Pharmacology of serotonin receptors   The great number of serotonergic receptor subtypes has hindered the design of subtype-specific agonists and antagonists. Thus far researchers have failed to develop compounds that are perfectly selective for one subtype. Yet numerous drugs that bind to serotonin receptors currently have clinical applications. **Buspirone** and **gepirone,** which are partial 5-HT$_{1A}$ agonists, are used to treat **generalized anxiety disorder** (**GAD**) but exhibit only modest efficacy. They are less effective than **benzodiazepines** (see Chapters 7 and 15) but are still used because

unlike benzodiazepines they do not cause drowsiness or dependence. **Sumatriptan,** a 5-HT$_1$ agonist that exerts somewhat selective effects on the 5-HT$_{1D}$ receptor, has been used since 1993 as a highly effective treatment for **migraine** headaches. Based on its success, many pharmaceutical companies have launched second-generation triptan drugs that are designed to treat this common syndrome (see Chapter 19).

All known **hallucinogenic** compounds are partial agonists at 5-HT$_{2A}$ receptors (Box 9–3). Conversely, many antipsychotic drugs, especially the more recently released medications such as **clozapine, risperidone,** and **olanzapine,** exert potent antagonist actions at 5-HT$_{2A}$ receptors in addition to their D$_2$ dopamine antagonist properties. Highly selective 5-HT$_{2A}$ antagonists, such as **MDL 100907,** are currently under evaluation for the treatment of **schizophrenia** (see Chapter 17).

Ondansetron, granisetron, and other 5-HT$_3$ antagonists are **antiemetics** and are used clinically to minimize chemotherapy-induced nausea and vomiting. In animals, these compounds also appear to have memory-enhancing and anxiolytic properties. The 5-HT$_4$ receptor

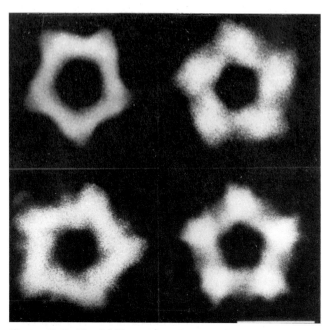

Figure 9–5. The 5-HT$_3$ receptor. Purified 5-HT$_3$ receptors from mice were examined with an electron microscope to determine the receptor's structure. Mathematical analysis of the receptor's rotational symmetry enabled the generation of images of individual receptors. Subsequently, each receptor was modeled as a pentameric cylinder with an outer diameter of 8 nm, a cavity diameter of 3 nm, and a length of 11 nm. (Reproduced with permission from Boess FG, Beroukhim R, Martin IL. 1995. *J Neurochem* 64:1404.)

agonist **metoclopramide,** whose many actions include potent antagonism of dopamine D$_2$ receptors, also alleviates nausea and vomiting. Pharmacologic agents that target the more recently cloned serotonin receptors (i.e., 5-HT$_5$, 5-HT$_6$, and 5-HT$_7$) are currently under development. Based on studies of animal models, it has been proposed that agonists for these receptors may exert antidepressant activity (see Chapter 15); however, this hypothesis remains speculative.

The cloning of the various serotonin receptor subtypes has produced several surprises. Clinically effective compounds known to act at other molecular targets also have been determined to act at serotonin receptors. Tricyclic antidepressants such as **amitriptyline,** whose ability to block norepinephrine and serotonin transporters is well-established, also antagonize 5-HT$_6$ and 5-HT$_7$ receptors. Whether actions at these receptors contribute to the antidepressant effects of such drugs is not yet known. Similarly, the SSRI **fluoxetine** recently has been proven to antagonize 5-HT$_{2C}$ receptors. These discoveries are humbling because they complicate our understanding of antidepressant action, and yet they are exciting because they suggest new targets for agents designed to treat depression and related disorders.

ACETYLCHOLINE

Based on studies by Dale, Loewi, Feldberg and others during the first half of the twentieth century, acetylcholine (ACh) was the first molecule to be identified as a neurotransmitter. First termed *vagusstoff* (German for vagus nerve substance) because of its actions in the autonomic nervous system, ACh subsequently was shown to function as a neurotransmitter at the neuromuscular junction and in the CNS. Within the CNS, ACh is produced by projection neurons, whose cell bodies are located in the brain stem and forebrain, and also is synthesized in interneurons intrinsic to many brain regions, including the striatum. ACh elicits its effects both in the peripheral nervous system and in the CNS by means of two very different classes of receptors: the *nicotinic receptors,* which are ligand-gated channels, and *muscarinic receptors,* which are G protein-coupled. ACh is implicated in the regulation of learning, memory, control of movement, and mood. The loss of memory function associated with **Alzheimer disease** has been attributed partly to the degeneration of the cholinergic system.

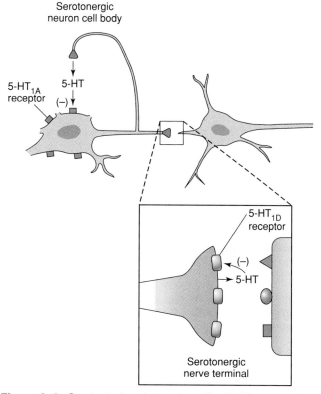

Figure 9–6. Serotonergic autoreceptors. The 5-HT$_{1A}$ receptor resides on the cell body and on dendrites and regulates cell firing as well as the synthesis and release of serotonin. The 5-HT$_{1D}$ receptor is localized in nerve terminals and regulates the synthesis and release of serotonin. The 5-HT$_{1B}$ receptor, not shown, is the rodent homolog of the human 5-HT$_{1D}$ receptor.

Box 9-3 Psychedelic Drugs

Several drugs that bind to serotonin receptors are unlikely to find clinical applications. Among these is D-lysergic acid diethylamide, or LSD, a nonselective 5-HT agonist that is one of the most potent psychedelic drugs known (see Chapter 17). LSD was first synthesized in 1943 by Albert Hoffman, who accidentally ingested the compound and discovered its powerful psychotomimetic properties. The ingestion of this indolamine hallucinogen is associated with sensory distortions, elation, paranoia, depression, and sometimes severe anxiety (popularly referred to as a bad trip). After its widespread abuse in the 1960s and 1970s, popular interest in LSD appeared to decline for many years. However, reports indicate that its use is currently on the rise.

Although LSD is a nonselective serotonin receptor ago-nist, its psychedelic effects are believed to be mediated through partial agonist effects on 5-HT$_{2A}$ receptors. Indeed the effects of many psychedelic agents—including those of other indolamine hallucinogens (e.g., *N,N*-dimethylamine [DMT] and psilocybin) and those of phenethylamines (e.g., mescaline and dimethoxymethylamphetamine [DOM])—can be traced to their actions at these receptors. Moreover, the actions of such agents in animal models can be blocked by selective 5-HT$_{2A}$ receptor antagonists. These findings have stimulated interest in determining whether the 5-HT$_{2A}$ receptor is involved in the pathophysiology of psychotic disorders. Research is also directed toward determining whether 5-HT$_{2A}$ receptor antagonists may be used in the treatment of schizophrenia (see Chapter 17).

SYNTHETIC AND DEGRADATIVE PATHWAYS

Acetylcholine is synthesized in a reversible reaction whereby choline acetyltransferase (ChAT) transfers an acetyl group from acetyl coenzyme A (CoA) to choline (Figure 9–7; Table 9–4). Its synthesis is regulated by the rate-limiting availability of choline. Choline is transported into neuronal terminals, either in its free form or bound to membrane phospholipids, by means of distinct high-affinity and low-affinity transport mechanisms that are discussed in the next section of this chapter. Most ACh is synthesized in terminals, which are rich in mitochondria and ChAT; mitochondria are essential components of this process because they are the site of acetyl CoA synthesis.

The synaptic actions of ACh are terminated by the enzyme acetylcholinesterase (AChE), which hydrolyzes ACh into acetate and choline (see Table 9–4). AChE is an extraordinarily efficient enzyme that is capable of hydrolyzing 1000 ACh molecules per second per molecule of enzyme. This enzyme occurs in the cytoplasm and in the outer cell membrane; thus it can metabolize ACh both intracellularly and extracellularly. **Anticholinesterases,** which inhibit AChE, cause released ACh to accumulate extracellularly; their effect is equivalent to the overstimulation of ACh receptors throughout the nervous system. Reversible inhibitors, such as **physostigmine** and **neostigmine,** inactivate AChE for as many as 4 hours and are used clinically to treat **glaucoma, myasthenia gravis,** and **smooth muscle dysfunction** of the bladder and intestines. Unlike physostigmine, neostigmine cannot enter the brain because it is a quaternary ammonium compound and thus is too highly charged to cross the blood–brain barrier. Central-acting anticholinesterases, such as **tacrine** and **donepezil,** are used to increase central ACh concentrations in patients with **Alzheimer dis-**

ease. However, anticholinesterases are only modestly efficacious in the treatment of this disease; although they may delay symptomatic deterioration, they do not produce dramatic clinical improvement (see Chapter 20).

Irreversible anticholinesterases phosphorylate AChE and thereby completely inhibit ACh breakdown; afterward normal AChE activity requires new AChE synthesis. These irreversible inhibitors are used as insecticides, which are highly toxic if ingested by humans. These agents also represent a major class of nerve gases. Thus, just before World War II, first German and then Allied

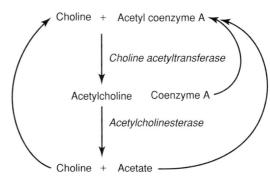

Figure 9–7. Biosynthesis of acetylcholine. Choline and acetyl coenzyme A produce acetylcholine in a reversible reaction catalyzed by choline acetyltransferase. After it is synthesized, acetylcholine is rapidly metabolized by acetylcholinesterase into choline and free acetate. Subsequently both metabolites may be recycled to produce more acetylcholine.

Table 9–4 Enzymes in Acetylcholine Synthesis and Catabolism

Enzyme (amino acid residues)	Substrate	Product	Inhibitors
Choline acetyltransferase 748 aa	Choline + acetyl CoA	Acetylcholine + CoA	Unknown
Acetylcholinesterase 614 aa	Acetylcholine	Acetate + choline	Physostigmine; neostigmine; tacrine; sarin; WIN8077

scientists began to explore potential uses for organophosphorus agents in chemical warfare. Their efforts resulted in the development of several extraordinarily lethal compounds, including **sarin, soman,** and **tabun.** Any one of these substances, commonly referred to as nerve gases, can cause death within 5 minutes of exposure. The primary cause of death is respiratory failure, which typically is preceded by cognitive impairment and numerous autonomic symptoms. Treatment for exposure to these toxins includes the administration of a muscarinic receptor antagonist, such as **atropine,** in conjunction with a nicotinic receptor antagonist, such as **pralidoxime**.

FUNCTIONAL ANATOMY

ACh is synthesized in interneurons and in long projection neurons. In marked contrast, the monoamines are rarely synthesized in interneurons—with the notable exception of dopamine in the retina.

Projecting cholinergic neurons arise from eight nuclei that are clustered in two areas, the basal forebrain and the upper brain stem (Figure 9–8). The basal forebrain comprises the medial septal nucleus (designated cholinergic nucleus-1 [Ch1] in the rat), the vertical nucleus of the diagonal band (Ch2), the horizontal limb of the diagonal band (Ch3), and the nucleus basalis of Meynert (Ch4). The last of these nuclei undergoes notable degeneration in patients with Alzheimer disease. Because neurons in this nucleus depend on nerve growth factor (NGF) for trophic support, NGF and drugs aimed at NGF signaling pathways are putative treatment for this disease; however, their efficacy remains unproved (see Chapters 11 and 20). Brain stem cholinergic nuclei include the pedunculopontine nucleus (Ch5), the laterodorsal tegmental nucleus (Ch6), the medial habenula (Ch7), and the parabigeminal nucleus (Ch8). The primary targets of both groups of projecting nuclei are listed in Table 9–5.

Among regions in brain that receive cholinergic input are the cerebral cortex and hippocampus. The dense innervation of the sensory and limbic cortices, which arises predominantly from the nucleus basalis

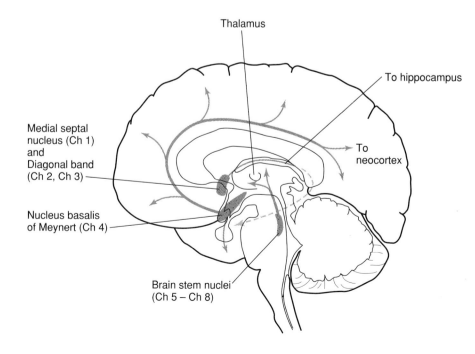

Figure 9–8. Cholinergic systems in the brain. Eight small nuclei in the forebrain and brain stem, designated Ch 1–8, supply cholinergic input to the brain. Most cholinergic innervation of the CNS is provided by the nucleus basalis of Meynert (Ch 4) and a complex that includes the medial septal nucleus (Ch 1) and diagonal band (Ch 2,3).

Table 9-5 Cholinergic Nuclei in Brain

Cholinergic Nucleus	Location	Principal Projection Target
Medial septal nucleus (Ch1)	Basal forebrain	Hippocampus
Vertical nucleus of the diagonal band (Ch2)	Basal forebrain	Hippocampus
Horizontal limb of the diagonal band (Ch3)	Basal forebrain	Olfactory bulb
Nucleus basalis of Meynert (Ch4)	Basal forebrain	Cerebral cortex
Pedunculopontine nucleus (Ch5)	Midbrain	Thalamus
Laterodorsal tegmental nucleus (Ch6)	Midbrain	Thalamus
Medial habenula (Ch7)	Caudal diencephalon	Interpeduncular nucleus
Parabigeminal nucleus (Ch8)	Midbrain	Superior colliculus

and the diagonal band, is believed to influence emotional state and cortical responsiveness to sensory input. Dense cholinergic projections to the hippocampus arise from the medial septal nucleus and vertical nucleus of the diagonal band, and are believed to be important for learning and memory.

The basal ganglia receive cholinergic input from the nucleus basalis, the pedunculopontine nucleus, and the laterodorsal tegmental nucleus. The most significant cholinergic innervation in the striatum, however, is intrinsic. Innervation in this region arises from large cholinergic interneurons, which are critical components of the complex circuitry that underlies extrapyramidal motor control and certain forms of implicit memory (see Chapter 14). In patients with **Parkinson disease,** the loss of dopaminergic input to the striatum from the substantia nigra leads to a profound motor disorder. Muscarinic cholinergic antagonists such as **trihexyphenidyl** and **benztropine** are prescribed to such patients to improve symptoms in the early stages of this disease, or to supplement the use of other drugs, such as L-dopa. These antimuscarinic agents also are used to treat the Parkinson disease-like side effects of antipsychotic drugs that are D_2 dopamine receptor antagonists. Muscarinic cholinergic antagonists are believed to act at muscarinic receptors on striatal medium spiny neurons, where they partially compensate for the decreased dopaminergic signaling in striatal neuronal circuits.

STORAGE, RELEASE, AND REUPTAKE

ACh is concentrated in storage vesicles in the presynaptic terminal (Figure 9–9). The mechanism by which it is transported into these vesicles is unknown; however, the drug **vesamicol** inhibits such transport and induces the depletion of ACh from cholinergic vesicles.

The vesicular pool of ACh, like that of other neurotransmitters, is released into the synaptic cleft in response to the depolarization of a nerve terminal. Several toxins are known to interfere selectively with the normal vesicular release of ACh into the synapse. **Botulinum toxin A** and **tetanus toxin,** which prevent ACh release from cholinergic motor neuron terminals, cause paralysis. These toxins are zinc endoproteases that appear to exert their effects on ACh release through the proteolytic cleavage of proteins critical to exocytosis, such as synaptobrevin, syntaxin, and SNAP 25 (see Chapter 4). **Black widow spider venom,** which contains **α-latrotoxin,** promotes massive vesicular release of ACh and a subsequent overstimulation of postsynaptic sites. It exerts its effects in part by uncoupling Ca^{2+} signals from the release process. Two putative receptors for this toxin are neurexin and a recently cloned novel G protein-coupled receptor. Toxins that interfere with ACh release have served as critical tools for elucidating the molecular processes that underlie normal neurotransmitter release.

Unlike monoamines, which are removed from the synapse by reuptake transporters, synaptically released ACh is broken down by AChE (see Figure 9–9). Because AChE metabolizes ACh rapidly, the duration of ACh signaling is very brief. Accordingly, diffusion from the synapse is negligible. As mentioned previously, potent anticholinesterases inhibit AChE activity and prolong the duration of ACh signaling.

Because ACh is not returned to the presynaptic terminal, unlike most other nonpeptide neurotransmitters, it cannot be recycled. Instead, choline, the metabolite produced by the breakdown of ACh, is transported with high affinity back into cholinergic nerve terminals, where it is used to synthesize new transmitter. Choline transport is the primary regulatory mechanism for controlling ACh concentrations in the synapse; thus choline transport inhibitors such as **hemicholinium** and **vesamicol** can be used to deplete neuronal stores of ACh. Despite the development of such inhibitors, the protein transporter responsible for choline reuptake has not yet been cloned.

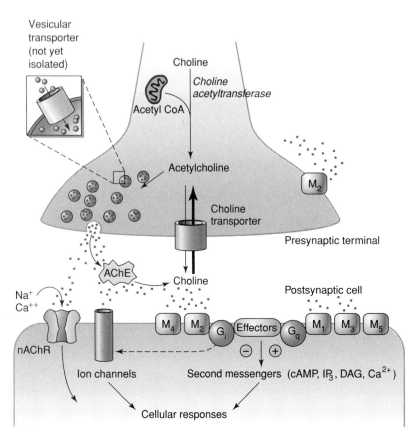

Figure 9–9. Model of a cholinergic synapse. Several interesting features of this synapse distinguish it from monoamine synapses (see Figure 9–4 and Chapter 8). First, the vesicular transporter for acetylcholine is distinct from the vesicular monoamine transporter (VMAT). Second, the reuptake transporter does not return neurotransmitter to the synapse but rather recycles its metabolite (choline). Third, the presence of mitochondria is especially important because these organelles supply the acetyl coenzyme A necessary for acetylcholine synthesis. In addition, both G protein-coupled receptors, such as muscarinic subtypes M_1–M_5, and ligand-gated ion channels, such as nicotinic receptors (nAChRs), may be present, as they are in serotonergic synapses.

ACETYLCHOLINE RECEPTORS

ACh acts on two major types of receptors (see Figure 9–9), which were named for the natural substances that selectively activate them. Muscarinic receptors, which are members of the G protein-coupled receptor super-family, represent one of these types. ACh also acts on nicotinic receptors, which are members of the ligand-gated ion channel superfamily; these include the 5-HT_3 receptor described in this chapter and the glutamate, GABA, and glycine receptors discussed in Chapter 7. The structural similarities among these receptor iono-phores are represented in Figure 9–10. Drugs that act on cholinergic receptors are important in the pharma-cologic manipulation of the autonomic nervous system, as discussed in Chapter 12.

Muscarinic receptors   Muscarinic receptors were first noted for their ability to bind **muscarine,** a com-pound derived from the poisonous mushroom *Amanita muscaria.* They are located in peripheral tissues, in the autonomic nervous system, and in the CNS. Five sub-types have been cloned, each of which displays the canonical seven membrane-spanning domains and alternating cytoplasmic and extracellular loops that characterize G protein-coupled receptors (Table 9–6).

All five subtypes are expressed in brain, and can be sub-grouped based on their patterns of G protein coupling: M_1, M_3, and M_5 receptors couple to G_q proteins, and M_2 and M_4 receptors couple to G_i proteins. Electro-physiologic responses elicited by the activation of any given subtype can vary from one cell to another, de-pending on the second messenger systems and ion channels expressed in the cell. M_1, M_3, and M_5 recep-tors produce their effects by stimulating or inhibiting activation of the phosphatidylinositol system. As with most other G_i-linked receptors, M_2 and M_4 receptors elicit mostly inhibitory responses; they act by activating inwardly rectifying K^+ channels, inhibiting voltage-gated Ca^{2+} channels, and inhibiting adenylyl cyclase.

M_1, M_3, and M_4 receptors are primarily located in the cerebral cortex and hippocampus, where their activity may mediate some of the effects of ACh on learning and memory. In the striatum, M_1 and M_4 subtypes occur in abundance and are believed to mediate cholinergic signaling in extrapyramidal motor circuits. M_2 receptors are concentrated in the basal forebrain, the site of sev-eral cholinergic nuclei; it is believed they act as autore-ceptors to control ACh synthesis and release from forebrain cholinergic neurons. The M_5 receptor is the least abundant of the muscarinic receptors and is expressed in very small quantities throughout the brain.

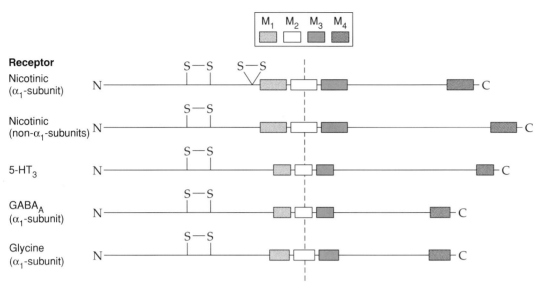

Figure 9–10. Ligand-gated ion channel receptors. Considerable structural similarity characterizes the receptors in this family. Each receptor subunit has an extracellular N terminus, four membrane-spanning domains (M1–M4), and a short extracellular C terminus. A single disulfide bond is conserved among all members of this family, with the exception of nicotinic α_1 subunits, which possess two disulfide bonds.

Muscarinic receptor pharmacology Few muscarinic receptor agonists and antagonists are subtype-selective, and none of the selective agents are used clinically. General muscarinic agonists include several alkaloids, such as **muscarine, pilocarpine,** and **arecoline,** and many synthetic compounds, such as **carbachol** and **oxotremorine.** **Arecoline** is an ingredient of betel leaves and is used for recreational purposes in some Asian cultures. All of these centrally acting agonists produce excessive salivation and sweating in addition to cortical arousal. None are subtype-selective or used to treat disorders of the CNS. However, muscarinic cholinergic agonists are used clinically to treat **glaucoma** and **urinary retention,** and also are effective in ameliorating the symptoms of **Sjögren syndrome,** a disorder characterized by autoimmune degeneration of the salivary glands.

Prototypical muscarinic antagonists include **atropine** and **scopolamine.** Neither of these is subtype-selective. Atropine is a derivative of **belladonna,** whose name (beautiful woman) reflects its cosmetic use as a pupillary dilator in decades past. Produced by the deadly nightshade plant, this muscarinic antagonist continues to be used in ophthalmic practice to enhance examinations of the retina. Related antagonists, such as **benztropine,** are commonly used to treat **Parkinson disease** and the Parkinson-like symptoms sometimes precipitated by antipsychotic drugs. Scopolamine, administered in a slow-release transdermal patch, is effective in preventing motion sickness. Many psychotropic drugs, including **tricyclic antidepressants** and low-potency **antipsychotic drugs** (e.g., **chlorpromazine**), are known to antagonize muscarinic cholinergic receptors in addition to producing their intended effects; this antago-

Table 9–6 Muscarinic Cholinergic Receptors

Receptor (amino acid residues)	Agonists[1] (carbachol, arecoline, pilocarpine, oxotremorine)	Antagonists[1] (atropine, scopolamine)	G-protein	Localization[2]
M1 (460 aa)	McN-A-343	Pirenzepine telenzepine	$G_{q/11}$	Cortex; hippocampus; striatum
M2 (466 aa)	—	AF-DX-116	$G_{i/o}$	Basal forebrain; thalamus
M3 (590 aa)	—	Hexhydrosiladifenidol	$G_{q/11}$	Cortex; hippocampus; thalamus
M4 (479 aa)	—	Himbacine; tropicamide	$G_{i/o}$	Cortex; striatum; hippocampus
M5 (532 aa)	—	4-DAMP	$G_{q/11}$	Substantia nigra

[1]Very few selective agonists and antagonists are available for muscarinic receptor subtypes. Some nonspecific or general agents are given in parentheses.
[2]mRNA expression for these receptors has been determined in rat brain, the distribution of each subtype may differ in human tissue.
4-DAMP, 4-diphenylacetoxy-N-methylpiperidine; McN-A-343, 4-(3-chlorophenylcarbamoyl-oxy)2-butynyltrimethylammonium chloride

nistic action is believed to contribute to the unwanted side effects (e.g., dry mouth and constipation) of some of these agents. Muscarinic antagonists can cause a characteristic **delirium** that tends to occur in geriatric patients treated with high doses of these agents or when combinations of drugs that share anticholinergic properties are used (see Chapter 20).

Nicotinic receptors   Nicotinic ACh receptors (nAChRs) are located in neuromuscular junctions, autonomic ganglia, the adrenal medulla, and the CNS. These ligand-gated ion channels were first character-ized based on their ability to bind **nicotine** isolated from the tobacco plant *Nicotiana tabacum.* Their activation by ACh leads to the rapid influx of Na^+ and Ca^+ and sub-sequent cellular depolarization. A prominent feature of nAChRs is their very rapid desensitization. Unlike de-sensitization of G protein-coupled receptors, which requires the actions of other proteins as described in Chapter 8, desensitization of nAChRs is an intrinsic property of the receptors themselves. The same may hold true for other ionotropic receptors. This latter type of desensitization may be similar to inactivation of voltage-gated Na^+ channels (see Chapter 3). However, the rate of desensitization of nAChRs can be regulated by the phosphorylation of receptor subunits. nAChRs expressed in neurons and those expressed in muscle differ in their subunit composition.

Muscular nAChRs are not described further in the section that follows, but their connection with **myasthe-nia gravis,** a rare neuromuscular disorder, deserves mention. This disease illustrates a pathophysiologic mechanism that occurs in several neurologic and psy-chiatric disorders. This unusual syndrome marked by weakness and muscle fatigue was first documented in 1877 and later called myasthenia gravis (Latin for mus-cle weakness). Although this disease was studied exten-sively, a century passed before its underlying cause was elucidated. For reasons that remain unknown, patients with this disease develop autoantibodies to muscular nAChRs. These antibodies sterically hinder ACh inter-action with receptors at neuromuscular junctions. In addition, they induce increased receptor turnover and degradation. Such actions result in a reduction in nAChRs at neuromuscular junctions, which in turn leads to decreased cholinergic signaling and severe muscle weakness. The standard treatment for myasthenia gravis involves the administration of AChE inhibitors, which prolong the duration of ACh in the synapse and increase its chance of activating remaining receptors. In some cases, glucocorticoids or other agents also may be administered to suppress immune function. With these therapies, myasthenia gravis is no longer life-threatening; however, definitive treatment will require a better understanding of the underlying autoimmu-nity that characterizes this disorder.

Neuronal nAChRs are composed of five subunits or-ganized around a central pore (Figure 9–11). Most recep-tors are believed to comprise heterologous subunits, of which at least twelve have been identified to date. Eight are classified as alpha subunits (α_2–α_9), and three as beta subunits (β_2–β_4); α_1 and β_1 subunits are expressed in muscle. Like other members of the ligand-gated ion channel family, each subunit has four membrane-spanning domains and disulfide loops (see Figure 9–10). The second transmembrane (M2) region of each subunit

A

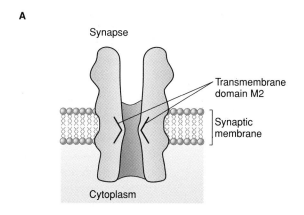

B

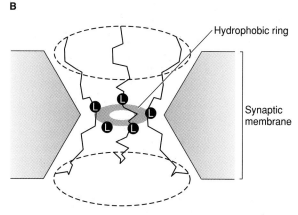

Figure 9–11. Model of the nicotinic acetylcholine receptor. Crystallized synaptic membranes were examined with an electron microscope to predict the three-dimensional structure of this receptor. **A.** A cylindrical membrane-embedded structure with a central pore is shown. The second transmembrane domain (M2) of each subunit lines the pore and bends inward to block ion flow through the channel. **B.** A highly conserved leucine residue (L) in the M2 bend of each subunit is believed to protrude into the pore to form a tight hydrophobic ring, which may act as a barrier to the flow of hydrated ions across the channel. (Adapted with permission from Unwin N. 1993. *J Mol Biol* 229:1118–1120.)

in each pentameric receptor lines the pore of the channel to regulate its gating properties (see Figure 9–11).

Most neuronal nAChRs contain both α and β subunits, and their stoichiometry is such that the ratio of these subunits typically is 2 to 3. However, some nAChRs are homomeric; α_7 subunits, for example, are capable of forming functional channels in vitro without the presence of other subunits. Because of the myriad combinations of subunits that might conceivably constitute a pentameric nAChR, it has been difficult to identify the combinations that occur naturally in the brain. Nevertheless, the distribution of individual subunits in the brain has been characterized (Table 9–7). In addition, several major types of nAChR complexes have been identified based on their affinities for certain toxins; for example, one population of receptors (i.e., α_7 homomeric receptors) binds **α-bungarotoxin** with high affinity and nicotine with low affinity, whereas most other populations bind nicotine with high affinity and are insensitive to bungarotoxin. α-Bungarotoxin also antagonizes muscle nAChRs.

Recent research in knockout mice indicates that the predominant nAChR in most brain regions may be composed of a β_2 subunit coupled with any of several α subunits; this receptor also may be responsible for the reinforcing and cognition-enhancing effects of nicotine. In contrast, homomeric α_7 receptors have been implicated in the effects of nicotine on sensory gating, whereas receptors containing the α_4 subunit mediate nicotine's analgesic effects.

Nicotinic receptor pharmacology   Only a small number of ligands bind at nAChRs. **Curare,** a poison that causes paralysis, blocks muscular, and to a lesser extent, neuronal nAChRs. **Succinylcholine,** a paralytic agent that is used clinically during anesthesia, acts as a weak partial agonist; it mildly activates nAChRs and subsequently induces their prolonged desensitization. Several blocking agents, including **hexamethonium** and **mecamylamine,** inhibit nAChRs that mediate neurotransmission in ganglia in both the sympathetic and parasympathetic branches of the autonomic nervous system (see Chapter 12). Very few antagonists that are selective for subtypes of neuronal nAChRs have been developed. Perhaps the most selective antagonist available is **methyllycaconitine,** which preferentially antagonizes α_7 homomeric receptor complexes. Although selective agonists for neuronal nAChRs might be of value in the treatment of several neuropsychiatric disorders, such agents have yet to be introduced into clinical practice. The selective agonist **epibatidine,** for example, binds with high affinity at nicotinic receptors but has been used only for experimental purposes (e.g., as an antinociceptive agent).

nAChRs possess several binding sites in addition to those that recognize ACh and bungarotoxin; for example, the AChE inhibitor **physostigmine** also binds to a channel activator site to increase the flow of ions through the receptor channel. A wide range of other compounds, including **phencyclidine** (**PCP**), **chlorpromazine,** and some anesthetics, also interact with nAChRs. Some act

Table 9–7 Distribution of nAChR Binding Sites and Subunit mRNAs in Rat Brain

	Ligand Binding		Subunit mRNA Distribution								
			α_2	α_3	α_4	α_5	α_6	α_7	β_2	β_3	β_4
						Amino Acid Residues					
Region	Nicotine	BgT	529 aa	503 aa	627 aa	468 aa	494 aa	502 aa	502 aa	458 aa	498 aa
Forebrain											
Cortex	+++	++	(+)	++	+++	+	−	+	+	−	+
Hippocampus	+	+++	(+)	+	++	++	−	+++	++	−	++
Thalamus	+++	(+)	−	++	+++	−	++	+	+++	++	++
Hypothalamus	+	+++	−	(+)	+	−	+	++	+	−	+
Amygdala	++	(+)	−	(+)	++	−	+	−	+	−	(+)
Septum	++		(+)	−	++	−	−	+	+	−	(+)
Brain stem											
Motor nuclei	++	−	−	+++	+	−	−	−	++	+	++
LC	++	++	−	+++	(+)	−	+	−	++	−	+
IPN	+++	+++	+++	+	+	++	−	−	++	−	++
Cerebellum	(+)	(+)	−	−	++	(+)	−	+	++	−	(+)
Cortex	+	++	−	+	+	−	−	++	++	−	+

Autoradiographic analysis with radiolabeled nicotine and bungarotoxin (BgT) reveals the distribution of receptor binding sites in the brain. In situ hybridization was used to determine the mRNA distribution of the various receptor subunits.

−, not detectable; (+), very weak signal; +, weak signal; ++, moderate signal; +++, strong signal; IPN, interpeduncular nucleus; LC, locus coeruleus.

Adapted with permission from Aneric SP, Sullivan JP, Williams, M. 1995. Neuronal nicotinic acetylcholine receptors. In: Bloom FE, Kupfer DJ, (eds). *Psychopharmacology: The Fourth Generation of Progress.* New York: Raven Press, p. 101.

as noncompetitive blockers to shorten the time that a channel remains open, while others accelerate receptor desensitization. Certain steroids inhibit nAChR activity by binding to an as yet unidentified site. More research is needed to determine whether such actions can be exploited for the development of novel pharmacotherapeutic agents.

As their name implies, nAChRs bind nicotine, which is a highly addictive substance. The addictive nature of nicotine and other drugs is discussed in Chapter 16; here nicotine is discussed in connection with other reported properties, which may be described as beneficial. Through mechanisms that have yet to be determined, the activation of central nAChRs by nicotine increases vigilance, improves memory, and enhances learning (Chapter 20). Nicotine also exerts antinociceptive effects; thus researchers hope that nicotinic agonists may be developed for use in the treatment of pain (Chapter 19). Interestingly, clinical studies reveal that systemic nicotine administration improves cognitive performance in patients with **Alzheimer disease;** moreover, recent epidemiologic studies indicate that smoking reduces the likelihood of developing this disease. Equally startling is evidence that smoking may decrease the incidence of **Parkinson disease.** Such findings seem to confirm speculation regarding the neuroprotective effects of nicotine.

Unfortunately, the use of nicotine or tobacco products is fraught with complications. First, as previously mentioned, nicotine is highly addictive. Second, it can have many adverse effects on health; high doses can damage the gastrointestinal tract and elevate blood pressure, and in some cases can precipitate myocardial infarction. In addition, tobacco products are responsible for a large number of deaths–approximately 500,000 each year in the United States alone. Thus the costs in terms of lives and health care dollars far outweigh the potential benefits of nicotine. However, novel nicotinic agonists yet to be developed may provide the purported clinical benefits of nicotine without its many harmful side effects.

HISTAMINE

Histamine occurs in abundance outside the nervous system, where it plays a central role in the secretion of gastric acid and in immune responses to allergens. Recent research indicates that it also serves important functions in the CNS. It has been determined that histamine is produced in the brain and that it is released synaptically throughout the CNS, where it acts on at least three receptor subtypes; however, details regarding this neurotransmitter's actions in the nervous system remain to be established.

SYNTHETIC AND DEGRADATIVE PATHWAYS

Histamine is produced in a one-step process involving the decarboxylation of the amino acid histidine by histidine decarboxylase, a 662-amino acid protein. Histidine also can be decarboxylated by L-aromatic amino acid decarboxylase (AADC), which, as previously discussed, is involved in the generation of catecholamines and serotonin. A recently developed inhibitor of histidine carboxylase, **α-fluoromethylhistidine,** is currently being examined for its in vivo effects in animal models.

Histamine is metabolized into methyl histidine by histamine methyl transferase. Alternatively, diamine oxidase may convert the neurotransmitter into imidazoleacetaldehyde. These pathways are represented in Figure 9–12.

The mechanisms underlying the storage, release, and reuptake of histamine remain poorly defined. It is presumed that histamine is concentrated in synaptic vesicles, yet the vesicular transporter responsible for such localization has not been determined. When histamine is released from nerve terminals in response to electrical stimulation, it acts on presynaptic and postsynaptic histamine receptors. However, it is not clear whether histamine is transported back into presynaptic terminals; the responsible transporter has yet to be characterized or isolated. An alternative possibility is that synaptically released histamine is degraded enzymatically.

FUNCTIONAL ANATOMY

Within the brain, histamine appears to be produced exclusively in the tuberomammillary nucleus of the posterior hypothalamus. Approximately 64,000 histaminergic neurons per nucleus exist in humans (Figure 9–13). These cells project to regions throughout the brain and spinal cord. Areas that receive especially dense projections include the cerebral cortex, hippocampus, neostriatum, nucleus accumbens, amygdala, and hypothalamus.

The widespread occurrence of histaminergic terminals in the brain is suggestive of many functions. Yet only histamine's influence on arousal has been well characterized (see Chapter 18). Many over-the-counter cold and allergy remedies that are known to cause drowsiness contain antihistamines (more specifically, H_1 receptor antagonists) as active ingredients. Newer antihistamines used as allergy medications are nonsedating because they do not cross the blood–brain barrier. Centrally acting antihistamines are the active ingredi-

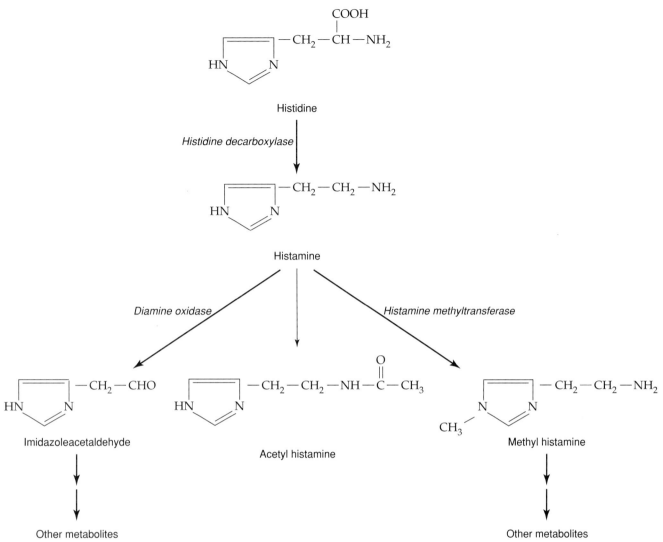

Figure 9–12. Biosynthesis and metabolism of histamine. Histamine is produced from the decarboxylation of the amino acid histidine and is subsequently metabolized into one of three products. Diamine oxidase converts histamine into imidazoleacetaldehyde, and histamine methyl transferase converts the neurotransmitter into its other major metabolite, methyl histamine. Acetyl histamine is a minor metabolite. These primary metabolites may be further processed into inactive forms.

ent in many over-the-counter sleep aids. Moreover, many psychotropic medications, including the antidepressants **mianserin** and **doxepin** and the antipsychotic **clozapine,** cause sedation partly because they are potent histamine H_1 receptor antagonists. Accordingly, it has been determined that the firing rate of histaminergic neurons in the tuberomammillary nucleus is strongly correlated with states of arousal. Firing is fastest during periods of wakefulness and slower during sleep; indeed, these cells fall silent during slow-wave sleep.

Histamine also has been implicated in the regulation of pituitary hormone secretion, perception of pain, control of appetite, and prevention of motion sickness and vertigo. With the advent of new centrally acting histaminergic drugs, our understanding of this neurotransmitter system in CNS function should become clearer.

HISTAMINE RECEPTORS

Three histamine receptors (H_1 to H_3) have been identified; all are members of the G protein-coupled receptor superfamily (Table 9–8). H_1 receptors couple to G_q proteins and H_2 receptors couple to G_s

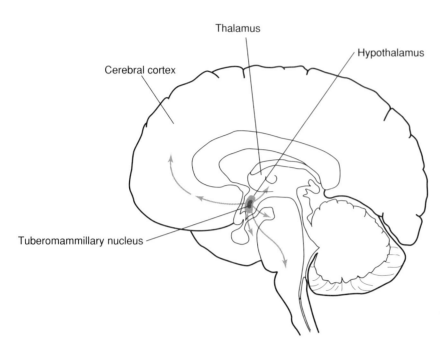

Thalamus

Hypothalamus

Cerebral cortex

Tuberomammillary nucleus

Figure 9-13. Histaminergic system in the brain. In the CNS, histamine is produced exclusively in the tuberomammillary nucleus of the hypothalamus. This small bilateral nucleus provides histaminergic input to most brain regions and to the spinal cord.

proteins. The H_3 receptor, only recently cloned, has been characterized in the CNS largely on the basis of radioligand binding with subtype-specific compounds; it is believed that this receptor couples to G_i proteins and acts as an autoreceptor, functionally analogous to the α_2-adrenergic, dopamine D_2, and 5-HT_{1a} receptors. H_3 receptors also function as heteroreceptors and regulate the release of other neurotransmitters from nerve terminals.

Antihistamines in over-the-counter products are histamine H_1 antagonists. Such drugs may be used to treat cold and allergy symptoms, to produce sedation, or to treat nausea and vomiting. Commonly used H_1 antagonists include **diphenhydramine, meclizine,** and **dimenhydrinate.** All of these drugs, which are called first-generation H_1 antagonists, penetrate the blood–brain barrier. Second-generation compounds, such as **loratadine** and **terfenadine,** are excluded from the brain and are prescribed as nonsedating allergy medications.

Most agents that are selective for the histamine H_2 receptor are not able to cross the blood–brain barrier. These agents inhibit the secretion of gastric acid and are used most often to control reflux, heartburn, and ulcers; commonly used examples include **cimetidine** and **ranitidine.** Such agents have been determined to cause confusion in a small percentage of patients.

H_3 selective agents are under current investigation for several possible therapeutic uses. Antagonists, such as **thioperamide,** increase wakefulness and are being evaluated for the treatment of cognitive deficits and obesity. Agonists, such as **R-α-methylhistamine,** promote sleep and may be useful in the treatment of insomnia.

Table 9-8 The Histamine Receptor Family

Receptor (amino acid residues)	Agonists	Antagonists	G protein	Localization
H1 487 aa		Mepyramine[1]; triprolidine; diphenhydramine; dimenhydrinate	$G_{q/11}$	Cortex; hippocampus; nucleus accumbens; thalamus
H2 359 aa	Dimaprit[1]	Ranitidine[1]; cimetidine[1]	G_s	Basal ganglia; hippocampus; amygdala; cortex
H3 445 aa	R-α-methylhistamine[1]; imetit[1]	Thioperamide[1]	Unknown (?$G_{i/o}$)	Basal ganglia; hippocampus; cortex

[1]Selective agonists or antagonists.

SELECTED READING

Alexander SPH, Peters JA. 2000. 2000 Receptor and ion channel nomenclature supplement. *Trends Pharmacol Sci* (suppl).

Blakely RD, Ramamoorthy S, Schroeter S, et al. 1998. Regulated phosphorylation and trafficking of antidepressant-sensitive serotonin transporter proteins. *Biol Psychiatry* 44:169–178.

Brunner D, Hen R. 1997. Insights into the neurobiology of impulsive behavior from serotonin receptor knockout mice. *Ann NY Acad Sci* 836:81–105.

Burns CM, Chu H, Rueter SM, et al. 1997. Regulation of serotonin-2C receptor G-protein coupling by RNA editing. *Nature* 387:303–308.

Caulfield MP. 1993. Muscarinic receptors: Characterization, coupling, and function. *Pharmacol Ther* 58:319–379.

Cooper JR, Bloom FE, Roth RH. 1996. *The Biochemical Basis of Neuropharmacology,* 7th ed. New York: Oxford University Press.

Cordero-Erausquin M, Marubio LM, Klink R, Changeux J-P. 2000. Nicotinic receptor function: new perspectives from knockout mice. *Trends Pharmacol* Sci 21:211–217.

Fitzpatrick PF. 2000. The aromatic amino acid hydroxylases. *Adv Enzymol* 74:235–294.

Heninger GR. 1997. Serotonin, sex, and psychiatric illness. *Proc Natl Acad Sci USA* 94:4823–4824.

Hill SJ, Ganellin CR, Timmerman H, et al. 1997. Classification of histamine receptors. *Pharmacol Rev* 49:253–278.

Hoffman BB, Lefkowitz RJ, Taylor P. 1996. Neurotransmission. The autonomic and somatic motor nervous systems. In Hardman JG, Limbird LE, Molinoff PB, et al (ed). *Goodman and Gilman's The Pharmacological Basis of Therapeutics,* 9th ed. New York: McGraw-Hill, pp. 105–139.

Hoyer D, Clarke DE, Fozard JR, et al. 1994. International Union of Pharmacology. Classification of receptors for 5-hydroxytryptamine serotonin. *Pharmacol Rev* 46:157–203.

Julius D. 1998. Serotonin receptor knockouts: A moody subject. *Proc Natl Acad Sci USA* 95:15153–15154.

Lena C, Changeux JP. 1998. Allosteric nicotinic receptors, human pathologies. *J Physiol* (*Paris*) 92:63–74.

Leurs R, Blandina P, Tedford C, Timmerman H. 1998. Therapeutic potential of histamine H_3 receptor agonists and antagonists. *Trends Pharmacol Sci* 19:177–183.

Lovenberg TW, Roland BL, Wilson SJ, et al. 1999. Cloning and functional expression of the human histamine H_3 receptor. *Mol Pharmacol* 55:1101–1107.

Martinez-Mir MI, Pollard H, Moreau J, et al. 1990. Three histamine receptors (H_1, H_2, and H_3) visualized in the brain of human and non-human primates. *Brain Res* 526: 322–327.

Mesulam MM. 1996. The systems-level organization of cholinergic innervation in the human cerebral cortex and its alterations in Alzheimer's disease. *Prog Brain Res* 109: 285–297.

Ni YG, Miledi R. 1997. Blockage of $5-HT_{2C}$ serotonin receptors by fluoxetine (Prozac). *Proc Natl Acad Sci USA* 94: 2036–2040.

Orr-Urtreger A, Goldner FM, Saeki M, et al. 1997. Mice deficient in the alpha7 neuronal nicotinic acetylcholine receptor lack alpha-bungarotoxin binding sites and hippocampal fast nicotinic currents. *J Neurosci* 17:9165–9171.

Picciotto MR, Zoli M, Rimondini R, et al. 1998. Acetylcholine receptors containing the beta2 subunit are involved in the reinforcing properties of nicotine. *Nature* 391:173–177.

Ramamoorthy S, Giovanetti E, Qian Y, Blakely RD. 1998. Phosphorylation and regulation of antidepressant-sensitive serotonin transporters. *J Biol Chem* 273:2458–2466.

Ricaurte GA, Yuan J, McCann UD. 2000. *(+/−)*3,4-Methylenedioxymethamphetamine ("Ecstasy")-induced serotonin neurotoxicity: studies in animals. Neuropsychobiology 42:5–10.

Rueter LE, Fornal CA, Jacobs BL. 1997. A critical review of 5-HT brain microdialysis and behavior. *Rev Neurosci* 8: 117–137.

Rouse ST, Marino MJ, Potter LT, et al. 1999. Muscarinic receptor subtypes involved in hippocampal circuits. *Life Sci* 64:501–509.

Sargent PB. 1993. The diversity of neuronal nicotinic acetylcholine receptors. *Annu Rev Neurosci* 16:403–443.

Schwartz J-C, Arrang J-M, Garbarg M, Traiffort E. 1995. Histamine. In Bloom FE, Kupfer DJ (ed). *Psychopharmacology: The Fourth Generation of Progress.* New York: Raven Press, pp. 397–405.

Sturman G. 1996. Histaminergic drugs as modulators of CNS function. *Eur J Physiol* (*suppl*) 431:R223–R224.

Taylor P. 1996. Anticholinesterase agents. In Hardman JG, Limbird LE, Molinoff PB (ed). *Goodman and Gilman's The Pharmacological Basis of Therapeutics,* 9th ed. New York: McGraw-Hill, pp. 161–176.

Unwin N. 1993. Nicotinic acetylcholine receptor at 9 Angstrom resolution. *J Mol Biol* 229:1101–1124.

Chapter 10

Neuropeptides and Purines

KEY CONCEPTS

- Neuropeptides are small proteins that serve neurotransmitter-like functions in the nervous system; other signaling peptides such as growth factors and cytokines are considered to be a distinct class even though they may have some overlapping functions.

- Like the monoamines and acetylcholine, the neuropeptides serve primarily modulatory roles in the nervous system and generally interact with G protein-coupled receptors.

- The synthesis of neuropeptides, like that of all proteins, requires the transcription of DNA and translation of the resulting mRNA into protein.

- Neuropeptides are synthesized as large precursor polypeptides that undergo extensive posttranslational processing that includes cleavages into smaller peptides and subsequent enzymatic modification.

- Neuropeptides contain an N-terminal signal sequence that directs the transport of a newly synthesized protein from ribosomes to the lumen of the endoplasmic reticulum.

- As a result of alternative RNA splicing and cleavage of propeptides, a single gene can give rise to diverse signaling peptides with distinct functions.

- Unlike classic small-molecule neurotransmitters, which are packaged in small synaptic vesicles, neuropeptides are packaged in large dense core vesicles; both types of vesicles may be found in the same neuron.

- Neuropeptides may diffuse for long distances within the extracellular space before binding to their specific receptors.

- The designation of a group of neurotransmitters as purines is a misnomer; in fact, purinergic signaling molecules are the nucleoside and nucleotide derivatives of purine and pyrimidine bases.

- The two principal purinergic signaling molecules are adenosine and ATP, which also serve modulatory roles in the nervous system.

- ATP is stored in small synaptic vesicles and released in response to action potentials in a calcium-dependent fashion whereas adenosine is released from nonvesicular cytoplasmic stores, likely via bidirectional nucleoside transporters.

- Purine receptors form a relatively large and diverse group and have been categorized as P_1 and P_2 receptors.

- P_1 receptors, also called adenosine receptors, bind adenosine and its analogs and are G protein-coupled receptors.

- The important stimulant drugs of the methylxanthine family, including caffeine, are antagonists of adenosine receptors.

This chapter introduces two classes of signaling molecules that were discovered after the principal neurotransmitters discussed in previous chapters. Like the monoamines and acetylcholine, the neuropeptides and purines serve primarily modulatory roles in the nervous system. Although we know that neuropeptides act as neurotransmitters, many of their functions are not as well established as those of other transmitters. Thus this chapter focuses on general aspects of neuropeptide transmission and describes a small number of neuropeptide systems in detail to illustrate these concepts. Several peptides are discussed at greater length in subsequent chapters; for example, hypothalamic peptides are considered in conjunction with the regulation of neuroendocrine function, stress responses, and eating behavior (Chapter 13), and opioid peptides and substance P are considered in connection with the regulation of nociception (Chapter 19).

Purinergic neurotransmitters, primarily adenosine and adenosine triphosphate (ATP), are discussed in the second half of this chapter. These molecules were long considered improbable mediators of neurotransmission because of their central involvement in intermediary metabolism. However, we now know that they are concentrated at certain synapses, that they are released in response to synaptic stimulation, and that they activate families of receptors to produce important responses in target neurons. It is also established that purinergic receptors mediate the actions of several pharmacologic agents, most notably **caffeine**.

CHARACTERISTICS OF NEUROPEPTIDES

When research first revealed that neuropeptides serve as signaling molecules in the nervous system, a revolution in neuropharmacology was anticipated. The drug industry viewed neuropeptides and their receptors as new targets for drugs that might influence a wide range of neural functions and in turn treat many neuropsychiatric disorders. The discovery also spawned further study of neuropeptides that has, in the past 25 years, revealed a great deal about normal neuronal functioning. Yet our ability to exploit neuropeptide systems pharmacologically is still in its infancy.

Peptides are small proteins and are therefore composed of amino acids covalently linked to each other by peptide bonds (Figure 10–1). The term *neuropeptide* is reserved for small proteins that serve neurotransmitter-like functions in the nervous system. Other signaling peptides, such as growth factors and cytokines (see Chapter 11), are traditionally distinguished from the neuropeptides even though they may have overlapping functions. Some neuropeptides mediate signaling between neurons only in the CNS; others are also utilized in the peripheral nervous system. In addition to their transmitter functions, some neuropeptides are released directly into the blood by neurons and act as hormones; many others act as hormones secreted by endocrine glands. A variety of molecules that are categorized as neuropeptides are listed in Table 10–1; however, this list is not exhaustive, and more peptides are likely to be discovered. Although most of these molecules exhibit features similar to those of classic neurotransmitters,

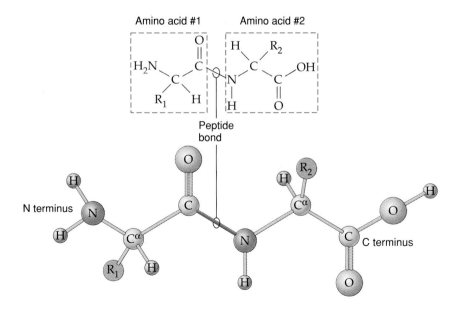

Figure 10–1. Peptide bond. Peptides are linear strings composed of the 20 different amino acids, the sequences of which are encoded by individual genes and mRNA (see Chapter 6). These amino acids are joined at peptide bonds, where the free carboxy group (C terminus) of one amino acid forms an amidoester bond with the free amino group (N terminus) of an adjacent amino acid. All amino acids share a common structure distinguished by their side chain (R_1 and R_2).

neuropeptides are synthesized differently and are distinguished by a wide range of other characteristics.

PRECURSOR PROTEINS

Many classic small-molecule neurotransmitters are derived from the step-wise enzymatic modification of a single amino acid that typically is transported into neurons from the general circulation. Serotonin, for example, is derived from the enzymatic modification of tryptophan (see Chapter 9). In contrast, the synthesis of neuropeptides, like that of all proteins, requires the transcription of DNA sequences and the translation of mRNA into protein (see Chapter 6). The protein product released by the ribosome is not a signaling molecule, but a large precursor polypeptide that undergoes extensive posttranslational processing that converts it into an active peptide. The steps in neuropeptide synthesis are represented in Figure 10–2 and also in Figure 10–3, which traces the processing of proopiomelanocortin (POMC). POMC is termed a *prepropeptide* and is the precursor of many active peptides, including adrenocorticotropic hormone (ACTH), melanocyte-stimulating hormone (α-MSH), and β-endorphin. Prepropeptides contain an N-terminal signal sequence that directs the transport of a newly synthesized protein from ribosomes to the lumen of the endoplasmic reticulum (ER). After a protein has been transported into the ER, the signal sequence is cleaved by a signal peptidase, which transforms the prepropeptide into a propeptide. The propeptide is subsequently transferred to the Golgi complex and packaged in large dense core vesicles, within which the protein undergoes further processing, and is transported from the cell body to the synapse.

PROTEOLYTIC PROCESSING

Propeptide precursors are converted into active neuropeptides by a series of steps, which include cleavages and modifications to particular amino acid residues (see Figure 10–3). During this process, endoproteases recognize and cleave dibasic amino acid pairs (Lys–Arg, Lys–Lys, Arg–Arg, or Arg–Lys) to liberate peptides that are further processed by exopeptidases and modifying enzymes (Table 10–2). The two key endoproteases involved in the processing of POMC and many other precursors are prohormone convertases 1 and 2 (PC1 and PC2), which are members of a larger family of prohormone convertases. Neuropeptide-processing enzymes such as those that cleave POMC generally act in stepwise fashion, first cleaving certain dibasic residues, and then, depending on the tissue, making additional cleavages. Ultimately, the cleavage of POMC by

Table 10–1 Examples of Peptides in the Nervous System

Gut–Brain Peptides
Cholecystokinin
Galanin
Gastrin
Glucagon
Insulin
Gastrin releasing peptide
Neurotensin (NT)
Neuropeptide Y (NPY)
Substance P
Vasoactive intestinal peptide

Pituitary Hormones
Adrenocorticotropic hormone (ACTH)
Growth hormone (GH)
Follicle stimulating hormone (FSH)
Luteinizing hormone (LH)
α-Melanocyte-stimulating hormone (α-MSH)
Oxytocin
Prolactin
Thyrotropin (thyroid-stimulating hormone or TSH)
Vasopressin

Hypothalamic Releasing Factors
Corticotropin-releasing factor (CRF)
Gonadotropin-releasing hormone (GnRH)
Growth hormone-releasing hormone (GHRH)
Somatostatin
Thyrotropin-releasing hormone (TRH)

Opioid Peptides
β-Endorphin
Dynorphin
Leu-enkephalin
Met-enkephalin

Other Peptides
Angiotensin
Bradykinin
Calcitonin
Calcitonin gene-related peptide
Neuromedin K

Peptides are traditionally grouped by function or by the regions in which their functions were first characterized. Gut–brain peptides, for example, are those that have been found not only in the nervous system but also in the gastrointestinal tract. As we learn more about each peptide, however, conventional classification schemes become less useful. ACTH and α-MSH, which are listed as pituitary hormones, are also found in nonneuroendocrine neurons and have nonendocrine functions. CRF, one of the hormones released from the hypothalamus, also functions in many other brain regions. Thus this table should be regarded merely as a starting point for understanding peptide function.

PC1 and PC2 yields smaller peptides whose C or N termini contain Lys or Arg residues. Another enzyme, carboxypeptidase E, removes basic C-terminal residues, and an aminopeptidase that has yet to be identified removes basic N-terminal residues.

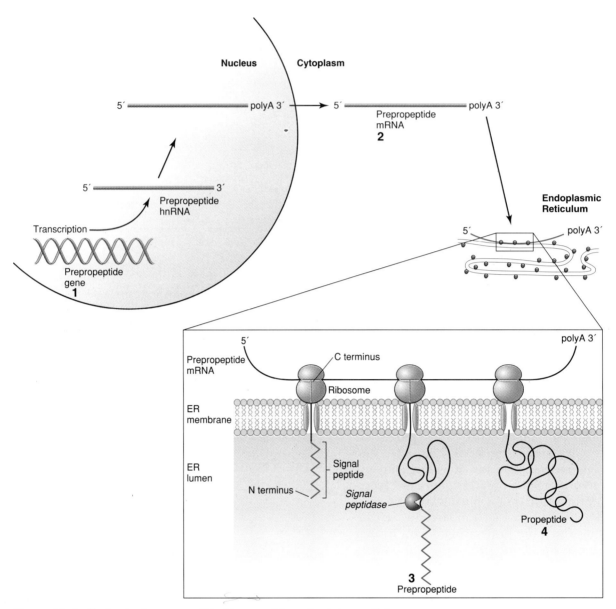

Figure 10–2. Synthesis of a neuropeptide. Neuropeptide synthesis is a multistep process that begins with (**1**) transcription of the prepropeptide gene in the nucleus, and (**2**) subsequent ribosomal translation of the prepropeptide mRNA in the cytoplasm. The N terminus of the growing prepropeptide (**3**) contains a signal sequence, a short stretch of amino acids that enables the peptide to be translocated into the lumen of the endoplasmic reticulum. After such translocation, the signal peptide is cleaved by a signal peptidase, and the remaining product is called the propeptide (**4**). The propeptide is not bioactive; further enzymatic modification is required to liberate its bioactive moieties.

Many neuropeptides undergo two additional modifications after convertase and peptidase action has taken place. N-terminal acetylation often serves to regulate the bioactivity of a peptide; for example, acetylation of α-MSH significantly enhances its biologic activity. Conversely, when β-endorphin is acetylated, its activity is markedly reduced. Peptides with a C-terminal glycine, such as α-MSH, also undergo α-amidation. The enzyme responsible for this modification is peptidylglycine α-amidating monooxygenase (PAM).

Thus the synthesis of a bioactive neuropeptide is a multistep process whereby a prepropeptide is converted into a propeptide, which subsequently yields bioactive peptides in response to the actions of endoproteases, exopeptidases, and other modifying enzymes. Drugs aimed at modifying these various

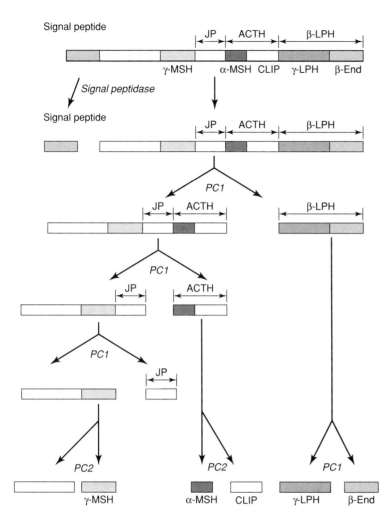

Figure 10–3. Proteolytic processing of proopiomelanocortin (POMC). After the signal peptide is removed from pre-POMC, the remaining peptide undergoes an ordered process of endoproteolysis by proconvertase 1 and 2 (PC1 and PC2) at dibasic residues between adjoining domains. PC1 is involved in the early steps of POMC processing and liberates the bioactive peptides adrenocorticotropic hormone (ACTH), β-endorphin (β-End), and γ-lipotropic hormone (γ-LPH). PC2 cleaves ACTH into corticotropin-like intermediate lobe peptide (CLIP) and α-melanocyte stimulating hormone (α-MSH) and also releases γ-MSH from the N-terminal portion of the propeptide. The joining peptide (JP) is the region of the precursor between ACTH and γ-MSH. Note that some of the peptides are amidated and/or acetylated before they become fully active.

enzymatic processes could be useful pharmacotherapeutic agents (Box 10–1).

GENERATION OF DIVERSITY

A single propeptide, such as POMC, is capable of generating several bioactive neuropeptides (see Figure 10–3); however, the steps by which such proteolytic processing occurs are tissue-specific. In the anterior lobe of the pituitary gland, for example, POMC typically is converted into ACTH. In the intermediate lobe of this gland and in neurons that express POMC, α-MSH and β-endorphin are the major end products. Variations in the cellular expression of prohormone convertases can determine which peptides are synthesized in each tissue. In addition, because much of the processing of peptides occurs after they are packaged in large dense core vesicles, and because convertases are highly sensitive to pH and Ca^{2+}, convertase activity is regulated by alterations in vesicular pH and Ca^{2+} concentrations.

Diverse neuropeptides also can be generated by alternative RNA splicing (Chapter 6). Calcitonin and calcitonin gene-related peptide (CGRP) were the first peptides known to be produced by alternative splicing. Tachykinins, a family of neuropeptides discussed later in this chapter, include several members that are derived from two preprotachykinin genes. One of the genes is alternatively spliced and subsequently translated into at least three distinct prepropeptides (Figure 10–4), which in turn are posttranslationally processed to produce five distinct bioactive peptides, including neurokinin A and substance P.

STORAGE AND RELEASE

The synaptic regulation of neuropeptides is distinguished from that of classic neurotransmitters by several key features represented in Figure 10–5. First, as previously described, peptides are synthesized by transcription, translation, and posttranslational modification in the cell body and axon. This is in marked contrast to

Box 10–1 Peptide-Processing Enzymes as Drug Targets?

A key step in the generation of a biologically active neuropeptide is its posttranslational processing. Neuropeptides are synthesized as parts of larger proteins; thus their precursors, called *prohormones* or *propeptides*, must be cleaved into smaller neuropeptide fragments. Proopiomelanocortin (POMC) is a prohormone whose structure contains the neuropeptides ACTH, α-MSH, and β-endorphin. Proteolytic enzymes known as prohormone convertases (PC1 and PC2) catalyze the rate-limiting step in the processing of prohormones such as POMC.

In contrast to classic neurotransmitters, whose components are readily available at synapses, neuropeptide precursors must be synthesized de novo in cell soma by means of DNA transcription and mRNA translation. Moreover, because no presynaptic reuptake mechanism exists for neuropeptides, these transmitters are not recycled after release. Hence, rapid replenishment of neuropeptides during synaptic activity relies heavily on the regulation and activity of PC1 and PC2, which act on stores of prohormones present in neurons.

PC1 and PC2, which have been cloned and extensively characterized, are expressed only in the brain and in neuroendocrine structures. This pattern of expression, which is consistent with their restricted role in neuropeptide function, suggests that drugs aimed at these enzymes would be unlikely to produce peripheral side effects. Several investigators have demonstrated that factors that alter prohormone expression, such as stress, similarly affect PC1 and PC2 expression. This finding indicates that prohormone and convertase expression may be highly coordinated. Computational modeling of interactions between prohormone convertases and their substrates, and the isolation of small peptides that antagonize these enzymes, have advanced our understanding of PC1 and PC2 and have pointed to the types of small molecules that eventually may be synthesized and used to alter their activity. Such agents may provide us with the pharmacologic means to alter proconvertase activity and, in turn, the rate of neuropeptide synthesis in the nervous system.

The angiotensin converting enzyme (ACE) inhibitors represent one class of drugs that act on peptide processing enzymes. These inhibitors, which include **captopril,** are widely used to treat **hypertension**. ACE cleaves a decapeptide angiotensin precursor to yield the biologically active octapeptide. Because angiotensin normally functions to increase vascular tone, ACE inhibitors, by reducing circulating levels of angiotensin, potently decrease blood pressure.

Table 10–2 Enzymes Involved in Neuropeptide Synthesis

Enzyme	Function
Amino acid residues (aa)	
Prohormone convertase 1 (PC1) 753 aa	Endoproteolysis of peptide bonds between dibasic residues in propeptides
Prohormone convertase 2 (PC2) 638 aa	Endoproteolysis of peptide bonds between dibasic residues in propeptides
Carboxypeptidase E (CPE) 451 aa	Exoproteolysis of carboxy terminal basic residues on peptides arising from convertase activity
Aminopeptidases	Exoproteolysis of amino terminal basic residues on peptides arising from convertase activity
Peptidyl glycine α-amidating monooxygenase (PAM) 938 aa	Amidation of carboxy terminal glycine residues; optimal activation of some peptides
N-acetyltransferases	Addition of acetyl group to N termini of some peptides to control their activity

Listed are the principal enzymes required for the processing of POMC and other propeptides. Additional processing enzymes, including some convertases and acetyltransferases, may be required for other neuropeptide systems.

noradrenergic, dopaminergic, and many other neurotransmitters, which can be synthesized in the presynaptic terminal. Likewise, neuropeptides are processed and stored in large dense core vesicles that are assembled in the Golgi apparatus and transported to the synapse, whereas norepinephrine, dopamine, glutamate, γ-aminobutyric acid (GABA), and other classic transmitters are stored in small clear synaptic vesicles that can be constructed in the terminal region. Both types of synaptic vesicles are located in the nerve terminals of many neuronal cell types. In fact, a hallmark of neuropeptides is their co-localization with classic neurotransmitters; for example, the presence of one or more neuropeptides is commonly detected in a single catecholaminergic or serotonergic neuron (Table 10–3).

Although large dense core vesicles containing neuropeptides and small synaptic vesicles containing classic neurotransmitters can be stored in the same synapses, the two types of transmitters are released by different mechanisms, and consequently may be released under different conditions. Large dense core and small synaptic vesicles are generally segregated in synaptic terminals such that the smaller vesicles are clustered in active zones abutting the synaptic cleft—zones from which the larger vesicles are excluded (see Chapter 4). The exocytosis of small synaptic vesicles occurs in response to

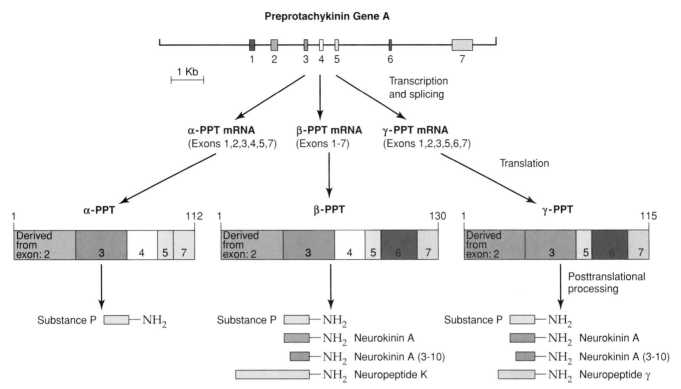

Figure 10–4. Alternative splicing of preprotachykinin (PPT) gene A. This gene, also called *PPT gene I* or *substance P–neurokinin A gene*, contains seven exons (numbered boxes), which are alternatively spliced into three prepropeptides (α, β, and γ PPT). The number shown above each PPT splice variant represents its amino acid length after translation. After translation and proteolytic processing, all three PPT splice variants liberate substance P, which is encoded in exon three. Neuropeptide K is encoded in exons 3–6 and thus is derived only from β-PPT. Neuropeptide γ is encoded in exons 3, 5, and 6, which occur together only in γ-PPT. Neurokinin A and the neurokinin A fragment (3-10) can be synthesized from either β- or γ-PPT. (Adapted with permission from Helke CJ, Krause JE, Mantyh PW, et al. 1990. *FASEB J* 4:1608.)

large, transient increases in intracellular Ca^{2+}, whereas the exocytosis of large dense core vesicles requires increases in Ca^{2+} of lesser magnitude but longer duration, so that the Ca^{2+} can diffuse in adequate concentrations to reach these vesicles. Typically, a single action potential causes small synaptic vesicles to fuse with the cell membrane, but a rapid train of action potentials may be required to trigger the release of a neuropeptide. Thus specific patterns of electrical activity in a neuron may lead to the preferential release of a neuropeptide or a small-molecule neurotransmitter, or may prompt the release of both.

The functional role of co-localization of classic neurotransmitters with neuropeptides within individual neurons is not clear. Several studies have documented the modification of a postsynaptic action of a small-molecule transmitter by a co-localized neuropeptide. In these cases the neuropeptide either facilitates or opposes the function of its co-localized transmitter. Accordingly, because neuropeptides tend to be re-

leased under conditions of sustained synaptic activity, they may regulate strongly stimulated synapses by providing positive or negative feedback.

LONG-DISTANCE SIGNALING BY NEUROPEPTIDES

One of the most interesting differences between neuropeptide signaling and that of classic neurotransmitters becomes evident after a neuropeptide is released from a presynaptic neuron. When a small-molecule neurotransmitter such as dopamine is released into a synapse, most of it is rapidly taken up and returned to the presynaptic cell by means of its corresponding transporter; among such transmitters only acetylcholine differs in that it is metabolized before its choline metabolite is actively transported back into cholinergic nerve terminals (see Chapter 9). In contrast, neuropeptides are not rapidly cleared from the synapse. Their action is terminated by endopeptidases and exopeptidases that

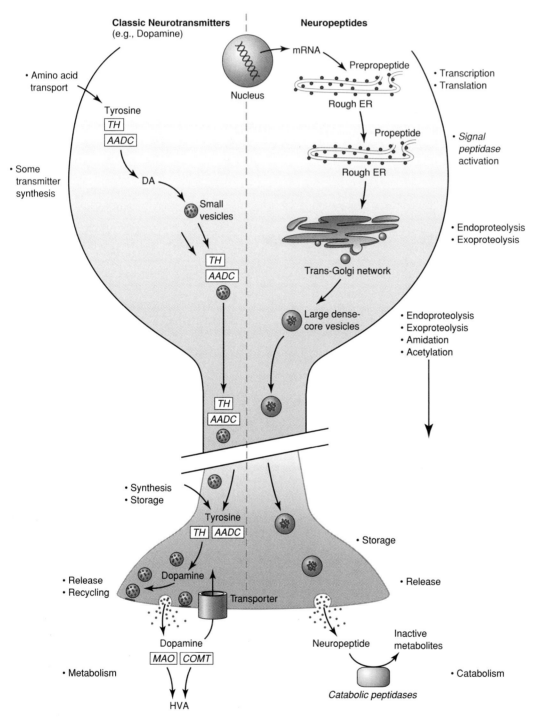

Figure 10–5. Comparison between classic neurotransmitter and neuropeptide systems. Dopamine is used here to represent a classic neurotransmitter. The principal difference between these two systems is the cellular location of their synthesis. Although some dopamine is synthesized in the cell body, most is produced in nerve terminals. In contrast, neuropeptide synthesis begins in the cell body and continues as it is transported down the axon. Unlike dopamine, which is stored in small clear synaptic vesicles, neuropeptide is stored in large dense core vesicles. Both dopamine and the neuropeptide are enzymatically degraded, but only dopamine is transported back into the nerve terminal, where it is repackaged for subsequent release. ER, endoplasmic reticulum; TH, tyrosine hydroxylase; AADC, aromatic amino acid decarboxylase; DA, dopamine; MAO, monoamine oxidase; COMT, catechol-O-methyltransferase; HVA, homovanillic acid.

Table 10-3 Examples of Co-localized Neuropeptides and Small-Molecule Neurotransmitters

Peptide	Small Molecule	Sites of Co-localization
NPY	NE	Neurons of the locus ceruleus; sympathetic postganglionic neurons
Dynorphin; substance P; enkephalin	GABA	Striatal GABAergic projection neurons
VIP	ACh	Parasympathetic postganglionic neurons
CGRP	ACh	Spinal motor neurons
Neurotensin; cholecystokinin	DA	Neurons of the substantia nigra

NE, norepinephrine; GABA, γ-aminobutyric acid; VIP, vasoactive intestinal peptide; ACh, acetylcholine; CGRP, calcitonin gene-related peptide; DA, dopamine.

Now envision a peptide such as neuropeptide Y (NPY), which is 36 amino acids in length. How does such a large molecule fit into the binding pocket of a G protein-coupled receptor? Which conformation has the highest affinity for the receptor, and which amino acid residues are critical for binding? Most importantly from a pharmacologic point of view, how might non-peptide analogs be developed to mimic or antagonize NPY binding? All of these questions are difficult to answer and currently are the focus of intensive investigation (Box 10–2). Although modified peptide analogs have been synthesized to bind to neuropeptide receptors, peptides are far from ideal pharmacotherapeutic agents. Synthetic peptides are subject to proteolysis by ubiquitous peptidases, and, more importantly, they cannot cross the blood–brain barrier; thus nonpeptide

cleave peptide bonds and thereby render peptides inactive. The peptidases involved in such catabolism are different from the convertases involved in propeptide processing and reside on extracellular membranes.

Accordingly, peptides can travel relatively large distances to activate receptors, and this may explain why the anatomic locations of many neuropeptides do not correspond precisely to the locations of their receptors. A striking example of this mismatch between neuropeptides and their receptors, which represents one of the more perplexing findings in neuroanatomy, is illustrated in Figure 10–6. The figure shows high levels of substance P in the substantia nigra, yet indicates a virtual absence of substance P receptors in the same region.

Most neuropeptide receptors belong to the superfamily of G protein-coupled receptors; a possible exception is a newly discovered neurotensin receptor described later in this chapter. Like small-molecule neurotransmitters, a given neuropeptide may have several receptor subtypes, as indicated in Table 10–4. However, the receptors for neuropeptides bind their ligands with much greater affinities than do the receptors for small-molecule transmitters; for example, acetylcholine binds to its receptors in the 100 μM–1 mM range, whereas neuropeptides can bind with nanomolar affinity.

The interactions between neuropeptides and their receptors are quite complex. Imagine a small molecule such as norepinephrine interacting with the binding pocket of its receptor. Only so many atoms of the norepinephrine molecule can possibly interact ionically or sterically with the receptor; thus the molecular modeling of feasible interactions is relatively straightforward.

A

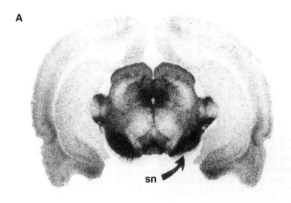

B

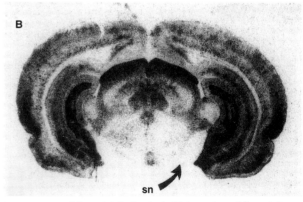

Figure 10-6. Mismatch in the tachykinin system. Mismatch refers to the disparity between the location of a neuropeptide and the location of its receptors. **A.** Substance P in rat, as detected by peptide antibodies. This neuropeptide is highly concentrated in the substantia nigra (sn) among other regions. **B.** Autoradiography of receptor binding indicates that substance P receptors are virtually nonexistent in the substantia nigra, despite their density in regions where the neuropeptide is scarce. (Adapted with permission from Herkenham M. 1987. *Neuroscience* 23:8.)

Box 10–2 Molecular Modeling of Neuropeptides

Before the interactions between a neuropeptide and its receptor can be characterized, the three-dimensional structure of the neuropeptide must be elucidated. Ultimately it is important to determine the precise conformation that the neuropeptide must assume in order to associate with its membrane-bound receptor. However, the aqueous–membrane interface that characterizes such binding presents a challenge. Peptides are flexible polymers whose structure in water is dynamic. In fact, many peptides are flexible enough to be considered structureless in an aqueous solution. Thus crystallographic analysis of these molecules is nearly impossible, and more creative means are required to elucidate their structures.

The mixed hydrophilic–hydrophobic environment in which a peptide binds to its receptor can be approximated when a peptide is placed in a solvent containing small membranous spheres known as micelles, which are composed of lipids (see Chapter 3). Subsequently NMR spectroscopy can be used to determine the conformations of the peptide as it associates with these spheres. When galanin, a 29-amino-acid peptide, is placed in such a solution, NMR calculations indicate that the peptide, even in association with hydrophobic membranes, is a highly flexible molecule. Indeed, galanin is capable of at least 32 random conformations (see part A of figure).

Peptide structures also may be elucidated in nonaqueous solutions that approximate a hydrophobic membrane environment yet stabilize peptide structure. When galanin is placed in trifluoroethanol, for example, it assumes a stable helical conformation (see part B of figure). The N terminus of galanin forms a hydrogen bond with Glu 271 of the galanin receptor; the peptide's second residue (tryptophan 2) interacts with His 264 and His 267 of the receptor; and its ninth residue (tyrosine 9) interacts with the receptor's Phe 282. Currently, models derived from such methods are best guesses that rely on numerous assumptions about the conformations of the peptide and its receptor. More sophisticated structural analyses should enable us to refine these basic models and gain a better understanding of neuropeptide–receptor interactions.

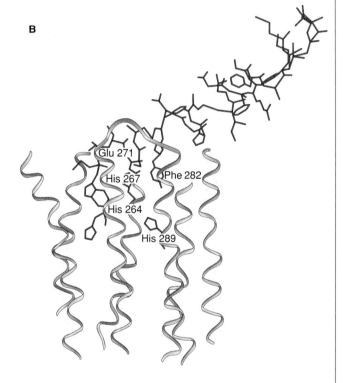

A   N terminus

C terminus

Reproduced with permission from Kask K, Berthold M, Kahl U, et al. 1996. *EMBO J* 15:241.

agents are essential for the treatment of disorders that affect the CNS. Consequently rational drug design and high-throughput screening are being used to find novel neuropeptide receptor agonists and antagonists (see Chapter 1); recent successes related to these efforts are mentioned in the sections that follow.

RECEPTOR TYPES AND SUBTYPES

Neuropeptide receptors are too numerous to describe individually (see Table 10–4). Therefore, a few families are highlighted in this chapter to illustrate the following important points. First, some neuropeptides,

Table 10–4 Examples of Human Neuropeptide Receptor Families

Neuropeptide	Receptor Subtype				
Bradykinin	B_1	B_2			
Amino acid residues (aa)	353 aa	364 aa			
G protein coupling	$G_{q/11}$	$G_{q/11}$			
Cholecystokinin	CCK_1	CCK_2			
Amino acid residues (aa)	428 aa	447 aa			
G protein coupling	$G_{q/11}, G_s$	$G_{q/11}$			
Corticotropin-releasing factor	CRF_1	CRF_2			
Amino acid residues (aa)	415 aa	411 aa			
G protein coupling	G_s	G_s			
Galanin	GAL_1	GAL_2	GAL_3		
Amino acid residues (aa)	349 aa	387 aa	368 aa		
G protein coupling	$G_{i/o}$	$G_{i/o}, G_{q/11}$	$G_{i/o}$		
Melanocortin (ACTH, MSH)	MC_1	MC_2	MC_3	MC_4	MC_5
Amino acid residues (aa)	317 aa	297 aa	360 aa	332 aa	325 aa
G protein coupling	G_s	G_s	G_s	G_s	G_s
Neuropeptide Y	Y_1	Y_2	Y_4[1]	Y_5	Y_6[2]
Amino acid residues (aa)	384 aa	381 aa	375 aa	445 aa	290 aa
G protein coupling	$G_{i/o}$	$G_{i/o}$	$G_{i/o}$	$G_{i/o}$	$G_{i/o}$
Neurotensin	NTS_1	NTS_2			
Amino acid residues (aa)	418 aa	410 aa			
G protein coupling	$G_{q/11}$	$G_{q/11}$			
Opioids	μ	δ	κ		
Amino acid residues (aa)	372 aa	380 aa	400 aa		
G protein coupling	$G_{i/o}$	$G_{i/o}$	$G_{i/o}$		
Somatostatin	SST_1	SST_2	SST_3	SST_4	SST_5
Amino acid residues (aa)	391 aa	369 aa	418 aa	388 aa	363 aa
G protein coupling	$G_{i/o}$	$G_{i/o}$	$G_{i/o}$	$G_{i/o}$	$G_{i/o}$
Tachykinins (Substance P; neuromedin K)	NK_1	NK_2	NK_3		
Amino acid residues	407 aa	398 aa	465 aa		
G protein coupling	$G_{q/11}$	$G_{q/11}$	$G_{q/11}$		
Thyrotropin-releasing hormone	TRH_1	TRH_2			
Amino acid residues (aa)	398 aa	not cloned			
G protein coupling	$G_{q/11}$	$G_{q/11}$			
Vasoactive Intestinal Peptide[3]	$VPAC_1$	$VPAC_2$	PAC_1		
Amino acid residues (aa)	457 aa	438 aa	525 aa		
G protein coupling	G_s	G_s	G_s		
Vasopressin and oxytocin[4]	V_{1A}	V_{1B}	V_2	OT	
Amino acid residues	418 aa	424 aa	371 aa	389 aa	
G protein coupling	$G_{q/11}$	$G_{q/11}$	G_s	$G_{q/11}$	

[1]Evidence supports a Y_3 receptor subtype, but it has not yet been cloned.
[2]The NPY Y_6 receptor gene in primates contains a frame shift mutation that renders it nonfunctional.
[3]VIP receptors bind both vasoactive intestinal peptide and pituitary adenylate cyclase activating peptide (PACAP).
[4]Vasopressin and oxytocin, which are structurally similar peptides, both bind to the same receptors. Vasopressin binds with higher affinity to all subtypes except the OT receptor.

such as thyrotropin-releasing hormone (TRH), bind to only one known receptor, whereas others, such as somatostatin, bind to as many as five receptor subtypes. Second, within a given receptor family, each subtype exhibits its own pattern of expression in the central and peripheral nervous systems. The two corticotropin-releasing factor (CRF) receptors (CRF$_1$R and CRF$_2$R) exhibit particularly interesting distributions in the brain. Each receptor subtype is most highly concentrated in regions in which the other is absent or nearly undetectable. The two receptors also show different lig-and-binding properties. CRF$_1$R shows high affinity for both CRF and a related peptide urocortin, whereas CRF$_2$R binds preferentially to urocortin. These observations suggest that the spatial segregation of these receptors has important physiologic consequences.

As illustrated by the CRF receptors, an important feature of some neuropeptide receptors is their ability to bind to more than one peptide. This ability is particularly notable among the members of the melanocortin receptor family; each of these receptors, termed MC$_{1-5}$R, is activated by ACTH, α-MSH, and γ-MSH with varying degrees of potency. Interestingly, MC$_4$R also can be antagonized by a distinct endogenous peptide called *agouti*–related peptide; indeed, it was the first receptor determined to have both agonists and antagonists that are expressed in the brain (see Chapter 13).

Until recently, the ligand specificity of neuropeptide receptors was believed to be determined solely by their intrinsic properties. Multiple regions of a receptor along various extracellular and transmembrane domains are known to form highly specific ligand recognition sites. However, newly discovered receptor activity modifying proteins, termed RAMPs, have been shown to regulate the transport of the calcitonin gene-related peptide (CGRP) receptor to the plasma membrane as well as its glycosylation. RAMP also determines the specificity of the receptor for CGRP or for adrenomedullin, a related but distinct peptide. Whether RAMPs, or related proteins, similarly regulate the ligand specificity of other G protein-coupled receptors remains unknown.

Although neuropeptide receptors tend to be localized in synapses, they also have been detected on the plasma membranes of axons, cell bodies, and dendrites. In fact, some of these receptor subtypes are hypothesized to reside primarily in extrasynaptic locations. In direct contrast, the ligand-gated channels that subserve fast excitatory and inhibitory neurotransmission tend to reside in synapses. However, both synaptic and extra-synaptic localization has been described for other G protein-coupled receptors, including those for certain small-molecule neurotransmitters, such as dopamine.

Neuropeptide receptors, like most G protein-coupled receptors, undergo internalization after sustained bind-ing to a ligand; subsequently, the internalized receptors are either recycled to the plasma membrane or degraded (see Chapter 8). Interestingly, for several neuropeptide receptors, such as neurotensin receptors, this type of cycling is exceptional in that the receptor–neuropeptide complex is transported from the synapse to the cell body. In fact, receptor–neuropeptide complexes have been detected near the nucleus, which suggests that either the receptor or the neuropeptide might be involved in the regulation of gene transcription, although such involvement remains hypothetical.

NEUROPEPTIDE FUNCTIONS

The functions of most classic neurotransmitters have been discovered partly because of the availability of small-molecule agonists and antagonists. Such agents have enabled investigators to ascertain the cellular and behavioral effects of these transmitters by mimicking or blocking their actions. In contrast, a lack of pharmacologic tools has been a major handicap in functional investigations of neuropeptide systems. Indeed only a small number of peptide agonists and antagonists that cross the blood–brain barrier are known.

It has been similarly difficult to interpret measurements of neuropeptide concentration in nervous tissue. When neuronal activity is inhibited, for example, the tissue levels of a neuropeptide may increase because peptides tend to accumulate in quiescent cells. Conversely, sustained neuronal activation can lead to the depletion of peptide stores. Although it remains difficult to determine whether the level of neuropeptidergic transmission is increased or decreased by a particular type of manipulation, in vivo microdialysis has enabled extracellular levels of a neuropeptide within a given brain region to be directly measured.

Because of obstacles to neuropeptide measurement, much work on neuropeptide function in the CNS has required the injection of peptides or synthetic peptide analogs into specific regions of the brain and spinal cord and subsequent physiologic or behavioral observation. The microinjection of milligram quantities of these peptides has raised concerns about the physiologic significance of observed effects, given the nanomolar affinity of their receptors; yet this approach has yielded first-order insight into the functions of neuropeptides, including their complex behavioral effects.

New tools of molecular biology—in particular, genetically engineered mice that lack or overexpress a given neuropeptide or receptor—have begun to significantly improve our understanding of neuropeptide function. Studies employing these tools have confirmed the results of earlier work and also have uncovered pre-

Box 10–3 The Body's Own Opiates

Historically, three types of observations suggested the presence of endogenous opiate-like substances, or opioids, in the human body by indicating the presence of a small number of corresponding receptors in the nervous system. First, opiate analgesics such as morphine produce effects at extremely low concentrations; for example, a few milligrams of morphine can produce clinically significant analgesia. Second, opiate drugs exhibit stereoselectivity. Third, at least one competitive antagonist of opiates (**naloxone**) was identified in early studies. Moreover, in the 1970s, four laboratories headed by Goldstein, Simon, Snyder, and Terenius used modern methods for identifying the binding sites of radiolabeled drugs in synaptic membranes (see Chapter 1) to produce direct evidence of opioid receptors in neural tissues.

The discovery of these receptors caused researchers to speculate about the existence of one or more endogenous ligands. Hughes, Kosterlitz, and colleagues searched for signs of endogenous opiate-like activity in the extracts of porcine brain. They used a sensitive bioassay to purify a minute amount of a putative endogenous opioid from large amounts of brain tissue. The bioassay was based on observations that opiate drugs inhibit the contraction of stimulated guinea pig ileum (indeed opiates that are used clinically have constipating properties). In 1975 these investigators reported the discovery of two pentapeptides with opioid activity; they named these peptides enkephalins (Greek for *in the head*). Subsequently, it has been determined that three separate genes encode at least 18 endogenous peptides with opiate-like activity.

---

viously unpredicted functions associated with these neurotransmitters. Discoveries relating to the possible roles of opioid peptides, CRF, substance P, neurotensin, and NPY in normal CNS function and in neuropsychiatric disorders are discussed in the sections that follow.

NEUROPEPTIDE SYSTEMS

OPIOID PEPTIDES

Primarily because of their potent analgesic properties, but also because of their antitussive and antidiarrheal effects, **opiates** have long ranked among the most important drugs in the pharmacopoeia. Indeed, of the drugs commonly used today, **morphine** is one of a small number that were available in the nineteenth century. The great need for opiate analgesics (see Chapter 19), combined with the serious risks related to dependence and addiction that they pose (see Chapter 16), has produced a continuing search for nonaddictive forms of these drugs. To date, it has not been possible to separate the most effective aspects of opiate analgesia from the addictive properties of these drugs. However, intense research has yielded many significant findings; for example, it resulted in the discovery of lipophilic, small-molecule opioid receptor antagonists, such as **naloxone** and **naltrexone,** which have been critical tools for investigating the physiology and behavioral actions of opiates. The term *opioid* refers to endogenous peptides with opiate-like pharmacology, whereas opiate refers to morphine and related nonpeptide analogs. Naloxone is effective in the treatment of opiate overdoses, and naltrexone, which is longer-acting,

is used in the treatment of **opiate addiction** and **alcoholism.** Perhaps most exciting, however, have been discoveries of opioid receptors and endogenous opioid peptides in the nervous system (Box 10–3).

All known opioid peptides are products of three large precursors, each of which is encoded by a separate gene (Figure 10–7A). These precursors include POMC, from which the opioid peptide β-endorphin and several nonopioid peptides are derived; proenkephalin, from which met-enkephalin and leu-enkephalin are derived; and prodynorphin, which is the precursor of dynorphin and related peptides. Although they are synthesized from different precursors, opioid peptides share significant amino acid sequence identity. Specifically, all of the well-validated endogenous opioids contain the same four amino acids (Tyr-Gly-Gly-Phe) at their N terminus, followed by either Met or Leu (see Figure 10–7B). It is believed that morphine-like opiate alkaloids, originally derived from the opium poppy, mimic the conformation of the N-terminal tyrosine in endogenous peptides.

Molecular cloning studies have confirmed the existence of three types of opioid receptors, designated μ, κ, and δ (see Table 10–4). However, some pharmacologic and biochemical data suggest that additional subtypes may be generated and that heterodimers may form between μ and δ receptors. The three known opioid receptors belong to the G protein-coupled receptor superfamily and are linked to the $G_{i/o}$ family of G proteins. Morphine-like opiates preferentially bind to μ receptors, which are concentrated in regions associated with descending analgesic pathways, such as the periaqueductal gray matter, rostroventral medulla, medial

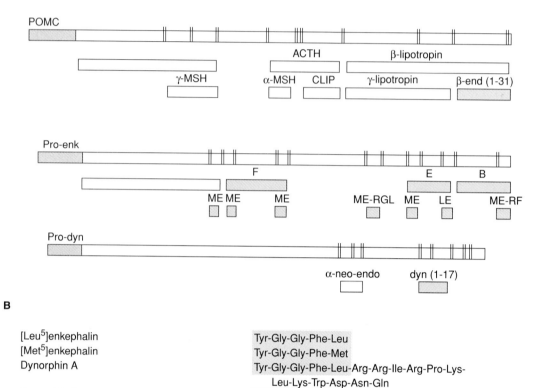

Figure 10–7. Opioid peptides. **A.** Structures of the three opioid precursors. Proopiomelanocortin (POMC) gives rise to the opioid β-endorphin and other nonopioid peptides, including melanocyte-stimulating hormones (MSH), adrenocorticotropin (ACTH), and corticotropin-like intermediate lobe peptide (CLIP). Proenkephalin (Pro-enk) gives rise to multiple copies of the pentapeptide met-enkephalin (ME), one copy of the pentapeptide leu-enkephalin (LE), and several extended enkephalin-containing peptides, including two extended versions of met-enkephalin, ME-Arg-Gly-Leu (ME-RGL) and ME-Arg-Phe (ME-RF). Other large enkephalin fragments are designated peptides E, F, and B. Prodynorphin (Pro-dyn) gives rise to dynorphin and α-neo-endorphin. **B.** Shared opioid peptide sequences. Although they vary in length from as few as five amino acids (enkephalins) to as many as thirty-one (β-endorphin), the endogenous opioid peptides shown here contain a shared N-terminal sequence followed by either Met or Leu.

thalamus, and dorsal horn of the spinal cord (see Chapter 19). These receptors also reside in other regions, such as the ventral tegmental area of the midbrain and the nucleus accumbens, where they are responsible for the reinforcing effects of opiates (Chapter 16). In addition, μ receptors occur in the striatum, which is important for motor control, and in the locus ceruleus, which mediates many somatic effects of opiate dependence and withdrawal. Among opioid receptors, the μ receptor appears to play the most significant role in supraspinal analgesia. However, barring the discovery of another subtype of this receptor, it is unlikely that investigators will succeed in separating μ receptor agonists from their addictive properties.

Enkephalins, rather than opiate alkaloid drugs, are the molecules for which δ opioid receptors exhibit the greatest affinity. These receptors are concentrated not only in the dorsal horn of the spinal cord but also in brain regions that have no clear association with pain. Clinical uses for selective δ receptor agonists have not been determined. κ Opioid receptors have a strong affinity for members of the benzomorphan class of opioid drugs, such as **pentazocine**. These receptors are found in the dorsal horn of the spinal cord, in the dorsal striatum and nucleus accumbens, in deep cortical layers, and in many other brain regions.

Among the endogenous opioid peptides, β-endorphin binds preferentially to μ receptors, enkephalins tend to bind to δ receptors, and dynorphin has the greatest affinity for κ receptors. However, these peptides do not bind exclusively to the receptors for which they have the strongest affinity; in vivo binding is also influenced by a peptide's proximity to each type of receptor.

A new class of neuropeptides has attracted interest in recent years because of its association with surprising anti-opioid-like effects. These peptides, termed *nociceptins*, or *orphanins*, bind to G protein-coupled receptors that share considerable homology with opioid receptors. However, for many years the nociceptin receptor was described as an orphan receptor because it did not have a known ligand (hence the term *orphanin*). Because nociceptins promote the perception of painful stimuli, there is current interest in the development of nociceptin receptor antagonists for use in the treatment of pain (see Chapter 19).

CORTICOTROPIN-RELEASING FACTOR

Corticotropin-releasing factor (CRF) is a 41-amino-acid peptide that was first isolated as a hypothalamic releasing factor that induces ACTH secretion from the anterior lobe of the pituitary gland, a capability that it shares with vasopressin. CRF is synthesized by a subset of neurons in the paraventricular nucleus (PVN) of the hypothalamus, from which it is released into the portal–hypophyseal circulation, which carries it to pituitary corticotrophs (see Chapter 13). However, CRF is not only delivered into the portal circulation; PVN neurons that express CRF also project to structures within the brain. Moreover, CRF is synthesized by neurons in regions outside the hypothalamus, including the central nucleus of the amygdala. The recent development of CRF antagonist drugs and the use of transgenic and knockout mice have confirmed that CRF has significant extrahypothalamic functions. CRF released in the amygdala appears to play a critical role in the brain's response to stress, and is also believed to contribute to states of fear and anxiety (see Chapter 15). In addition, CRF appears to partly mediate the negative affective state that characterizes withdrawal from drugs of abuse (Chapter 16). Other potential roles for CRF are just beginning to emerge; for example, studies have suggested that it may be involved in cerebellar long-term depression, a form of synaptic plasticity.

As stated above, two subtypes of CRF receptors have been cloned. The CRF_1R receptor is expressed widely in the brain. Several CRF_1R antagonists are currently under evaluation as anti-anxiety and antidepressant medications (Chapter 15). The CRF_2R receptor exhibits a much narrower distribution in brain and tends to be concentrated in lateral septal nuclei of the forebrain. The lateral septum has been strongly linked to emotionality, fear, and cognitive function. As previously mentioned, the endogenous ligand for CRF_2R is not CRF, but urocortin. Recently, another family member, tentatively named *urocortin II*, has been identified.

SUBSTANCE P

Substance P, neurokinin A (NKA; previously known as substance K), and neurokinin B (NKB) are members of the tachykinin peptide family, all of which share the C-terminal sequence Phe-X-Gly-Leu-Met-NH_2. Substance P and NKA are encoded by the preprotachykinin-A gene, and are produced by alternative splicing, as previously described. NKB is encoded by the preprotachykinin-B gene. The three known tachykinin receptors are G protein-coupled and are designated NK_1, NK_2, and NK_3. Substance P binds with highest affinity to the NK_1 receptor, NKA preferentially binds to the NK_2 receptor, and NKB tends to bind to NK_3.

Substance P has been a subject of particular interest because of its role as a pronociceptive peptide; indeed, in the late 1970s it was believed that substance P might be the chief pain transmitter. Primary afferent nociceptors that synapse in the dorsal horn of the spinal cord (see Chapter 19) express a complex array of neuropeptides, of which the most abundant are calcitonin gene-related peptide (CGRP), substance P, and NKA. Substance P is co-localized with glutamate in the synaptic terminals of a class of nociceptors called C fibers. As might be expected, substance P and other peptides are contained within large dense core vesicles in these fibers, and glutamate is stored in small synaptic vesicles. Release of substance P from the large dense core vesicles appears to require a stronger stimulus than does the release of glutamate. Substance P is released not only in the dorsal horn but also in retrograde fashion from the free nerve endings of nociceptive neurons; the latter type of release contributes to the phenomenon of **neurogenic inflammation**, whereby substance P interacts with the peptide known as bradykinin (see Chapter 19).

Given these physiologic findings, studies of knockout mice lacking preprotachykinin-A or NK$_1$ receptor genes have yielded some surprises. Neurogenic inflammation is largely absent in these mice, yet nociceptive responses are diminished in only a subset of pain models; for example, these mice exhibit no changes in inflammation-induced mechanical hypersensitivity. Overall, these animals appear to have deficits in nociception only in response to stimuli with a narrow range of intensities. This finding suggests that other neurotransmitters can significantly, although not entirely, compensate for the absence of substance P in pain pathways. Moreover, clinical trials have revealed that nonpeptide substance P antagonists exhibit little effect on pain in humans.

Substance P and NK$_1$ receptors also are concentrated in the amygdala. Interestingly, **MK-869,** an NK$_1$ receptor antagonist, blocks the amygdala-based behavior of distress vocalization in guinea pig pups separated from their mothers. Based on this type of preclinical research, NK$_1$ receptor antagonists are currently being tested as **antidepressants** and as **anti-anxiety** medications (see Chapter 15). These antagonists also have shown promise in the treatment of chemotherapy-induced **nausea**. Many chemotherapeutic agents induce intense nausea both at the time of administration and during a second, delayed-onset phase. Although 5-HT$_3$ antagonist drugs such as **odansetron** block the early phase of nausea (Chapter 9), NK$_1$ antagonists, which in early trials appear to block both the early and late phases, may prove to be more effective.

NEUROTENSIN

Neurotensin (NT) is a 13-amino-acid peptide derived from a larger precursor that also contains neuromedin N (NN), a 6-amino-acid peptide that is similar to neurotensin. Neurotensin is expressed in tissues of the brain, adrenal gland, and gut in slightly different forms; its C terminus contains one of three different Lys–Arg sequences, which are differentially cleaved depending on the tissue in which neurotensin is processed. In the brain, the precursor gives rise to both neurotensin and neuromedin N, whereas in the adrenal gland, neurotensin, a larger form of neuromedin N, and a larger form of neurotensin sequence are produced. In the gut, the most common products are neurotensin and large neuromedin N. Central administration of neurotensin produces hypothermia and analgesia.

Molecular cloning has led to the identification of three subtypes of neurotensin receptors. Two of these, NTS$_1$ and NTS$_2$, are G protein-coupled receptors. NTS$_1$ mRNA is expressed in the substantia nigra, but not in the striatum; however, the protein is targeted to dopaminergic nerve terminals in the striatum, which suggests that striatal neurotensin may assist in modulating dopaminergic neurotransmission. In the striatum, neurotensin mRNA is induced by D$_2$ receptor antagonists—many of which are **antipsychotic** drugs—in striatopallidal neurons, and by psychostimulant drugs such as **cocaine** and **amphetamine** in striatonigral neurons. Therefore it has been hypothesized that neurotensin influences dopamine signaling and perhaps contributes to the plasticity induced by drugs that act on dopamine systems in the brain. A putative NTS$_3$ receptor unrelated to NTS$_1$ or NTS$_2$ has been cloned; if verified, it will represent a new type of neuropeptide receptor with a single transmembrane domain.

NEUROPEPTIDE Y

As previously mentioned, NPY is one of a series of related peptides that comprise the pancreatic polypeptide family (Table 10–5). Other members of this family include pancreatic polypeptide (PP) and polypeptide YY (PYY). NPY is the most abundant neuropeptide in the cerebral cortex. It also is concentrated in the dorsal horn of the spinal cord and in the hypothalamus. In addition, we know that NPY is co-localized with norepinephrine in the CNS and in the sympathetic nervous system (see Table 10–3). Yet despite our ability to track the location of this peptide, its precise physiologic function remains poorly described.

NPY and related peptides act on a series of receptors, designated Y$_1$ to Y$_6$, which exhibit varying selectivity for NPY, PP, and PYY (see Table 10–4). These receptors also are characterized by marked region-specific distributions in the brain and are located on both postsynaptic and presynaptic sites. Activation of the Y$_1$ receptor is speculated to cause a decrease in anxiety-like behavior, perhaps at the level of the amygdala and cortex. This hypothesis has generated considerable interest in exploring the use of Y$_1$ agonists for the treatment of **anxiety disorders**. Y$_1$ agonists also may exert a mild antinociceptive effect and thus may be useful in the control of **pain**. In contrast, activation of the Y$_5$ receptor has been proven to stimulate feeding, presumably at the level of the hypothalamus; accordingly, Y$_5$ antagonists may be useful medications for the treatment of **obesity** (see Chapter 13). All of these

Table 10–5 Pancreatic Polypeptide Family

Peptide	Amino Acid Sequence
NPY	YPSKPDNPGEDAPAEDMARYYSALRHYINLITRQRY–NH$_2$
PP	APLEPVYPGDNATPEQMAQYAADLRRYINMLTRPRY—NH$_2$
PPY	YPIKPEAPGEDASPEELNRYYASLRHYLNLVTRQRY–NH$_2$

applications of NPY pharmacology show promise yet remain conjectural.

Although less is known about neuropeptides than about many classic neurotransmitters, our knowledge of the former is expanding rapidly. We understand the biochemical steps necessary to synthesize peptides; we have determined their location in large dense core vesicles and are beginning to understand their release and their ability to act extrasynaptically; we have cloned many—perhaps most—of the neuropeptide receptor subtypes and have determined their regional distribution in the brain; and we are finally succeeding in attempts to develop nonpeptide receptor ligands. Thus we have reached an exciting stage in which neuropeptide systems are being manipulated at the molecular level and in turn novel therapies for neuropsychiatric illnesses are being evaluated.

PURINES

Most students who have studied biochemistry and molecular biology know that purines act as building blocks of RNA and DNA, as metabolic cofactors, and as second messengers, for example, cAMP and cGMP. Yet what is often overlooked or poorly understood is the role that these molecules play in the signaling between neurons. In the sections that follow this role is discussed in conjunction with other principal features of this interesting class of neurotransmitters.

BIOCHEMISTRY

Our practice of referring to these signaling molecules as purines is to some degree a misnomer. Purines are ring-structured basic compounds that are primarily represented by adenine and guanine. These particular compounds are not neurotransmitters; nor are pyrimidines, which include uracil, thymidine, and cytosine. So-called purinergic signaling molecules are in fact the nucleoside and nucleotide derivatives of purine bases (Figure 10–8; see also Chapter 6). The two principal neurotransmitters in this family are adenosine and ATP. Related to these are the adenine dinucleotides, which consist of two adenosine molecules covalently linked by a chain of two to six phosphate groups. Adenine dinucleotides are represented by the abbreviation ApnA, wherein n equals the number of phosphates between the two adenosines (see Figure 10–8). ApnA molecules are released by neurons and thus may be considered part of the purinergic signaling family. There is also evidence that nucleoside and nucleotide derivatives of pyrimidine bases may serve as transmitter substances in the nervous system, although this remains less well characterized.

STORAGE AND RELEASE

Despite their similarities, adenosine and ATP have distinct properties. ATP, and ApnA, are stored in small synaptic vesicles and are released in response to action potentials in a Ca^{2+}-dependent process similar to the release process for classic neurotransmitters (Chapter 4). Indeed, ATP and classic neurotransmitters often can be detected in the same synapses and even in the same synaptic vesicles.

In contrast, adenosine is released from nonvesicular cytoplasmic stores and most likely reaches the extracellular space by one of two means. First, any of several bidirectional nucleoside transporters can secrete adenosine into the extracellular space, including the synapse. Second, ATP is very rapidly metabolized into adenosine once it is released from a cell. A membrane-bound ectodiphosphohydrolase converts ATP into ADP and AMP, and subsequently a membrane-associated or soluble ecto-5′-nucleotidase converts AMP into adenosine. Because the conversion of ATP to adenosine takes place in less than a second, the synaptic release of ATP should be regarded as an important source of extracellular adenosine.

The schematic representation of the purinergic cascade in Figure 10–9 shows that the release of ATP can lead to the production of other purinergic compounds and to the subsequent activation of several different receptors. It should be noted that ApnA is hydrolyzed much more slowly than ATP and can reside in the synaptic cleft for longer periods of time.

TRANSPORTERS

Nucleoside transporters are membrane-bound proteins that shuttle purine and pyrimidine nucleosides into and out of many cells, including neurons. They are distinguished by their substrate specificity in that they are purine- or pyrimidine-selective, and they also are differentiated by their thermodynamic properties. Some act to concentrate the nucleosides in a cell in a Na^+-dependent fashion. Others transport nucleosides down their concentration gradients. Pharmacologic studies indicate that there are at least seven nucleoside transporters, four of which have been cloned (Table 10–6). Although not much is known about the structure and function of these proteins, they have been exploited in the development of powerful therapeutic agents. A number of cancer chemotherapeutic drugs such as **gemcitabine** and several potent antiviral compounds such as **zidovudine** (**AZT**), which are used in the treatment of **AIDS,** are nucleoside analogs that enter target cells by means of nucleoside transporters. Given the powerful effects that adenosine exerts on

A

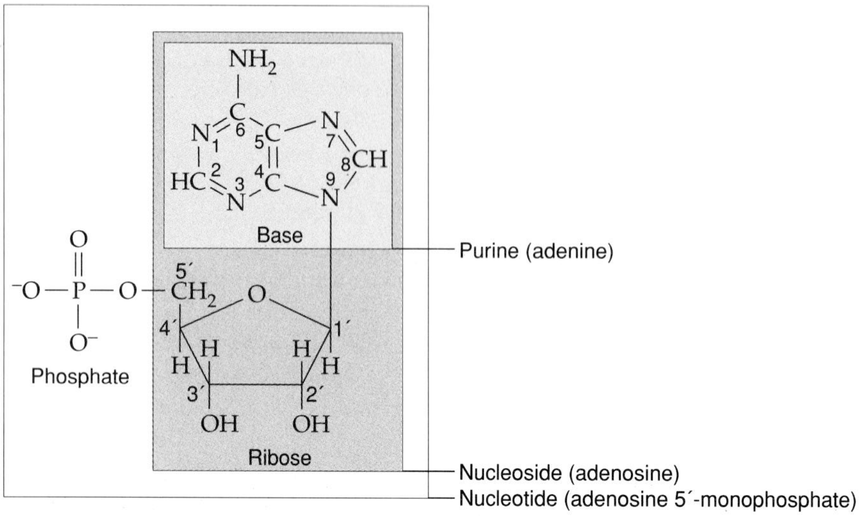

Purine (adenine)

Nucleoside (adenosine)
Nucleotide (adenosine 5′-monophosphate)

B

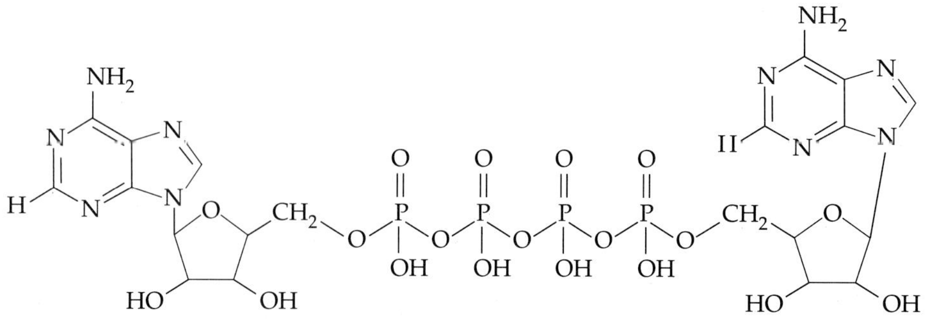

Adenine dinucleotide (Ap4A)

Figure 10–8. Structures of purinergic compounds. **A.** Purines, such as adenine, are basic ring-structured molecules, often referred to as bases. Nucleosides are molecules composed of a pentose sugar, such as ribose, covalently linked to a nitrogen atom in the base. Nucleotides are nucleosides whose mono-, di-, or triphosphate groups are linked to the 5′ carbon of a pentose sugar. Adenine's nucleosides and nucleotides are neurotransmitters, but adenine is not involved in neurotransmission. **B.** Adenine dinucleotides are two nucleosides linked by two to six phosphate groups. Ap4A signifies a diadenosine molecule with four intervening phosphate groups.

brain function, it is possible that drugs that regulate nucleoside transporters might prove useful in the treatment of neuropsychiatric disorders.

RECEPTORS

Purine receptors form a relatively large and diverse group of proteins that comprise two main subgroups, referred to as P_1 and P_2 receptors. Characteristics of both of these receptor families are discussed here and are summarized in Table 10–7.

P_1 receptors, also known as adenosine receptors (A_1 and A_2), bind adenosine and its analogs and are cou-

pled to G proteins. Four subtypes have been cloned and characterized, and each displays the canonical seven transmembrane domains found in other members of the G protein-coupled receptor superfamily. The A_1 receptor subtype is the most widely expressed in the brain and spinal cord and has the highest affinity for adenosine. Its activation has been implicated in the putative anxiolytic, anticonvulsant, analgesic, and sedative properties of adenosine. Conversely, antagonism of A_1 receptors by **methylxanthines** such as **caffeine** and similar drugs results in stimulatory effects, including increased alertness at low doses and anxiety and irritability at much higher doses (Box 10–4).

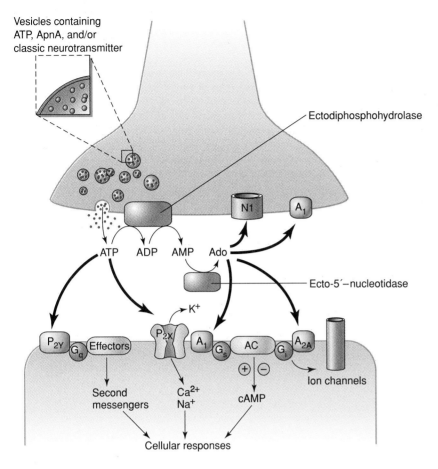

Vesicles containing ATP, ApnA, and/or classic neurotransmitter

Figure 10–9. A purinergic synapse. Adenosine triphosphate (ATP) and ApnA typically are co-localized with a classic neurotransmitter and are released into the synaptic cleft in a Ca^{2+}-dependent fashion. After it is released, ATP can directly activate P_{2Y} and P_{2X} receptors. P_{2Y} receptors are coupled to G proteins and activate second messenger systems. Most are coupled to G_q and activate phospholipase C (PLC) and the phosphatidylinositol pathway. P_{2X} receptors are ligand-gated channels that depolarize the postsynaptic membrane. ATP remaining in the synapse is rapidly converted into adenosine (Ado) by the actions of an ectodiphosphohydrolase and an ecto-5'-nucleotidase. Subsequently Ado is able to activate presynaptic and postsynaptic G protein-coupled P_1 receptors (A_1 and A_2) and regulate adenylyl cyclase (AC) and the cAMP pathway, and in turn can be recycled into the presynaptic cell by means of a Na^+-dependent transporter (N1).

Two subtypes of the A_2 receptor, A_{2A} and A_{2B}, have been cloned, both of which have a somewhat lower affinity for adenosine than do A_1 receptors. The A_{2B} receptor is ubiquitous in the human body yet is expressed only at very low levels in the brain and spinal cord. In contrast, the A_{2A} receptor is highly concentrated in the dorsal striatum, nucleus accumbens, and olfactory tubercle—three brain regions that receive rich dopaminergic innervation (see Chapter 14). Indeed the actions of adenosine and dopamine are interrelated in these regions. In the striatum, A_{2A} re-

ceptor agonists inhibit dopamine D_2 receptor-mediated behaviors, and A_{2A} antagonists mimic D_2 receptor agonists; these actions most likely contribute to the stimulant properties of methylxanthines among other effects. The inverse relationship between adenosine and dopamine has led to speculation that A_{2A} antagonists might be useful in the treatment of **Parkinson disease,** as discussed in the next section of this chapter.

The A_3 receptor is expressed at low levels in the brain, and its function is not yet known. It is distinguished from the other subtypes in that it has a much lower affinity for adenosine. Whereas A_1 and A_2 receptors bind adenosine with nanomolar affinity, micromolar concentrations are necessary to activate A_3 receptors.

The P_2 receptor family is intriguing because it comprises both G protein-coupled receptors (the P_{2Y} family) and ligand-gated ion channels (the P_{2X} family). Five P_{2Y} receptors have been cloned and characterized. These receptors display unique pharmacologic profiles, and bind purine and pyrimidine nucleotide diphosphates and triphosphates, as well as ApnA molecules, with varying potencies (see Table 10–7). The P_{2Y1} receptor, for example, binds ATP and ADP but not UTP or UDP. In contrast, the P_{2Y2} receptor is activated by ATP and UTP with equal potency. Both P_{2Y1}

Table 10–6 Nucleoside Transporters

Name	Equilibrative		Concentrative	
	es	ei	N1	N2
Substrate	pu = py	pu > py	pu > py	py > pu
Amino acid (residues)	456 aa	456 aa	658 aa	650 aa

Nucleoside transporters are currently classified by their thermodynamic properties and are divided into equilibrative (e) and concentrative, Na^+-dependent (N) subtypes. Although N3, N4, and N5 transporters have been identified pharmacologically, they have not yet been cloned. pu, purine nucleosides; py, pyrimidine nucleosides that serve as substrates for the transporters.

Box 10–4 Java Nation

Although most people have never heard of the term **methylxanthines,** almost everyone is familiar with several of these drugs and their behavioral effects. One of these agents, 1,3,7-trimethylxanthine, is better known to most of us as **caffeine,** a drug that is used more often than any other psychoactive substance. Caffeine is found in coffee, tea, cocoa, chocolate, and many soft drinks; in mild doses it decreases fatigue and enhances cognition. It is believed that the stimulatory properties of caffeine and of its structural analogs, **theophylline** (found in tea) and **theobromine** (found in cocoa), are caused primarily by the antagonism of adenosine receptors, particularly the A_1 receptor.

The average daily dose of caffeine in the United States is approximately 200 mg, which is equivalent to two cups of coffee or approximately four cans of cola. These relatively high doses are not generally considered dangerous and do not produce significant side effects in most individuals. However, prolonged use of products containing methylxanthines can lead to tolerance to the stimulatory properties of the drug, and to physical dependence. As anyone who has habitually consumed large volumes of coffee knows, quitting the habit suddenly can lead to withdrawal symptoms that include headaches, drowsiness, and nausea. In addition, consuming high doses of caffeine (400 mg or more per day) can lead to anxiety and nervousness and can trigger panic symptoms in vulnerable individuals.

and P_{2Y2} subtypes have been detected in the brain. Studies of the regional distribution and functional significance of P_{2Y} receptors in the CNS are in progress.

Seven P_{2X} receptor subtypes have been cloned and characterized. Each is an ATP- or ApnA-gated cation channel composed of multiple subunits. Although the exact stoichiometry of P_{2X} receptors is unknown, functional homomeric receptors have been constituted in vitro. Because these receptors have multiple subunits, each of the cloned proteins in Table 10–7 should be regarded as a subunit rather than as a complete receptor. P_{2X} receptor activation leads to rapid Na^+, K^+,

and Ca^{2+} flux and subsequent membrane depolarization. These fast-acting channels have been detected in the peripheral nervous system, neuromuscular junction, spinal cord, and many brain regions, yet the biologic effects of their activation remain incompletely characterized.

PURINE FUNCTIONS

The recent cloning of the P1 and P2 receptor families has opened up numerous avenues for investigating purine function in the nervous system. Receptor-selective

Table 10–7 Purine Receptor Families

	Receptor Subtype				
P_1 (Adenosine) Receptor	A_1	A_{2A}	A_{2B}	A_3	
Amino acid residues (aa)	326 aa	412 aa	332 aa	318 aa	
G protein coupling	$G_{i/o}$	G_s	G_s	$G_{i/o}$	
P_{2Y} Receptor	P_{2Y1}	P_{2Y2}	P_{2Y4}	P_{2Y6}	P_{2Y11}
Amino acid residues (aa)	372 aa	377 aa	352 aa	?	371 aa
G protein coupling	$G_{q/11}$	$G_{q/11}, G_{i/o}$	$G_{q/11}, G_i$	$G_{q/11}$	?
Substrate specificity	ADP, ATP, ApnA	ATP = UTP	UTP > ATP	UDP	ATP $\gg$ ADP
P_{2X} Receptor (ionotropic)	P_{2X1}	P_{2X2}	P_{2X3}	P_{2X4}	P_{2X5}
Amino acid residues (aa)	399 aa	Unknown	397 aa	388 aa	422 aa
Substrate specificity	ATP > ADP	ATP	ATP	ATP > CTP	ATP
	P_{2X6}	P_{2X7}			
Amino acid residues (aa)	Unknown	595 aa			
Substrate specificity	Unknown	ATP			

Purine receptors have only recently been cloned, and several subtypes have yet to be isolated from human sources. P_2 receptors can be further divided into P_{2X} ligand-gated channels and P_{2Y} G protein-coupled receptors. Jumps in the numbering of receptors e.g., no P_{2Y5} receptor is listed) stem from the incorrect initial identification of cloned proteins as purine receptor subtypes. These incorrectly identified entities subsequently have been withdrawn. For some subtypes, such as the P_{2X6} receptor, no information is provided because the human variant has not yet been isolated.

agonists and antagonists are being developed, and transgenic animals that underexpress or overexpress individual receptor subtypes are being generated. These pharmacologic and genetic tools are significantly enhancing our understanding of purines and are enabling us to examine their potential relevance to clinical neuroscience. Although many putative roles for nucleosides and nucleotides have been hypothesized, only a handful have been clearly established.

Adenosine has both anxiolytic and hypnotic properties, and the administration of adenosine receptor antagonists dramatically confirms these findings. Caffeine and other methylxanthine compounds, by blocking endogenous adenosine action, increase alertness and improve cognitive performance. The cognition-enhancing properties of these drugs are particularly interesting, partly because of the wide use of caffeine, and partly because adenosine receptor antagonists may prove useful, at least as symptomatic treatment, in ameliorating the cognitive deficits associated with **Alzheimer disease** and other forms of dementia (see Chapter 20).

Adenosine also is being investigated for its neuroprotective effects, and it is hoped that these properties might be exploited in the treatment of **stroke**. It is believed that stroke is characterized by an ischemia-induced increase in glutamate release—followed by an overstimulation of glutamate receptors and the subsequent massive influx of Ca^{2+} into neurons—that unleashes a cascade of cytotoxic events (see Chapter 21). Thus an ideal neuroprotective agent would inhibit glutamate release presynaptically and prevent postsynaptic membrane depolarization and subsequent Ca^{2+} influx. Adenosine can accomplish both feats. Adenosine activation of presynaptic A_1 receptors inhibits the release of glutamate and other neurotransmitters. Activation of postsynaptic A_1 receptors opens K^+ and Cl^- channels, and thereby hyperpolarizes neurons and counters the excitatory effects of glutamate. The net result is believed to be decreased Ca^{2+} influx and decreased neuronal death. Experiments in animal models support this hypothesis. The administration of selective A_1 agonists just before or during an ischemic event in animals significantly reduces neuronal loss and protects against subsequent memory deficits. Conversely, the administration of A_1 antagonists augments ischemic brain damage.

It is important to note that ischemia dramatically increases adenosine levels in the brain. Although adenosine's activation of A_1 receptors may provide some measure of neuroprotection, its actions at other receptor subtypes may exert the opposite effect. Its activation of A_2 receptors, for example, has had deleterious effects on animals in models of stroke. Conversely, A_2-selective antagonists are known to produce neuropro-

tective effects. Acute activation of A_3 receptors with A_3-selective agonists also profoundly increases brain damage and mortality in animal models. In contrast, long-term administration of these same drugs has the opposite effect and dramatically improves survival. Adenosine's actions on vascular tone and platelet function likely contribute to these various observations. The interplay that occurs among adenosine receptor subtypes during ischemia requires further investigation, but adenosine systems may be important targets for future therapeutic agents designed to treat acute episodes of stroke.

Adenosine systems also may prove to be promising targets for drugs designed to treat **Parkinson disease**. As discussed in Chapter 14, this disease is caused by a loss of dopaminergic innervation to the striatum, which leads to a variety of motor abnormalities. The striatum, as previously mentioned, expresses high levels of adenosine A_{2A} receptors. A_{2A} receptor agonists produce biochemical and behavioral effects that mimic those associated with Parkinson disease: A_{2A} receptor activation decreases dopamine neurotransmission in the striatum and significantly decreases motor activity. Accordingly, it is believed that the blocking of A_{2A} receptors might have the opposite effect; that is, dopamine function in the striatum and motor activity might be expected to increase.

Several orally active compounds that selectively block A_{2A} receptors have been described. When used in animal models of Parkinson disease, these drugs significantly reverse motor deficits while inducing little if any dyskinesia, a side effect associated with L-dopa therapy (see Chapter 14). Moreover, when coadministered with L-dopa, A_{2A} antagonists diminish L-dopa-induced dyskinesia. Although these particular drugs have not been examined in humans, a nonselective A_1 and A_2 antagonist, **theophylline,** has been found to ameliorate symptoms in some patients with Parkinson disease.

Adenosine also has been reported to exhibit anticonvulsant, anxiolytic, and antidepressant activity, as well as both analgesic and pain-enhancing properties. Although these purported functions require further investigation, they point to the therapeutic potential of selective adenosine receptor agonists and antagonists.

SELECTED READING

Alexander SPH, Peters JA. 1999. 1999 Receptor and ion channel nomenclature supplement. *Trends Pharmacol Sci (supplement)*.

Bischofberger N, Jacobson KA, VonLubitz DKJE. 1997. Adenosine A_1 receptor agonists as clinically viable agents for treatment of ischemic brain disorders. *Ann NY Acad Sci* 825:23–29.

Castro MG, Morrison E. 1997. Post-translational processing of proopiomelanocortin in the pituitary and in the brain. *Crit Rev Neurobiol* 11:35–57.

Chalmers DT, Lovenberg TW, DeSouza EB. 1995. Localization of novel corticotropin-releasing factor receptor CRF2 mRNA expression to specific subcortical nuclei in rat brain: comparison with CRF1 receptor mRNA expression. *J Neurosci* 15:6340–6350.

Fan W, Boston BA, Kesterson RA, et al. 1997. Role of melanocortinergic neurons in feeding and the agouti obesity syndrome. *Nature* 385:165–168.

Feldman RS, Meyer JS, Quenzer LF. 1997. Peptide Neurotransmitters. In *Principles of Neuropsychopharmacology*, pp. 455–491. Sunderland, MA: Sinauer Associates.

Fredhold BB, Battig K, Holmen J, et al. 1999. Actions of caffeine in the brain with specific reference to factors that contribute to its widespread use. *Pharmacol Rev* 51:83–133.

Gehlert DR. 1998. Multiple receptors for the pancreatic polypeptide (PP-fold) family: Physiology implications. *Proc Soc Exp Biol Med* 218:7–22.

Gomes I, Jordan BA, Gupta A, et al. 2000. Heterodimerization of μ and δ opioid receptors: a role in opiate synergy. *J Neurosci* 20:RC110(1–5)

Grondin R, Bédard PJ, Tahar H, et al. 1999. Antiparkinsonian effect of a new selective adenosine A2A receptor antagonist in MPTP-treated monkeys. *Neurology* 52:1673–1677.

Kramer MS, Cutler N, Feighner J, et al. 1998. Distinct mechanism for antidepressant activity by blockade of central substance P receptors. *Science* 281:1640–1645.

Mains RE, Eipper BA. 1999. Peptides. In Siegel GJ, Agranoff B, Albers RW, Fisher SK, Uhler MD (eds): *Basic Neurochemistry: Molecular, Cellular, and Medical Aspects,* 6th ed, pp 363–382. Philadelphia: Lippincott-Raven.

Mansbach RS, Brooks EN, Chen YL. 1997. Antidepressant-like effects of CP-154,526, a selective CRF1 receptor antagonist. *Eur J Pharm* 323:21–26.

Nyce JW. 1999. Insight into adenosine receptor function using antisense and gene-knockout approaches. *Trends Pharmacol Sci* 20:79–83.

Ongini E, Adami M, Ferri C, Bertorelli R. 1997. Adenosine A2A receptors and neuroprotection. *Ann NY Acad Sci* 825:30–48.

Öhman A, Lycksell P-O, Juréus A, et al. 1998. NMR study of the conformation and localization of porcine galanin in SDS micelles. Comparison with an inactive analog and a galanin receptor antagonist. *Biochem* 37:9169–9178.

Pastor-Anglada M, Felipe A, Casado FJ. 1998. Transport and mode of action of nucleoside derivatives used in chemical and antiviral therapies. *Trends Pharmacol Sci* 19:424–430.

Perrin MH, Vale WW. 1999. Corticotropin releasing factor receptors and their ligand family. *Ann NY Acad Sci* 885:312–328.

Poyner D, Cox H, Bushfield M, et al. 2000. Neuropeptides in drug research. *Prog Drug Res* 54:121–149.

Ralevic V, Burnstock G. 1998. Receptors for purines and pyrimidines. *Pharmacol Rev* 50:413–492.

Richardson PJ, Kase H, Jenner PG. 1997. Adenosine A2A receptor antagonists as new agents for the treatment of Parkinson's disease. *Trends Pharmacol Sci* 18:338–344.

Rouillé Y, Duguay SJ, Lund K, et al. 1995. Proteolytic processing mechanisms in the biosynthesis of neuroendocrine peptides: The substilisin-like proprotein convertases. *Front Neuroendocrinol* 16:322–361.

Satoh S, Matsumura H, Hayaishi O. 1998. Involvement of adenosine A2A receptors in sleep promotion. *Eur J Pharmacol* 351:155–162.

Schulz DW, Mansbach RS, Sprouse J, et al. 1996. CP-154,526: A potent and selective nonpeptide antagonist of corticotropin releasing factor receptors. *Proc Natl Acad Sci USA* 93:10477–10482.

Seidah NG, Chretien M. 2000. Proprotein and prohormone convertases: a family of subtilases generating diverse bioactive peptides. *Brain Res* 848:45–62.

Stenzel-Poore MP, Heinrichs SC, Rivest S, et al. 1994. Overproduction of corticotropin-releasing factor in transgenic mice: A genetic model of anxiogenic behavior. *J Neurosci* 14:2579–2584.

Vincent J-P, Mazella J, Kitabgi P. 1999. Neurotensin and neurotensin receptors. *Trends Pharmacol Sci* 20:302–309.

VonLubitz DKJE. 1997. Adenosine A3 receptor and brain. *Ann NY Acad Sci* 825:49–67.

Williams M, Jarvis MF. 2000. Purinergic and pyramidinergic receptors as potential drug targets. *Biochem Pharmacol* 59:1173–1185.

Chapter 11

Neurotrophic Factors

KEY CONCEPTS

- Neurotrophic factors are peptides that support the growth, differentiation, and survival of neurons.

- In contrast to peptide neurotransmitters, neurotrophic factors produce their effects by activation of tyrosine kinases, which may be either intrinsic to their receptors or separate proteins.

- In the absence of appropriate neurotrophic signals many neurons die through a process of programmed cell death known as apoptosis.

- Apoptotic pathways involve a cascade of proteins including proteolytic enzymes of the caspase family.

- Target-derived growth factors such as NGF are secreted by target tissues in only limited amounts; thus only neurons that make appropriate synaptic contacts survive.

- Neurotrophic factors may also be released by neurons themselves and by glia, and may act in autocrine and paracrine fashion.

- Some functions of neurotrophic factors overlap with those of neurotransmitters; for example, brain-derived neurotrophic factor (BDNF) is reported to regulate synaptic transmission.

- The neurotrophin family, which comprises NGF, BDNF, neurotrophin-3 (NT-3) and neurotrophin-4

(NT-4, also known as NT-4/5), acts by binding to a family of receptors with intrinsic tyrosine kinase activity known as Trk receptors, TrkA, TrkB, TrkC.

- A protein known as p75 binds all neurotrophins with a lower affinity than Trk receptors; under some circumstances p75 is involved in the initiation of programmed cell death.

- Trophic factors are important therapeutic candidates for neurodegenerative diseases; as one example, glial-derived neurotrophic factor supports the survival of dopaminergic neurons in some model systems and is therefore of interest for the treatment of Parkinson disease.

- A number of cytokine-like peptide factors including ciliary neurotrophic factor, leukemia inhibitory factor, interleukin-6, growth hormone, interferons, leptin, and others are characterized by binding to receptors that activate a family of protein tyrosine kinases called Janus kinases (JAKs), which in turn activate transcription factors called signal transducers and activators of transcription (STATs).

- Chemokines are small proteins originally found to be involved in immune responses; in the brain chemokines are expressed predominately by microglia and to a lesser extent by astrocytes and some neurons.

The belief that extracellular signals can promote the growth and differentiation of nerve cells is more than half a century old, yet the molecular diversity of growth factors and of their intracellular signaling cascades did not become apparent until the past decade. Knowledge of growth factor signaling has dramatically enhanced our understanding of the ways in which the nervous system evolves during development and adapts throughout the adult life of an organism. Such knowledge also has provided insight into mechanisms responsible for neuronal survival, whose failure may underlie neurodegenerative disorders such as **Alzheimer disease, Parkinson disease, Huntington disease,** and **amyotropic lateral sclerosis.** Moreover, growth factors and their signaling proteins represent a large number of potential targets for the pharmacotherapeutic treatment of these and other neuropsychiatric disorders.

A discussion of neurotrophic factors requires the definition of several terms. Neurotrophic factors themselves are literally growth factors for nerve cells: they are agents that influence the growth, differentiation, and survival of neurons. A related term is *cytokine,* which is borrowed from the field of immunology and refers to molecules released by activated lymphoid cells to modulate the activity of other cells. Some authors apply the term *cytokine* to all growth-related factors, including neurotrophic factors; others use cytokine only to refer to growth factors that influence glial cells. As this chapter demonstrates, tremendous overlap exists among growth factors for neurons and glia. Thus in this book the term *neurotrophic factor* refers to any molecule that affects the nervous system by influencing the growth, differentiation, or cell cycles of neurons or glia. The term is restricted to proteins that serve these functions so that neurotrophic factors are distinguished from many nonpeptide molecules, including steroid hormones, retinoic acid, and neurotransmitters, that also can influence the growth and integrity of the nervous system.

Although neurotrophic factors originally were noted for their role in nervous system development, and neurotransmitters for their role in synaptic transmission in the adult, we now know that there is considerable overlap in the actions of these molecules. Accordingly, the distinction between neurotrophic factors and neurotransmitters is becoming increasingly blurred. Like neurotransmitters, many neurotrophic factors are synthesized by neurons and alter the functioning of other neurons; under some circumstances, they may even be released as a result of neuronal activity. Moreover, neurotrophic factors may produce rapid changes in target neurons that are indistinguishable from those elicited by conventional neurotransmitters associated with synaptic transmission. Likewise, many neurotransmitters not only elicit rapid changes in synaptic transmission but also can potently affect the growth and differentiation of neurons during development, the survival of such neurons, and the differentiation of adult phenotypes.

Yet certain key features of neurotrophic factors distinguish them from peptide neurotransmitters. Notably, neurotrophic factors tend to be larger molecules; for example, brain-derived neurotrophic factor (BDNF) is a 14-kDa protein, whereas peptide neurotransmitters typically are very small polypeptides (see Chapter 10). In addition, most neurotrophic factors produce their biologic effects through the regulation of protein tyrosine kinases, whereas most peptide neurotransmitters signal through G protein-coupled receptors and classic second messenger cascades (see Chapter 5).

FUNCTIONAL CHARACTERISTICS OF NEUROTROPHIC FACTORS

We know much less about the life cycles of most neurotrophic factors than we know about those of the neurotransmitter substances discussed in previous chapters. Neurotrophic factors are synthesized as proteins in the cell bodies of particular neurons and glia. Some are stored in these cells, perhaps in large dense core vesicles (see Chapter 4), and are transported either to nerve terminals or to dendritic extensions. The mechanisms controlling the release of neurotrophic factors are poorly understood. Many factors, such as interleukin-1 (IL-1), BDNF, and glial cell line-derived neurotrophic factor (GDNF) are the products of immediate early genes; thus the activity-dependent synthesis of these factors may be the major determinant of their release. The release of other neurotrophic factors can be triggered by depolarization, as previously mentioned. The major mechanism responsible for the termination of neurotrophic factor signals appears to be their proteolytic degradation; however, some factors—for example, BDNF—are sequestered by functionally inactive receptors that limit their diffusion and perhaps the duration of their action.

A major question in the field concerns the site of action of neurotrophic factors. A classic description of the synthesis and activity of nerve growth factor (NGF) has been developed. The first growth factor to be identified, NGF was discovered more than 40 years ago by Levi-Montalcini and Hamburger, who demonstrated that certain sympathetic and sensory neurons require this protein for their survival (see Figure 11–1 for NGF's dramatic effect on cultured neurons). Classic

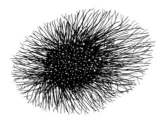

Figure 11–1. The effect of nerve growth factor (NGF) on cultured spinal neurons. (Adapted with permission from Levi-Montalcini R. 1987. *Science* 237:1157.)

studies conducted by these investigators revealed that NGF is synthesized by the target organs of these nerve cells and is needed to maintain the sympathetic and sensory neurons that innervate the organs. Because the supply of NGF is limited, competition for the factor exists among growing nerve fibers. Growing neurons that do not receive the NGF signal from their target do not survive. Likewise, only neurons that successfully respond to NGF survive and make appropriate connections with their targets. According to what is sometimes referred to as the *neurotrophic hypothesis*, these findings demonstrate that NGF is indispensable in the establishment of suitable nerve–target connections during development (Figure 11–2).

Although such patterns of synthesis and action of NGF appear to predominate in the peripheral nervous system, different patterns emerge in the brain and spinal cord (see Figure 11–2). In these areas, a target neuron may supply neurotrophic factor for an innervating neuron, but many neurotrophic factors and their receptors are synthesized by the same neuron; thus factors in the brain and spinal cord may serve additional autoregulatory, or autocrine, functions. Furthermore, evidence suggests that certain neurotrophic factors can be anterogradely transported to axon terminals, where they act on the cell bodies or nerve terminals of other nerve cells immediately after their release. Evidence also indicates that neurotrophic factor–receptor complexes, formed on the plasma membrane of nerve terminals, can be retrogradely transported back to cell bodies, where they exert some of their biologic effects.

Glia further complicate the production of neurotrophic factors. Some factors are synthesized by both neurons and glia and act on receptors expressed by both cell types. Such patterns of synthesis and activity result in highly complex forms of intercellular communication among neurons and glia that investigators have yet to disentangle.

FAMILIES OF NEUROTROPHIC FACTORS

Although neurotrophic factors comprise numerous families, these have yet to be categorized according to a generally accepted system. Indeed, their classification has been complicated partly by their history. The names of many neurotrophic factors were based on the actions with which they were originally associated. Thus interleukins were given their name because initially they were identified as proteins that mediate communication among white blood cells, even though they are also produced by glia. Likewise, GDNF originally was identified as a factor derived from a glial cell line, even though it is also made by many types of neurons; fibroblast growth factor (FGF) was regarded as a growth factor for fibroblasts, even though it is also produced by glia; and ciliary neurotrophic factor (CNTF) was named for its contribution to the growth and maintenance of ciliary ganglion neurons in the eye, even though it is also generated by glia and may be produced by several neuronal cell types.

Currently neurotrophic factors can be categorized based on their homologies and on the shared signal transduction mechanisms through which they produce their biologic effects (Table 11–1). The remainder of this chapter focuses on three families of neurotrophic factors that have been grouped according to such characteristics: the neurotrophins, GDNF and related factors, and CNTF-related factors. Among neurotrophic factors, these families are the best characterized; how-

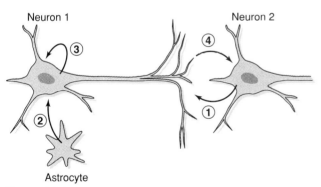

Figure 11–2. Modes of intercellular communication subserved by neurotrophic factors. **1.** In this classic model, a target-derived neurotrophic factor acts on an innervating nerve terminal. **2.** Paracrine transmission. A neurotrophic factor released from a neighboring cell (neuron or glial cell, such as astrocyte) acts on many nearby neurons in the absence of formal synaptic connections. **3.** Autocrine transmission. A neurotrophic factor acts on the neurons that release it. **4.** Anterograde transmission. A neurotrophic factor released from the terminals of a nerve cell acts on the synaptic targets of these terminals. The mode of transmission that predominates in the adult brain and spinal cord has yet to be determined.

Table 11-1 Examples of Neurotrophic Factors and Their Receptors

Neurotrophic Factor Family and Representative Examples	Receptor Family and Representative Examples

Neurotrophins
  NGF, BDNF, NT-3, NT-4
	Trk (R-PTKs)
	  TrkA, TrkB, TrkC[1]

GDNF family
  GDNF, neurturin, persephin
	Coupled to Ret
	  GFRα1, GFRα2, unknown

CNTF family
  CNTF, LIF, IL-6
	Coupled to Janus kinase (JAK)
	  GP130, CNTFRα, LIFRα

Ephrins	Eph (R-PTKs)
EGF family EGF, TGFα, neuregulins[2]	ErbB (R-PTKs)
Other growth factors insulin, IGF, FGF, PDGF	R-PTKs
Interleukins and related cytokines	
Interleukin-1 (IL-1)	IL-1R coupled to PS/TK
IL-2	R-PTK
IL-3, IL-5	Coupled to JAK
TNFα, TNFβ	Related to p75[3]
TGF family TGFβ	R-PS/TKs
Other cytokines	
interferons (IFNα, β, γ)	Coupled to JAK
m-CSF	R-PTKs
gm-CSF	Coupled to JAK
Chemokines	G protein-coupled receptors
CC chemokines (IL-8)	CC_1-CC_8R
CXC chemokines (MIP, MCP)	CXC_1-CXC_4R
CX₃C chemokines (neurotactin)	Cx_3C_1R

[1]Specificity of neurotrophins for the various Trk receptors is shown in Figure 11–4.
[2]Neuregulins are also referred to as ARIA, heregulin, or neu differentiation factor.
[3]TNF receptors couple to so-called "death receptors" of the TRADD and related families (see Box 11–5).
BDNF, brain-derived neurotrophic factor; NT-3 and -4, neurotrophin-3 and -4; GDNF, glial cell line-derived neurotrophic factor; GFR, GDNF-neurturin receptor; CNTF, ciliary neurotrophic factor; LIF, leukemia inhibitory factor; EGF, epidermal growth factor; R-PTK, receptor-associated protein tyrosine kinase; IGF, insulin-like growth factor; FGF, fibroblast growth factor; PDGF, platelet-derived growth factor; TNF, tumor necrosis factor; IL, interleukin; R-PS/TK, receptor-associated protein serine/threonine kinase; TGF, transforming growth factor; IFN, interferon; m-CSF, macrophage colony stimulating factor; gm-CSF, granulocyte-monocyte CSF; MIP, macrophage inflammatory protein; MCP, monocyte chemoattractant protein.

ever, many other families are believed to be important not only in nervous system development but also in the regulation of nervous system function in the adult, under both normal and pathophysiologic conditions.

NEUROTROPHINS

The neurotrophin family of neurotrophic factors comprises NGF and subsequently identified factors that employ some of the same signaling mechanisms, including BDNF, neurotrophin-3 (NT-3), and neurotrophin-4

(NT-4; also known as neurotrophin-4/5). Although it has been identified only in fish, neurotrophin-6 (NT-6) also is considered a member of this family. All neurotrophins are small proteins; BDNF, for example, has a molecular mass of approximately 14 kDa. Another common feature of neurotrophins is that they produce their physiologic effects by means of the Trk receptor family.

Neurotrophins produce effects on a wide range of neurons. As previously mentioned in connection with NGF, their role in ensuring the survival of neurons in the peripheral nervous system is well established. NGF, for example, is present in target fields of small sympathetic and sensory neurons that have nociceptive and temperature-sensing functions, and the NGF receptor is expressed in these neurons. BDNF is produced in skeletal muscle that is innervated by motor neurons; BDNF, NT-4, and NT-3 each support the survival of a subset of peripheral sensory neurons.

Although neurotrophins similarly affect the survival and maintenance of some neurons in the CNS, their role in the brain and spinal cord is less clear. NGF is believed to promote the survival of cholinergic neurons in the septal nuclei of the basal forebrain. Cholinergic septal neurons innervate hippocampal neurons, which express NGF at high levels (Figure 11–3). According to one hypothesis, acetylcholine released from septal nerve terminals activates hippocampal neurons, causing an

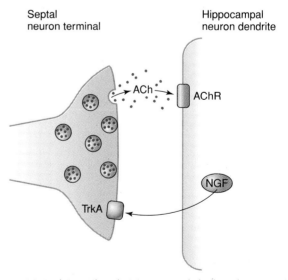

Figure 11-3. Interactions between septal cholinergic neurons and target hippocampal neurons. Acetylcholine (ACh) released from a septal nerve terminal activates a target neuron in the hippocampus. Such activation stimulates an increase in the synthesis and release of nerve growth factor (NGF) from the neuron, which then acts on TrkA receptors on the septal nerve terminals to enhance neuronal survival.

increase in the synthesis and release of NGF. NGF in turn acts on the nerve terminals to promote the survival of the cholinergic neurons. This positive feedback scheme enables the survival of neurons that have made appropriate connections and that are physiologically active. Other neurotrophins also support neurons in the CNS. BDNF, NT-3, and NT-4 have been shown to promote the survival of some cortical motor and hippocampal neurons, and of noradrenergic, dopaminergic, and serotoninergic neurons located in the brain stem. Together these findings have suggested the possible use of NGF in the treatment of **Alzheimer disease** and the use of other neurotrophins in the treatment of **Parkinson disease**; however, clinical trials have not supported such applications.

How neurotrophins might contribute to the development of the brain has yet to be determined. Whether their primary function is target-derived support of afferent neurons (a function analogous to their role in the peripheral nervous system), the support of efferent neurons, or the generation and maintenance of differentiated characteristics of neurons in specific circuits remains under investigation. Research also is directed toward determining whether neurotrophins continue to play a role in the adult brain, where evidence has suggested that they support the survival and plasticity of fully differentiated neurons and may contribute to synaptic transmission.

TRK RECEPTORS

All neurotrophins bind to a class of highly homologous receptor tyrosine kinases known as Trk receptors, of which three types are known: TrkA, TrkB, and TrkC. These transmembrane receptors are glycoproteins whose molecular masses range from 140 to 145 kDa. Each type of Trk receptor tends to bind specific neurotrophins; for example, TrkA is believed to be the receptor for NGF, TrkB the receptor for BDNF and NT-4, and TrkC the receptor for NT-3. However, some overlap in the specificity of these receptors has been noted (Figure 11–4).

The characteristic structural domains of the Trk receptor are represented in Figure 11–5. The extracellular portion contains the binding site for the neurotrophin and consists of leucine-rich segments believed to be im-

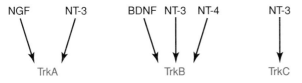

Figure 11–4. Specificity of various Trk receptors for members of the neurotrophin family. NGF, nerve growth factor; NT, neurotrophin; BDNF, brain-derived neurotrophic factor.

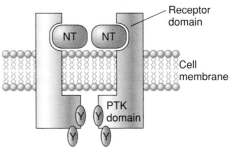

Figure 11–5. Structure of the Trk tyrosine kinase receptor. This receptor contains two major domains: an extracellular neurotrophin-binding domain and an intracellular protein tyrosine kinase (PTK) domain. Here, a neurotrophin (NT) dimer binds to a Trk receptor dimer. Receptor dimerization is required for autophosphorylation of the receptor at specific tyrosine residues (Y). Such autophosphorylation 1) enables phosphorylation of other substrates, such as PLCγ, and 2) forms docking sites, or SH2 domains, for other signaling proteins such as Shc and Grb2 (see Chapter 5).

portant for protein–protein interactions, cysteine-rich clusters, and two immunoglobulin (Ig)-like domains. The intracelluar portion contains the protein tyrosine kinase catalytic domain, which is required for signal transduction.

The binding of neurotrophin to the Trk receptor causes activation of the receptor's catalytic domain. Neurotrophins bind as dimers, and in turn cause the dimerization of Trk molecules, which results in the autophosphorylation of Trk on several key cytoplasmic tyrosine residues. Such autophosphorylation initiates intracellular signaling cascades that lead to many of the biologic effects of receptor activation (see Chapter 5). Intracellular signaling occurs because phosphorylated tyrosine residues form a recognition sequence for the SH2 domains that are present on several types of cellular proteins. SH2 domains on Shc and Grb2, for example, eventually link Trk receptors to the activation of the small G protein Ras, which in turn triggers the activation of the microtubule-associated protein (MAP)-kinase cascade. Genetic abnormalities in Ras-related proteins cause **neurofibromatosis** in humans, which involves excessive growth of Schwann cells (Box 11–1).

Other biologic effects of Trk receptor activation result from the phosphorylation of different signaling proteins on tyrosine residues. The most important of these are phospholipase Cγ (PLCγ), which triggers the phosphatidylinositol cascade, and insulin receptor substrate (IRS), which leads to activation of the phosphatidylinositol-3-kinase cascade. Interestingly, mutations in the ATM gene, which encodes one subtype of phosphatidylinositol-3-kinase, have been shown to cause **ataxia-telangiectasia**, a disease characterized by progressive

Box 11–1 Neurofibromatosis: A Disease of Ras Signaling Pathways

Defects in the intracellular signaling pathways activated by neurotrophic factors can lead to the overproliferation of cells, and in turn can give rise to various disorders. The best established of these is **neurofibromatosis,** an inherited disease caused by mutations in a Ras modulatory protein.

As explained in Chapter 5, Ras is a key protein in neurotrophin signaling cascades that switches between an inactive GDP-bound state and an activated GTP-bound state. If Ras remains in its GTP-bound state, cell growth pathways remain constitutively active and may spur an overproliferation of cells. Indeed, mutations in Ras are believed to be responsible for a large percentage of human **cancers.** Oncogenic Ras genes have mutations that cause Ras to remain in its constitutively active state by 1) lowering the intrinsic GTPase activity of Ras, or 2) rendering Ras insensitive to regulation by GTPase activating proteins (GAPs). GAPs accelerate the intrinsic rate of GTP hydrolysis and thereby promote Ras inactivation.

Neurofibromatosis type I (NF1), which is caused by mutations in a certain form of GAP, is an autosomal dominant disorder that affects 1 in 3500 people. Its primary manifestations are changes in skin pigmentation, called *cafe au lait spots,* and tumors that derive from cells of neural crest origin, such as neurofibromas and malignant neurofibrosarcomas. When the NF1 gene was cloned, it was discovered that its encoded protein, termed *neurofibromin,* was homologous to several known GAPs. Subsequently, investigators determined that neurofibromin indeed functions as a GAP, and therefore as a primary negative regulator of Ras. Yet why the loss of NF1, which is expressed rather broadly in mammalian tissues, results in the overproliferation of only certain types of cells remains unknown.

Loss-of-function mutations in the NF1 gene result in a loss of neurofibromin and in turn cause the hyperfunction of Ras. Interestingly, tumor cell lines derived from schwannomas of patients with NF1 exhibit very low levels of NF1 expression and elevated levels of GTP-bound Ras. When the catalytic region of GAP is transfected into these cells, GTP-bound Ras decreases to near-normal levels, and tumor cells show morphologic signs of differentiation. These exciting findings suggest that anti-Ras therapies may be developed for the treatment of NF1-related malignancies.

degeneration and atrophy of several brain regions, particularly that of the cerebellum. The various intracellular signaling cascades activated by the neurotrophins and their Trk receptors are discussed in greater detail in Chapter 5.

Trk receptors display multiple splice variants, yet the functional significance of this diversity requires investigation. The best understood splice variants are the TrkB and TrkC isoforms that contain normal extracellular ligand-binding domains but lack the catalytic tyrosine kinase domain. As previously discussed, such truncated Trk receptors may limit the scope and duration of neurotrophin activity.

THE p75 RECEPTOR

The first neurotrophin receptor to be cloned was not a Trk receptor, but p75, a 75-kDa protein that is currently described as the low-affinity neurotrophin receptor. p75 binds to all neurotrophins with roughly equal affinity. It also appears to modulate Trk signaling, although Trk receptors can mediate functional responses to neurotrophins in the absence of p75. Cultured MAH cells, derived from a neuronal progenitor cell line that expresses TrkA and p75, exhibit significantly greater phosphorylation of, and may exhibit increased activation of, TrkA compared with cells that express TrkA alone. In addition, although p75 knockout mice have only slight neurologic defects, the survival of trigeminal sensory ganglion neurons in these mice requires four times more NGF than is required by wildtype mice. Thus, p75 may allow Trk receptors to respond to lower concentrations of NGF and other neurotrophins—a highly desirable trait in a receptor that competes for limited quantities of growth factor. Yet the mechanism by which p75 exerts this effect remains elusive. Surprisingly, p75 also is believed to be a key player in cell death pathways, as discussed in a subsequent section of this chapter.

NEUROTROPHIN AND Trk RECEPTOR KNOCKOUT MICE

To learn about the functions of neurotrophins and their corresponding receptors, researchers have used mice in which the genes that encode these proteins have been deleted. Reliance on mutant mice has been necessary because the pharmacologic tools that have been used to study neurotransmitters, such as small-molecule agonists or antagonists, generally are not available for use in the study of neurotrophic factors. By examining the populations of neurons that die in neurotrophin or Trk knockout mice, researchers have attempted to determine which neurotrophins and Trks support the survival of particular classes of neurons.

Some of these studies have confirmed in vitro observations that neurotrophins mediate the survival of many neurons in the peripheral nervous system and

Box 11-2 Neurotrophin and Trk Receptor Knockout Mice

Because small-molecule agonists and antagonists of Trk receptors are not yet available, studies of neurotrophin systems have depended on the use of mice engineered to lack a particular neurotrophin or Trk receptor. Mice in which the genes encoding NGF or TrkA have been inactivated exhibit a loss of sympathetic neurons as well as sensory neurons in dorsal root ganglia of the trigeminal system. Such findings are consistent with what is known about NGF's role during development. NGF and TrkA knockout mice also exhibit a partial loss of the cholinergic neurons in the basal forebrain that project to the hippocampus and cerebral cortex. Because these neurons have been implicated in the symptoms of **Alzheimer disease** (see Chapter 20), it is believed that TrkA agonists may have some utility in the treatment of this illness and other disorders of memory.

The analysis of TrkB knockout mice has been complicated by the fact that NT-4, BDNF, and to a lesser degree, NT-3, can stimulate the TrkB receptor. TrkB knockout mice exhibit the death of cranial motor neurons, trigeminal ganglion neurons, and nodose ganglion neurons; thus TrkB signaling most likely is necessary for the survival of these cells. In accord with the partial overlap in function of neurotrophin ligands, the phenotype of BDNF knockout mice is less severe than that of TrkB knockouts. BDNF and NT-4 double-knockout mice exhibit more cell loss than mice that lack only one of these factors.

Because BDNF has been proven to support motor neuron survival in vitro and in vivo, BDNF knockout mice might be expected to exhibit significant motor neuron loss. Such findings would have great clinical significance because diseases such as **amyotrophic lateral sclerosis** are characterized by the degeneration of cortical and spinal motor neurons. However, BDNF knockouts exhibit no loss of facial or spinal motor neurons. In contrast, TrkB knockouts show significant motor neuron loss. Thus it is likely that another neurotrophin, such as NT-4 or combination of neurotrophins may be important for motor neuron survival during development.

NT-3 and TrkC knockout mice are characterized by a loss of the dorsal root ganglion proprioceptive neurons that project to motor pools; consequently these mice display defects in the movement and positioning of their limbs. A loss of cochlear and trigeminal ganglia neurons also is evident in NT-3 knockouts. Moreover, large myelinated Ia sensory afferent fibers from muscle are absent from both NT-3 and TrkC knockout mice. Although NT-3 is highly expressed in embryonic muscle, motor neurons appear intact in NT-3 knockouts, possibly because motor neurons express both TrkB and TrkC and therefore may respond to BDNF and NT-4 as well as to NT-3. Indeed motor neuron survival is better supported by BDNF and NT-4 than by NT-3 in vitro.

The use of neurotrophin and Trk knockout mice has demonstrated the difficulty of assigning precise functions to specific neurotrophin or Trk receptors and has suggested that neurotrophins and Trks have overlapping and redundant physiologic actions.

---

of certain neurons in the CNS. Moreover, examination of the knockout mice used in these studies has supported the belief that neurotrophins have both distinct and overlapping functions in the nervous system. Yet the use of these mutant animals requires complex analyses that are at times difficult to reconcile. Furthermore their use in the study of neurotrophins in the adult brain is limited because many of these mice do not survive into adulthood. A brief overview of findings and limitations associated with the study of neurotrophin and Trk knockout mice is provided in Box 11-2.

NEUROTROPHINS AND SYNAPTIC PLASTICITY

Studies of the formation of ocular dominance columns in the developing visual cortex have confirmed that neurotrophins mediate forms of synaptic plasticity. As axons from the lateral geniculate nucleus (LGN) of the thalamus grow into the cortex and synapse with primary visual cortical neurons, they segregate into eye-specific, alternating patches known as ocular dominance columns in layer 4 of the cortex.

Monocular deprivation experiments, such as those involving the suturing of one eyelid, have revealed that this process is activity dependent; LGN neurons that receive inputs from the deprived eye exhibit weakened synaptic connections. NT-4 can rescue these neurons from such plastic changes. Because BDNF and NT-4 are expressed in the visual cortex and TrkB is expressed by certain LGN neurons, it is possible that LGN neurons might compete for TrkB ligands and that this competition might be crucial for the formation of ocular dominance columns. Indeed, the infusion of excess BDNF or NT-4 into the visual cortex blocks both the segregation of LGN axons and the formation of ocular dominance columns. A later study revealed that endogenous neurotrophins are necessary for this process by demonstrating that the infusion of a neurotrophin antagonist can block the formation of ocular dominance columns. The neurotrophin antagonist used was TrkB–IgG, a fusion protein of the ligand-binding domain of the TrkB receptor coupled to an immunoglobulin molecule, which binds to and prevents the biologic activity of endogenous neurotrophins.

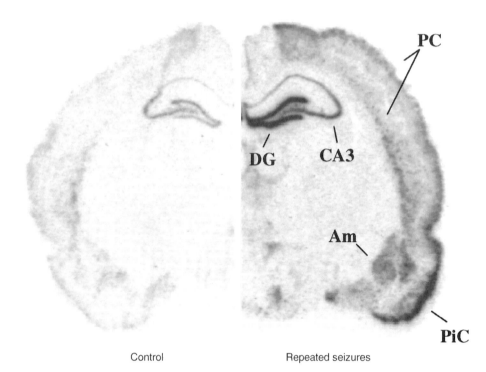

Figure 11-6. Regulation of BDNF mRNA in the hippocampus, cerebral cortex, and amygdala by repeated electroconvulsive seizures. Single seizures were induced with an electrical stimulus each day for 10 days, and rats were analyzed 18 hours after the last seizure. Control rats underwent sham treatment. Levels of BDNF mRNA subsequently were determined by in situ hybridization. CA3, pyramidal cell layer in hippocampus; DG, dentate gyrus of hippocampus; PC, parietal cortex; Am, amygdala; PiC, piriform cortex. (Borrowed with permission from L. Tolbert and R. S. Duman, Yale University.)

Accumulating evidence suggests that neurotrophins also are involved in regulating synaptic plasticity in the fully differentiated adult brain. To begin with, neuronal activity dramatically and rapidly regulates the expression of certain neurotrophins and their Trk receptors in adult neurons. The induction of BDNF and TrkB, for example, has been observed in neurons of the hippocampus and cortex in response to seizures (Figure 11–6); in neurons of the hippocampus in response to trains of synaptic stimuli (including those associated with the formation of long-term potentiation [LTP]; see Chapters 7 and 20); and in neurons of the locus ceruleus in response to opiate withdrawal. Conversely, the expression of BDNF can be reduced by exposure to hyperpolarizing stimuli such as γ-aminobutyric acid (GABA)$_A$ receptor agonists. The rapidity of BDNF induction in some systems is consistent with that of other immediate early genes, such as c-fos (see Chapter 6); indeed the induction of BDNF is mediated by the activation of pre-existing transcription factors such as CREB.

Increasing evidence suggests that neurotrophins can modulate synaptic transmission and regulate the formation and strengthening of synapses. Such actions most likely are mediated by cross-talk between neurotrophin signaling pathways and mechanisms of neurotransmitter release and receptor signaling; for example, in cell cultures NT-3 has been shown to rapidly enhance synaptic transmission at the neuromuscular junction, typically within 10 minutes. Because NT-3 increases the frequency of spontaneous synaptic currents but not their amplitude, it most likely enhances transmission by increasing the probability that quantal acetylcholine release from the presynaptic neuron will occur. Moreover, its effects appear to be mediated by Trk receptors; indeed they can be blocked by the putative, but not highly specific, Trk receptor inhibitor known as **K252a**.

Neurotrophins also have been reported to regulate synaptic transmission in the hippocampus, although such accounts remain controversial. BDNF or NT-3, but not NGF, is reported to increase the size of excitatory postsynaptic potentials at the Schaeffer collateral–CA1 synapse for as long as 2 to 3 hours. Accordingly, BDNF knockout mice exhibit reduced basal synaptic transmission at this synapse. In addition, hippocampal slices from these mice are reportedly deficient in LTP, and when slices of hippocampus from wildtype mice are treated with TrkB–IgG, the magnitude of the late phase of LTP decreases. Furthermore, adult heterozygous BDNF knockout mice exhibit reduced sprouting of hippocampal granule cells in response to seizures. Although these data clearly implicate the involvement of BDNF in hippocampal function in the adult, they are drawn from studies (particularly those on LTP) that have not been universally replicated. Thus further research is needed to support these findings.

GDNF FAMILY

GDNF, a glycosylated protein of approximately 18 kDa, was first isolated from a glial cell line that supports the survival of dopaminergic neurons from the midbrain in culture. Subsequently GDNF was proven to support these neurons after toxic injury in vivo. Because **Parkinson disease** is caused by the degeneration of dopaminergic neurons in the midbrain (see Chapter 14), GDNF has received considerable attention as a potential therapeutic agent for this disease.

More recently, GDNF has been proven to support the survival of many other neuronal cells, including those of the myenteric plexus of the gut. Yet despite this factor's significant involvement in neuronal development, the most profound abnormality observed in GDNF knockout mice is maldevelopment of the kidney, which causes these mutants to die shortly after birth. This finding demonstrates that GDNF serves as a critical growth factor outside of the nervous system.

Like the neurotrophins, GDNF produces its biologic effects through the activation of a protein tyrosine kinase, but such activation is achieved indirectly through an intervening receptor protein (Figure 11–7). A GDNF dimer binds to a specific receptor, termed GFRα1, a protein of approximately 40 kDa, which is anchored to the plasma membrane by glycophosphatidylinositol (GPI). GDNF binding triggers the association of GFRα1 with Ret, a transmembrane protein tyrosine kinase of about 150 kDa. This association results in Ret activation, which is believed to lead to many of the biologic effects of GDNF by triggering the phosphorylation of specific substrates. Although such substrates have yet to be identified, it is possible that Ret activation leads to the perturbation of MAP-kinase cascades. Loss-of-function mutations in Ret are associated with **Hirschsprung disease** in humans, a disorder characterized by abnormal gut motility. This association is consistent with neurotrophic effects of GDNF on gut neurons and Hirschsprung-like abnormalities in GDNF knockout mice. In contrast, gain-of-function mutations in Ret are associated with neural crest malignancies in humans, such as **multiple endocrine neoplasias** and **medullary thyroid carcinoma**.

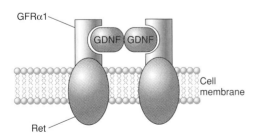

Figure 11–7. GDNF receptor complex. A GDNF dimer binds to GFRα1, which subsequently associates with tyrosine kinase Ret, a transmembrane protein. This association triggers Ret activation and the phosphorylation of specific substrates, which in turn produce the biologic effects of GDNF. Most of the specific substrates involved in this process remain unknown. GDNF, glial cell line-derived neurotrophic factor.

Also considered members of the GDNF family of neurotrophic factors are neurturin and persephin, both of which signal by means of Ret. Like GDNF, each binds to a specific Rα subunit, which subsequently converges on Ret. Also like GDNF, neurturin can support the survival of dopaminergic neurons in the midbrain. This latter finding has sparked interest in this factor as another possible treatment for **Parkinson disease**.

An understanding of the cell–cell communication mediated by the GDNF family of neurotrophic factors has come from the analysis of midbrain dopaminergic systems. In these systems, striatal medium spiny neurons express GDNF but lack GFRα1 and Ret. In contrast, dopaminergic neurons lack GDNF but express high levels of GFRα1 and Ret. These findings support a scheme, analogous to that previously described for NGF in the peripheral nervous system, wherein dopaminergic neurons are supported by GDNF supplied by their target striatal neurons. Yet whether GDNF is released predominantly in the striatum, where it may act on GFRα1–Ret in dopaminergic nerve terminals, or whether it is anterogradely transported by striatal neurons to the midbrain, where it may be released on the dendrites and cell bodies of dopaminergic neurons, remains unknown (see Chapter 14 for further information about these striatal circuits.)

Because GDNF, like BDNF, can be induced in the brain after intense synaptic stimulation, it may assist in synaptic transmission and plasticity. However, further research is needed to confirm this hypothesis.

CNTF FAMILY

Ciliary neurotrophic factor belongs to an important family of growth factors whose members also include leukemia inhibitory factor (LIF), interleukin-6 (IL-6), prolactin, growth hormone, leptin, interferons, and oncostatin-M, among others (see Table 11–1). This family is defined by the shared signaling mechanisms described in the next section of this chapter. Most members of the CNTF family are best known for their roles outside of the nervous system—hence their designation as cytokines. Yet several of these factors, including CNTF, LIF, and IL-6, have been associated with the dramatic regulation of neuronal survival or phenotype and thus can be considered neurotrophic factors.

The actions of CNTF, a protein approximately 24 kDa in size, are best characterized for neuronal cells. As previously mentioned, CNTF initially was studied as a survival factor for chick ciliary ganglion neurons and was known to up-regulate choline acetyltransferase (see Chapter 9) in these cells. More recently, CNTF has been proven to regulate the survival or differentiation of many other neuronal cells, including preganglionic sympathetic neurons, sensory neurons, motor neurons, cultured hippocampal neurons, and dopaminergic neurons in the midbrain. Its effects on motor neurons are perhaps the most dramatic: CNTF not only supports the survival of these neurons in vitro, it also prevents their degeneration after axotomy and improves some motor defects in murine models of motor neuron disease. Consequently, CNTF has been tested as a therapeutic agent in the treatment of motor neuron disease in humans, but produced serious side effects.

LIF and IL-6 are believed to similarly regulate neuronal growth, differentiation, and lineage commitment, although the mechanisms by which they achieve such regulation are not as well established. IL-6, for example, promotes the survival of septal cholinergic, mesencephalic catecholaminergic, and hypothalamic neurons in culture, and induces the neural differentiation of PC12 cells. The actions of LIF are best established in the hypothalamus in vivo. In vitro, LIF and CNTF can suppress the adrenergic phenotype of sympathetic neurons and induce a cholinergic, parasympathetic phenotype (see Chapter 12 for a discussion of sympathetic and parasympathetic neurons).

Glial cells are generally believed to be the primary or sole source of CNTF, LIF, and IL-6 in the brain, although neural expression of these factors has not been ruled out. However, the receptor signaling mechanisms for these factors are clearly expressed by both neuronal and glial cell types. Thus these factors may mediate critical effects of glial cells on their neighboring neurons, particularly after injury. Yet it is important to emphasize that the details of such involvement in cell–cell communication remain largely unknown.

CNTF SIGNALING PATHWAYS

CNTF and related family members exert their effects through a distinct signaling pathway. The CNTF receptor complex consists of three components: the signaling transducers known as LIF receptor (LIFR) and glycoprotein of 130 kDa (gp130), and the CNTF-binding protein CNTFRα (Figure 11–8). CNTFRα is an ~80-kDa protein that is anchored to the plasma membrane by means of GPI. The binding of CNTF to CNTFRα triggers its association with gp130 and subsequently its association with LIFR. The formation of this tripartite receptor complex triggers signaling steps—namely, the activation of Janus kinase (JAK) and of related protein tyrosine kinases, such as Tyk—which subsequently mediate biologic effects such as activation of the STAT family of transcription factors (see Chapters 5 and 6).

Other members of the CNTF family signal through related mechanisms (see Figure 11–8). In a manner analogous to CNTF's binding of CNTFRα, IL-6 binds to a specific protein termed IL-6Rα, which in turn associates with a gp130 dimer. The resulting complex triggers the activation of JAK and subsequent signaling cascades. LIF binds to a dimer of LIFR (hence its name) and gp130, and in turn triggers the activation of JAK. Thus certain components of these receptors, such as CNTFRα and IL-6Rα, are specific for a particular factor, whereas others, including LIFR and gp130, are shared by receptors for several factors.

Surprisingly, CNTF knockout mice develop normally, exhibiting only mild motor neuron defects during adulthood. Also surprising is a related finding in humans. Approximately 2.5% of the Japanese population are homozygous for inactivating mutations of CNTF and thus are, in a sense, human CNTF "knockouts"; like CNTF knockout mice, these individuals develop without obvious deficits. In contrast, mice lacking the CNTF-binding protein CNTFRα lose almost all of their motor neurons and die within 24 hours of birth. The striking discrepancies between CNTF and CNTFRα knockout mice suggest the existence of another endogenous ligand for CNTFRα that has yet to be discovered.

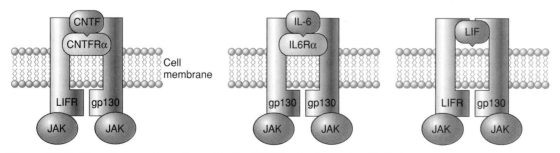

Figure 11–8. Receptor complexes formed by the CNTF family of neurotrophic factors. CNTF binds to CNTFRα, which in turn forms a tripartite complex with gp130 and LIFR. The resulting trimer induces the biologic effects of CNTF by binding to the protein tyrosine kinase JAK. Interleukin-6 (IL-6) binds to IL-6Rα, which subsequently associates with two gp130 molecules; the resulting trimer associates with JAK. LIF associates with JAK by binding to a gp130-LIFR dimer. CNTF, ciliary neurotrophic factor; LIFR, leukemia inhibitory factor receptor; JAK, Janus kinase.

IMMUNE-RESPONSE CYTOKINES AND THE CNS

As alluded to previously, the best studied effects of many cytokines are their actions on the immune system. Only recently has it emerged that some of these factors, particularly IL-1 and IL-6, tumor necrosis factor-α (TNFα), and transforming growth factor-β (TGFβ), also mediate CNS responses to immunologic challenges.

Cytokines implicated in immune function appear to be critical for systemic homeostasis. Any insult or change in the normal homeostasis of the body—such as might be induced by stress or sickness—causes a defense response that aids in the body's recovery. This response involves processes that are mediated in part by the CNS, such as fever, reduced appetite, cardiovascular changes, sleep disturbances, and malaise. A more detailed discussion of these processes is provided in Chapter 13; the section that follows is devoted to the general schemes by which cytokines affect brain function, whether they are generated in the CNS or peripherally.

The impact that immune-response cytokines can have on the brain is exemplified by the fever—which is mediated by the brain—that occurs in animals and humans in response to the peripheral injection of IL-1. How do systemically administered cytokines gain access to the brain? Although the blood–brain barrier is believed to limit cytokine entry to most of the brain, some cytokines can enter at sites where the blood–brain barrier is incomplete, such as certain periventricular areas (see Chapter 13). Cytokines also may induce lipophilic signals, such as prostaglandins, within endothelial cells, which subsequently diffuse from the vasculature into the brain parenchyma.

Substantial evidence suggests that the brain itself can synthesize immune-response cytokines. Such cytokines are believed to be synthesized exclusively in glia—particularly in microglia, the CNS equivalent of macrophages—and in astrocytes; however, expression of some of these cytokines by neurons has not been ruled out. Receptors for these cytokines are expressed primarily in glia, although expression in at least some neuronal cell types appears likely. After almost any dramatic perturbation, such as brain infection, injury, hypoxia, toxins, or head trauma, activated microglia and astrocytes produce many such cytokines, including IL-1, IL-6, TNFα, and TGFβ, among others. An effect of these factors may be to further activate glial cells and in turn stimulate gliosis—the generation of new astrocytes and microglia. The activated glia presumably help the brain recover by restoring normal homeostasis. The molecular mechanisms mediating these protective effects are poorly understood.

However, excessive levels of these cytokines can contribute to neural injury. This phenomenon is demonstrated dramatically in mutant mice that overexpress specific factors such as IL-1 or IL-6; such mice exhibit significant neurodegeneration in the vicinities of cytokine overexpression. Moreover, elevated levels of immune-response cytokines have been associated with several neurodegenerative disorders, including **Alzheimer disease**. Elevated cytokine levels are also observed in individuals with **multiple sclerosis,** an autoimmune disease that results in the degeneration of myelin sheaths around axons (Box 11–3). Interestingly, the immune-response cytokine known as **interferon-β** (IFN-β) has shown promise as a treatment for this disease, although its precise mechanism of action remains obscure.

In some cases, immune-response cytokines produce effects similar to those produced by CNTF. As previously discussed, IL-6 supports the survival of certain neuronal cell types. IL-1 enhances survival of neurons of the spinal cord, forebrain, and hippocampus in culture. TGFβ, like CNTF, appears to be important for neural crest cell differentiation during development. Moreover, like other neurotrophic factors, these cytokines may directly affect neurons in the adult brain. Receptors for IL-1, IL-6, TNFα, and TGFβ are most densely concentrated in the hippocampus and hypothalamus, where some of their corresponding factors have been proven to influence synaptic plasticity; for example, IL-1 is reported to attenuate the generation of hippocampal LTP. Immune-response cytokines also may mediate the rate of neurogenesis and the survival of newly formed neurons in the dentate gyrus of the adult hippocampus (Box 11–4). More research will be required to better characterize the direct effects of these cytokines on neurons, and to explore their possible role in the regulation of synaptic transmission and other aspects of neuronal function.

CHEMOKINES

Chemokines represent a growing family of small (8–10 kDa) proteins that originally were characterized in terms of their involvement in immune responses. In particular, they have been noted for their recruitment of leukocytes to sites of infection and their role in inflammation. More recently, studies have revealed that many chemokines and their receptors—all of which belong to the G protein-coupled receptor superfamily—are expressed in the brain. These chemokines are expressed predominantly by microglia, and to a lesser extent by astrocytes and certain neurons.

Chemokines comprise several categories based on the spacing between two required cysteine residues in their primary structure. Some have contiguous (CC) residues, some have one intervening residue (CXC), and others have several intervening residues (CX_3C). Receptors for these chemokines also are named according to these

Box 11–3 Multiple Sclerosis

Multiple sclerosis (MS) is a relatively common inflammatory demyelinating syndrome of the CNS. Its presentation is highly variable, depending on the neural circuits affected, but may include impaired vision, paresthesias (sensations of pins and needles or burning), and muscle weakness. Cognitive function and affect also may be affected. These symptoms are caused by the demyelination of corresponding nerve fibers; as mentioned in Chapters 2 and 3, myelin sheaths, generated from oligodendrocytes, are required for the efficient transduction of nerve impulses along most axons. Demyelination currently can be detected by high-resolution magnetic resonance imaging (MRI), which has become an indispensable tool in the diagnosis of this disease.

MS is believed to be an autoimmune illness. This belief originally was based on studies of laboratory animals, in which subcutaneous injections of myelin fractions triggered immune responses. The immune reaction to these injected proteins led to a demyelination syndrome called **experimental autoimmune encephalomyelitis,** whose characteristics resemble certain features of MS in humans. Indeed, patients with MS show autoimmunity to some myelin proteins, such as oligodendrocyte glycoprotein; however, the proteins that serve as antigens most likely vary in different patients. Immune responses to such antigens appear to be both humoral and cellular.

Like other autoimmune illnesses, MS is associated with particular immune response genes. In particular, it is associated with genes that encode HLA antigens. The mechanism that triggers the autoimmune response to myelin-associated proteins remains unknown. According to one hypothesis, this process can be attributed to molecular mimicry; that is, an immune response mounted toward a bacterial or viral pathogen cross-reacts with an endogenous protein, leading to autoimmunity. As discussed in Chapter 14, a similar process is involved in neuropathologic reactions to strepto-

coccal infections, wherein antibodies to the bacterium cross-react with cardiac valve proteins, resulting in **rheumatic fever,** or with striatal neuronal proteins, resulting in **Sydenham chorea** and perhaps some cases of **obsessive-compulsive disorder**.

There has been considerable interest in determining whether cytokines play a role in the etiology of MS, and in turn whether others might be used to treat the illness. Interferon-γ (INF-γ) and tumor necrosis factor-α (TNF-α) are two cytokines that have been implicated in the pathophysiology of MS. Both are secreted by peripheral lymphocytes or macrophages as well as by central microglia. Moreover, both cytokines have been detected in MS plaques but not in healthy white matter. Cytokines may contribute to the pathophysiology of MS by 1) activating central microglia, which may enhance the immune response to central antigens such as myelin-associated proteins, or 2) exerting direct toxic effects on oligodendrocytes.

The treatment of MS has depended primarily on the use of antiinflammatory agents, yet recent trials involving the use of interferon-β have been promising. INF-β ameliorates clinical symptoms of the illness, reduces the number and size of plaques detectable by MRI, and appears to decrease the rate at which acute exacerbations recur. Although the mechanism by which INF-β exerts these effects is unclear, it has been proven to reduce the production of INF-γ in vitro and to exert general antiinflammatory effects in vitro and in vivo. Such actions may occur both peripherally and centrally. Moreover, INF-β may act to restrict the movement of peripheral lymphocytes across the blood–brain barrier and in turn may further reduce the immune response to myelin-associated proteins. Regardless of the mechanism of action by which INF-β improves the symptoms of MS, its application represents the first widespread use of a neurotrophic factor for the treatment of a neuropsychiatric disorder.

---

categories (see Table 11–1). Although approximately 15 chemokine receptors have been cloned thus far, very little is known about their molecular pharmacology.

The functions undertaken by chemokines and their receptors in the brain remain incompletely understood. As previously mentioned, chemokines may mediate part of the brain's inflammatory response. Indeed, the most dramatic activation of chemokines and their receptors occurs in response to inflammatory stimuli, such as the lipopolysaccharides derived from the cell walls of gram-negative bacteria such as *Escherichia coli,* which dramatically induce increased expression of specific chemokines and chemokine receptors in microglia. Chemokines may be involved in several human disorders, including **multiple sclerosis, brain tumors,** and **stroke**. In addition, chemokine receptors, in particular CC_5R and perhaps other subtypes, are required for HIV entry into cells.

Whether treatment of these diseases can be facilitated by agents directed against particular chemokine receptors will depend partly on whether receptor-specific ligands can be developed.

Chemokines also may play a role in regulating the migration of neurons during development and in attracting growing nerve fibers toward target neurons, for example, in axonal guidance. Recent work with knock-out mice has supported such hypotheses; for example, mice that lack the chemokine receptor CXC_4R exhibit abnormal migration of cerebellar granule cells during late stages of development. Investigators also have speculated that chemokines may assist in regulating neuron–neuron interactions during adulthood. According to this hypothesis, which requires further investigation, chemokines may contribute to the formation or retraction of synapses in the context of long–term plasticity.

Box 11–4 Neurogenesis in the Adult Brain

During development, neurons originate from the proliferation of pluripotent stem cells concentrated in specialized regions of the brain, such as the subventricular zones that generate cerebral cortical neurons. The newly formed cells subsequently differentiate into either neurons or glia and migrate to their appropriate locations in the brain. For decades neuroscientists have believed that the formation of new neurons, or neurogenesis, in mammals is completed before birth and that no new neurons are formed in the adult brain. However, recent findings have shattered this view.

Strong evidence currently suggests that the adult brain contains highly localized regions that remain capable of neurogenesis throughout life. Among these regions, the dentate gyrus of the hippocampus has received the greatest attention. This region contains large numbers of dividing granule cell precursors, some of which differentiate into mature neurons, receive afferent synaptic inputs, and form efferent connections with neuronal targets in the mossy fiber pathway. Such neurogenesis has been documented in rodents, in nonhuman primates, and most recently in humans. It is estimated that as many as several hundred to a thousand new hippocampal neurons are formed each day; thus a significant turnover of these neurons may occur throughout life.

Prolonged exposure to antidepressant treatment increases neurogenesis in the hippocampus, as shown in the figure (newly born cells in the rat dentate gyrus are labeled with bromodeoxyuridine [BrdU] and appear darkly stained). An increase in the number of such cells occurs after repeated administration of three standard antidepressant therapies: electroconvulsive seizures (ECS); fluoxetine, a selective serotonin reuptake inhibitor; or tranylcypromine, a monoamine oxidase inhibitor (see Chapter 15).

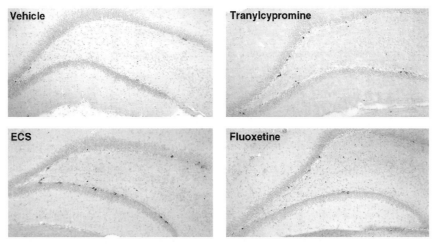

(Borrowed with permission from J. Malberg and R. Duman, Yale University.)

The functional significance of adult neurogenesis—for example, its relationship to cognitive function or to the formation of memory—remains completely unknown. However, research has revealed that stress, including sychosocial stress, interferes with the formation of new neurons, in part through the actions of adrenal glucocorticoids. In contrast, hippocampal-based learning facilitates the creation of neurons. Endogenous agents other than glucocorticoids that control the rate of neurogenesis are poorly understood, but most likely include neurotrophic factors.

The discovery of neurogenesis in humans has prompted investigators to explore the use of progenitor cells in the treatment of neurodegenerative disorders. Such cells might be engineered to express exogenous proteins, such as neurotrophic factors and subsequently might be injected into target regions of the nervous system. Clearly this is an exciting avenue of research that remains in the earliest stages of development.

NEURONAL INJURY AND DEATH

In the absence of appropriate signals, neurons die. As previously indicated, this phenomenon occurs primarily during development, when in many systems only cells that receive appropriate target-derived trophic support survive. However, a cell's fate also is determined by the balance between signals controlling life and death. Thus neuronal cell death is induced by two general mechanisms: 1) neurotrophic factor withdrawal and the subsequent inactivation of vital signaling pathways, or 2) the activation of distinct pathways that trigger cell death. Because of the devastation associated with human diseases that involve neuronal cell death, interference with pathways that lead to the death of neurons has been a prime strategy in drug innovation.

During development, most neurons that die do so by programmed cell death, or *apoptosis*, which is charac-

Box 11–5 Cell Death Pathways

Tremendous progress has been made toward identifying the key elements of intracellular signaling pathways responsible for programmed cell death, or apoptosis, in neurons (see figure; see also Chapter 21). Our evolving knowledge has required a growing understanding of the dynamic balance between death signals (grey in figure) and survival signals (blue in figure). Many details of apoptotic mechanisms remain unclear and may vary according to experimental paradigms and cell types; thus the figure shown here is necessarily oversimplified.

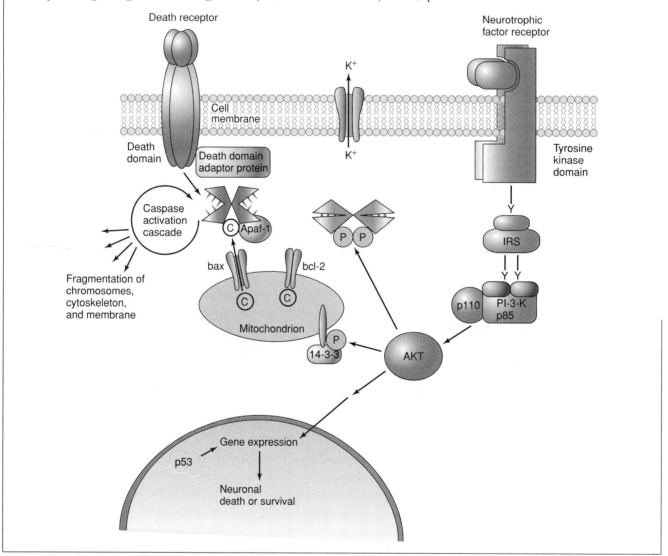

terized morphologically by cell shrinkage and nuclear and cytoplasmic condensation (see Chapter 21). Apoptosis occurs by means of several pathways, the key features of which are still being investigated (Box 11–5). The p75 receptor described previously in this chapter has been implicated as a key player in one cell death pathway, despite evidence that this receptor can also enhance neurotrophin and Trk function and promote cell survival under some conditions. p75 has a region that has been described as a death domain, analogous to similar domains in the TNFα receptor, through which it activates apoptosis by the generation of ceramide from sphingolipids in the cell membrane. Ceramide in turn may cause cell death by activating NF-κB or various stress-activated protein (SAP)-kinase-regulated transcription factor pathways. Direct evidence suggests that p75 mediates death in several cell types. In neuroblastoma cells, for example, p75 triggers apoptosis in response to the withdrawal of NGF. Programmed death of cholinergic neurons in the basal forebrain also

Apoptosis is triggered by transmembrane receptors, such as Fas, TNFα, and p75, that contain a conserved death domain that recruits and activates caspases by means of death-domain adaptor proteins such as the TNF receptor-associated death domain (TRADD) and the Fas-associated death domain (FADD). As mentioned in this chapter, caspases are a family of proteases that inactivate prosurvival proteins and activate proapoptotic proteins, including other caspases, in an amplifying cascade that leads to the eventual fragmentation of cell structures.

Caspase-9, for example, is autoproteolytically activated after oligomerization in a complex that includes the protein known as apoptotic protease activating factor (Apaf-1), which is bound to cytochrome C (cytC). CytC is released from mitochondria when apoptosis is triggered. The B-cell lymphoma (Bcl) protein family, which contains both proapoptotic and prosurvival elements, also is involved in the fate of neurons. Proapoptotic Bax homologs dimerize in the mitochondrial membrane and enhance cytC release; Bcl-2 prosurvival homologs interfere with Bax action and inhibit cytC release.

One of the prototypical triggers for apoptosis, at least in vitro, is the withdrawal of neurotrophic factors. Neurotrophic factor receptors, such as the TrkA receptor for NGF or the IGF-I receptor for insulin-like growth factor, activate prosurvival signaling cascades; as in the figure, these involve the sequential activation of insulin receptor substrate (IRS), phosphatidylinositol-3'-kinase (PI-3-K), and AKT kinase. AKT phosphorylates proapoptotic proteins such as Bad (a Bax homolog) and caspase-9, inhibiting their apoptotic action. K^+ efflux through membrane channels also contributes to apoptosis by means of unclear mechanisms.

Both prosurvival and proapoptotic signaling pathways lead to altered gene expression in the nucleus; accordingly, apoptosis often can be blocked by inhibitors of transcription or translation. Beyond its function in development, apoptosis offers a protective mechanism by which an organism can rid itself of damaged and potentially carcinogenic cells. p53, for example, is a tumor suppressor, a transcription factor that activates proapoptotic gene expression in response to DNA damage that might lead to cell transformation.

Thus programmed cell death must be viewed as a mechanism that is essential for the survival of an organism. In the nervous system, it enables the pruning of excess neurons during development, and the formation of anatomically precise and correct connections between nerve cells. However, increasing evidence indicates that apoptotic mechanisms of neuronal death also may contribute to several neurodegenerative disorders and to decrements in brain function associated with aging. Consequently, considerable attention is focused on developing medicinal agents that might interfere with these processes.

appears to be mediated by p75 because an increase in the number of these neurons has been detected in p75 knockout mice. Moreover, retinal cells that express p75 but not TrkA undergo cell death that can be prevented by the introduction of anti-NGF antibodies.

Jun N-terminal kinase (JNK), a type of SAP-kinase, also has been implicated in cell death. It is activated by cell stress, which can be produced by a variety of agents and environmental factors, including ultraviolet radiation, ceramide, anisomycin, some cytokines, osmotic shock, and anoxia. As explained in Chapter 5, JNK is a protein serine–threonine kinase that is involved in one branch of the MAP-kinase cascades. Activation of specific forms of MAP-kinase kinases (MEK kinases), a process that depends on the Ras-like small G protein Rac, leads to activation of various MEKs and ultimately to the activation of JNK or the related SAP-kinase p38. In vitro studies have indicated that the p38 pathway kinases may be involved in cell death by demonstrating that the transfection of PC12 cells with a dominant negative form of p38 rescues cells from death caused by NGF deprivation. In vivo studies have yielded similar evidence with observations of reduced hippocampal apoptosis in JNK knockout mice after kainate-induced injury (see Chapter 7 for a discussion of kainate activation of glutamate receptors). A primary target of JNK is the activation of transcription factors c-Jun and ATF2. c-Jun levels are elevated in the CNS after excitotoxic injury and also in cerebellar granule cells undergoing apoptosis. Such increases in c-Jun may reflect the activation of c-Jun-ATF2 heterodimers bound to the c-Jun promoter; that is, c-Jun activates its own expression when phosphorylated by JNK (see Chapter 6). Dominant negative forms of c-Jun rescue NGF-deprived cells from death.

The cell death signaling pathways described here ultimately converge at so-called death genes, which mediate the balance between cell survival and death. Studies of cell death in the model organism *C. elegans* has contributed greatly to our understanding of these genes. Because loss-of-function mutations in *C. elegans* genes ced-3 and ced-4 lead to cell survival, it has been determined that these genes are positive regulators of cell death. In contrast, ced-9 is a negative regulator of cell death because gain-of-function mutations on this gene have been proven to block cell death.

The mammalian homologue of ced-9 is Bcl-2. In several studies, both in vitro and in vivo, overexpression of Bcl-2 has rendered several types of neurons—including hippocampal, sympathetic, dorsal root ganglion, and mesencephalic neurons—resistant to apoptosis. Conversely, neurons in mice that lack Bcl-2 are more susceptible to apoptosis. Other proteins related to Bcl-2, such as Bcl-x, also protect neurons from cell death. However, some members of this protein family, such as Bag-1, Bak, and Bad, promote death by interacting with Bcl-2 to decrease its protective activity.

The vertebrate homolog of ced-3 is the interleukin-1B coverting enzyme (ICE). Inhibition of ICE, a member of the cysteine aspartate protease (caspase) family, can block programmed cell death of neurons in vitro and in vivo; for example, inhibition of ICE can block motor neuron cell death triggered by trophic factor withdrawal. Because such findings indicate that caspases assist in cell death, the development of clinically useful caspase inhibitors has received much attention.

Our knowledge of cell death pathways indicates that neurotrophic factors can prevent cell death 1) by blocking the expression of death effector genes, or 2) by increasing the expression of survival promoting genes. The ways in which such genes are regulated and the factors that control their level of expression have yet to be determined with certainty; however, these processes most likely are influenced by interactions between the products of death genes and protective genes. It is hoped that a greater understanding of the individual proteins involved in cell death and the molecular basis of their interactions will provide a rich source of targets for the development of neuroprotective medications (Box 11–6).

OXIDATIVE STRESS

Oxidative stress is a major source of neuronal injury and death. Reactive oxygen species such as superoxide anions (O_2^-) and hydroxyl radicals (OH^-) are generated by normal processes of cellular metabolism. However, if these species are not cleared or decomposed, their potent chemical reactivity can result in lipid peroxidation and subsequent membrane destruction, and can directly damage DNA. Such reactivity is implicated in the neuronal cell death associated with stroke, ischemia, and certain neurodegenerative disorders.

The formation of reactive oxygen species is a downstream effect of excitotoxicity, which is caused primarily by the excessive activation of glutamate receptors (see Chapter 21 for a discussion of stroke and excitotoxicity). As discussed in Chapter 7, some types of glutamate receptors, such as *N*-methyl-D-aspartate (NMDA) receptors, trigger the entry of Ca^{2+} into cells. Among many other actions, Ca^{2+} entry activates phopholipase A, which in turn releases arachidonic acid and results in the generation of O_2^-. Arachidonic acid and O_2^- can further enhance glutamate release and inhibit its uptake, which in turn leads to the accumulation of reactive oxygen species and to the perpetuation of the excitotoxic cycle. The overstimulation of glutamate receptors also can lead to increases in superoxide and nitric oxide, which can combine to form the neurotoxic agent known as peroxynitrite ($OONO^-$) (see Chapter 21). Moreover, Ca^{2+} promotes cell death through the activation of certain caspases—an observation that underscores the overlap among cellular pathways that control cell death and survival.

Cells combat oxidative stress by means of several mechanisms. Antioxidants such as **vitamin E** (α-tocopherol) and **vitamin C** (ascorbic acid) have been proven to protect cells. Vitamin E is considered a chain-breaking antioxidant because of its ability to donate hydrogens to reactive oxygen species and in turn prevent lipid peroxidation. Because vitamin E is recycled by cells, it is a particularly effective antioxidant that has been used with some success in the treatment of oxidative stress in newborns. However, its efficacy in the treatment of neurodegenerative disorders has not been demonstrated. Some neurotrophic factors also prevent oxidative damage by mechanisms that are not yet understood.

Cellular enzymes such as superoxide dismutases (SODs) degrade reactive oxygen species. Among these enzymes, the most abundant in the brain is the cytosolic Cu/Zn SOD termed *SOD1*. Mutations in this enzyme and consequent increases in oxidative stress cause a familial form of **amyotrophic lateral sclerosis** (**ALS**), also known as **Lou Gehrig disease**. This neurodegenerative disease is characterized by the progressive and selective degeneration of upper and lower motor neurons. Interestingly, each family affected by familial ALS exhibits distinct missense mutations in this enzyme. Why motor neurons are selectively killed by an enzymatic defect expressed in many tissues is not clear. Transgenic mice with SOD1 mutations exhibit motor neuron degeneration and death even though SOD1 catalytic activity is normal in these animals. This finding suggests that such cell death may be caused by the toxic effects of SOD1 mutations rather than by a reduction in the activity of the enzyme. SOD1 mutations may, for example, result in mitochondrial damage, which in turn may trigger apoptosis. The involvement of apoptosis in this process is supported by recent observations that loss of motor neurons in mutant SOD transgenic mouse models is blocked with overexpression of Bcl-2 or inhibition of caspases, such as by the caspase inhibitor **zVAD-fmk** (*N*-benzyloxycarbonyl-Val-Asp-fluoromethylketone). Whether such mechanisms operate in humans with familial ALS remains unclear.

Box 11–6 Therapeutic Agents Directed at Neurotrophic Factors and Their Signaling Pathways

Because neurotrophic factors support neuronal cell survival and rescue neurons from cell death, they would appear to be ideal candidates for use in the treatment of neurodegenerative disease. Yet clinical trials designed to support the use of such agents have been disappointing. Such setbacks can be attributed in part to inadequate animal models of many human neurodegenerative diseases. Moreover, because neurotrophic factors are relatively large proteins, their delivery to the CNS is particularly challenging. The delivery of quantities large enough to ensure bioavailability can result in serious side effects. Consequently small-molecule ligands of Trk and other receptors are needed.

Clinical experience with neurotrophic factors is reviewed only briefly here. As previously mentioned in this chapter, BDNF, CNTF, and IGF-1 have been proven to support motor neuron survival in vitro and in vivo. In addition, treatment with BDNF, CNTF, or a combination of these factors has been shown to slow or arrest the progression of motor neuron degeneration in the *wobbler* mouse. Encouraged by these results, investigators have used these factors in human clinical trials involving patients with **amyotrophic lateral sclerosis**. In such trials, BDNF has been well tolerated, but has generally produced only modest clinical effects. IGF-1 has produced only a modest decrease in clinical progression of the disease.

Clinical trials involving CNTF in amyotrophic lateral sclerosis have proven to be even more problematic. Although treatment with CNTF slowed deterioration of muscle strength, it produced severe toxicity in most patients—especially in those receiving higher doses. Yet such high doses are 30 times lower than the effective dose (corrected for body weight) in *wobbler* mice. In addition, patients treated with this neurotrophic factor can develop neutralizing antibodies to CNTF that limit its bioavailability.

The therapeutic use of neurotrophic factors in the treatment of other diseases has been equally disappointing. Because NGF supports the survival of many sensory neurons, investigators have attempted to treat sensory neuropathy with this factor. However, as in studies of motor neuron therapies, humans have not been able to tolerate the highest doses of NGF, although such doses are 10,000 times lower than effective doses used in animal models.

Because BDNF, GDNF, and other factors have enhanced the survival of dopaminergic neurons in animal models, the use of neurotrophic factors in the treatment of **Parkinson disease** is a top research priority (see Chapter 14). Likewise, because cholinergic afferent systems, whose function appears to be supported by NGF, may be important for memory function, investigators are exploring the use of NGF as a treatment for **Alzheimer disease** (see Chapter 20). Indeed, after treatment with NGF, aged rats have exhibited improvement in their ability to perform memory tasks.

However, the need to deliver such therapeutic factors directly to targeted neurons of the CNS represents a significant challenge. Intracranial injection of these factors in slow-release preparations and injection of cultured cells or viral vectors that overexpress these factors are currently under evaluation. Ideally, a systemically administered vector would be targeted to the appropriate area of the brain; however, a great deal of research will be necessary before such viral vectors are ready for human use.

The challenges associated with administering neurotrophic factors have inspired hopes of developing small molecules that might promote neurotrophic factor function. Small-molecule agonists of neurotrophic factor receptors or even small molecules that assist postreceptor signaling proteins in mediating the actions of neurotrophic factors would be quite valuable. Inhibitors of proteins that promote cell death, such as caspases and JNKs, would be similarly useful. Progress along these lines has been limited. Indeed, it might be quite difficult to devise a small molecule that mimics BDNF (a 14-kDa protein) at what is likely to be a large ligand-binding domain on the TrkB receptor. More creative approaches to such research may be necessary; for example, small molecules that promote the dimerization and hence activation of TrkB, or that promote the association of the Shc-Grb2-Sos linker proteins in the TrkB signaling cascade, might be developed. Such strategies represent major challenges in drug development.

SELECTED READING

Arenas E. 1996. GDNF, a multispecific neurotrophic factor with potential therapeutic applications in neurodegenerative disorders. *Mol Psychiatry* 1:179–182.

Asensio VC, Campbell IL. 1999. Chemokines in the CNS: plurifunctional mediators in diverse states. *Neurosciences* 22:504–512.

Baloh RH, Enomoto H, Johnson EM Jr, Milbrandt J. 2000. The GDNF family ligands and receptors—implications for neural development. *Curr Opin Neurobiol* 10:103–110.

Black IB. 1999. Trophic regulation of synaptic plasticity. *J Neurobiol* 41:108–118.

Bonni A, Greenberg ME. 1997. Neurotrophin regulation of gene expression. *Can J Neurol Sci* 24:272–283.

Cabelli RJ, Shelton DL, Segal RA, Shatz CJ. 1997. Blockade of endogenous ligands of TrkB inhibits formation of ocular dominance columns. *Neuron* 19:63–76.

Datta SR, Greenberg ME. 1998. Molecular mechanisms of neuronal survival and apoptosis. *Hormones and Signaling* 1:257–306.

D'Mello SR. 1998. Molecular regulation of neuronal apoptosis. *Curr Opin Dev Biol* 39:187–213.

Ernfors P, Lee KF, Jaenisch R. 1994. Mice lacking brain–derived neurotrophic factor develop with sensory deficits. *Nature* 368:147–150.

Ewing C, Bernard CC. 1998. Insights into the aetiology and pathogenesis of multiple sclerosis. *Immunol Cell Biol* 76: 47–54.

Farinas I, Jones KR, Backus C, et al. 1994. Severe sensory and sympathetic deficits in mice lacking NT-3. *Nature* 369: 658–661.

Gage FH. 2000. Mammalian neural stem cells. *Science* 287: 1433–1438.

Gould E, Tanapat P. 1999. Stress and hippocampal neurogenesis. *Biol Psychiatry* 46:1472–1479.

Hefti F. 1997. Pharmacology of neurotrophic factors. *Annu Rev Toxicol* 37:239–267.

Hjelmstrom P, Juedes AE, Ruddle NH. 1998. Cytokines and antibodies in myelin oligodendrocyte glycoprotein-induced experimental allergic encephalomyelitis. *Res Immunol* 149: 794–804.

Ibanez CF. 1998. Emerging themes in structural biology of neurotrophic factors. *Trends Neurosci* 21:438–444.

Kong J, Xu Z. 1998. Massive mitochondrial degeneration in motor neurons triggers the onset of amyotrophic lateral sclerosis in mice expressing a mutant SOD1. *J Neurosci* 18: 3241–3250.

Levi-Montalcini R. 1987. The nerve growth factor 35 years later. *Science* 237:1154–1162.

Li M, Ona VO, Guegan C, et al. 2000. Functional role of caspase-1 and caspase-3 in an ALS transgenic mouse model. *Science* 288:335–339.

Malberg JE, Eisch AJ, Nestler EJ, Duman RS. 2000. Chronic antidepressant treatment increases neurogenesis in adult rat hippocampus. *J Neurosci* 20:9104–9110.

Martino G, Furlan R, Brambilla E, et al. 2000. Cytokines and immunity in multiple sclerosis: the dual signal hypothesis. *J Neuroimmunol* 109:3–9.

Mehler MF, Kessler JA. 1997. Hematolymphopoietic and inflammatory cytokines in neural development. *Trends Neurosci* 20:357–365.

Mennicken R, Maki R, de Souza EB, Quirion R. 1999. Chemokines and chemokine receptors in the CNS: A possible role in neuroinflammation and patterning. *Trends Pharmacol Sci* 20:73–78.

Milligan CE, Prevette D, Yaginuma H, et al. 1995. Peptide inhibitors of the ICE protease family arrest programmed cell death of motoneurons in vivo and in vitro. *Neuron* 15: 385–393.

Nebrada R, Porras A. 2000. p38 MAP kinases: beyond the stress response. *Trends Biochem Sci* 25:257–260.

Nijhawan D, Honarpour N, Wang XD. 2000. Apoptosis in neural development and disease. *Annu Rev Neurosci* 23:73–87.

Oppenheim RW. 1997. Related mechanisms of action of growth factors and antioxidants in apoptosis: An overview. *Adv Neurol* 72:69–78.

Pettmann B, Henderson CE. 1998. Neuronal cell death. *Neuron* 20:633–647.

Reiter RJ. 1995. Oxidative processes and antioxidative defense mechanisms in the aging brain. *FASEB J* 9:526–533.

Rosen DR, Siddique T, Patterson D, et al. 1993. Mutations in the Cu/Zn superoxide dismutase gene are associated with familial amyotrophic lateral sclerosis. *Nature* 362:59–62.

Rothwell NJ, Luheshi G, Toulmand S. 1996. Cytokines and their receptors in the central nervous system: Physiology, pharmacology, and pathology. *Pharmacol Ther* 69:85–95.

Schuman EM. 1999. Neurotrophin regulation of synaptic transmission. *Curr Opin Neurobiol* 9:105–109.

Skaper SD, Walsh FS. 1998. Neurotrophic molecules: Strategies for designing effective therapeutic molecules in neurodegeneration. *Mol Cell Neurosci* 12:179–193.

Song Z, Steller H. 1999. Death by design: mechanism and control of apoptosis. *Trends Cell Biol* 9:M49–M52.

Steiner JP, Hamilton GS, Ross DT, et al. 1997. Neurotrophic immunophilin ligands stimulate structural and functional recovery in neurodegenerative animal models. *Proc Natl Acad Sci USA* 94:2019–2024.

Troy CM, Derossi D, Prochiantz A, et al. 1996. Downregulation of Cu/Zn superoxide dismutase leads to cell death via the nitric oxide–peroxynitrite pathway. *J Neurosci* 16:253–261.

Turnley AM, Bartlett PF. 2000. Cytokines that signal through the leukemia inhibitory factor receptor-beta complex in the nervous system. *J Neurochem* 74:889–899.

Xu B, Zang K, Ruff NL, et al. 2000. Cortical degeneration in the absence of neurotrophin signaling: Dendritic retraction and neruonal loss after removal of the receptor TrkB. *Neuron* 26:233–245.

Xu GF, Lin B, Tanaka K, et al. 1990. The catalytic domain of the neurofibromatosis type 1 gene product stimulates ras GTPase and complements ira mutants of *S. cerevisiae*. *Cell* 63:835–841.

Yong W, Chabot S, Stuve O, Williams G. 1998. Interferon beta in the treatment of multiple sclerosis. *Neurology* 51:682–689.

Yuen EC, Mobley WC. 1996. Therapeutic potential of neurotrophic factors for neurological disorders. *Ann Neurol* 40: 346–354.

PART 3

Neuropharmacology of Specific Neural Functions and Related Disorders

Chapter 12

Autonomic Nervous System

KEY CONCEPTS

- The autonomic nervous system, which has two major functional divisions—the sympathetic nervous system and the parasympathetic nervous system—plays a critical role in maintaining homeostasis and permitting adaptation for almost every organ in the body.

- The sympathetic and parasympathetic nervous systems produce functionally opposite effects in most organs of the body and are thus viewed as physiologic antagonists.

- The sympathetic nervous system is activated in response to changes in the environment; it usually discharges as a whole, orchestrating a coordinated response to a threat.

- The parasympathetic nervous system is generally continuously active, coordinating the function of multiple organs in accord with the physiologic state of the organism, thereby facilitating such functions as digestion and excretion.

- Because of its importance to the physiology of the organism the autonomic nervous system is a target for many pharmacologic interventions.

- The autonomic nervous system, a division of the peripheral nervous system, has a two-neuron arrangement, with a pre- and post-ganglionic neuron; in both sympathetic and parasympathetic

ganglia, neurotransmission is carried by a cholinergic signal that interacts with a nicotinic receptor pharmacologically distinct from that found in the brain or at the neuromuscular junction.

- Acetylcholine is the main neurotransmitter used by postganglionic neurons in the parasympathetic nervous system; its target receptors are muscarinic acetylcholine receptors, which are G protein coupled.

- With few exceptions, the postganglionic neurons in the sympathetic nervous system release norepinephrine, which acts on α- and β-adrenergic receptors located on end organs.

- Chromaffin cells in the adrenal medulla are developmentally related to sympathetic ganglia, are activated via nicotinic acetylcholine receptors, and release epinephrine.

- Agonists and antagonists of peripheral sympathetic function are important in medicine; agonists are known as sympathomimetics and antagonists, sympatholytics.

- β-Adrenergic antagonists such as propranolol play an important role in the treatment of heart disease and hypertension; β-adrenergic agonists such as terbutaline are used to treat obstructive pulmonary disease.

The autonomic nervous system is a functional division of the peripheral nervous system that innervates virtually every organ in the body. The other major division of the peripheral nervous system, known as the somatic nervous system, comprises motor nerves that innervate skeletal muscle and primary sensory nerve fibers.

Through the integration and control of vital processes such as blood pressure, fluid and electrolyte balance, and body temperature, the autonomic nervous system maintains homeostasis in the body. It also regulates the locally driven activities of smooth muscle, car-

diac muscle, and some glands. Moreover, it integrates the visceral systems and coordinates these with somatic motor function. Under ordinary circumstances, the organ systems that are governed by the autonomic nervous system function independently of volitional control—that is, below the level of consciousness—yet they can be influenced to some degree by volition and emotion. Without autonomic innervation, such organs continue to function but cannot adapt to changing environmental and emotional conditions.

Based on anatomy and constituent neurotransmitter systems, the autonomic nervous system is divided into

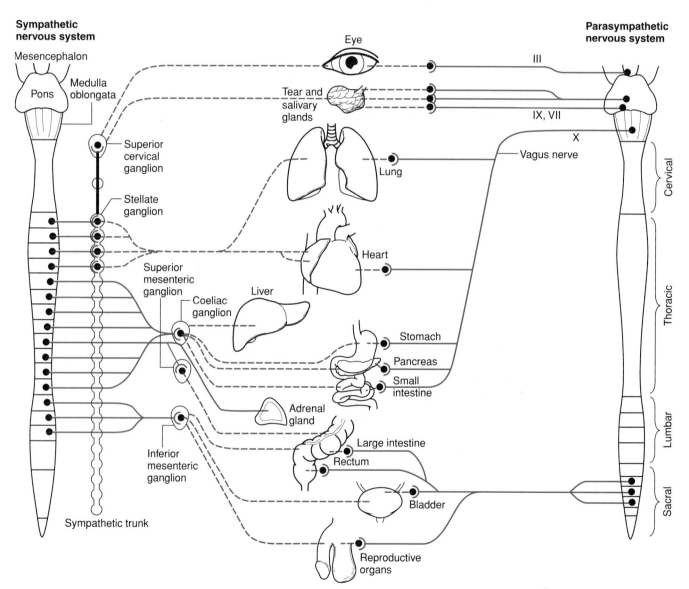

Figure 12–1. Autonomic nervous system. Solid lines indicate preganglionic axons; dashed lines indicate postganglionic axons. Sympathetic innervation of blood vessels, sweat glands, and piloerector muscles is not shown. Roman numerals denote cranial nerves. (Adapted with permission from Bannister R, Mathias CJ (eds). 1992. *Autonomic Failure,* p. 107. New York: Oxford University Press.)

two functional components: the sympathetic nervous system and the parasympathetic nervous system. Most organs are innervated by both. The sympathetic and parasympathetic systems usually produce opposite functional effects and thus are viewed as physiologic antagonists. Because they also are regulated independently, their combined actions result in an especially fine degree of control of organ function (Figure 12–1; Table 12–1).

The autonomic nervous system reaches its effector organs by means of a two-neuron chain. The primary or presynaptic neuron, also known as the preganglionic neuron, is located in the intermediolateral cell column of the brain stem and spinal cord. The secondary, postsynaptic, or postganglionic neuron is located in a ganglion lying outside the CNS that innervates the end organ directly. Sympathetic ganglia are located some distance from end organs, whereas parasympathetic ganglia are located in close proximity—often within the parenchyma of such organs. Consequently, postganglionic sympathetic nerves typically are much longer than postganglionic parasympathetic nerves (Figure 12–2).

The sympathetic nervous system, which is characterized by episodic activity, assists an organism in adjusting to changes in the environment, such as occur during periods of danger or stress. It usually discharges as a whole, orchestrating a coordinated, multiorgan response to a threat. Activation of this system is associated with increases in the force and rate of heart contractions, an increase in blood pressure, a shift in blood flow from the skin and viscera to skeletal muscle, an increase in blood glucose, and dilation of the bronchial tree. These responses prepare an organism for fight or flight in response to a threatening or appetitive stimulus. Yet such adaptive responses become symptoms when they occur out of proportion to environmental stimuli as in **panic disorder, posttraumatic stress disorder,** or forms of **social anxiety** such as **stage fright** (see Chapter 15). Each of these **anxiety** disorders involves an inappropriate discharge of the sympathetic nervous system.

In contrast, the parasympathetic nervous system is characterized by graded activity in anatomically discrete segments that serves to coordinate the functioning of

Table 12-1 Prominent Actions of the Autonomic Nervous System

End Organ	Sympathetic Function[1]	Parasympathetic Function[2]
Eye	Mydriasis (pupillary dilation) (α_1)	Miosis (pupillary constriction) Accommodation (contracts ciliary muscle)
Lacrimal gland	No appreciable effect	Stimulates secretion
Salivary gland	No appreciable effect	Stimulates secretion
Skin		
Sweat glands	Stimulates secretion[3]	Stimulates secretion
Pilomotor muscles	Stimulates piloerection (α_1)	No appreciable effect
Nasopharyngeal glands	Inhibits secretion (α_1)	Stimulates secretion
Heart	Increases heart rate and contractility	Decreases heart rate and contractility
Blood vessels	Dilates (β_1) or constricts (α_1) cardiac and skeletal muscle vessels Constricts vessels of the skin and GI tract (α_1)	No appreciable effect
Lung	Dilates bronchial tree (β_2)	Constricts bronchial tree
GI tract		
Gut wall	Decreases motility (β_2)	Increases motility and secretion
Sphincters	Contracts (α_1)	Relaxes
Bladder		
Muscle	Relaxes (β_2)	Contracts
Sphincter	Contracts (α_1)	Relaxes
Penis	Ejaculation (α_1)	Erection
Liver	Increases glycogenolysis (β_2)	No appreciable effect
Skeletal muscle	Increases glycogenolysis (β_2)	No appreciable effect
Fat cells	Increases lipolysis (β_1 and β_3)	No appreciable effect
Pancreatic β-cells	Increases insulin secretion (β_2)	No appreciable effect

[1]The adrenergic receptor that predominantly mediates each effect is shown in parentheses.
[2]All of these actions are mediated by muscarinic ACh receptors. Although five subtypes (M_1–M_5) have been identified, little is known about their selective roles in the responses listed (see Chapter 9).
[3]This effect, mediated by postganglionic sympathetic neurons that are cholinergic, is responsible for sweating at localized sites, such as the palms of the hands.

Sympathetic nervous system

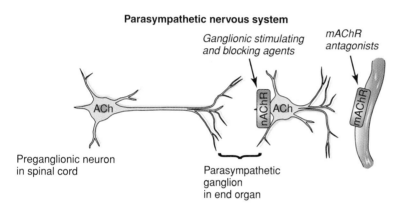

Parasympathetic nervous system

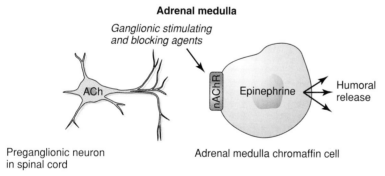

Adrenal medulla

Figure 12–2. Patterns of innervation in sympathetic and parasympathetic nervous systems. Both systems comprise preganglionic neurons, which originate in the CNS, and postganglionic neurons, which originate in the peripheral nervous system. Sympathetic ganglia generally are located far from their end organs, whereas parasympathetic ganglia are located in close proximity to their end organs. Preganglionic neurons in both the sympathetic and parasympathetic nervous systems are cholinergic and act by means of nicotinic cholinergic receptors (nAChR) on postganglionic cells. Transmission at these synapses can be modified by nicotinic cholinergic agonists and antagonists (ganglionic stimulating and blocking agents, respectively). With a few exceptions, which are mentioned in this chapter, postganglionic sympathetic neurons are noradrenergic and affect end organ function by means of α_1, β_1, and β_2 adrenergic receptors (AR). Presynaptic α_2 receptors generally function as inhibitory autoreceptors. Postganglionic parasympathetic neurons are cholinergic and affect end organ function by means of muscarinic cholinergic receptors (mAChR). Adrenal medulla chromaffin cells may be regarded as an extension of the sympathetic nervous system. These cells are stimulated by preganglionic cholinergic neurons that act on nicotinic receptors and secrete epinephrine into the general circulation. Such activity regulates most of the end organs influenced by postganglionic sympathetic neurons.

individual organs with the physiologic state of an organism. This system assists in maintaining the organism by facilitating functions such as digestion and excretion. In addition, it decreases the rate and force of heart contractions and blood pressure.

Because of its anatomic accessibility and its robust regulation of peripheral organ functions, the autonomic nervous system was among the first components of the mammalian nervous system to be studied. Consequently, many of the principles of neuropharmacology currently applied to studies of the CNS

originally were derived from classic studies of autonomic systems. Such studies enabled investigators to establish the chemical basis of neurotransmission, identify acetylcholine and norepinephrine as neurotransmitters, explore the pharmacology of cholinergic and adrenergic receptors, and discover the role of inhibitory presynaptic autoreceptors in neurotransmission. Indeed, many of the pharmacologic agents studied during the past century originally were characterized according to their actions on the autonomic nervous system.

ANATOMY OF THE AUTONOMIC NERVOUS SYSTEM

SYMPATHETIC NERVOUS SYSTEM

The sympathetic division of the autonomic nervous system consists of fibers that arise in the intermediolateral cell column of the thoracolumbar (T1 to L2–3) spinal cord (Figure 12–3). Myelinated preganglionic fibers leave the spinal cord with the motor fibers of ventral roots, but soon separate to form white rami communicantes. The white rami carry the preganglionic fibers from the thoracic and upper lumbar segments to the sympathetic trunk, which comprises the paired, ganglionic chains of nerve fibers that extend along either side of the vertebral columns from the base of the skull to the coccyx. Some of the fibers of the white rami synapse with postganglionic neurons in the chain ganglion nearest their point of entrance to the chain, whereas other fibers pass up or down the chain to terminate in a ganglion situated above or below the point of entrance. Thus the cervical, lower lumbar, and sacral ganglia of the chain receive preganglionic fibers that have traveled up or down the trunk from thoracolumbar levels. Postganglionic fibers are nonmyelinated. Some of these form gray rami communicantes, which deliver postganglionic fibers to blood vessels, erector pili muscles in the skin, and sweat glands. Thirty-one gray rami—one for each spinal nerve—are located on each side of the body.

Cervical ganglia receive their preganglionic input from cells in spinal cord segments T1 to T5. Axons of these cells enter the sympathetic chain in the thorax

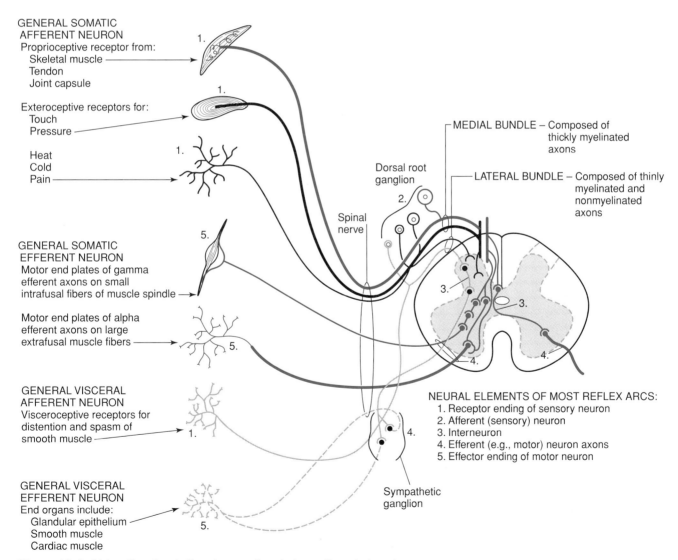

GENERAL SOMATIC AFFERENT NEURON
Proprioceptive receptor from:
  Skeletal muscle
  Tendon
  Joint capsule

Exteroceptive receptors for:
  Touch
  Pressure

  Heat
  Cold
  Pain

GENERAL SOMATIC EFFERENT NEURON
Motor end plates of gamma efferent axons on small intrafusal fibers of muscle spindle

Motor end plates of alpha efferent axons on large extrafusal muscle fibers

GENERAL VISCERAL AFFERENT NEURON
Visceroceptive receptors for distention and spasm of smooth muscle

GENERAL VISCERAL EFFERENT NEURON
End organs include:
  Glandular epithelium
  Smooth muscle
  Cardiac muscle

MEDIAL BUNDLE – Composed of thickly myelinated axons

LATERAL BUNDLE – Composed of thinly myelinated and nonmyelinated axons

Dorsal root ganglion

Spinal nerve

Sympathetic ganglion

NEURAL ELEMENTS OF MOST REFLEX ARCS:
1. Receptor ending of sensory neuron
2. Afferent (sensory) neuron
3. Interneuron
4. Efferent (e.g., motor) neuron axons
5. Effector ending of motor neuron

Figure 12–3. Major afferent and efferent connections between the spinal cord and peripheral tissues. (Adapted with permission from Carpenter MB. 1976. *Human Neuroanatomy,* p. 232. Baltimore: Williams and Wilkins.)

and ascend through the cervical trunk. The superior cervical ganglion cells give rise to the carotid plexus, a network of postganglionic fibers that follow the ramifications of the carotid arteries and furnish the sympathetic innervation of the entire head. Some fibers end in blood vessels and sweat glands of the head and face; others supply the lacrimal and salivary glands. The eye receives sympathetic fibers that innervate the dilator muscles of the pupil and the smooth muscle fibers that help raise the eyelid. The lower cervical ganglia supply the viscera of the neck.

Thoracic viscera receive postganglionic innervation from cells in the upper thoracic chain ganglia. These fibers also enter the plexus of the heart and lungs. The abdominal and pelvic viscera are supplied by thoracic splanchnic nerves, which carry mainly preganglionic fibers from spinal cord levels T5 through T12 to the sympathetic ganglia of the abdomen. These ganglia include the celiac, superior mesenteric, and aorticorenal ganglia located at the roots of arteries. The lumbar splanchnic nerves carry preganglionic fibers from the upper lumbar spinal cord to inferior mesenteric and hypogastric ganglia, from which postganglionic fibers reach end organs in the lower abdomen and pelvis.

PARASYMPATHETIC NERVOUS SYSTEM

The preganglionic fibers of the parasympathetic nervous system originate in the brain stem and in the sacral region of the spinal cord. The former travel in cranial nerves III, VII, IX, X, and XI. The latter arise from cell bodies in the intermediolateral cell column of sacral segments 2 through 4 and form the pelvic splanchnic nerves. Parasympathetic preganglionic neurons have relatively long myelinated axons that synapse with postganglionic neurons in the many small ganglia located close to or within target organs (see Figure 12–2). Thus, as stated earlier, postganglionic parasympathetic fibers are generally shorter than the postganglionic axons of the sympathetic nervous system. In the pelvic region, the parasympathetic system is primarily involved with sexual function and with emptying of the bladder and bowel. Under the influence of strong emotional stimuli, these fibers may discharge in conjunction with a generalized sympathetic response and produce involuntary emptying of these organs.

NEUROTRANSMITTERS OF THE AUTONOMIC NERVOUS SYSTEM

PRINCIPAL NEUROTRANSMITTERS

The autonomic nervous system functions predominantly through the actions of acetylcholine (ACh) and norepinephrine (see Figure 12–2). As discussed in Chapter 9, ACh is the neurotransmitter released at the neuromuscular junction. In addition, ACh is used by all preganglionic neurons in both the sympathetic and parasympathetic nervous systems. Accordingly, all of the efferent fibers that leave the CNS are cholinergic. In both sympathetic and parasympathetic ganglia, the cholinergic signal from a preganglionic neuron is transmitted to a postganglionic neuron by means of nicotinic ACh receptors. These receptors differ in pharmacology from those at the neuromuscular junction, based on differences in their constituent subunits (see Chapter 9). ACh also is the main neurotransmitter used by postganglionic neurons in the parasympathetic nervous system (see Figure 12–2). The cholinergic signal from postganglionic parasympathetic fibers is transmitted to target organs primarily through muscarinic ACh receptors.

In contrast, norepinephrine is used by most of the postganglionic neurons of the sympathetic nervous system. The norepinephrine signal acts on several α- and β-adrenergic receptors located on target organs. There are some exceptions to the rule that postganglionic sympathetic neurons are noradrenergic. Postganglionic sympathetic neurons that innervate some sweat glands and certain regions of vasculature are cholinergic and act by means of muscarinic ACh receptors. Moreover, chromaffin cells of the adrenal medulla are developmentally related to sympathetic ganglia and may be seen as an extension of the sympathetic nervous system (see Figure 12–2). They receive innervation from preganglionic sympathetic cholinergic fibers that act through nicotinic ACh receptors. In response to stimulation, chromaffin cells release epinephrine, which, like norepinephrine, acts on α- and β-adrenergic receptors located on end organs. Accordingly, the adrenal medulla typically is activated in concert with other components of the sympathetic nervous system.

NEUROPEPTIDES

Most sympathetic and parasympathetic neurons express, in addition to their principal neurotransmitters, a variety of neuropeptides. Neuropeptide Y (NPY) is most often coexpressed with norepinephrine in postganglionic sympathetic neurons, and vasoactive intestinal peptide (VIP) is typically coexpressed with ACh in postganglionic parasympathetic neurons. Other peptides expressed more sparingly in the autonomic nervous system include galanin, enkephalin, somatostatin, and substance P.

As discussed in Chapter 10, the co-localization of peptide transmitters with small-molecule transmitters appears to be common throughout the central and peripheral nervous systems. However, our knowledge of the functional role played by such peptide cotransmitters remains rudimentary. Most evidence suggests that, at least in the autonomic nervous system, peptide transmitters act synergistically with small-molecule transmitters; for example, VIP promotes salivary gland secretion by itself, and the effect is intensified when VIP is coupled with ACh. Similarly, NPY increases vascular smooth muscle contraction by itself, and produces synergistic increases in vascular tone when coupled with norepinephrine. These synergistic actions are significant because outside of the autonomic nervous system, peptide cotransmitters sometimes antagonize the actions of small-molecule transmitters.

Data obtained from the study of several neuronal cell types indicate that peptide cotransmitters, which appear to be stored independently of small-molecule transmitters in the same nerve terminals, typically require more intense stimulation to be released (see Chapter 10). Thus peptide cotransmitters may serve to facilitate sympathetic or parasympathetic drive during periods of extreme need. Moreover, their anatomic distribution and physiologic actions suggest that drugs directed at VIP, NPY, or other peptide receptors, although not yet available clinically, might be used in the future to modulate autonomic function.

PHARMACOLOGY OF THE AUTONOMIC NERVOUS SYSTEM

As previously mentioned, pharmacologic studies of the autonomic nervous system in many ways defined the field of neuropharmacology during the past 100 years. Indeed, the number and variety of pharmacologic agents that influence autonomic function are vast and well beyond the scope of this book. The sections that follow provide a concise summary of the classes of drugs that affect the autonomic nervous system and an overview of their physiologic actions.

GANGLIONIC STIMULATING AND BLOCKING AGENTS

Because cholinergic transmission through sympathetic and parasympathetic ganglia is mediated by means of nicotinic cholinergic receptors, it is not surprising that nicotinic cholinergic agonists and antagonists have profound effects on the functioning of all end organs that are regulated by the autonomic nervous system. Nicotinic cholinergic agonists are often called ganglionic stimulating drugs; antagonists are called ganglionic blocking drugs.

The best characterized ganglionic stimulating drugs are **nicotine** and **lobeline** (Figure 12–4). Nicotine, also

discussed in Chapters 9 and 16, is a natural alkaloid of the tobacco plant. Lobeline is a natural alkaloid of Indian tobacco. Both drugs are agonists at nicotinic cholinergic receptors, although their actions are complicated by the fact that they can rapidly desensitize these receptors. The initial effects of nicotine and lobeline are consistent with the activation of autonomic ganglionic transmission. Such effects include increased heart rate and blood pressure (in response to predominant activation of the sympathetic system and of the adrenal medulla); increased contractile activity of the gut that may lead to nausea, vomiting, and diarrhea (in response to predominant activation of the parasympathetic nervous system); and increased salivation (caused by the activation of both systems). Prolonged exposure to nicotine causes the desensitization of nicotinic receptors, which results in the sustained inhibition of autonomic activity. Such desensitization is dose-dependent: the higher the dose, the more rapid and complete the desensitization and subsequent depression of autonomic activity.

A small number of synthetic nicotinic cholinergic agonists, such as **tetramethylammonium,** have been identified (Figure 12–5). However, the clinical usefulness of such agents is limited. Most efforts in nicotinic cholinergic pharmacology have focused on the use of agonists that selectively activate nicotinic receptors in the brain and spinal cord for cognitive enhancement or analgesia (see Chapters 9, 19, and 20). Other efforts have been directed toward the treatment of nicotine addiction (see Chapter 16).

Among ganglionic blocking agents, **tetraethylammonium** was the first to be identified; other examples include **trimethaphan, hexamethonium,** and **mecamylamine** (see Figure 12–5). The net effect of these agents on end organ function depends on whether sympathetic or parasympathetic regulation of the organ pre-

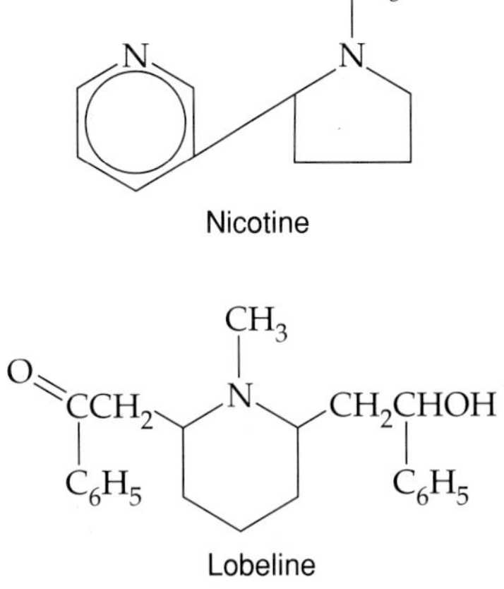

Figure 12–4. Chemical structures of nicotine and lobeline.

Nicotinic agonist

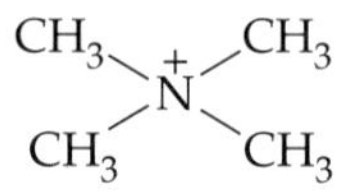

Tetramethylammonium (TMA)

Nicotinic antagonists

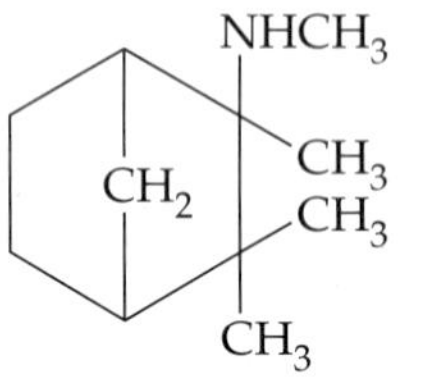

Mecamylamine

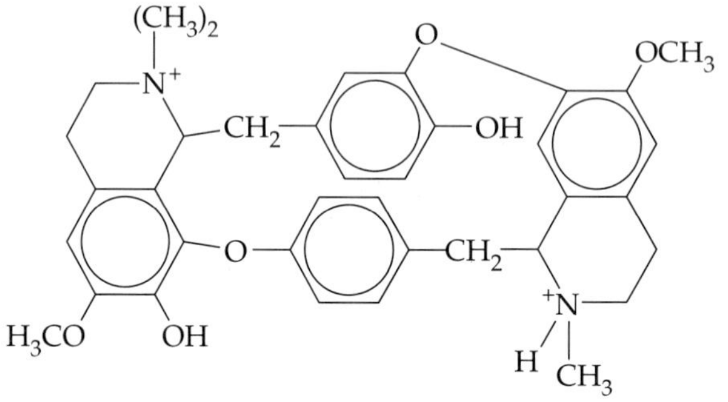

Tubocurarine

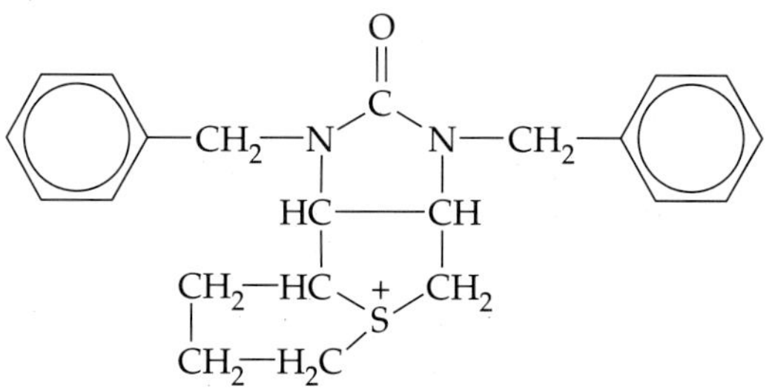

Trimethaphan

Figure 12-5. Chemical structures of representative nicotinic cholinergic agonists and antagonists.

dominates and on the physiologic state of the organism (Table 12–2). These principles can be illustrated by a consideration of blood pressure, which is regulated by sympathetic tone. Under normal conditions, when an individual is reclining, the maintenance of blood pressure does not require an appreciable level of sympathetic activity. In contrast, when an individual is sitting or standing, the maintenance of blood pressure depends

Table 12-2 Predominance of Sympathetic or Parasympathetic Tone at Various End Organs and Effects of Autonomic Ganglionic Blockade

Site	Predominant Tone	Effect of Ganglionic Blockage
Arterioles	Sympathetic	Vasodilation; increased peripheral blood flow; hypotension
Veins	Sympathetic	Dilation; peripheral pooling of blood; decreased venous return; decreased cardiac output
Heart	Parasympathetic	Tachycardia
Iris	Parasympathetic	Mydriasis
Ciliary muscle	Parasympathetic	Cycloplegia—loss of accommodation
Gastrointestinal tract	Parasympathetic	Reduced tone and motility; constipation; decreased gastric and pancreatic secretions
Urinary bladder	Parasympathetic	Urinary retention
Salivary glands	Parasympathetic	Xerostomia
Sweat glands	Sympathetic[1]	Anhidrosis

[1]This effect is mediated by cholinergic sympathetic fibers.

on increased sympathetic tone. Accordingly, ganglionic blocking agents have little effect on blood pressure when an individual is reclining but can cause a precipitous decline in blood pressure when administered to someone sitting or standing.

Ganglionic blocking agents were used clinically to treat hypertension several decades ago but for the most part have been replaced by medications that exhibit fewer side effects. They continue to be used to achieve very rapid decreases in blood pressure in emergency situations and to reduce blood flow during certain surgical procedures. They also are used to treat rare autonomic diseases, some of which are discussed in this chapter. Other nicotinic cholinergic antagonists, such as **curare** (see Figure 12–5), act on nicotinic receptors at both autonomic ganglia and the neuromuscular junction, although actions at the latter site, such as muscular paralysis, predominate. Several related snake venoms, typified by **α-bungarotoxin,** exert curare-like effects at the neuromuscular junction and at autonomic ganglia; they also affect central nicotinic ACh receptors that contain the α_7 subunit (see Chapter 9). So-called depolarizing agents, such as **succinylcholine,** exert effects primarily on the nicotinic ACh receptors in skeletal muscle. Initially, they activate nicotinic receptors, resulting in muscle contractions, but quickly cause paralysis through sustained depolarization of end plates (postsynaptic specializations on muscle cells) and subsequent depolarization blockade (see Chapter 3).

ADRENERGIC RECEPTOR AGONISTS AND ANTAGONISTS

Agonists and antagonists at various adrenergic receptors exert profound effects on the functioning of many organs by mimicking or antagonizing, respectively, sympathetic innervation. Agonists often are termed **sympathomimetics,** and antagonists are referred to as **sympatholytics.** The effects of these agents vary, depending on the tissue in which the particular receptor subtype is expressed. Further information on adrenergic agonists and antagonists is provided in Chapter 8.

Much of our early knowledge of adrenergic function was obtained from studies of natural plant alkaloids that potently affect sympathetic nervous system activity. A prominent example of such an alkaloid is **reserpine,** which is synthesized from *Rauwolfia serpentina,* a shrub found on the Indian subcontinent (Figure 12–6). Reserpine is a potent sympatholytic agent, which acts by depleting body stores of norepinephrine and other monoamines, including dopamine and serotonin. As discussed in Chapter 8, this effect is mediated through the inhibition of the vesicular monoamine transporter (VMAT), which is responsible for concentrating mono-

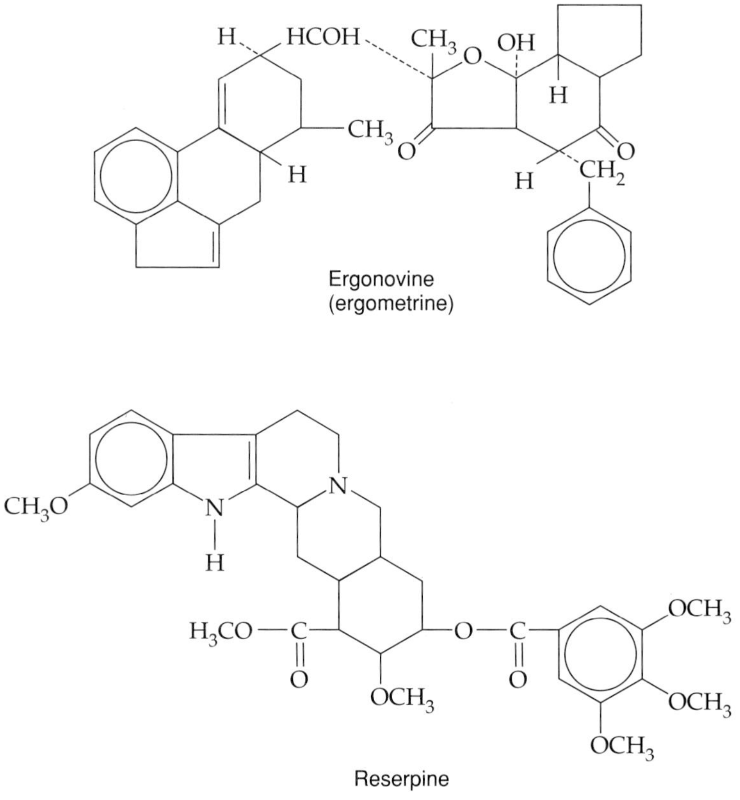

Ergonovine
(ergometrine)

Reserpine

Figure 12–6. Chemical structures of ergonovine, an ergot alkaloid, and reserpine.

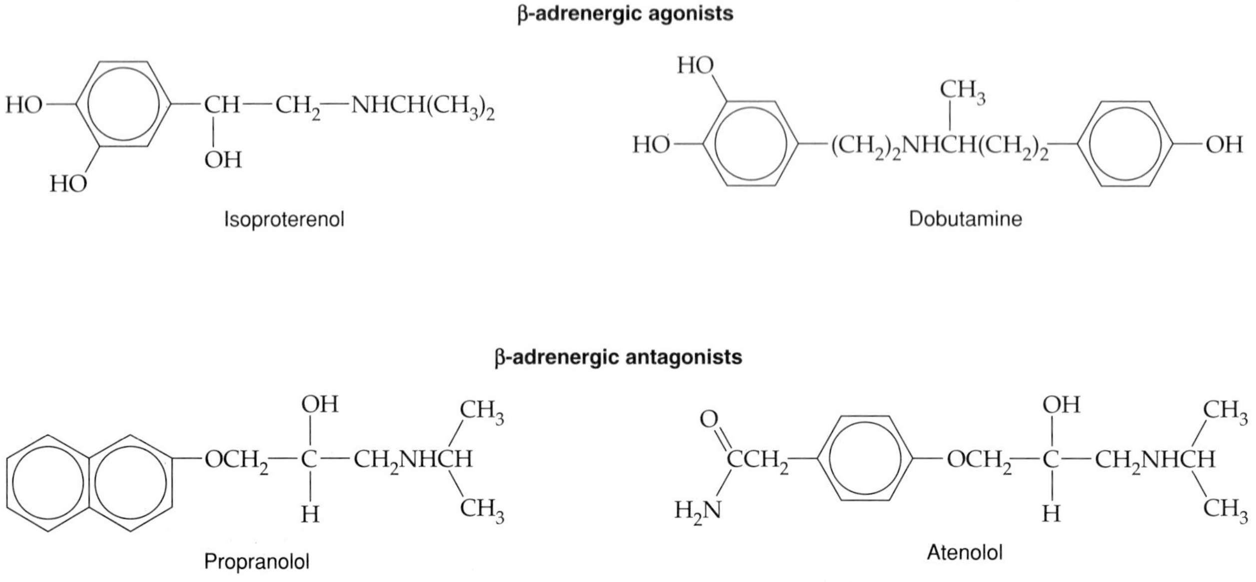

β-adrenergic agonists

Isoproterenol

Dobutamine

β-adrenergic antagonists

Propranolol

Atenolol

Figure 12–7. Chemical structures of representative β-adrenergic agonists and antagonists.

amines into synaptic vesicles. Although reserpine was one of the first **antihypertensive** and **antipsychotic** agents used clinically, its use has been supplanted by that of more specific, and hence safer, medications.

Early information about adrenergic function also was drawn from studies of **ergot** alkaloids, which are produced by *Claviceps purpurea,* a fungus that grows on rye and other grains (see Figure 12–6). Ergot-containing preparations have been used medicinally for more than two millennia for indications as varied as **uterine bleeding** and **headache.** During the twentieth century, a large number of ergot derivatives were prepared; these exerted a variety of effects on the adrenergic system, including receptor agonist and antagonist activity. Such compounds served as invaluable tools in the pharmacologic characterization of different subtypes of adrenergic receptors and in the delineation of their physiologic functions. Some ergot derivatives, such as **lysergic acid diethylamide** (**LSD**), affect the serotonin system (see Chapter 17). Others affect the dopamine system; an example is **bromocriptine,** an agonist at D_2 dopamine receptors that is used in the treatment of **Parkinson disease** (see Chapter 14) and **prolactin-secreting pituitary tumors.**

β-Adrenergic ligands β-Adrenergic agonists have profound effects on many peripheral organs; clinically, their most important targets are the organs that comprise the cardiovascular and pulmonary systems. The activation of β-adrenergic receptors increases the force and rate of heart contractions, and also can lead to the relaxation of vascular smooth muscle. The net effect is a large increase in cardiac output and a relatively mod-

est increase in blood pressure. β-Adrenergic receptor activation causes relaxation of bronchial smooth muscle in the lungs, which increases pulmonary function and facilitates respiration. β-Adrenergic antagonists exert opposite effects. Chemical structures of representative β-adrenergic agonists and antagonists are shown in Figure 12–7.

In cardiovascular medicine, β-adrenergic agonists such as **dobutamine** are used clinically only under extraordinary circumstances; for example, they may be used to stimulate a failing heart in an intensive care setting. The prototypical β-adrenergic agonist is **isoproterenol;** it is the agonist most often used in preclinical studies, although it is rarely used clinically. However, β-adrenergic antagonists such as **propranolol** continue to be mainstays in the treatment of **ischemic heart disease** and **hypertension.** In the lungs, β-adrenergic stimulation increases pulmonary function, as previously mentioned. Accordingly, β-adrenergic agonists are one of the primary agents used to treat **asthma** and other **chronic obstructive pulmonary diseases.** The expression of different subtypes of β-adrenergic receptors in the heart (β_1) and lung (β_2) has enabled the development of relatively selective adrenergic agents. Selective β_1-adrenergic antagonists such as **atenolol** can be used to treat ischemic heart disease and hypertension without causing excessive bronchoconstriction; likewise, selective β_2-adrenergic agonists such as **terbutaline** can be used to treat obstructive pulmonary disease without causing excessive tachycardia. β-Adrenergic antagonists are also used clinically to reduce sympathetic activity in individuals with **stage fright,** a type of **social anxiety disorder** (see Chapter 15). Interestingly, the attenuation of peripheral symptoms of social anxiety—including increased heart rate, palpitations, sweating, and flushing of skin—that occurs in response to the administration of a β antagonist is often sufficient to improve an individual's performance dramatically.

α-Adrenergic ligands   α-Adrenergic agonists and antagonists also are potent modulators of sympathetic nervous system activity. The predominant effect of α_1-adrenergic agonists is the constriction of arterial smooth muscle, which in turn causes an increase in blood pressure. α_1-Adrenergic agonists such as **methoxamine** and **phenylephrine** are used infrequently in clinical practice to increase blood pressure during severe hypotensive episodes. Phenylephrine and related α_1-adrenergic agonists are also widely used as nasal decongestants; their

decongestive action may be mediated by the constriction of blood flow to nasal mucosa or by a reduction in airway secretions. α_1-Adrenergic antagonists are used as **antihypertensive** drugs and to treat **benign prostatic hypertrophy**. The chemical structures of some of these agents, including the prototypical α_1-adrenergic antagonist **prazosin,** are shown in Figure 12–8.

α_2-Adrenergic receptors appear to function as inhibitory autoreceptors on noradrenergic neurons; thus it is not surprising that α_2-adrenergic agonists such as **clonidine** and **guanfacine** reduce sympathetic nervous system activity. Yet it is believed that such agents produce this effect by acting not on nerve terminals of postganglionic sympathetic neurons, but on neurons of the CNS. Indeed α_2-adrenergic agonists have been proven to inhibit the firing of noradrenergic neurons

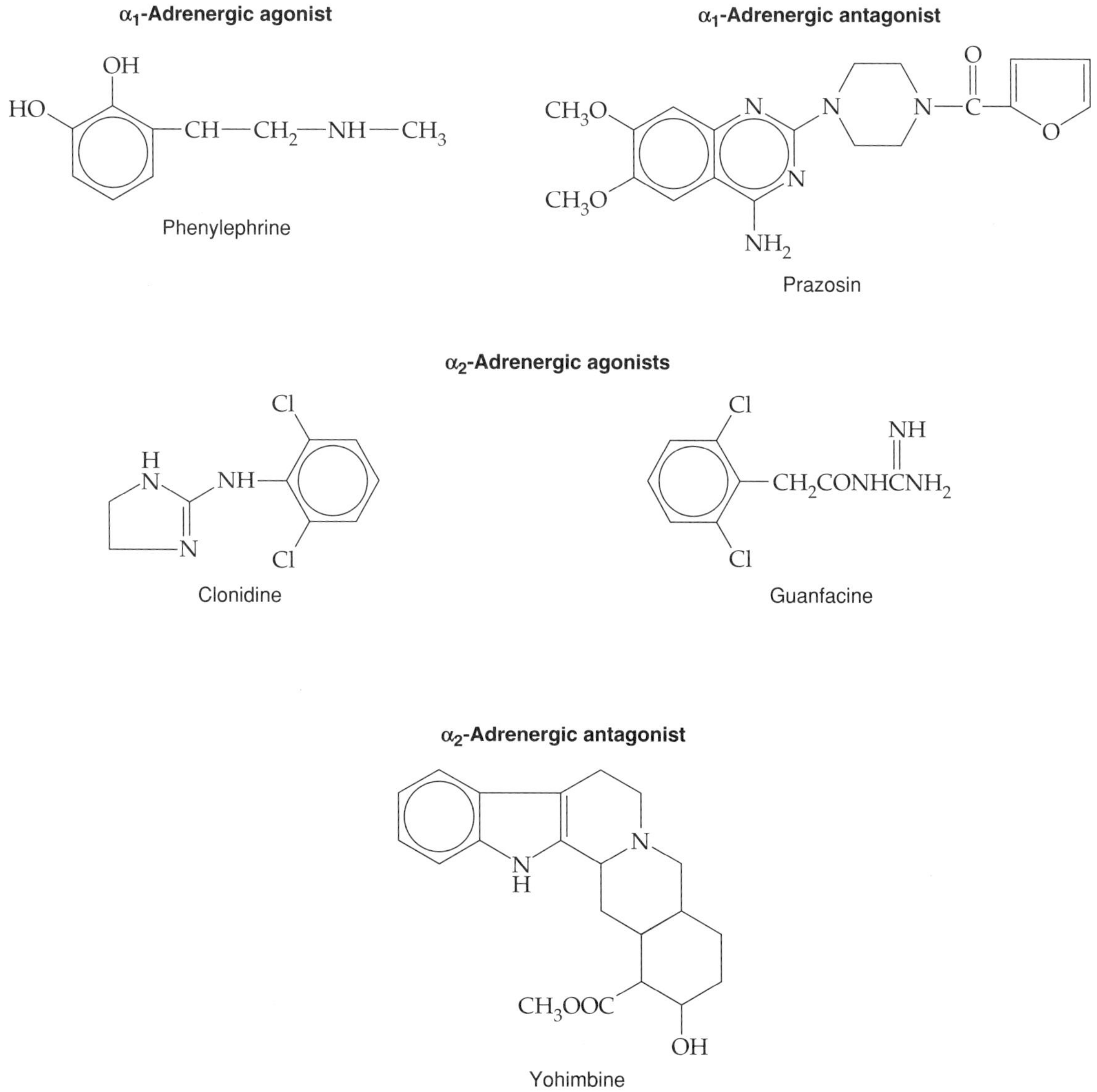

Figure 12–8. Chemical structures of representative α-adrenergic agonists and antagonists.

in the CNS, such as those in the locus ceruleus, which in turn leads to reduced sympathetic activity. Such agonists are commonly used in the treatment of hypertension and of several neuropsychiatric disorders associated with the CNS, such as **opiate withdrawal, attention deficit disorder,** and **Tourette syndrome** (see Chapters 14 and 16). α_2-Adrenergic antagonists such as **yohimbine** exert opposite effects: they stimulate sympathetic activity by activating noradrenergic neurons of the CNS.

MUSCARINIC CHOLINERGIC RECEPTOR AGONISTS AND ANTAGONISTS

Muscarinic cholinergic agonists and antagonists exert profound effects on the autonomic nervous system and on many regions of the brain (see Chapter 9 for a more detailed discussion of these compounds). Prototypical muscarinic agonists include synthetic agents such as **carbachol** and **bethanechol,** and natural plant products such as **arecoline, pilocarpine,** and **muscarine** (Figure 12–9). These agents affect the peripheral nervous system by slowing the heart and reducing blood

pressure; in the CNS, they exert a characteristic cortical activation. Because they stimulate emptying of the bladder, the major clinical use of muscarinic agonists is in the treatment of **urinary retention**. These drugs are also sometimes used to stimulate motility of the gastrointestinal tract and to stimulate salivary gland secretion. In addition, they have nonmedicinal uses in several Eastern cultures; for example, arecoline is used recreationally on the Indian subcontinent.

The effects of muscarinic cholinergic antagonists can be predicted based on their blockade of postganglionic parasympathetic transmission. Muscarinic antagonists decrease the rate and force of cardiac contractions and cause blurred vision, hot and dry skin, pupillary dilation and reduced accommodation, and decreased gastrointestinal motility. Independent of their effects on the autonomic nervous system, these drugs profoundly affect the CNS and result in pervasive delirium, including confusion, disorientation, and hallucinations. Prototypical muscarinic antagonists include **atropine** and **scopolamine** (see Figure 12–9). Muscarinic antagonists were once widely used in the treatment of gastrointesti-

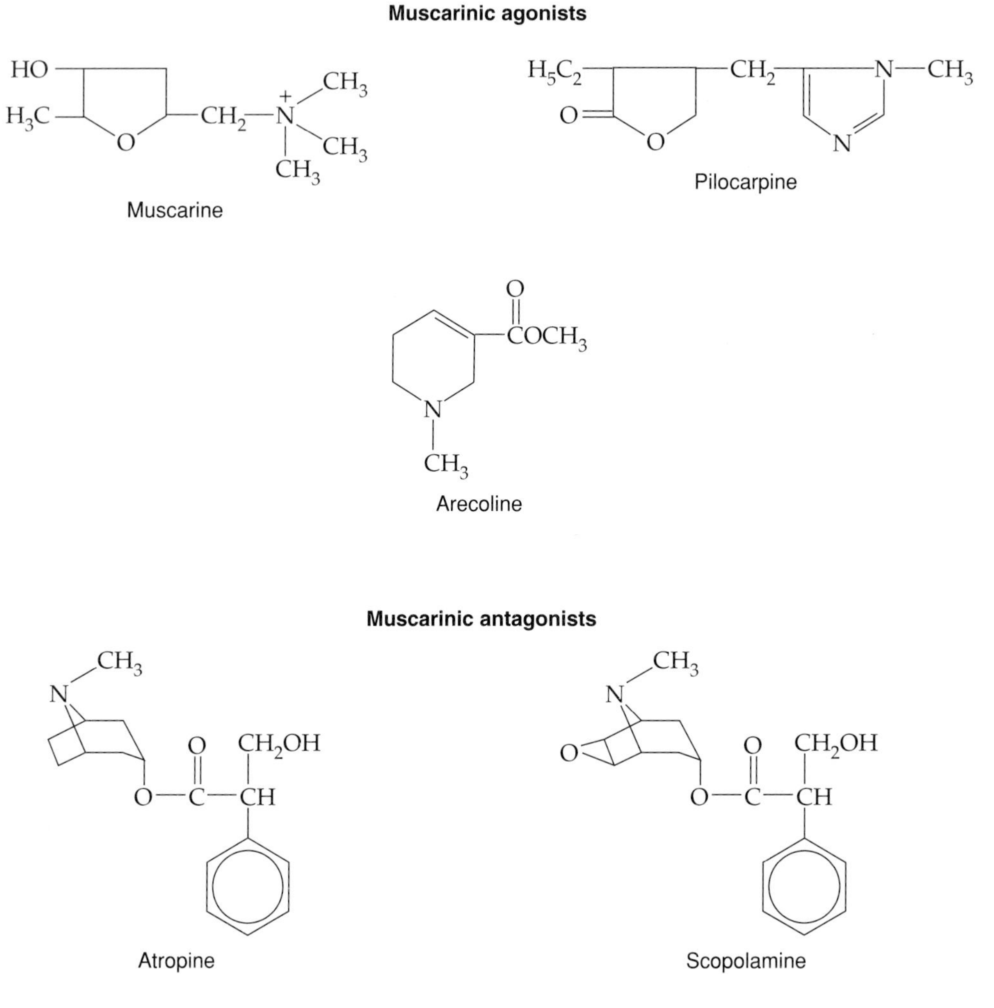

Figure 12–9. Chemical structures of representative muscarinic cholinergic agonists and antagonists.

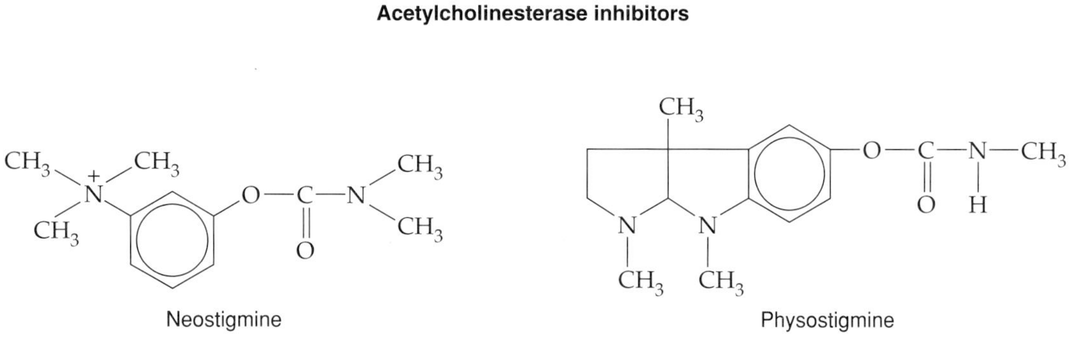

Acetylcholinesterase inhibitors

Neostigmine

Physostigmine

Figure 12–10. Chemical structures of representative acetylcholinesterase inhibitors.

nal symptoms, but for the most part have been supplanted by newer agents with fewer side effects. Regular clinical use of muscarinic antagonists occurs in ophthalmology; for example, these drugs are used in routine eye examinations to produce mydriasis. These agents also are used as adjuncts in anesthesia to reduce pharyngeal and bronchial secretions. Another common use of muscarinic cholinergic antagonists is in the treatment of **Parkinson disease** and in the management of parkinsonian side effects associated with D_2 antagonist **antipsychotic** drugs. Interestingly, the use of many psychotropic medications, including **tricyclic antidepressants** and **phenothiazine antipsychotic** agents, is limited by side effects such as blurred vision, dry mouth, and delirium that are caused by muscarinic cholinergic antagonism.

Cholinergic transmission can be enhanced not only by cholinergic receptor agonists, but also by acetylcholinesterase inhibitors. As mentioned in Chapter 9, acetylcholinesterase is the enzyme responsible for the degradation of ACh. Inhibitors of this process in current clinical use include **physostigmine, pyridostigmine, neostigmine,** and **edrophonium** (Figure 12–10). These agents are used for a variety of ophthalmic and gastrointestinal indications as well as for the treatment of **atonic bladder** and **myasthenia gravis.** Other acetylcholinesterase inhibitors, including **tacrine** and **donepezil,** are used to diminish cognitive symptoms of **Alzheimer disease,** although their effectiveness is limited (see Chapter 20).

CENTRAL CONTROL OF THE AUTONOMIC NERVOUS SYSTEM

The sympathetic and parasympathetic divisions of the autonomic nervous system are closely integrated and regulated by the central autonomic network. This network is involved in the control of visceromotor, neuroendocrine, complex motor, and pain modulating systems that ultimately are responsible for homeostasis and responses to stressors. It consists of a group of interconnected areas in the hypothalamus, midbrain, pons, and medulla that are responsible for integrating inputs from other brain areas as well as inputs from baroreceptors, chemoreceptors, and other sensory receptors in the skin, muscle, and viscera. The components of the central autonomic network include 1) the insular and medial prefrontal cortices, 2) the central nucleus of the amygdala and the bed nucleus of the stria terminalis, 3) the hypothalamus, 4) the periaqueductal gray matter in the midbrain, 5) the nucleus tractus solitarius (NTS), and 6) the medullary reticular zone (Figure 12–11).

Tight regulation of autonomic response is dependent on reciprocal connections among all components of the central autonomic network. Parallel anatomic pathways from the hypothalamus and ventral medulla to the intermediolateral cell column control the patterns of activity of preganglionic neurons.

NUCLEUS TRACTUS SOLITARIUS

The NTS is located in the dorsomedial region of the medulla, ventral to the dorsal motor nucleus of the vagus nerve. It is one of the most important structures of the brain stem component of the central autonomic network. It receives afferent taste fibers as well as visceral sensory afferent signals from the cardiovascular, respiratory, and gastrointestinal systems, which convey important information related to the control of cardiac rhythm and contractility, peripheral vascular tone, respiration, and gastrointestinal motility and secretion (Figure 12–12). Axons originating from the NTS innervate neurons of the reticular formation of the ventrolateral medulla, which in turn project to the intermediolateral cell column of the lateral horn of the spinal cord. NTS neurons also send efferent fibers to higher brain stem, hypothalamic, and limbic structures, to the vagus nerves, and to respiratory centers of the spinal cord. Reciprocal connections occur between the NTS and more rostral nuclei, including the amygdala, paraventricular nucleus, bed nucleus of the stria terminalis, periaqueductal gray matter, and raphe nuclei. The NTS also receives sensory afferents from the dorsolateral spinal cord and spinal trigeminal lemniscus, which permit the NTS to serve as a site of integration for autonomic and somatic sensory information. Thus the NTS plays a vital role in the maintenance of body homeostasis.

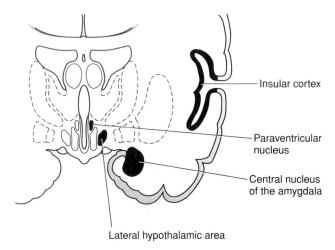

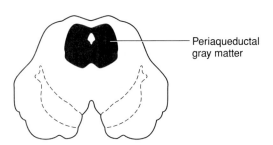

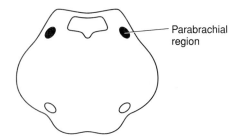

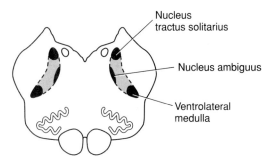

Figure 12–11. Significant areas of the central autonomic network. (Adapted with permission from Benarroch EE. 1993. *Mayo Clin Proc* 68:989.)

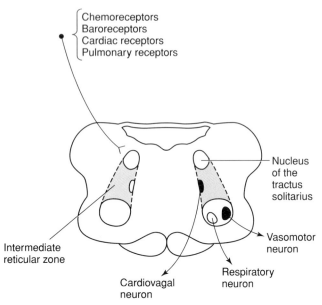

Figure 12–12. Principal areas of the medulla. Included are areas that mediate tonic and reflex control of vasomotor, cardio-vagal, and respiratory functions. (Adapted with permission from Benarroch EE. 1993. *Mayo Clin Proc* 68:989.)

HYPOTHALAMUS

The hypothalamus is the control center for the autonomic nervous system and is considered its highest level of integration. It also appears to integrate autonomic responses with the processing of emotion (see Chapter 15) and with neuroendocrine control (see Chapter 13). The hypothalamus is under the descending control of the cerebral cortex, hippocampus, and amygdala. It gains ascending visceral and somatic sensory information and receives ascending input from monoamine systems. In addition, it contains a complex network of internal connections.

Autonomic activity is initiated and regulated by the hypothalamus. Experimentally, sympathetic responses are most readily induced by stimulation in posterolateral regions, whereas parasympathetic responses are most often induced by anterior regions (Figure 12–13). Fibers from the hypothalamus descend in the lateral tegmentum of the midbrain, pons, and medulla to the intermediolateral cell column of the spinal cord. Stimulation or lesions of specific hypothalamic regions result not in isolated effects on smooth muscle, cardiac muscle, or glands but in coordinated actions involving all of these systems. Stimulation of the posterior hypothalamus, for example, may result in the conservation of body heat and in elevated body temperature caused by the constriction of cutaneous blood vessels and relative uncoupling of oxidative phosphorylation in the body's tissues. Such findings attest to the highly coordinated

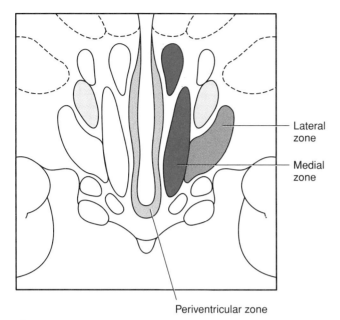

Figure 12–13. Three functional longitudinal zones of the hypothalamus. The periventricular zone controls biologic rhythms and endocrine and autonomic function. The medial zone initiates responses related to homeostasis and reproduction. The lateral zone controls arousal and motivated behavior. (Adapted with permission from Benarroch EE. 1993. *Mayo Clin Proc* 68:989.)

Lateral zone

Medial zone

Periventricular zone

nature of hypothalamic control of the autonomic nervous system.

OTHER CONTROL CENTERS

Empirical evidence indicates that other regions of the brain also assist in controlling the autonomic nervous system. Such evidence is primarily drawn from experiments involving electrophysiologic stimulation and the effects of tissue ablation on autonomic function. Autonomic responses have been obtained from several neocortical regions, including the superior frontal gyrus, the cortex of the insula, and the primary sensorimotor cortex. The specific neural pathways that mediate these responses are unknown. However, perturbation of these brain regions causes alterations in blood pressure, changes in cardiac and respiratory rates, piloerection, pupillary dilation, alterations in gastric motility, and changes in peristaltic activity, salivation, and adrenal secretion. Similarly, stimulation of the cerebellum affects heart rate and blood pressure, although a cerebellar contribution to the nerve fibers of the autonomic nervous system has not been detected. The area postrema, located in the midline dorsal surface of the caudal medulla oblongata, is involved in emetic, cardiovascular, and gustatory functions. The

locus ceruleus contains the densest aggregate of norepinephrine-containing neurons, which have efferent projections throughout the brain and spinal cord (see Chapter 8); it is involved in the control of blood pressure and neuroendocrine responses, and in the modulation of behavioral activation and attention.

DISORDERS OF THE AUTONOMIC NERVOUS SYSTEM

Autonomic dysfunction, or **dysautonomia,** occurs in a large number of diseases that involve primary disorders of either the central or peripheral nervous systems (Table 12–3 provides a classification of autonomic disorders). Such dysfunction may involve either the sympathetic nervous system or the parasympathetic nervous system, or both; thus, autonomic disorders may be localized or generalized. Because many simultaneous and diverse responses may occur as a result of sympathetic activation, a disorder that is primarily sympathetic may render the body incapable of dealing appropriately with strenuous physical or emotional stimulation. In contrast, parasympathetic dysfunction may result in more circumscribed symptoms such as bowel or sexual dysfunction. A comprehensive description of dysautonomias is beyond the scope of this text; however, a small number of illustrative examples are included in the following sections of this chapter. Some of the methods used to diagnose autonomic disorders are described in Box 12–1.

GENETIC CAUSES OF DYSAUTONOMIA

Dopamine β-hydroxylase deficiency Congenital absence of the enzyme dopamine β-hydroxylase (DBH), which converts dopamine into norepinephrine (see Chapter 8), results in sympathetic adrenergic failure, with preserved sympathetic cholinergic and parasympathetic function. The clinical syndrome consists of childhood onset of orthostatic hypotension, hypothermia, and hypoglycemia, which progresses in adulthood to marked hypotension, bilateral ptosis, decreased sweating, retrograde ejaculation, reduced vaginal secretions, and hyporeflexia.

Individuals with DBH deficiency have abnormally elevated levels of dopamine but a virtual absence of circulating norepinephrine and epinephrine. Results of parasympathetic tests of heart rate control and sympathetic cholinergic sweat tests are normal. Skin biopsies can be used to demonstrate the absence of the enzyme. **D,L-dihydroxyphenylserine** can dramatically improve the symptoms of this enzyme deficiency; converted by aromatic amino acid decarboxylase directly into

Table 12–3 Classification of Peripheral Autonomic Disorders

Acute dysautonomia
  Acute pandysautonomia
  Acute cholinergic dysautonomia
  Acute sympathetic dysautonomia

Hereditary neuropathies
  Familial amyloid polyneuropathy
  Hereditary sensory and autonomic neuropathy, type III (Riley-
    Day syndrome)
  Hereditary sensory and autonomic neuropathy, type IV
    (Swanson type)
  Dopamine-beta-hydroxylase deficiency
  Hereditary sensory and autonomic neuropathy, types I, II, and V
  Hereditary motor and sensory neuropathy, types I and II
    (Charcot-Marie-Tooth disease)
  Fabry disease
  Multiple endocrine neoplasia, type 2b (MEN 2b)
  Navajo neuropathy, type B

Inflammatory neuropathies
  Acute inflammatory polyneuritis (Guillain-Barré syndrome)
  Chronic inflammatory demyelinative polyradiculoneuropathy
    (CIDP)

Infections
  Leprosy   Diphtheria
  Human immuno-   Lyme disease
    deficiency virus (HIV)   Botulism
  Chagas disease

Metabolic disorders
  Diabetes   Chronic liver disease
  Primary amyloidosis   Vitamin B_{12} deficiency
  Acute intermittent and   Thiamine deficiency
    variegate porphyria   (Wernicke-Korsakoff
  Chronic renal failure   syndrome)

Alcohol Abuse

Disorders precipitated by cancer
  Direct infiltration of nerves   Enteric neuronopathy
  Paraneoplastic dysautonomia   Lambert-Eaton myasthenic
  Subacute sensory   syndrome
    neuronopathy

Connective tissue disorders
  Rheumatoid arthritis   Sjögren syndrome
  Systemic lupus erythematosus   Systemic sclerosis
  Mixed connective tissue disease

Inflammatory bowel disease
  Crohn disease   Ulcerative colitis

Chronic lung disease

Multiple symmetric lipomatosis (Madelung disease)

Drugs and toxins
  Vincristine   Arsenic
  Cisplatin   Inorganic mercury
  Taxol   Organic solvents
  Amiodarone   Hexacarbons
  Perhexiline   Acrylamide
  Thallium   Vacor

Central nervous system
  Parkinson disease   Brain stem tumors
  Spinal cord lesions   Multiple sclerosis
  Wernicke encephalopathy   Adie syndrome
  Cerebrovascular disease   Tabes dorsalis

From Bannister R, Mathias CJ, (editors) 1992. *Autonomic Failure,* New York:
Oxford University Press, p. 107.

noradrenaline, it bypasses the DBH step and thus restores adrenergic function (Figure 12–14).

Familial dysautonomia   Familial dysautonomia, also known as **Riley-Day syndrome** or type-II hereditary sensory neuropathy, is an autosomal recessive disease that occurs primarily in children of Jewish descent. The heterozygous parents of these children typically are asymptomatic. The disease is associated with degenerative changes in the CNS and peripheral autonomic system that commence in infancy. The main clinical features are decreased or absent lacrimation, transient skin blotching, hyperhidrosis or erratic sweating, episodes of hypertension and labile blood pressure, episodes of hyperpyrexia and vomiting, impaired taste discrimination, and relative insensitivity to pain. Areflexia, corneal insensitivity and abrasions, loss of fungiform tongue papillae, poor motor coordination, and emotional instability also occur. Poor feeding and recurring aspiration-induced pulmonary infections and dehydration are the usual causes of death during infancy and childhood. During adolescence most autonomic symptoms decrease, with the exception of postural hypotension. Early diagnosis and better management of complications have increased the life expectancy of patients with this disease.

The pathogenesis of familial dysautonomia is believed to involve the presence of abnormal neural crest cells, and in turn the abnormal development and maintenance of certain neural crest derivatives. Preganglionic neurons in the intermediolateral columns are reduced in number, as are small myelinated fibers in the ventral roots. Because reduced amounts of nerve growth factor (NGF) have been detected in cultured human fibroblasts and in the serum of patients with familial dysautonomia, investigations have attempted to determine whether the disease is linked to NGF-related defects. Changes in the levels of certain neurotransmitters also have been detected in patients with the disease. Moreover, levels of vanillylmandelic acid (VMA), a urinary norepinephrine and epinephrine metabolite, are decreased in patients with familial dysautonomia, while levels of homovanillic acid (HVA), a dopamine metabolite, are normal; thus an abnormal VMA to HVA ratio may be a sign of this disease.

Porphyria   Acute hepatic porphyrias, including **acute intermittent porphyria, variegate porphyria,** and **hereditary coproporphyria,** result from autosomal dominant defects of enzymes in heme biosynthetic pathways. Such diseases manifest as severe, acute, or subacute neuropathies that are sometimes life-threatening and are caused by excess porphyrins and porphyrin precursors (Figure 12–15). It is believed, for example, that aminolevulinic acid and porphobilinogen

Box 12–1 Evaluation of Autonomic Dysfunction

Common manifestations of autonomic dysfunction include orthostatic hypotension, cardiac dysregulation, loss of sweating, bladder or bowel dysfunction, penile impotence, and pupillary abnormalities. When autonomic neuropathy is suspected, clinical and laboratory investigations may be used to confirm its presence and to determine which pathway is involved. Initially, noninvasive tests of autonomic function are performed at a patient's bedside. Common tests involve assays of cardiovascular function, sweating, and the function of special organs such as the skin, pupils, and bladder (Table 12–4). Other screening tests measure changes in blood pressure and heart rate in response to exercise or change in posture, heart rate variation during breathing, pupillary function, and plasma norepinephrine.

Plasma norepinephrine, which originates predominantly from postganglionic sympathetic synaptic terminals, can be a crude but useful index of postganglionic sympathetic activity. Screening tests measure only the norepinephrine that has escaped enzymatic breakdown or reuptake and has diffused into the bloodstream—a small portion of the norepinephrine

released from sympathetic nerve terminals. Moreover, plasma norepinephrine levels are affected by many factors including emotion, exercise, eating, smoking, caffeine, time of day, blood volume, and hypoglycemia. In normal individuals, plasma norepinephrine increases during standing and also increases with age. Patients with neuropathies that cause postganglionic autonomic abnormalities often have subnormal levels of plasma norepinephrine. Plasma levels in patients with preganglionic failure are normal when such patients are supine but fail to undergo normal increases during standing. Plasma norepinephrine alone typically cannot be used to diagnose the site of a lesion because considerable overlap exists between preganglionic and postganglionic abnormalities in individual patients. Although quantities of norepinephrine or its metabolites in plasma or urine have long been used in the evaluation of neuropsychiatric disorders, such data are more likely to reflect peripheral sympathetic nervous system activity than CNS function (see Chapter 15).

Autonomic testing also may involve techniques that are more complex and more invasive. A patient's response to the Valsalva maneuver, measured with an intraarterial catheter, can be used to evaluate the afferent and efferent segments of the baroreflex arc. Baroreflex sensitivity can be measured as changes in blood pressure induced by pharmacologic agents that have no direct effect on heart rate. The infusion of pressor drugs such as norepinephrine usually can be used to elevate blood pressure and to slow heart rate; excessive responses indicate sensitivity caused by denervation. Other tests, which focus on specific organs, include measurement of tear production, electromyography, and gastrointestinal motility studies; pupillography also may be used to determine pupillary abnormalities.

Table 12–4 Screening Tests for Autonomic Dysfunction

Heart Rate Tests
  Response to deep breathing
  Response to standing or tilting
  Response to Valsalva maneuver

Blood Pressure Tests
  Response to standing or tilting
  Response to sustained hand grip

Sweat Test
  Sympathetic skin response

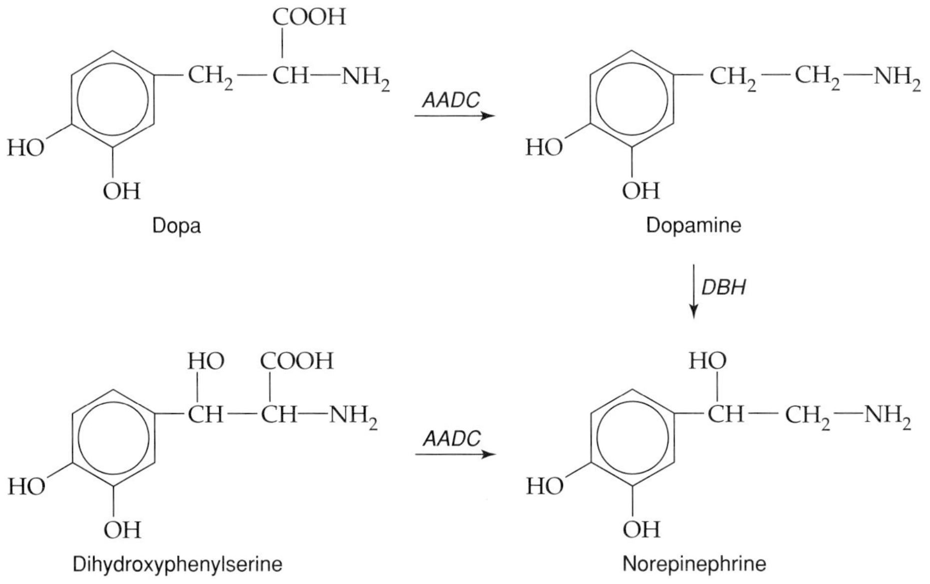

Figure 12–14. Alternative pathway for the generation of norepinephrine. Normally, dopa is converted to dopamine by the aromatic amino acid decarboxylase (AADC); subsequently dopamine is converted to norepinephrine by dopamine-β-hydroxylase (DBH) (see Chapter 8). In patients with DBH deficiency, this step can be bypassed with the administration of dihydroxyphenylserine, which is converted to norepinephrine by AADC.

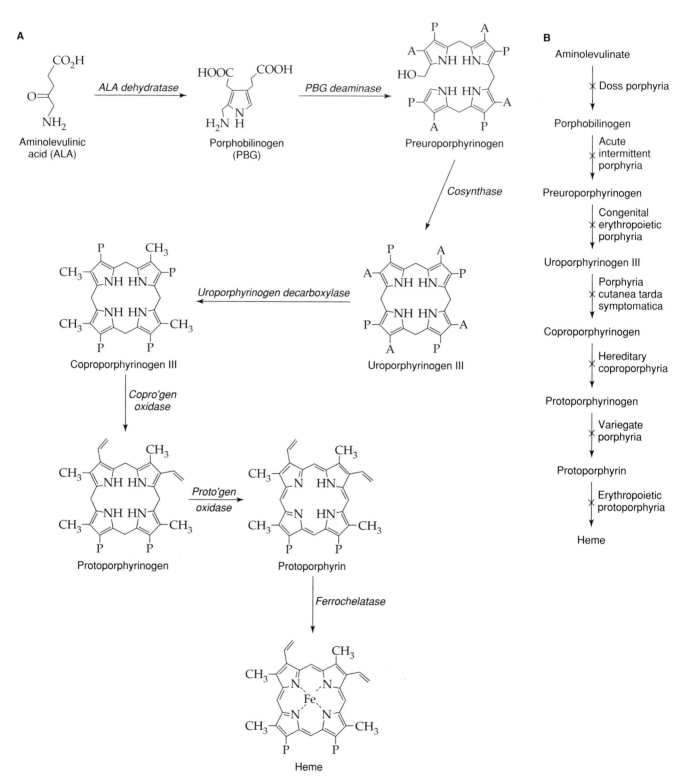

Figure 12–15. Heme biosynthetic pathways. **A.** Biosynthesis of heme from 5-aminolevulinic acid. The first three enzymes in the pathway build the macrocyclic structure, which is subsequently modified and aromatized. **B.** Porphyrias resulting from defects in any of the seven enzymes in the heme biosynthetic pathway.

are directly neurotoxic, although the molecular mechanism of such toxicity is unknown. Because heme biosynthesis is highly regulated by a variety of external factors, including drugs, hormones, nutritional status, and stress, the clinical symptoms of porphyrias can occur for hours to days in response to environmental stimuli.

Clinical presentations of porphyrias typically include peripheral neuropathy, which causes muscle weakness and autonomic dysfunction. Pathologic involvement of the autonomic nervous system can lead to acute attacks, which are characterized by abdominal pain, severe vomiting, constipation, intestinal dilation and stasis, persistent sinus tachycardia, labile hypertension, postural hypotension, hyperhidrosis, and sphincteric bladder problems. Porphyrias also are associated with CNS disturbances that result in symptoms as varied as headaches, seizures, psychosis, and delirium. Such disturbances most likely are directly related to the toxic effects of porphyrins and their precursors on neurons in the CNS.

Laboratory diagnoses of porphyrias are based on measurements of porphyrins or their precursors in urine or stool specimens or assessments of specific enzyme activities in erythrocytes. King George III is believed to have suffered from acute intermittent porphyria, based on a constellation of clinical symptoms that included bouts of madness and blue urine. The unusual color of urine results from the presence of excess porphyrins and oxidized pyrrole species. Treatment of porphyria is usually aimed at preventing acute attacks by avoiding starvation, dehydration, infection, and consumption of alcohol and precipitating medications. Treatment of acute attacks is aimed at addressing precipitating factors and managing specific symptoms individually. Intravenous **dextrose** suppresses the heme biosynthetic pathway, and β-adrenergic antagonists such as **propranolol** are helpful in treating associated hypertension and tachycardia. **Chlorpromazine** and other **phenothiazines** may be helpful in treating related abdominal and mental symptoms but have no effect on peripheral neuropathy.

SYSTEMIC DISEASES ASSOCIATED WITH AUTONOMIC DYSFUNCTION

Diabetes   Diabetes mellitus is the most common cause of autonomic neuropathy. Most studies indicate that 20–70% of individuals with diabetes exhibit abnormal autonomic function; estimates vary depending on the criteria examined. The likelihood of autonomic failure increases with the severity of hyperglycemia, the duration of the diabetes, and the age of the patient; failure also is more likely to occur in males.

The precise pathophysiologic mechanisms that underlie changes in the autonomic nervous system associated with diabetes are unknown. Proposed etiologic factors include localized endoneurial hypoxia, chronic hyperglycemia, episodic hyperglycemia, polyol accumulation, myoinositol deficiency, immune mechanisms, genetic predisposition, and impaired axonal transport. Manifestations of diabetic peripheral neuropathy are heterogeneous, but most commonly include distal sensory and sensorimotor involvement. Other clinical features include postural hypotension, impaired control of heart rate, peripheral edema, abnormal reflex vasoconstriction, impaired sweating (anhidrosis), pupillary abnormalities, esophageal and gastrointestinal motor abnormalities, diarrhea, atonic bladder, and penile impotence.

In patients with diabetes, clinical autonomic neuropathy has been associated with poor long-term prognoses and survival rates. It also is associated with an increased incidence of sudden death caused by decreased reactions to hypoglycemia, an increased incidence of silent cardiac arrest, and an increased incidence of cardiovascular complications during anesthesia. A large controlled clinical trial has indicated that long-term diabetic complications, including autonomic dysfunction, are delayed and slowed in response to tight glucose control. In addition, a number of trials have shown that **aldose reductase inhibitors** offer a slight benefit in halting or slowing the progression of neuropathy.

Vitamin B₁₂ deficiency   Vitamin B_{12} comprises a porphyrin ring and a central cobalt atom (Figure 12–16). It is not synthesized by animals or plants and thus must be derived microbially from meat, eggs, and dairy products. Vitamin B_{12} deficiency can cause severe pathologic and physiologic changes in several organs and degenerative changes in the peripheral (somatic and autonomic) and central nervous systems. Common symptoms include orthostatic hypotension, paresthesias of hands and feet, altered vibratory sensations, and confusional states. Like **thiamine deficiency,** vitamin B_{12} deficiency often is associated with **alcoholism,** a disease with which it produces synergistic damage both peripherally and centrally.

Toxin- or drug-induced neuropathies   Autonomic dysfunction occurs in some individuals exposed to environmental and pharmacologic toxins. Such dysfunction is best documented in association with exposure to organic solvents such as **carbon disulfide** and **heavy metals**. Workers exposed to aliphatic, aromatic, or other **hydrocarbons,** or to **alcohols, ketones, esters,** or **ethers** typically exhibit altered autonomic function. Industrial exposure to **acrylamide** has caused peripheral sensory

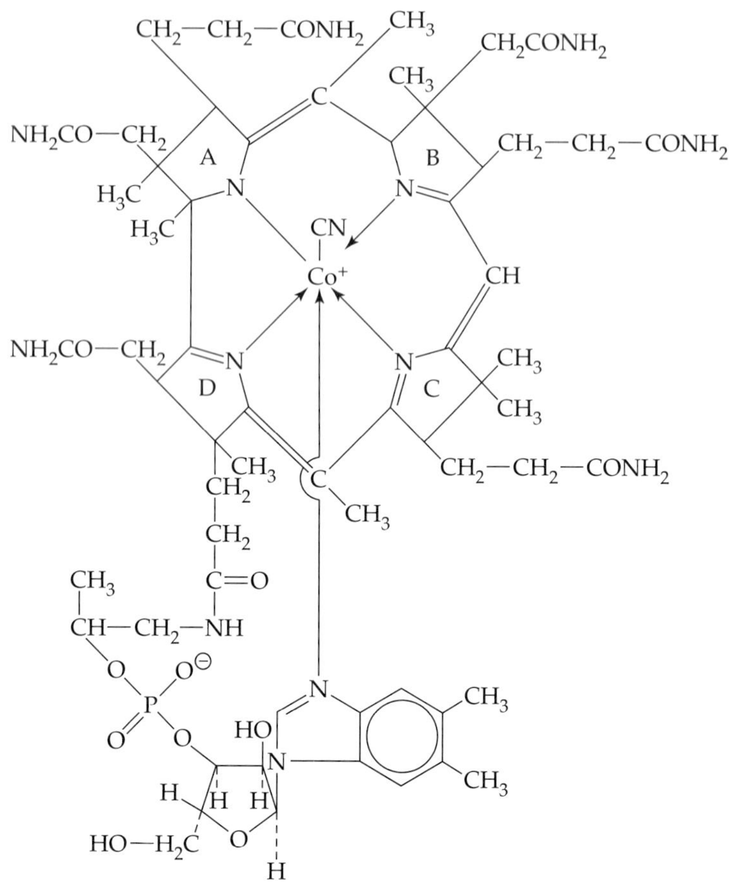

Figure 12–16. Structure of cyanocobalamin, or vitamin B_{12}.

polyneuropathy, which often is preceded by blue skin color and excessive sweating of the extremities. **Arsenic** also produces abnormal extremity sweating. **Mercury** poisoning, which is most common in children, leads to acrodynia, which is characterized by hypertension, tachycardia, and pain and redness of the fingers, toes, and ears. Acrodynia is effectively treated with **ganglionic blocking agents.** Ingestion of **vacor** (*N*-3-pyridylmethyl-*N'*-*p*-nitrophenylurea), a rat poison that antagonizes nicotinamide metabolism, results in acute hyperglycemic ketoacidosis and a combined somatic and autonomic neuropathy.

Some commonly used chemotherapeutic agents also cause a dose-dependent and cumulative effect on autonomic function. **Vincristine,** a natural product of vinca alkaloids used to treat lymphoma, leukemia, and other cancers, has limited applications because of its neurotoxic effects. Autonomic symptoms associated with its use include postural hypotension, constipation, abdominal pain, paralytic ileus, and urinary retention. Some evidence suggests that unmyelinated fibers are more susceptible than myelinated fibers to neurotoxic damage associated with vincristine. **Cisplatin,** a nonspecific cytotoxic agent that inhibits the cell cycle, causes ototoxicity, retrobulbar neuritis, and peripheral neuropathy.

Guillain-Barré syndrome This acute-onset, predominantly motor neuropathy commonly involves autonomic hypoactivity or hyperactivity. Approximately 65% of patients with Guillain-Barré syndrome have some dysautonomia, which is attributed to demyelination of the glossopharyngeal and vagus nerves and of the preganglionic fibers of the sympathetic nervous system. Afferent baroreflex abnormalities in individuals with this syndrome can cause intermittent episodes of orthostatic hypotension, and abrupt fluctuations in blood pressure may precede fatal arrhythmias. Adynamic ileus and atonic bladder also are symptoms of this syndrome. Many cases of Guillain-Barré syndrome occur in the context of a viral infection or occasionally after immunizations, and are thought to be mediated by an autoimmune mechanism. In most patients, the syndrome is self-limited and resolves spontaneously over time.

Acute pandysautonomia Acute panautonomic neuropathy, or acute pandysautonomia, is a rare and

Box 12–2 Lambert-Eaton Myasthenic Syndrome

The Lambert-Eaton myasthenic syndrome (LEMS) is one of the best understood paraneoplastic dysautonomias. It is an acquired disorder of neuromuscular transmission that is associated with a reduction in presynaptic quantal release of acetylcholine in the peripheral nervous system, including autonomic ganglia. More than half of all cases of LEMS occur in patients with small-cell lung cancer or other cancers, and involve antibodies that cross-react with voltage-gated Ca^{2+} channels and tumor-specific epitopes. LEMS frequently is associated with dry mouth, impotence, constipation, blurred vision, and impaired sweating. Some patients also may have orthostatic lightheadedness, difficulty with micturition, or tonic pupils. Approximately half of all patients demonstrate cholinergic and adrenergic hypersensitivity of the pupils when tested. Tear production also may be reduced. Variations in heart rate and blood pressure may occur in response to Valsalva maneuver or deep breathing.

Treatment of the underlying tumor substantially improves autonomic function. In patients who do not have an underlying malignancy, treatment is directed toward enhancing cholinergic function and immunosuppression. The enhancement of neuromuscular transmission is achieved most readily with the use of **acetylcholinesterase inhibitors,** which increase levels of acetylcholine at the neuromuscular junction and in autonomic ganglia (see Chapter 9). Indeed, a rapid diagnostic test for LEMS consists of determining whether a short-acting acetylcholinesterase inhibitor improves neuromuscular function. **Guanidine** increases the number of acetylcholine quanta released by increasing the duration of action potentials at the motor nerve terminal. Other agents that have been used to enhance the efficacy of transmission, such as **guanidine hydrochloride, 4-aminopyridine,** and **3,4-diaminopyridine,** lead to a reduction in voltage-dependent potassium conductances and thereby produce prolonged depolarizations (see Chapter 3). Such actions increase Ca^{2+} influx and in turn increase the quantal release of acetylcholine.

usually self-limiting syndrome, which is characterized by concomitant and widespread involvement of sympathetic and parasympathetic components of the autonomic nervous system but limited damage to somatic nerve fibers. Symptoms evolve over a few days to a few months in previously healthy individuals of all ages and both sexes. The disease most likely is mediated by the immune system and may involve a mechanism similar to Guillain-Barré syndrome. Affected individuals typically experience orthostatic hypotension, anhidrosis, cold or heat intolerance, reduced lacrimation and salivation, bowel disturbances (ileus, abdominal colic, diarrhea, and constipation), atonic bladder, impotence, and a fixed heart rate. Pure cholinergic neuropathy, which affects only postganglionic cholinergic neurons, most likely is a restricted expression of acute panautonomic neuropathy; it produces a markedly similar clinical picture, except that it does not result in orthostatic hypotension. No effective treatment for these conditions exists other than supportive therapy. Recovery usually is prolonged and incomplete.

OTHER AUTONOMIC SYNDROMES

Many diseases in addition to those previously discussed have been associated with autonomic dysfunction. **Paraneoplastic syndromes,** for example, involve antibodies generated against tumor-specific epitopes that cross-react with normal proteins expressed by neurons and damage those neurons. Such syndromes commonly affect cancer patients (see Box 12–2 for a discussion of the **Lambert-Eaton myasthenic syndrome**). Autonomic dysfunction also occurs in the context of certain pain syndromes, such as **causalgia** and **reflex sympathetic dystrophy,** which are discussed in Chapter 19.

EXPERIMENTAL MODELS OF AUTONOMIC NEUROPATHY

Dysautonomia has been investigated in animals with experimental forms of various diseases. Animal models of diabetes mellitus involving genetically diabetic animals or animals treated with pancreatic islet β-cell toxins such as **streptozin** and **alloxan** have exhibited impaired autonomic control of the heart, blood vessels, alimentary canal, and urinary bladder. Animals with **acrylamide**-induced neuropathy have been used to study previously mentioned toxic and nutritional neuropathies, such as those caused by alcoholism.

Experimental allergic neuritis has been induced in animals to create models of Guillain-Barré syndrome. Such models, which have been produced with injections of peripheral nerve tissue and adjuvants, closely resemble acute idiopathic polyneuritis in humans. The animal model is characterized by demyelination and axonal degeneration, and impaired control of heart rate caused by immune cell infiltrates in splanchnic and sympathetic nerves. Affected animals experience limb weakness and urinary and fecal incontinence.

Experimental sympathectomy has been achieved with **6-hydroxydopamine, guanethidine,** and antibodies to NGF or acetylcholinesterase. These agents, administered peripherally, selectively affect postganglionic sympathetic neurons but exert little or no effect on the parasympathetic nervous system or on enteric or peripheral nerves. Affected animals exhibit a shortened life span, decreased weight gain, low blood pressure, ptosis, and diarrhea.

SELECTED READING

Backonja MM. 1994. Reflex sympathetic dystrophy/sympathetically maintained pain/causalgia: The syndrome of neuropathic pain with dysautonomia. *Semin Neurol* 14: 263–271.

Bannister R, Mathias CJ (eds). 1992. *Autonomic Failure.* New York: Oxford University Press.

Barajas-Lopez C, Huizinga JD. 1993. New transmitters and new targets in the autonomic nervous system. *Curr Opin Neurobiol* 3:1020–1027.

Benarroch EE. 1993. The central autonomic network: Functional organization, dysfunction, and perspective. *Mayo Clin Proc* 68:989–1001.

Biaggioni I, Goldstein DS, Atkinson T, Robertson D. 1990. Dopamine-beta-hydroxylase deficiency in humans. *Neurology* 40:370–373.

Carpenter MB. 1972. *Core Text of Neuroanatomy.* Baltimore: Williams and Wilkins.

Fernandez A, Hontebeyrie M, Said G. 1992. Autonomic neuropathy and immunological abnormalities in Chagas' disease. *Clin Auton Res* 2:409–412.

Freeman R, Cohen JA. 1993. Autonomic failure and AIDS. In Low PA (ed): *Clinical Autonomic Disorders,* pp. 677–683. Boston: Little Brown.

Freeman R, Miyawaki E. 1993. The treatment of autonomic dysfunction. *J Clin Neurophysiol* 10:61–82.

Gibbins IL, Jobling P, Messenger JP, et al. 2000. Neuronal morphology and the synaptic organisation of sympathetic ganglia. *J Autonomic Nerv Sys* 81:104–109.

Hoffman BB, Lefkowitz RJ, Taylor P. 1996. Neurotransmission: The autonomic and somatic motor nervous systems. In Hardman JG, Limbird LE, Molinoff PB, et al (eds): *Goodman and Gilman's The Pharmacological Basis of Therapeutics,* 9th ed, pp 105–139. New York: McGraw-Hill.

Holmgren G, Ericzon BG, Groth CG, et al. 1993. Clinical improvement and amyloid regression after liver transplantation in hereditary transthyretin amyloidosis. *Lancet* 341: 1113–1116.

Hugdahl K. 1996. Cognitive influences on human autonomic nervous system function. *Curr Opin Neurobiol* 6:252–258.

Khurana RK. 1993. Paraneoplastic autoimmune dysfunction. In Low PA (ed): *Clinical Autonomic Disorders,* pp. 505–516. Boston: Little Brown.

Low PA. 1993. *Clinical Autonomic Disorders: Evaluation and Management.* Rochester, MN: Mayo Foundation.

Matikainen E, Juntunen J. 1985. Autonomic nervous system dysfunction in workers exposed to organic solvents. *J Neurol Neurosurg Psychiatry* 32:297–304.

McCombe PA, McLeod JG. 1984. The peripheral neuropathy of vitamin B12 deficiency. *J Neurol Sci* 66:117–126.

McDougall AJ, McLeod JG. 1996. Autonomic neuropathy. I. Clinical features, investigation, pathophysiology, and treatment. *J Neurol Sci* 137:79–88.

McDougall AJ, McLeod JG. 1996. Autonomic neuropathy. II. Specific peripheral neuropathies. *J Neurol Sci* 138:1–13.

McLeod JG, Tuck RR. 1987. Disorders of the autonomic nervous system: Part 2. Investigation and treatment. *Ann Neurol* 21:519–529.

Oh SJ, Dropcho EJ, GC Claussen. 1997. Anti-Hu-associated paraneoplastic sensory neuropathy responding to early aggressive immunotherapy: Report of two cases and review of literature. *Muscle Nerve* 20:1576–1582.

Pascuzzi RM, Kim YI. 1990. Lambert-Eaton syndrome. *Semin Neurol* 10:35–41.

Polinsky RJ. 1996. Biochemical and pharmacologic assessment of autonomic function. *Adv Neurol* 69:373–376.

Pourmand R. 1997. Diabetic neuropathy. *Neurol Clin* 15:569–76.

Rostami AM. 1993. Pathogenesis of immune-mediated neuropathies. *Pediatr Res* 33(suppl):S90–94.

Rubino FA. 1992. Neurologic complications of alcoholism. *Psychiatr Clin North Am* 15:359–372.

Schatz IJ, Low PA, Polinsky RJ. 1997. Disorders of the autonomic nervous system. *N Engl J Med* 337:278–280.

Tefferi A, Colgan JP, Solberg LA. 1994. Acute porphyrias: Diagnosis and management. *Mayo Clin Proc* 69:991–995.

Warren MJ, Jay M, Hunt DM, et al. 1996. The maddening business of King George III and porphyria. *Trends Biochem Sci* 21:229–232.

Chapter 13

Neuroendocrine Control of the Internal Milieu

KEY CONCEPTS

- Hormones are signaling molecules that reach their target cells via the bloodstream.

- The three major classes of hormones are peptides, small neurotransmitter-like molecules such as epinephrine (adrenaline), and steroids.

- Neuroendocrine regions of the hypothalamus play the key role in the brain's regulation of endocrine systems.

- The hypothalamus interacts closely with the pituitary gland, which in humans has two divisions. The posterior division, or neurohypophysis, contains axon terminals from the hypothalamus, and the anterior division, or adenohypophysis, is composed of endocrine cells.

- The hypothalamic–neurohypophyseal system secretes two peptide hormones, arginine vasopressin and oxytocin.

- In the adenohypophyseal system, peptide releasing factors, synthesized in hypothalamic neurons, are transported to nerve terminals in the median eminence, where they are released into the hypophyseal-portal circulation, which drains into the blood vessels of the anterior pituitary.

- Hypothalamic releasing factors stimulate or inhibit the release of anterior pituitary hormones into the systemic circulation.

- The hypothalamic–pituitary–adrenal axis is critical for stress responses. It comprises corticotropin-releasing factor, released by the hypothalamus;

adrenocorticotropic hormone, released by the anterior pituitary; and cortisol, released by the adrenal cortex.

- The hypothalamic–pituitary–thyroid axis consists of hypothalamic neurons that release thyrotropin-releasing hormone; the anterior pituitary hormone thyroid-stimulating hormone, also known as thyrotropin; and thyroid hormones T_3 and T_4.

- The hypothalamic–pituitary–gonadal axis comprises hypothalamic gonadotropin-releasing hormone, the anterior pituitary hormones, luteinizing hormone and follicle-stimulating hormone, and the gonadal steroids.

- Prolactin is synthesized and released by lactotrophs of the anterior pituitary gland and triggers lactation in females; it is under the inhibitory control of D_2 dopamine receptors.

- Growth hormone is released by the somatotrophs of the anterior pituitary; it is under the stimulatory control of growth hormone-releasing hormone and the inhibitory control of somatostatin.

- The hypothalamus contains a complex network of peptide-releasing cells involved in the regulation of energy balance, which involves the control of both food intake and energy expenditure.

- Leptin, the product of the *ob* gene, is released by adipocytes and is involved in regulating the long-term state of the body's energy reserves via its actions on the hypothalamus.

The brain controls bodily function and behavior through the motor system (see Chapter 14), the autonomic nervous system (see Chapter 12), and hormones released by neuroendocrine neurons. Hormones are signaling molecules that reach their target cells by means of the bloodstream. They comprise three major classes: peptides, neurotransmitter-like small molecules such as epinephrine, and steroid-like signals. Through the systematic control of these critical hormones, the brain maintains homeostasis, regulates growth and maturation, and permits the body to respond to environmental stressors, illness, and injury.

the periphery is required not only for responses to changes in the environment but also for the inhibition of subsequent neuroendocrine release and other appropriate feedback control.

The hippocampus, amygdala, and septum, all of which are involved in processing the salience of environmental events (see Chapters 15 and 16), provide substantial input to the hypothalamus. Such connections enable adaptive responses; for example, they allow the hypothalamus to alter hormonal release and autonomic output in response to a perceived threat. Communication between these regions and the hypothalamus is largely reciprocal; thus the hippocampus,

NEUROENDOCRINE HYPOTHALAMUS

AFFERENT SIGNALS

The synthesis and release of hormones occurs primarily in the neuroendocrine regions of the hypothalamus. Despite its small size, the hypothalamus has an extremely complex architecture that permits the processing of information from both the internal milieu and external environment. Located at the base of the diencephalon, it receives information about the external environment from higher brain centers, messages about the state of the body from brain stem nuclei that relay information gathered from peripheral sensory neurons, and input from the ascending noradrenergic, serotonergic, and cholinergic signals described in Chapters 8 and 9. The hypothalamus also receives nociceptive information directly from the dorsal horn of the spinal cord. In addition to such neural input, it gains information about the state of the internal milieu from thermoreceptors, osmoreceptors, and glucoreceptors.

Hypothalamic neurons also receive direct or indirect input from peptide hormones and cytokines circulating in the bloodstream. Peptides normally do not cross the blood–brain barrier, but may gain access to the brain in regions where the barrier is incomplete—for example, at the median eminence at the base of the hypothalamus, or near circumventricular organs, where the tight junctions of the blood–brain barrier give way to fenestrated capillaries that permit sampling of peripheral blood (see Chapter 2). In addition, receptors for cytokines (see Chapter 11) have been found on cerebral endothelial cells, which may respond to cytokine binding by releasing prostaglandins or other lipophilic signals. Because they are lipophilic, circulating steroid hormones may cross directly into the brain and bind receptors in the hypothalamus or may bind in brain regions, such as the hippocampus, which send substantial projections to the hypothalamus. Information from

Neurotransmitter

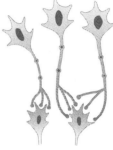

Neuroendocrine

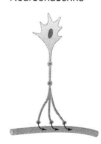

Endocrine

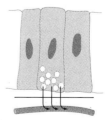

Figure 13–1. Types of secretion. Neurons secrete neurotransmitter into the synaptic space. Neuroendocrine neurons secrete hormones into the bloodstream through axon terminals embedded in capillaries. Endocrine cells secrete hormones into the bloodstream without the use of specialized terminals.

amygdala, and septum also receive input from the hypothalamus, which most likely permits information about the internal milieu to affect cognition and behavior. Accordingly, altered glucose metabolism and a trip to the refrigerator often go hand in hand. In addition to the many types of afferent signals directed toward the hypothalamus, there are extensive intrahypothalamic connections, which presumably are involved in coordinating the many hormonal and autonomic outputs of this brain region.

EFFERENT SIGNALS

The output of the neuroendocrine hypothalamus consists primarily of peptide hormones released into the circulation. Neuroendocrine neurons are specialized for the purpose of transducing neural signals into hormonal signals; in response to depolarization, they release peptides into the bloodstream by means of axons that terminate on capillaries rather than at synapses (Figure 13–1). Such peptides are considered hormones because, like all hormones, they travel in the bloodstream to influence a target distant from their point of release. Yet many of these same peptides are considered neurotransmitters when they are released from other neurons in the brain and diffuse across synapses or into the extracellular fluid of the brain until they bind receptors or are catabolized.

ORGANIZATION OF THE HYPOTHALAMIC–PITUITARY UNIT

The hypothalamus and pituitary gland may be seen as an interacting unit (Figure 13–2). In humans the pituitary has two divisions: the neurohypophysis or posterior pituitary, which contains axon terminals of some hypothalamic neurons, and the adenohypophysis or anterior pituitary, which is primarily composed of nonneuronal endocrine cells. Rodents also possess an intermediate lobe of the pituitary gland.

In the neurohypophyseal system, peptide hormones are synthesized in hypothalamic neurons and transported to capillary-associated nerve terminals in the posterior pituitary, where they are released directly into the systemic circulation. In the adenohypophyseal system, peptide releasing factors (Table 13–1), which are synthesized in hypothalamic neurons, are transported to nerve terminals in the median eminence; when the hypothalamic neurons are stimulated, peptide hormones are released into the hypophyseal–portal circulation, which drains into the blood vessels of the anterior pituitary. Such peptides act to stimulate or inhibit the release of anterior pituitary hormones into the systemic circulation (see Table 13–1). After reaching their targets, pituitary hormones cause the release of additional hormones, which subsequently act on diverse tissues of the body. Hypothalamic releasing factors that cause

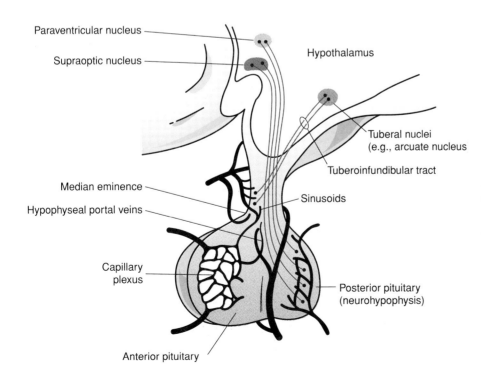

Paraventricular nucleus

Supraoptic nucleus

Hypothalamus

Tuberal nuclei (e.g., arcuate nucleus)

Tuberoinfundibular tract

Median eminence

Sinusoids

Hypophyseal portal veins

Capillary plexus

Posterior pituitary (neurohypophysis)

Anterior pituitary

Figure 13–2. Interrelationship of the hypothalamus and the pituitary gland. The anterior pituitary, or adenohypophysis, receives rich blood flow from the capillaries of the hypophyseal portal system. This system delivers releasing factors to the median eminence by means of hypothalamic neurons, such as those in the tuberal (arcuate) nuclei by means of the tuberoinfundibular tract. The posterior pituitary, or neurohypophysis, contains axon terminals of neurons projecting from the paraventricular and supraoptic nuclei of the hypothalamus.

Table 13-1 Hypothalamic Releasing Factors and Pituitary Hormones

Anterior Pituitary Hormone	Corresponding Hypothalamic Releasing Factors
Proopiomelanocortin products Adrenocorticotropic hormone (ACTH) α-Melanocyte stimulating hormone (α-MSH) β-Endorphin	Corticotropin releasing factor (CRF) (+)
Thyroid stimulating hormone (TSH)	Thyrotropin releasing hormone (TRH) (+) Somatostatin (−)
Luteinizing hormone (LH) Follicle-stimulating hormone (FSH)	Gonadotropin releasing hormone (GnRH) (+)
Growth hormone (GH)	Growth hormone releasing hormone (GHRH) (+) Somatostatin (−)
Prolactin (PRL)	TRH (+) Dopamine (−)

+, Stimulates release; −, inhibits release.

pituitary hormone release also have trophic influences on anterior pituitary cells; likewise, hormones of the anterior pituitary gland have trophic influences on their targets. Thus, hypersecretion of a hormone can lead to hypertrophy or hyperplasia of target endocrine cells, whereas the absence of a hormone can lead to the atrophy of such cells.

HYPOTHALAMIC–NEUROHYPOPHYSEAL SYSTEM

The hypothalamic–neurohypophyseal system secretes two major peptide hormones: arginine vasopressin (AVP), also known as antidiuretic hormone (ADH), and oxytocin. AVP and oxytocin are synthesized in distinct magnocellular neurons of the paraventricular nucleus (PVN) and supraoptic nucleus (SON) of the hypothalamus, respectively, and are carried by axoplasmic flow to nerve endings in the posterior pituitary. AVP also is synthesized in a distinct subset of PVN neurons; AVP from these cells influences anterior pituitary function, as described in the section of this chapter devoted to corticotropin-releasing factor. Like most peptide transmitters (see Chapter 10), AVP and oxytocin are derived from large precursor proteins, which are cleaved to form active peptides. Associated cleavage events also produce carrier proteins, or neurophysins, which are co-released with the peptides.

ARGININE VASOPRESSIN

Release of neurohypophyseal AVP occurs in response to inputs from the central and peripheral nervous systems that are responsible for monitoring both osmotic conditions and blood pressure. Action potentials generated within AVP-secreting neurons lead to depolarization and release by exocytosis into the systemic circulation at capillaries of the posterior pituitary. Stimuli such as pain, psychogenic stress, and exercise can lead to posterior pituitary AVP release. The primary peripheral action of AVP occurs at the distal nephron within the kidney, where it increases reabsorption of water across the collecting duct epithelium. Many drugs can interfere with AVP action. **Lithium** (Chapter 15) interferes with AVP in the kidney, possibly through the inhibition of adenylyl cyclase (renal AVP receptors signal through the cAMP pathway); such interference results in increased urine flow and may lead to nephrogenic **diabetes insipidus,** which is defined as the production of more than 3 liters of urine per day. Other drugs, including **nicotine** when taken in high doses, may cause a syndrome of inappropriate ADH secretion (**SIADH**), which results in water retention and can lead to seizure-producing **dilutional hyponatremia**.

AVP also influences the anterior pituitary gland and assumes other functions in the brain (Box 13–1).

OXYTOCIN

Oxytocin acts during parturition to cause uterine contractions. Synthetic forms of this hormone are used to induce labor. Oxytocin also mediates milk letdown in lactating mothers. Nipple stimulation causes oxytocin release, which in turn causes the myoepithelial cells of the nipple to contract, resulting in the ejection of milk. The release of oxytocin is subject to classical conditioning; thus a lactating mother may experience milk letdown in response to the cry of a baby.

Box 13–1 Vasopressin and Affiliative Behavior

A large body of research has implicated arginine vaso-pressin (AVP) and its V_{1a} receptor in the regulation of affil-iative behavior. It appears that species differences in the promoter of the V_{1a} receptor gene result in markedly dif-ferent patterns of receptor expression in the brain, which in turn lead to variations in behavioral responses to vaso-pressin. Indeed, V_{1a} receptor patterns affect male repro-ductive and social behavior in several rodent species, most notably in two types of voles. The male montane vole, whose V_{1a} receptor pattern is similar to that found in mice and most other rodents, tends to be asocial and promiscuous. In contrast, the male prairie vole, which exhibits more exten-

sive V_{1a} receptor expression in the brain, is highly social and monogamous. Studies of mice have provided direct evidence that such differences in V_{1a} receptor expression affect affiliative behavior. Transgenic mice that express the prairie vole V_{1a} receptor show prairie vole-like patterns of V_{1a} receptor distribution superimposed on their normal, endogenous expression of V_{1a} receptors. Such mice respond to vasopressin administration with an increase in affiliative behavior, whereas control mice do not exhibit this response. Thus it appears that the pattern of V_{1a} receptor expression in brain can mediate significant effects of AVP on affiliative behavior in some mammalian species.

HYPOTHALAMIC–PITUITARY–ADRENAL AXIS

The hypothalamic–pituitary–adrenal (HPA) axis (Figure 13–3) comprises a cascade of hormones involved in the stress response. These hormones include corticotropin releasing factor (CRF), a releasing hormone produced by the hypothalamus; adrenocorticotropic hormone (ACTH), a hormone produced by the anterior lobe of

the pituitary; and **cortisol** (corticosterone in the rat), a peripheral hormone secreted by the adrenal cortex. Basal release of CRF is controlled partly by the circa-dian pacemaker, located in the suprachiasmatic nucleus of the hypothalamus in mammals (see Chapter 18). Maximum secretion of this hormone occurs in the morn-ing in humans near the time of waking; maximum secre-tion in rodents, which are nocturnal, typically occurs in

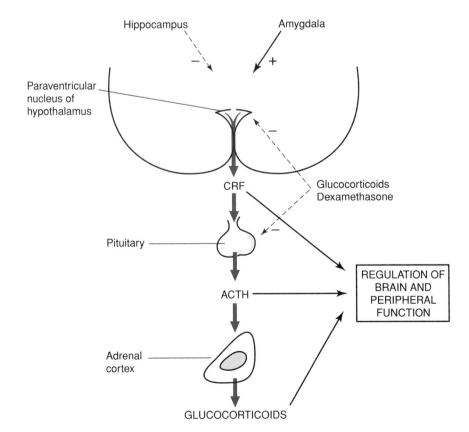

Figure 13–3. The hypothalamic–pituitary–adrenal axis. Corticotropin releasing factor (CRF) and arginine vasopressin are released from parvo-cellular neurons of the paraventricular nucleus of the hypothalamus into the hypophyseal portal system and act on the corticotrophs of the anterior pituitary to cause release of adrenocorticotropic hormone (ACTH). ACTH reaches the adrenal cortex by means of the bloodstream, where it stimulates the release of glucocorticoids. In addition to their diverse functions, glucocorticoids, including synthetic forms such as dexamethasone, repress CRF and ACTH synthesis and release. In this manner, glucocorticoids inhibit their own synthesis.

the early evening. Superimposed on normal circadian variation in CRF release is release precipitated by a variety of stressors both psychologic (e.g., an academic test) and physiologic (e.g., starvation, hypothermia, or inflammation). Stressors also stimulate release of AVP by PVN neurons. Like CRF, AVP is a secretagogue for ACTH. ACTH triggers cortisol release from the adrenal gland, which alters energy metabolism and other functions to prepare an organism to cope with a perceived crisis.

A complex array of afferent stress-related signals is integrated in the parvocellular neurons of the PVN, where they act to stimulate or inhibit CRF and AVP secretion. As previously mentioned, these signals include inhibitory inputs from the hippocampus and excitatory inputs from the amygdala (see Figure 13–3). Noradrenergic afferent signals from the brain stem, such as those from the locus ceruleus, are believed to play a particularly important role in conveying stress-related information to the PVN; however, serotonergic, cholinergic, and other types of input also contribute to this process. Parvocellular (small) neurons of the PVN, which synthesize and secrete both CRF and AVP, are distinct from magnocellular (large) neurons, which secrete AVP into the systemic circulation by means of the posterior pituitary. CRF and AVP are incorporated into the same secretory granules and are co-released in the capillaries of the median eminence. The role of the HPA axis in **stress** and **depression** is discussed in Chapter 15.

CORTICOTROPIN-RELEASING FACTOR AND ITS RECEPTORS

The biologic effects of CRF are mediated by two distinct G protein-coupled receptors, called CRF_1R and CRF_2R. CRF_1R is expressed in the pituitary gland, cerebral cortex, medial septum, cerebellum, and brain stem. CRF_2R is expressed in the hypothalamus and medial septum in the brain, but is expressed more widely outside the brain. In all of its locations, it binds not only CRF but also a closely related peptide known as **urocortin**. Because the affinity with which CRF_2R binds urocortin is 40 times greater than the affinity with which it binds CRF, it is believed that urocortin may be the endogenous ligand of CRF_2R. Knockout mice lacking CRF_1R have normal basal levels of ACTH but cannot mount a significant ACTH response to restraint stress. Mice lacking CRF_2R are, in contrast, hyperresponsive to stress, with ACTH and cortisol elevations occurring more rapidly than in wildtype mice.

CRF plays a major role not only in neuroendocrine (pituitary) responses to stress, but also in behavioral responses, such as anxiety, that may be related to stress. CRF_1R knockout mice display markedly reduced anxiety-like behaviors compared with controls in tests of anxiety such as the elevated plus maze (see Chapter 15). Such mice also exhibit low levels of corticosterone; however, normalization of corticosterone levels by means of external supplementation does not restore normal anxiety responses. This finding suggests that the reduction in anxiety seen in these mice is not mediated by changes in circulating glucocorticoids; rather, it reflects a reduction of CRF function in the CNS. Indeed, in normal animals, intracerebral administration of CRF into brain regions such as the amygdala stimulates anxiety-like behavior, whereas administration of CRF_1R antagonists exerts the opposite effect. Other converging evidence also indicates that CRF and CRF_1R play critical roles in anxiety states. Consequently, CRF_1R antagonists are being tested in clinical trials as potential **anxiolytics** (anti-anxiety agents) and **antidepressants** (see Chapter 15). As discussed in Chapter 16, CRF also may be involved in aversive symptoms associated with withdrawal from drugs of abuse.

ACTH AND GLUCOCORTICOIDS

CRF and AVP promote the secretion of ACTH through their actions on the corticotrophs of the anterior pituitary gland. The processing of ACTH, which is a product of the proopiomelanocortin (POMC) gene, is described in detail in Chapter 10. ACTH released into the systemic circulation stimulates the adrenal cortex—through high-affinity G_s-coupled ACTH receptors—to synthesize and secrete adrenal glucocorticoids, including **cortisol,** the most important of these steroids in humans, and **corticosterone,** the most significant steroid in rodents. A cAMP-mediated intracellular signal maintains adrenal steroidogenesis by controlling transcription of the major enzymes in the steroid synthetic pathway. Most secreted cortisol becomes associated with one of three carrier proteins: corticosteroid-binding-globulin, transcortin, or albumin. Free cortisol, which is biologically active, represents less than 5% of circulating cortisol. ACTH also stimulates the secretion of other adrenocortical steroids, including **aldosterone,** 17α-hydroxyprogesterone, and adrenal androgens.

GLUCOCORTICOID SYNTHESIS

Dietary **cholesterol** is the primary component in the biosynthesis of glucocorticoids and other adrenal steroids (Figure 13–4). Uptake of cholesterol by the adrenal cortex is mediated by low-density lipoprotein (LDL) receptors. Cholesterol enters one of three

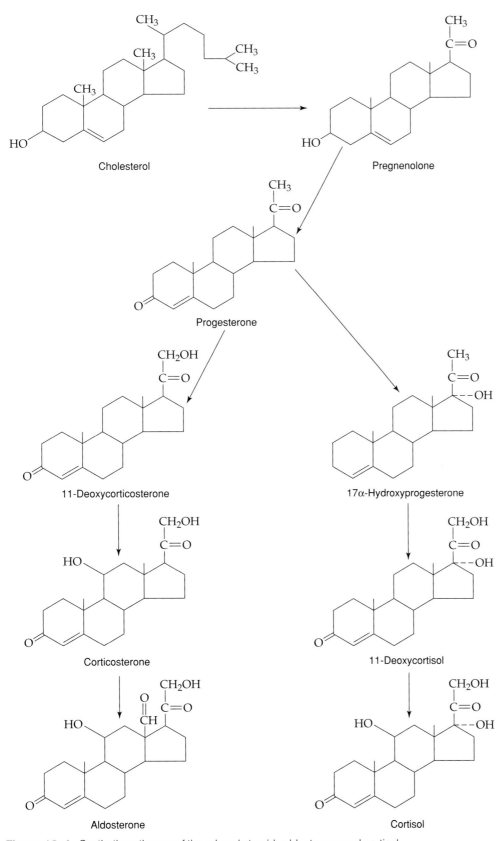

Figure 13-4. Synthetic pathways of the adrenal steroids aldosterone and cortisol.

Box 13–2 Neuroactive Steroids

Most steroid hormones produce their physiologic effects at the level of the cell nucleus, where they regulate gene transcription. In contrast, some steroids, may interact directly with neurotransmitter receptors on cell surfaces to produce allosteric modifications; when these are synthesized in the brain, they are called *neurosteroids* (or neuroactive steroids). Such compounds include the reduced metabolites of progesterone and deoxycorticosterone, such as **3α- and 5α-tetrahydroprogesterone (3α- and 5α-THP)** and **allopregnanolone, 3α- and 5α-tetrahydrodeoxycorticosterone (3α- and 5α-THDOC), pregnenolone sulfate (PS)**, and **dehydroepiandrosterone sulfate (DHEA-S)**.

In vitro, 3α- and 5α-THP and 3α- and 5α-THDOC enhance GABA-mediated Cl⁻ conductance and increase binding of benzodiazepines to GABA$_A$ receptors; thus they are considered positive allosteric regulators of GABA$_A$ receptors. In contrast, PS and DHEA-S are reported to be negative allosteric regulators of these receptors. Some pharmacologic evidence suggests that neuroactive steroids interact with the GABA$_A$ receptor near the barbiturate-binding site,

but such interaction has not been demonstrated with certainty (see Chapter 7). Several members of this class of steroids also have been reported to produce positive or negative modulation of NMDA and AMPA-kainate glutamate receptors and negative regulation of nicotinic acetylcholine and 5-HT$_3$ serotonin receptors. However, the degree to which neuroactive steroids influence GABA$_A$ receptors or other ligand-gated channels in vivo remains controversial.

Because of conflicting evidence, controversy also exists as to whether these compounds exert significant behavioral effects. Thus whether pregnenolone and DHEA-S enhance hippocampal-dependent memory functions, whether progesterone and other steroids have anxiolytic or hypnotic actions, and whether some members of this class exhibit antidepressant or anticonvulsant properties remain undetermined. Research has been hampered by an inability to isolate interactions between neurosteroids and target channels; indeed, these steroids appear to exhibit a panoply of effects. Consequently unequivocal data regarding the biologic impact of neurosteroids awaits further research.

---

biosynthetic pathways in the adrenal cortex, which lead to the production of glucocorticoids (cortisol), mineralocorticoids (aldosterone), and adrenal androgens (dehydroepiandrosterone). Cells within different zones of the adrenal cortex express distinct synthetic enzymes that catalyze the production of these specific hormones.

GLUCOCORTICOID PHYSIOLOGY

Glucocorticoids produce their biologic effects by binding to one of two cytosolic receptors: the glucocorticoid receptor (GR) or the mineralocorticoid receptor (MR), both of which are members of the large superfamily of steroid hormone (nuclear) receptors (see Chapter 6). Compared with the GR, the MR has a much higher affinity for glucocorticoids; however, MR binding sites may be saturated under physiologic conditions. In contrast, the occupancy of GR binding sites varies in response to changes in circulating glucocorticoid levels. Certain metabolites of glucocorticoids not only bind to these cytosolic receptors but also are reported to exert direct effects on the cell membrane (Box 13–2).

The GR is expressed in essentially every tissue in the body. It is concentrated in the hippocampus and also is

expressed at varying levels in other areas of the brain, depending on each region's constituent cell types. MR expression is more restricted; in addition to the brain it is expressed in the kidney, gut, and heart. As discussed in Chapter 6, some actions of GRs and MRs are DNA-binding dependent and others occur independently of DNA binding. After they bind hormone, these receptors are freed from an inactive cytosolic complex, which contains heat shock proteins, and are subsequently translocated to the nucleus (Figure 13–5). Heat shock proteins are considered chaperone proteins because they sequester receptors in the cytoplasm until they are activated by hormone. In the nucleus the receptors may directly bind to their specific glucocorticoid response elements (GREs) in the regulatory regions of genes; alternatively they may inhibit or enhance the functions of other transcription factors by means of protein–protein interactions. Thus glucocorticoid receptors may inhibit the actions of AP-1, CREB, NF-κB, and other transcription factors.

Mutations in mice have confirmed that some GR feedback activity occurs independently of DNA binding. A mutation of the GR gene that impedes the receptor's ability to bind DNA does not interfere with the viability of affected mice. In contrast, a mouse with a complete knockout of the GR gene is not able to inflate

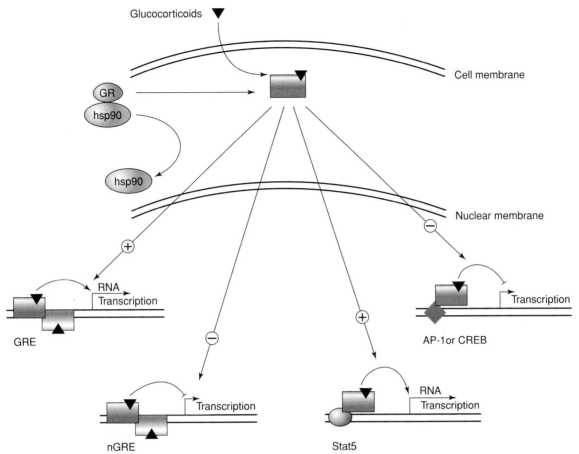

Figure 13–5. Glucocorticoid receptor (GR) function. After entering a cell, glucocorticoids bind to their receptors, which subsequently are released from their associations with chaperones such as heat shock proteins (hsp90). Ligand-bound GRs translocate to the nucleus, where they bind as dimers to positive GREs to activate gene expression or bind to negative GREs (nGRE) to repress gene expression. Alternatively, a ligand-bound GR can interact with other transcription factors to repress AP-1 or CREB-mediated transcription. Interaction with Stat5 can enhance the activation of target gene expression (see Chapter 6).

its lungs at birth. Such mutations have established that GR feedback that inhibits CRF synthesis is DNA-binding independent. Because CREB binding to a CRE in the CRF gene is critical for CRF expression, an inhibitory protein–protein interaction of the GR with CREB might be responsible for GR-mediated feedback repression. In contrast, GR feedback inhibition of POMC expression is DNA-binding dependent. POMC mRNA expression is highly up-regulated in the anterior pituitary of mutant mice lacking the GR gene, as is the expression of prolactin, another anterior pituitary hormone. Although the synthesis of POMC and its cleav-

age product, ACTH, are increased, secretion of ACTH, which is also under the control of glucocorticoids, is unaltered compared with basal levels.

As their name suggests, glucocorticoids increase plasma glucose levels during periods of stress, including starvation; thus they exert catabolic effects on target tissues. Glucocorticoids also suppress the immune system by decreasing the synthesis and release of cytokines. In addition, they appear to affect the brain by rapidly increasing alertness and enhancing cognition. As described in Chapter 15, chronic excessive glucocorticoid release, as may occur in individuals with

Box 13–3 Cushing and Addison Syndromes

Cushing syndrome develops in response to sustained **hypercortisolemia**. Hypercortisolemia may be caused by adrenal tumors or by cancers associated with the ectopic production of ACTH; it also may occur as a reaction to exogenous steroids, such as **prednisone** or **dexamethasone**, that are used to treat inflammatory conditions, autoimmune disease, and some types of cancer. When it is caused by microadenomas (small ACTH-secreting tumors) of the corticotroph cells of the anterior pituitary gland, it is called **Cushing disease**. Cushing syndrome is characterized by many symptoms but classically involves trunkal obesity, thinning skin, osteoporosis, and proximal muscle weakness. A substantial proportion (30–50%) of patients with this syndrome have some depressive or manic symptoms. Insomnia also is common among affected individuals.

Secondary adrenocortical insufficiency, or hypocortisolemia, caused by a lack of ACTH secretion results in **Addison syndrome**. This disorder most commonly occurs after discontinuation of long-term steroid treatment; such treatment leads to atrophy of corticotrophs and of the adrenal gland caused by glucocorticoid-mediated feedback inhibition. Classic symptoms include anorexia, nausea, and hypotension; in addition, hyperpigmentation often occurs in response to unrestrained POMC expression, which results in high levels of α-MSH. Apathy, fatigue, and irritability also are common among affected individuals. Moreover, sleep, appetite, and cognitive performance may be affected. **Addison disease** results from primary adrenocortical insufficiency, which is most often caused by an idiopathic autoimmune process that leads to destruction of the adrenal gland.

Cushing syndrome (Box 13–3) and **major depression**, may cause damage to the hippocampus.

HYPOTHALAMIC–PITUITARY–THYROID AXIS

The synthesis and release of thyroid hormones are controlled by the hypothalamic–pituitary–thyroid (HPT) axis (Figure 13–6). Hypothalamic neurons synthesize and release thyrotropin-releasing hormone (TRH), a peptide consisting of only three amino acids. TRH is stored in axon terminals in the median eminence of the hypothalamus until it is released into the pituitary portal circulation. Normal TRH release is pulsatile and occurs in a circadian pattern; in humans, the highest levels of this hormone are released during the night. In the anterior pituitary gland, TRH binds to its receptors on thyrotroph cells and stimulates the release of the peptide hormone thyrotropin, also called thyroid-stimulating hormone (TSH). Neurons of the neuroendocrine hypothalamus synthesize and release somatostatin, a peptide that inhibits release of TSH and of growth hormone from the anterior pituitary (see Table 13–1). Somatostatin also functions as a neurotransmitter in many brain regions.

Because biologically active TSH requires glycosylation, it is described as a glycoprotein hormone. It is composed of two subunits; the α subunit is identical to that of two other pituitary hormones, luteinizing hormone (LH) and follicle-stimulating hormone (FSH). The β subunit is unique to each of these dimeric hormones and provides specificity for receptor binding. TRH stimulates the synthesis of both α and β chains of TSH in thyrotroph cells.

After TRH releases TSH into the portal circulation, the latter exerts—by means of G_s-coupled TSH receptors—trophic effects on cells of the thyroid gland, which in turn synthesize two thyroid hormones: triiodothyronine (T_3) and tetraiodothyronine, or **thyroxine** (T_4) (Figure 13–6B). T_4 is the predominant form of thyroid hormone secreted by the thyroid gland; it is subsequently converted to T_3 in target cells. All of the steps in the synthesis of these thyroid hormones are stimulated by TSH. Subsequently these hormones are released into the circulation to act on all tissues in the body. They also provide feedback control of transcription of the pre-pro-TRH gene by hypothalamic neurons and of the two subunits of TSH within pituitary thyrotrophs. Low levels of thyroid hormone stimulate transcription, and high levels lead to inhibition. Of the two thyroid hormones, T_3 exerts the more potent effects; consequently, altered rates of conversion of T_4 to T_3 can regulate the activity of the HPT axis. The most common forms of **hypothyroidism** are caused by failure of the thyroid gland and are best detected through the measurement of serum TSH levels. These may become elevated to drive a failing thyroid gland before levels of T_4 and T_3 become abnormal. Hypothyroidism caused by hypothalamic or pituitary failure is characterized by low levels of TSH. **Hyperthyroidism** is indicated by elevated levels of T_4 and T_3, which must be corrected to measure free thyroid hormone, because a considerable fraction of T_4 and T_3 in plasma is bound to thyroid-binding globulin or thyroglobulin (TBG) and is physiologically inactive.

Thyroid hormones exert genomic effects by regulating the transcription of target genes, and nongenomic effects by regulating intracellular ion concentrations

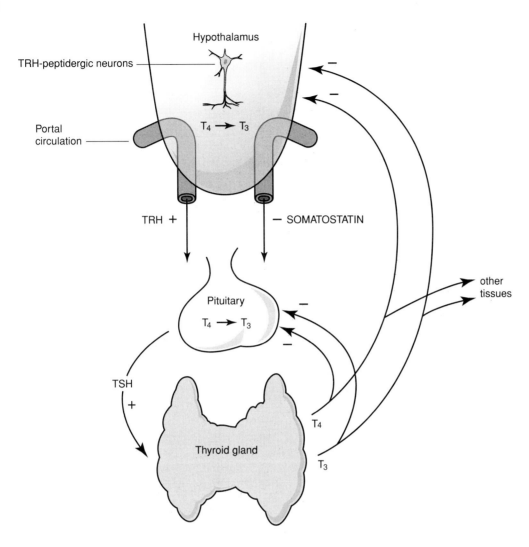

Thyroid Hormones

3,5,3'-Triiodothyronine (T₃) Thyroxine (T₄)

Figure 13–6. Hypothalamic–pituitary–thyroid axis. **A.** Thyrotropin-releasing hormone (TRH) stimulates and somatostatin inhibits release of TSH from anterior pituitary thyrotrophs. By means of the general circulation, TSH reaches the thyroid, where it stimulates the synthesis and release of triiodothyronine (T₃) and tetraiodothyronine or thryroxine (T₄) from the thyroid gland. **B.** The chemical structures of thyroid hormones T₃ and T₄.

and glucose transport. Genomic effects are mediated by two major thyroid hormone receptors: TRα-1 and TRβ-1; like GR and MR, these receptors are members of the steroid hormone receptor superfamily. Like other ligand-regulated transcription factors, TRα-1 and TRβ-1 bind to a specific DNA element, known as the thyroid hormone-responsive element (TRE), which is found in the promoter region of many genes. The receptors bind as homodimers or, with other nuclear proteins such as thyroid hormone receptor auxiliary proteins (TRAPs), as heterodimers to stimulate or repress the transcription of target genes.

FUNCTION OF THE HPT AXIS IN STRESS AND DEPRESSION

The adaptive response to stress previously described in relation to the HPA axis also involves the HPT axis. During stress or illness, thyroid axis function is suppressed, resulting in less secretion of TSH and reduced conversion of T_4 to T_3 in peripheral tissues. During acute and chronic illness, binding of T_4 to TBG also increases, in turn further decreasing levels of free hormone. These phenomena are believed to be adaptations aimed at conserving energy. Some of these adaptations are similar to those that occur during starvation.

Hyperthyroidism and hypothyroidism, which can result from lesions in any part of the HPT axis, are known to have profound effects on behavior. Several changes in the HPT axis have been documented in connection with **major depression,** although the percentage of individuals affected and the impact of such changes are smaller compared with changes in the HPA axis (see Chapter 15). Depression typically does not affect levels of thyroid hormones, but has been associated with a blunted TSH response to TRH infusion. Reports also have indicated a reduced diurnal variation of TSH release and a reduced rate of conversion of T_4 into T_3. The physiologic significance of such findings is unknown; however, some studies suggest that the administration of T_3 may increase the effectiveness of antidepressant treatment even in patients who are euthyroid. When administered alone, T_3 is not effective in the treatment of depression. Interestingly, prominent neuropsychiatric symptoms, including those of depression, can develop when free T_4 or T_3 levels are elevated, as occurs with **hyperthyroidism,** or when such levels are diminished, as occurs with **hypothyroidism**. Typical causes of hyperthyroidism include **Graves disease, toxic multinodular goiter,** and **thyroiditis**. Symptoms include tachycardia, weight loss, heat intolerance, and sweating. Most individuals with hyperthyroidism are anxious, tense, and unable to concentrate. Some patients, gener-

ally older individuals, may demonstrate an apathetic form of hyperthyroidism, characterized by a depressed mood and retarded psychomotor activity. Some cases of hyperthyroidism are caused by autoantibodies that bind to and activate the TSH receptor, resulting in sustained stimulation of the thyroid gland.

Most cases of hypothyroidism occur secondary to disease processes of the thyroid gland, which commonly are autoimmune in nature and result in destruction of thyroid tissue. Typical features of hypothyroidism include lethargy, weight gain, cold intolerance, dry skin, and constipation. Depressed mood, slowed speech, reduced initiative, and reduced memory capacity also are common. Rarely, individuals with severe forms of this disorder **(myxedema)** may experience delusions and hallucinations.

HYPOTHALAMIC–PITUITARY–GONADAL AXIS

Reproductive function is controlled by the hypothalamic–pituitary–gonadal (HPG) axis (Figure 13–7) through the release of gonadotropin-releasing hormone (GnRH), previously known as luteinizing hormone-releasing hormone (LHRH). Like CRF, TRH, and somatostatin, this peptide-releasing factor is released into the portal circulation by hypothalamic neurons, from axons that project to the median eminence. GnRH-expressing neurons are located in the medial basal hypothalamus and arcuate nucleus. GnRH acts on gonadotrophs of the anterior pituitary gland to stimulate the synthesis and release of the gonadotropins, luteinizing hormone (LH) and follicle-stimulating hormone (FSH). A long-acting GnRH agonist, **leuprolide,** which produces continuous stimulation of GnRH receptors, causes their desensitization and thereby inhibits release of LH and FSH. Leuprolide is used clinically to delay puberty in children who have precocious onset of puberty. A third gonadotropic hormone, chorionic gonadotropin, is secreted by the syncytiotrophoblast cells of the placenta during pregnancy; measurement of this hormone is the basis of many pregnancy tests.

All gonadotropins are dimeric glycoprotein hormones that consist of a common α subunit (identical to the α subunit of TSH) and unique β subunits. GnRH stimulates the synthesis of both types of subunit and the glycosylation step required for their biologic activity. GnRH release must be pulsatile to effectively activate pituitary gonadotrophs. Such release of GnRH in adults depends on an intrinsic pulse generator that releases the hormone in intervals of 60–100 minutes. Located in the medial basal hypothalamus, this generator functions even when the medial basal hypothala-

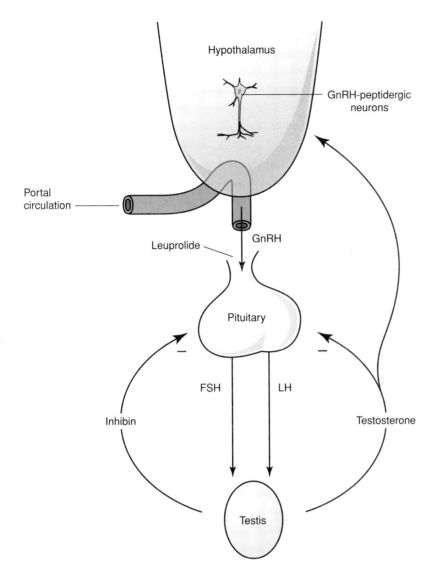

Figure 13–7. Hypothalamic–pituitary–gonadal axis. The male version of this axis is shown. Neurons that express gonadotropin-releasing hormone (GnRH) cause the pituitary to release luteinizing hormone (LH) and follicle-stimulating hormone (FSH), which in turn act on the testis (shown) or ovary. Gonadal steroids, such as testosterone or estrogen, inhibit both GnRH and LH release as part of a regulatory feedback process. The gonads also produce a peptide hormone known as inhibin, which inhibits FSH secretion. Leuprolide, a potent GnRH agonist, desensitizes the GnRH receptor and thereby inhibits this axis. It is used in the treatment of precocious puberty and to suppress testosterone secretion in prostate cancer. It also is used experimentally in the investigation and treatment of perimenstrual mood disorders.

mus is surgically isolated from the rest of the brain; however, its molecular basis remains obscure.

The targets of LH and FSH are the gonads. In the ovary, LH induces ovulation of the mature follicle and acts on theca cells to promote the synthesis of androgen precursors necessary for estrogen production (Figure 13–8A). Such precursors diffuse into nearby granulosa cells, where FSH stimulates the production of the steroid hormone estrogen. LH also sustains the ruptured follicle that forms the corpus luteum by stimulating progesterone synthesis; FSH stimulates development of the mature follicle. In the testes, LH stimulates testosterone biosynthesis in Leydig cells (see Figure 13–8B). FSH is believed to be a key factor in the development of the seminiferous tubules and in the initia-

tion of puberty; however, its physiologic importance in the adult male remains unclear.

Feedback control of gonadotropin secretion is complex, particularly in females, in whom such control varies during the different stages of the menstrual cycle. It comprises a complex integration of influences exerted by the gonadal steroids (estradiol, progesterone, and testosterone) and by the peptide hormones (inhibin and activin), which also are produced by the gonads. Moreover, GnRH release is influenced by several neurotransmitter and neuromodulatory agents, including catecholamines, endogenous opioids, γ-aminobutyric acid (GABA), neuropeptide Y, and possibly dopamine.

Among the actions that can be traced to gonadal steroids, their participation in gene transcription is best

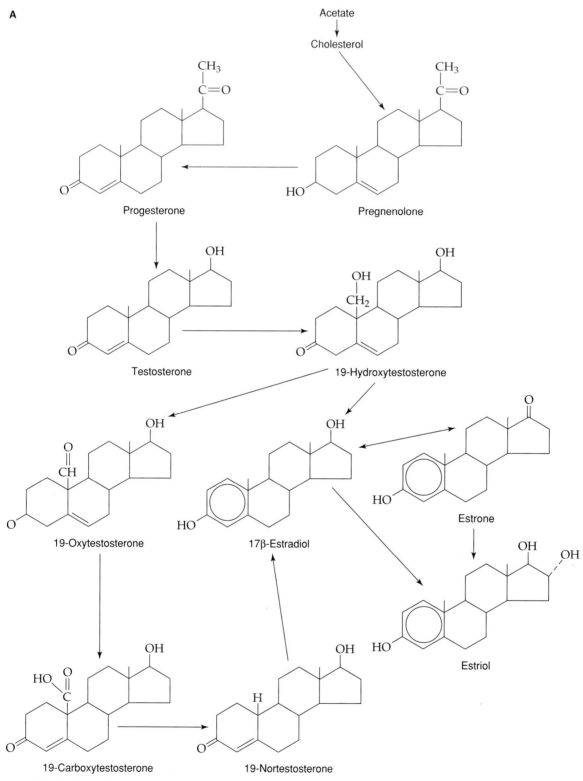

Figure 13-8. Gonadal steroid synthesis. **A.** Synthetic pathways in the female. Like all steroid hormones, gonadal steroids are derived from cholesterol.

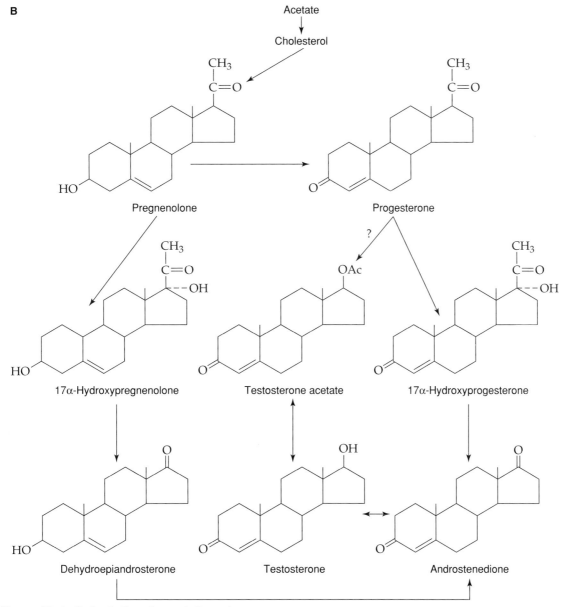

Figure 13–8. B. Synthetic pathways in the male.

understood. Like glucocorticoids, gonadal steroids can regulate transcription either directly or indirectly. In some cases they bind to estrogen or androgen response elements in the regulatory regions of specific target genes and thereby influence the expression of those genes. In other cases, gonadal steroids affect transcription by interacting with AP-1, CREB, or other transcription factor families and in turn altering the expression of genes controlled by those transcription factors. Gonadal steroids also produce some of their

physiologic effects by acting on cell surface proteins, as discussed in Box 13–2.

Gonadal steroids have significant effects on normal male and female development, which are not discussed in this book. Importantly, changing levels of gonadal steroids may have a profound impact on behavior in adults (Box 13–4); for example, **hydroxyprogesterone (Depo-Provera)** has been used to diminish sex drive in criminal sex offenders. Certain derivatives of gonadal steroids, called *neuroactive steroids*, are reported to have

Box 13–4 Disorders of Mood Related to Reproductive Function

Postpartum mood disorders

Many women develop transient blues after childbirth; however, a minority go on to develop serious **postpartum depression** or **postpartum mania.** Such disorders are believed to be triggered by the rapid and dramatic changes in hormonal levels that occur perinatally. Both estrogen and progesterone levels rise during pregnancy and fall rapidly after delivery. Moreover, estrogen stimulates the production of thyroid-binding globulin, which leads to reduced levels of free thyroid hormone. Prolactin and cortisol levels also rise during pregnancy and subsequently return to a normal range within weeks of delivery. Although the pathophysiology is not fully understood, these postpartum alterations in mood are, fortunately, highly responsive to standard **antidepressant** or **antimanic** medications (see Chapter 15).

Premenstrual disorders of mood

Many women with depression experience a premenstrual worsening of symptoms. Likewise, some women experience depressive or anxiety symptoms that occur reliably only during the luteal phase of the menstrual cycle and generally resolve shortly after the onset of menstruation. In a small percentage of women, symptoms are severe enough to interfere with social or occupational activities. In a study aimed at reducing such symptoms, the GnRH receptor agonist **leuprolide** was administered to women with severe premenstrual syndrome; it was discovered that this agent suppresses the menstrual cycle and in turn decreases symptoms significantly (see Figure 13–7). Moreover, in the presence of leuprolide, the addition of either estradiol or progesterone induces symptoms of mood disorder in women with a history of premenstrual syndrome, but does not trigger symptoms in women without such a history. Yet the endogenous levels of estradiol and progesterone are not abnormal in women with premenstrual syndrome. Consequently, it has been proposed that disorders of mood during the premenstrual period stem from abnormal receptor or postreceptor responses to normal levels of cycling gonadal steroids.

---

diverse effects on behavior, including the alleviation of anxiety, and thus may have future clinical applications (see Box 13–2). Effects of estrogens on neuronal morphology also have been documented. In female rats, for example, estradiol increases the density of dendritic spines on CA1 hippocampal pyramidal neurons. The physiologic and behavioral impact of these changes is currently under investigation (see Chapter 15). In addition, certain androgen derivatives, known as **anabolic steroids,** are used to increase muscle mass and athletic performance; such steroids often are used illegally and can produce deleterious effects on the CNS. Anabolic steroids appear to be reinforcing, and hence potentially addicting, in some individuals; moreover, they can induce psychotic symptoms after chronic use. Despite our awareness of these effects, much remains to be known about the cellular and molecular mechanisms by which gonadal steroids influence complex behaviors.

PROLACTIN

Prolactin, like growth hormone and placental lactogen, is considered a member of the somatotropic hormone family. It is synthesized and released by lactotrophs of the anterior pituitary gland. In males, serum prolactin levels normally are low throughout life. In females, such levels typically are only slightly higher but increase markedly during pregnancy. Pregnancy-related increases decline at term unless the mother breast feeds; suckling causes marked increases in prolactin levels, which serve to initiate lactation. Hypothalamic control of prolactin is primarily inhibitory. It is mediated by dopamine released into the portal circulation at the median eminence by neurons of the tuberoinfundibular dopaminergic system, which originates in the arcuate nucleus (Figure 13–9; see Chapter 8). In the pituitary, dopamine binds to D_2 dopamine receptors to inhibit prolactin synthesis and release. TRH from the hypothalamus and vasoactive intestinal peptide (VIP), which is produced locally in the pituitary, act to increase the release of prolactin. Moreover, the existence of a prolactin-releasing factor has been hypothesized.

Although it has been determined that prolactin is released in response to stress, both the mechanism and function of such release in humans remain unclear. **Hyperprolactinemia** is most commonly caused by tumors, or microadenomas, of pituitary lactotrophs or by D_2 dopamine receptor antagonists (**antipsychotic drugs**). It can result in galactorrhea and amenorrhea in females. In males, it may produce galactorrhea and impotence. Because prolactin is under inhibitory control of dopamine, hyperprolactinemia can be treated with dopamine D_2 receptor agonists, such as **bromocriptine** (see Chapter 14).

The prolactin receptor belongs to the family of glycophosphatidylinositol (GPI)-linked receptors, which modulate the actions of many cytokines, including ciliary neurotrophic factor, leukemia inhibitory factor, and leptin. As described in Chapter 11, these receptors are trimeric; each is composed of a ligand-binding protein that is hormone- or cytokine-specific and some common subunits. For all members of this receptor family, the net effect of receptor trimerization is activation of the cytoplasmic protein tyrosine kinase Janus kinase (JAK), which phosphorylates and activates the signal transducers and activators of transcription, or STAT transcription factors (see Chapters 6 and 11). Current efforts are aimed at identifying the genes that are regulated by STATs to mediate the physiologic actions of prolactin.

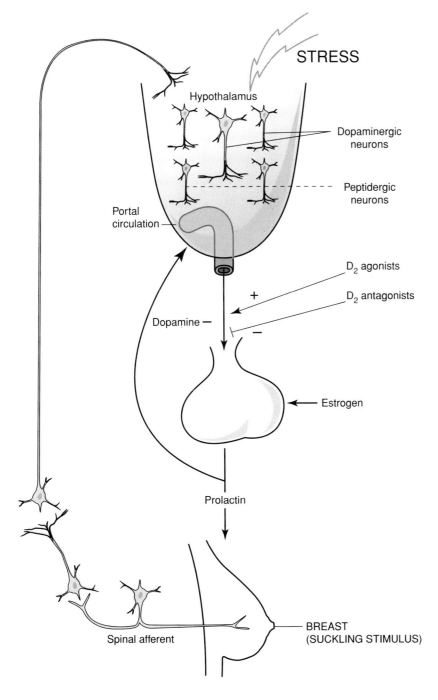

Figure 13–9. Prolactin secretion. Prolactin secretion is induced in lactotrophs of the anterior pituitary by thyrotropin-releasing hormone and perhaps other petidergic signals, and is inhibited by dopamine acting at D$_2$ dopamine receptors. Antipsychotic drugs that are potent D$_2$ antagonists (see Chapter 17) increase prolactin secretion. In lactating females, prolactin is strongly induced by suckling.

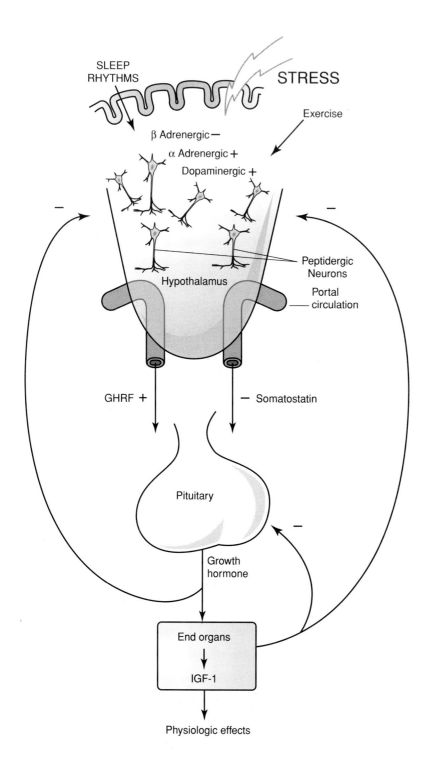

Figure 13–10. Growth hormone secretion. Growth hormone secretion is induced in somatotrophs of the anterior pituitary by growth hormone-releasing hormone (GHRH; also called *GHRF*) and is inhibited by somatostatin. Release of these hypothalamic peptides is modulated by adrenergic and dopaminergic systems. Growth hormone acts on peripheral tissues largely through production of insulin-like growth factor-1 (IGF-1).

GROWTH HORMONE

The production of growth hormone by the somatotrophs of the anterior pituitary is under the stimulatory control of growth hormone-releasing hormone (GHRH) and the inhibitory control of somatostatin (Figure 13–10). GHRH is produced by cells of the infundibular and arcuate nuclei of the hypothalamus and is released at the median eminence. It binds to its G protein-linked receptor on the somatotroph membrane and stimulates transcription of growth hormone mRNA and release of mature growth hormone. Somatostatin, produced by neurons of the anterior periventricular region of the hypothalamus, is also released into the portal circulation at the median eminence; it acts on somatotrophs to inhibit the release of growth hormone, but does not seem to affect its rate of synthesis. The secretion of growth hormone, which is pulsatile, is coordinated by somatostatin and GHRH. Growth hormone provides negative feedback by stimulating somatostatin release. Growth hormone also induces the production of insulin-like growth factor 1 (IGF-1) in target tissues in the periphery, which among other actions suppresses the release of growth hormone from the pituitary.

Growth hormone is released in response to phasic stressors, such as starvation, exertion, or emotional stress. It also is necessary for longitudinal growth, particularly during the later stages of childhood; accordingly, levels of this hormone are high in children, reach maximal levels during adolescence, and decline during adulthood. In addition to the growth of long bones, the metabolic effects of this hormone, which generally are anabolic in nature, lead to increased muscle mass and decreased body fat.

The growth hormone receptor, which contains a single transmembrane domain, has a large extracellular N terminus involved in hormone binding and a large intracellular C terminus. Hormone binding causes the receptor to dimerize and results in the activation of tyrosine kinase activity. Growth hormone has direct effects on some target tissues, and its induction of IGF-1 in peripheral tissues mediates some of its growth-promoting and anabolic effects.

CONTROL OF ENERGY BALANCE AND APPETITE

The regulation of energy balance involves the coordination of food intake and energy expenditure. Both are controlled by complex physiologic processes, which involve networks of neurotransmitter systems and hormonal signals regulated by the hypothalamus (Table 13–2). Since the cloning in 1994 of the leptin (*ob*) gene, which involved an inactivating mutation that produced a classic mouse model of obesity, enormous progress has been made in identifying the particular signaling molecules that comprise these networks (Box 13–5). Hormonal and neural signals from the periphery inform the brain of the body's energy status. Leptin, which is produced by adipocytes, and other signals are involved in regulating the long-term state of the body's energy reserves. Such regulation involves a delicate balance between food intake over time and the rate of energy expenditure. The latter is determined by levels of general motor activity and also by the efficiency of oxidative phosphorylation in mitochondria, which controls the amount of energy derived from energy sources such as fat. Other signals, which have short-term functions after food ingestion, are called satiety signals. Cholecystokinin (CCK), an important satiety signal, is synthesized in the gut wall and released into the circulation in response to the presence of certain nutrients in the gut. It stimulates G protein-coupled receptors located on the vagus nerve, which in turn transmit information to brain stem nuclei (e.g., to the nucleus of the solitary tract) and subsequently to the hypothalamus. Blockade of peripheral CCK receptors leads to increased food intake. Another satiety signal is provided by circulating levels of glucose.

Based on early studies, it was hypothesized that the lateral hypothalamus facilitates feeding because lesions in this area produced starvation. Conversely, the medial hypothalamus was believed to suppress feeding because corresponding lesions produced marked hyperphagia. More recent molecular studies are generally consistent with the data based on lesions in that the leptin receptor (Ob-R), which mediates leptin's suppression of feeding, is most densely concentrated in the medial hypothalamus—specifically in the arcuate nucleus and in parts of the ventromedial, dorsomedial, and ventropremammillary nuclei. Moreover, these nuclei are near the median eminence, a region of the brain where the

Table 13–2 Peptides[1] That Regulate Feeding

Peptides That Increase Feeding	Peptides That Decrease Feeding
NPY[2]	Leptin[3]
Orexin A and B[4]	CCK
Galanin	CART
MCH	α-MSH[5]
YY	CRF
ARP	Urocortin
	Bombesin
	Insulin
	GLP-1

[1] Released by or acting on the hypothalamus.
[2] By means of the Y_5 receptor.
[3] Leptin is released by adipocytes and may reach the hypothalamus through the median eminence.
[4] The actions of orexins (also known as hypocretins) on feeding are being reevaluated based on the role of these peptides in control of sleep; some actions may result from sleep cycle-mediated effects on behavior.
[5] By means of the MC-4 receptor.
ARP, agouti-related peptide (also known as ART, agouti-related transcript); CART, cocaine- and amphetamine-regulated transcript; CCK, cholecystokinin; CRF, corticotropin-releasing factor; GLP-1, glucagon-like peptide-1; MCH, melanin-concentrating hormone; α-MSH, α-melanocyte-stimulating hormone.

Box 13–5 Leptin

Much of what we currently know about the neurobiology of appetite and energy balance initially was derived from genetic studies of obesity and diabetes in mice. The obese (*ob*) mouse and the diabetic (*db*) mouse have identical phenotypes that stem from recessive mutations. Both strains are diabetic and their weights typically are more than three times those of normal mice, even when they are fed an identical diet. Classic parabiosis experiments, in which the circulation of *ob* and *db* mice were joined, suggested that the *ob* gene encodes a circulating factor and that the *db* gene encodes its receptor. Subsequently it was proven that the missing factor in the *ob* mouse is leptin and that the missing receptor in the *db* mouse is the leptin receptor (Ob-R). Obesity and diabetes occur in these mice because of a profound disruption in their metabolic state.

Leptin is expressed primarily by adipocytes and at lower levels in the gastrointestinal tract and immune system. Plasma levels of leptin correlate with adipose tissue mass; in both humans and rodents, such levels increase with increased

adipose tissue and decrease with weight loss (see Figure 13–11). Leptin levels do not change abruptly with meals; this finding distinguishes alterations in leptin levels from such short-term responses to feeding as changes in plasma levels of glucose, CCK, or amino acids. Administration of leptin over time results in a dose-dependent decrease in body weight.

Leptin appears to have several neuroendocrine functions that may be related to its influence on body weight. For example, *ob* mice exhibit many abnormalities characteristic of the starvation state, despite the animals' obesity and hyperphagia. Such mice exhibit decreased body temperature, decreased energy expenditure, infertility, and decreased immune function. Because leptin replacement corrects all of these abnormalities in the *ob* mouse, it is believed that leptin is a key factor in multiple neuroendocrine cascades. Related observations in humans appear to support this hypothesis; for example, starvation is known to delay puberty in girls, and some evidence suggests that endogenous leptin may be involved in regulating its onset.

blood–brain barrier is incomplete and therefore may allow the entry of circulating leptin.

Ob-R is a member of the cytokine receptor family previously mentioned in connection with prolactin (see Chapter 11). Leptin binding causes the activation of the JAK–STAT pathway, in particular that of JAK2 and STAT3 (see Chapter 6). Together with Ob-R, a peptide called the *suppressor of cytokine signaling-3* (SOCS-3) is expressed in the arcuate nucleus. SOCS-3 blocks leptin-induced phosphorylation of its receptor and thereby inhibits leptin signaling. Ob-R has five alternatively spliced forms, only one of which, Ob-Rb, has a cytoplasmic domain that is consistent with signaling. Rare mutations in leptin or in the leptin receptor in humans produce morbid obesity and failure to undergo puberty.

Leptin signaling in the medial hypothalamus suppresses feeding and thus is characterized as anorexigenic; several orexigenic peptides, which promote feeding, are expressed in the lateral hypothalamus. The precise physiologic functions of orexigenic peptides—for example, those of neuropeptide Y (NPY), melanin-concentrating hormone (MCH), and the orexins (also referred to as hypocretins)—are not yet completely understood. Levels of these peptides increase in the lateral hypothalamus in response to starvation and decrease in response to feeding or leptin administration. The most important orexigenic peptide appears

to be NPY, as discussed in the next section of this chapter. In addition, targeted deletion of the MCH gene results in decreased food intake and body weight. Orexin (from the Greek word for appetite) received its name because it stimulates feeding when injected. However, the theory that peptides expressed in the medial hypothalamus suppress feeding and peptides expressed in the lateral hypothalamus induce feeding has turned out to be overly simplistic. Inactivating mutations of the orexin or orexin receptor genes do not have a dramatic effect on feeding; rather, they surprisingly result in a phenotype that mimics human **narcolepsy** (Box 13–6). Further work is needed to better define the function of the orexin system in both feeding behavior and narcolepsy.

The role of the lateral hypothalamus is further complicated by the presence of peptides that suppress feeding, including melanotropin (also called α-*melanocyte-stimulating hormone*, or α-MSH) and CART (cocaine- and amphetamine-regulated transcript). CART was discovered based on its regulation by cocaine and amphetamines, yet its predominant function may be related to appetite. Although cocaine and amphetamine are known to suppress appetite, the role that hypothalamic CART plays in this psychostimulant effect has not yet been determined. Also expressed in lateral hypothalamic neurons is CRF, which produces anorexia when administered to the CNS. However, tar-

Box 13–6 Narcolepsy and the Orexin System

Narcolepsy is characterized by excessive daytime sleepiness, cataplexy (attacks of muscle weakness without impairment of consciousness, often precipitated by strong emotion), and sleep paralysis. These symptoms result from abnormalities in the mechanisms that produce rapid eye movement (REM) sleep, as described in greater detail in Chapter 18. In certain dogs, narcolepsy is transmitted as an autosomal recessive trait. However, this is not the case in humans, in whom patterns of transmission appear to be genetically complex.

After the canine narcolepsy gene (*canarc-1*) was cloned from Doberman pinschers, investigators were surprised to discover that it encoded the type-2 orexin (hypocretin) receptor. Orexin A and B are the active peptide products of a single precursor. Orexin A binds with high affinity to the type-1 orexin receptor, and both peptides bind with equal affinity to the type-2 orexin receptor. Interestingly, targeted deletion of the orexin gene produces a narcolepsy-like syndrome in mice (see Chapter 18).

The possibility that orexin peptides may be involved in the control of REM sleep is further supported by the fact that orexin neurons project from the lateral hypothalamus to the locus ceruleus, raphe nuclei, medullary reticular formation, paraventricular nucleus of the thalamus, and septal nuclei—brain regions implicated in sleep regulation. The possibility that abnormalities in the orexin system contribute to human narcolepsy is now supported by direct experimental evidence (see Chapter 18).

---

geted deletions of the CRF or CRF_1R gene do not produce obvious abnormalities in feeding.

POTENTIAL PATHWAYS OF LEPTIN ACTION

Despite investigation of the intercellular signaling cascades produced by leptin, much about leptin action (Figure 13–11) remains to be discovered. NPY (see Chapter 10), when bound to its Y_5 and perhaps Y_1 receptors, is believed to assist in mounting a response to low levels of leptin. When directly administered into the CNS, NPY is among the most potent orexigenic agents known. Leptin, which is abundant when adipocytes are increased, suppresses NPY expression and secretion. Yet the precise position of NPY in the cascade of events that control feeding is not yet clear. Knockout of the NPY gene attenuates the obesity of *ob* (leptin knockout) mice, but targeted deletion of the Y_5 receptor does not affect normal food intake, and deletion of the NPY gene does not decrease food intake or body weight in otherwise normal mice. The discrepancies between pharmacologic and knockout experiments are difficult to interpret because compensations may occur in response to the deletion of certain genes but not in response to the deletion of others.

Other genetic data that help explain the pathways that respond to high levels of leptin are more straightforward. α-MSH, which is derived from the POMC gene (see Chapter 10), acts at the melanocortin-4 receptor (MC_4R) to initiate physiologic and behavioral responses to increased plasma levels of leptin (see Figure 13–11). MC_4R is expressed in the paraventricular nucleus, dorsomedial hypothalamic nucleus, and lateral hypothalamus. Targeted deletion of MC_4R results in obesity in mice, and rare natural human mutations in this pathway also produce obesity. In *ob* mice, or fasted normal rodents (i.e., rodents in whom leptin is absent or insubstantial), POMC mRNA is decreased in the hypothalamus and is normalized by leptin administration. Moreover, anorexia produced by leptin administration can be inhibited if a melanocortin receptor antagonist is coadministered.

Studies of *agouti*, a strain of obese mice with yellow coats, have indicated that α-MSH is not the only protein that acts at MC_4R. Such work has revealed that the agouti protein acts as an endogenous antagonist of melanocortin receptors. Because the agouti protein blocks MC_1R, which controls pigment dispersion in melanocytes, it produces the yellow coat that is characteristic of *agouti;* it also causes obesity by blocking MC_4R. Although agouti protein is not normally expressed in the brain, an agouti-related peptide (ARP), also called *agouti-related transcript* (ART), is expressed in the brain. ARP is an endogenous antagonist at MC_4R. Overexpression of ARP produces obesity similar to that of *agouti* and MC_4R knockout mice.

Although the mechanisms underlying the chemical signaling and circuitry of weight control continue to challenge investigators, recent advances in our understanding have stimulated excitement and anticipation. The enormous health problems associated with **obesity** and its high prevalence continue to spur research. However, the treatment of obesity in humans will require sophistication. Obesity in human populations is not caused by inadequate plasma levels of leptin; rather, it often is associated with high levels of leptin and with leptin resistance. (Similarly, type 2 diabetes mellitus is associated with high levels of insulin and with insulin resistance.) Nevertheless, the wealth of information that has been obtained in recent years concerning hypothalamic mechanisms that control feeding behavior has provided clues to the many types of agents that may prove useful in the future treatment of obesity (see Table 13–2). Furthermore, our understanding of weight control should lead to the develop-

ment of therapy for eating disorders such as **anorexia nervosa** and **bulimia.**

DISORDERS OF APPETITE CONTROL

Anorexia nervosa is a syndrome characterized by self-starvation and a profoundly distorted body image. Affected individuals believe that they are overweight even when they are so thin that their lives are threatened. This

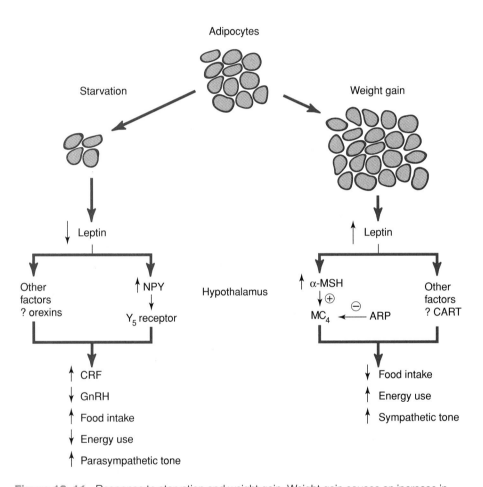

Figure 13–11. Response to starvation and weight gain. Weight gain causes an increase in adipocyte mass and the production of leptin. Starvation reduces adipocyte mass and leads to a corresponding reduction in leptin. Leptin acts as a feedback signal to maintain constant body mass; such signaling occurs in the hypothalamus in conjunction with other complex systems. Neuropeptide Y (NPY), acting primarily at Y_5 receptors, is believed to assist in the response to low leptin levels, but many other factors, including orexins and corticotropin-releasing factor (CRF), may be involved in ultimate behavioral and metabolic responses. α-Melanocyte stimulating hormone (α-MSH) acting at melanocortin receptors (e.g., MC_4R) mediates some of leptin's actions. *Agouti*-related peptide (ARP) antagonizes the effect of α-MSH at the MC_4R. Many other factors, such as cocaine- and amphetamine-regulated transcript (CART), may be involved in the metabolic and behavioral responses to weight gain. GnRH, gonadotropin-releasing hormone.

illness, which is more common among females than among males, results in multiple endocrine abnormalities that are typical of starvation. Amenorrhea is common in women with anorexia nervosa; moreover, growth hormone levels may be elevated, T_3 levels are reduced, and cortisol levels are high. Starvation may be severe enough to cause death; indeed, anorexia nervosa is associated with a 10% mortality rate. Bulimia, which also is more common among females, is characterized by binge eating and purging, the latter of which often occurs by means of induced vomiting, laxative abuse, or intense exercise. **Antidepressants,** particularly **SSRIs (serotonin selective reuptake inhibitors)**, have been used with some success to decrease the binging and purging associated with bulimia; however, pharmacologic treatment of anorexia remains unsatisfactory. Moreover, therapies based on leptin pathways may be difficult to develop. In patients with anorexia nervosa, leptin levels often are extremely low—even lower than might be predicted based on the extremely low fat content of the body. Furthermore, weight gain in response to treatment has been associated with increases in leptin that rise beyond appropriate levels. Such leptin signals may reduce appetite and increase energy expenditure and may in part explain the barriers to weight gain experienced by these patients. Because of the prevalence and seriousness of these eating disorders, the development of more effective medical treatment is a major goal of current research.

HYPOTHALAMIC RESPONSE TO INFECTION AND INFLAMMATION

Inflammatory stimuli represent a substantial threat to homeostasis; thus it is not surprising that the hypothalamus, which is indispensable in the response to stress, also assists in the response to infection and inflammation. Inflammatory stimuli induce the synthesis and release of a variety of cytokines from lymphocytes and other components of the immune system. Although cytokines are best understood in terms of their ability to mobilize the immune system, they also induce responses in the CNS that are primarily coordinated by the hypothalamus. CNS-mediated effects of cytokines include fever, anorexia, reduced activity, modified sleep patterns, and altered hormonal output, such as increased CRF secretion and suppressed GnRH release.

Bacterial endotoxins are glycolipid components of cell walls of gram-negative bacteria. Endotoxins play an important role in natural bacterial infections and also are used as experimental tools in the stimulation of inflammatory responses. They activate cells of the immune system to secrete cytokines, including inter-

leukin-1β(IL-1β), tumor necrosis factor-α (TNF-α), and interleukin-6 (IL-6). These cytokines are endogenous pyrogens, molecules produced by the body that are capable of inducing fever. The pyrogenic actions of exogenous agents are mediated primarily through the induction of endogenous pyrogenic cytokines. Cytokines also are believed to be responsible for the induction of a coordinated set of behaviors that typically accompany infection, including decreased activity, increased fatigue, depressed motivation and cognitive capacity, and lack of appetite.

The mechanisms by which cytokine signals affect CNS functions such as thermoregulation remain unknown. Cytokines are large proteins and cannot easily penetrate the blood–brain barrier. Although some evidence suggests the existence of cytokine-specific active transport mechanisms that enable cytokines to traverse the blood–brain barrier, the capacity of such mechanisms most likely would be insufficient to produce observed CNS effects. Some evidence indicates that immune signals may reach the CNS along neural pathways by stimulating peripheral sensory nerves. Cytokines also may act on neurons in circumventricular organs; as previously mentioned, these are brain structures in which neurons or their processes lie outside of the blood–brain barrier. It also has been hypothesized that cytokines interact with capillary endothelial cells on the blood side of the blood–brain barrier to produce lipophilic messengers, such as prostaglandins, that diffuse directly into the brain. Accordingly, fever is believed to result from the actions of prostaglandin PGE_2 near the preoptic area in the hypothalamus. In turn, the hypothalamus acts to induce heat generation through motor activity such as shivering, and also functions to decrease heat loss. Antipyretics, including salicylates such as **aspirin** and nonsteroidal anti-inflammatory drugs (NSAIDs) such as **ibuprofen,** block production of PGE_2 by inhibiting cyclooxygenase (COX), which is the critical biosynthetic enzyme necessary for the production of prostaglandins and related arachidonic acid metabolites (see Chapter 5). The chemical structures of some commonly used antipyretics and antiinflammatory agents are presented in Chapter 19.

One recent advance in the treatment of inflammation has involved the introduction of drugs that selectively inhibit type-2 cyclooxygenase (COX2). Examples include **celecoxib** and **rofecoxib**. Such drugs are antiinflammatory but do not produce some of the side effects, such as increased risk of peptic ulcers, that are caused by inhibition of the type-1 enzyme (COX1) (see Chapter 19). A variety of synthetic glucocorticoids, including **dexamethasone** and **prednisone,** also are commonly used in the treatment of inflammation (Figure 13–12); however, these drugs are not antipyretics.

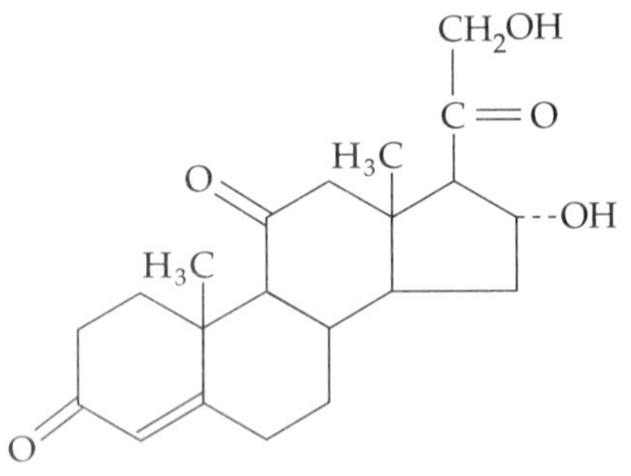

Figure 13-12. Chemical structures of representative synthetic glucocorticoids.

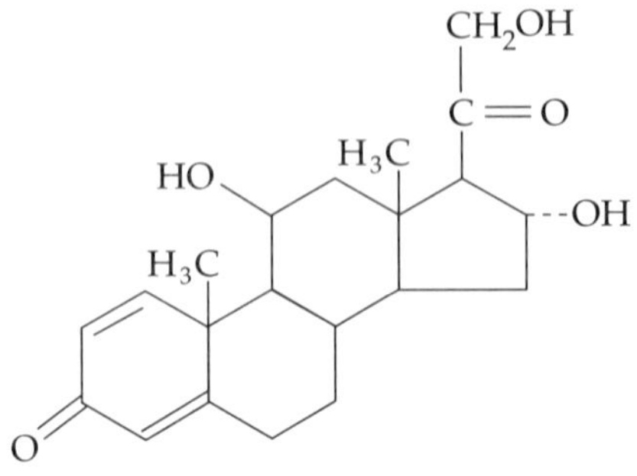

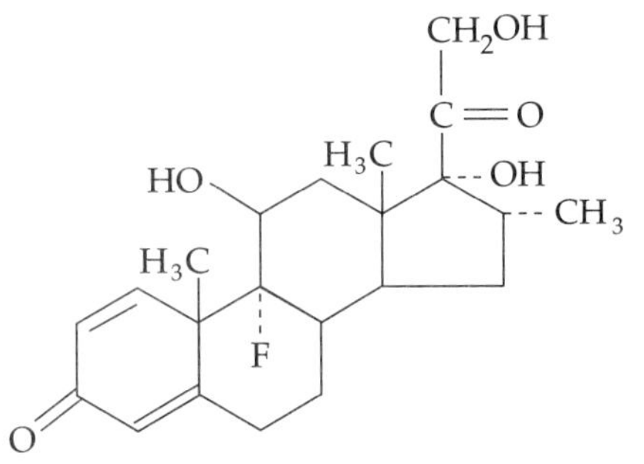

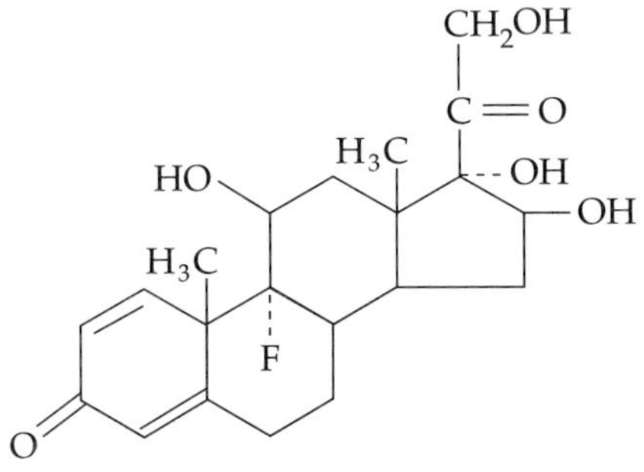

SELECTED READING

Ahima RS, Flier JS. 2000. Leptin. *Annu Rev Physiol* 62:413–437.

Bagatell CJ, Bremner WJ. 1996. Androgens in men: Uses and abuses. *New Engl J Med* 334:707–714.

Bradbury MJ, McBurnie MI, Denton DA, et al. 2000. Modulation of urocortin-induced hypophagia and weight loss by corticotropin-releasing factor receptor 1 deficiency in mice. *Endocrinology* 141:2715–2724.

Castro MG, Morrison E. 1997. Posttranslational processing of proopiomelanocortin in the pituitary and in the brain. *Crit Rev Neurobiol* 11:35–57.

Chambers J, Ames RS, Bergsma D, et al. 1999. Melanin-concentrating hormone is the cognate ligand for the orphan G-protein-coupled receptor SLC-1. *Nature* 400:261–265.

Chemelli RM, Eillie JT, Sinton CM, et al. 1999. Narcolepsy in orexin knockout mice: Molecular genetics of sleep regulation. *Cell* 98:437–451.

de Kretser DM, Meinhardt A, Meehan T, et al. 2000. The roles of inhibin and related peptides in gonadal function. *Mol Cell Endocrinol* 161: 43–46.

Drouin J, Sun YL, Chamberland M, et al. 1993. Novel glucocorticoid receptor complex with DNA element of the hormone-repressed POMC gene. *Embo J* 12:145–156.

Elmquist JK, Elias CF, Saper CB. 1999. From lesions to leptin: Hypothalamic control of food intake and body weight. *Neuron* 22:221–232.

Elmquist JK, Scammell TE, Saper CB. 1997. Mechanisms of CNS response to systemic immune challenge: The febrile response. *Trends Neurosci* 20:565–570.

Ericsson A, Arias C, Sawchenko PE. 1997. Evidence for an intramedullary prostaglandin-dependent mechanism in the activation of stress-related neuroendocrine circuitry by intravenous interleukin-1. *J Neurosci* 15: 166–179.

Fink G, Sumner BE, Rosie R, et al. 1996. Estrogen control of central neurotransmission: Effect on mood, mental state, and memory. *Cell Mol Neurobiol* 16:325–344.

Gasior M, Carter RB, Witkin JM. 1999. Neuroactive steroids: Potential therapeutic use in neurological and psychiatric disorders. *Trends Neurosci* 20:107–112.

Halaas JL, Friedman JM. 1998. Leptin and the regulation of body weight in mammals. *Nature* 395:763–770.

Halford JC, Blundell JE. 2000. Pharmacology of appetite suppression. *Prog Drug Res* 54:25–58.

Holsboer F, Rupprecht R. 1999. Neuroactive steroids: Mechanisms of action and neuropsychopharmacological perspectives. *Trends Neurosci* 22:410–416.

Inui A. 1999. Feeding and body-weight regulation by hypo-thalamic neuropeptides—mediation of the actions of lep-tin. *Trends Neurosci* 22:62–67.

Kuhar MJ, Dall Vechia SE. 1999. CART peptides: novel addic-tion- and feeding-related neuropeptides. *Trends Neurosci* 22:316–320.

Lin L, Faraco J, Li R, et al. 1999. The sleep disorder canine narcolepsy is caused by a mutation in the hypocretin orexin receptor 2 gene. *Cell* 98:365–376.

McEwen BS. 1999. Stress and hippocampal plasticity. *Annu Rev Neurosci* 22:105–122.

McEwen BS, Alves SE. 1999. Estrogen actions in the central nervous system. *Endocr Rev* 20:279–307.

Owens MJ, Nemeroff CB. 1991. Physiology and pharmacology of corticotropin releasing factor. *Pharmacol Rev* 43: 425–473.

Reichardt HM, Kaestner KH, Tuckermann J, et al. 1998. DNA binding of the glucocorticoid receptor is not essential for survival. *Cell* 93:531–541.

Reichardt HM, Schutz G. 1998. Glucocorticoid signaling: Multiple variations of a common theme. *Mol Cell Endocrinol* 146:1–6.

Rubinow DR, Schmidt PJ. 1995. The neuroendocrinology of menstrual cycle mood disorders. *Ann NY Acad Sci* 771: 648–659.

Salton SRJ, Hahm S, Mizuno TM. 2000. Of mice and MEN: What transgenic models tell us about hypothalamic con-trol of energy balance. *Neuron* 25:265–268.

Sapolsky RM. 1992. *Stress, the Aging Brain, and the Mechanisms of Neuron Death.* Cambridge, MA: MIT Press.

Smith GW, Aubry J-M, Dellu F, et al. 1998. Corticotropin-releasing factor receptor 1-deficient mice display decreased anxiety, impaired stress response, and aberrant neuroen-docrine development. *Neuron* 20:1093–1102.

Young LJ, Nilsen R, Waymire KG, et al. 1999. Increased affil-iative response to vasopressin in mice expressing the V_{1a} receptor from a monogamous vole. *Nature* 400: 766–768.

Chapter 14
Control of Movement

KEY CONCEPTS

- Motor outputs are controlled by two major systems, the corticospinal tract, which is also called the pyramidal system, because of the appearance of its descending projections as they traverse the brain stem, and the extrapyramidal system, a diverse group of structures that are often lumped together.

- The corticospinal and closely related corticobulbar pathways consist of upper motor neurons in the cerebral cortex that synapse on lower motor neurons with cell bodies in the anterior horn of the spinal cord or the brain stem, respectively.

- Lower motor neurons project to striated muscle.

- Upper motor neurons utilize glutamate as their neurotransmitter and lower motor neurons utilize acetylcholine.

- Prominent components of the extrapyramidal system include the basal ganglia, the cerebellum, and several brain stem nuclei.

- The basal ganglia are composed of the caudate nucleus, the putamen, and the globus pallidus, structures interconnected anatomically and functionally with each other and with the subthalamic nucleus, the substantia nigra, and the mediodorsal nucleus of the thalamus.

- The basal ganglia and thalamus form a large-scale circuit that receives and processes input from the cerebral cortex and subsequently provides feedback to the cerebral cortex; this circuit is involved in the integration of information that underlies the generation and initiation of voluntary movement and in the selection of responses to certain stimuli.

- The striatum also plays a key role in the development of certain types of implicit memory, including stimulus-response and habit-related memories.

- Loss of dopamine input to the basal ganglia causes the symptoms of Parkinson disease; restoration of dopamine function, for example, with the dopamine precursor L-dopa, remains the mainstay of therapy for Parkinson disease.

- Huntington disease is caused by a mutation in the gene for huntingtin; rare familial forms of Parkinson disease are caused by mutation in the genes for α-synuclein or parkin.

- The cerebellum is involved in the maintenance of posture, in producing accurate trajectories for movement, and in the maintenance of smooth motor movements.

- Disorders of the cerebellum are characterized by a type of incoordination known as ataxia.

Perhaps no output of the nervous system is more perceptible than movement. It is easily identifiable and measurable, and also can be elicited and studied readily in laboratory animals. Consequently, it has been possible to identify major neural pathways in the brain and spinal cord that govern normal movement and to understand the mechanisms by which principal classes of drugs affect motor function. During the past few decades great progress has been made toward understanding the pathophysiology of several human movement disorders, including **Parkinson disease** and **Huntington disease**. Observation of the motor effects of highly localized lesions in patients—produced, for example, by **stroke**—also has contributed to our understanding of the brain's control of movement.

We currently know a great deal more about movement than we do about the control of many neural functions discussed in subsequent chapters, including mood, motivation, and cognition. Yet important questions regarding movement, even under normal conditions, remain unanswered. How is sensory information processed, interpreted, and subsequently relayed to cortical motor areas? How does conscious thought initiate a motor task? How do the many subcortical regions that are critical for normal movement modulate cortical output to produce exquisitely coordinated motor activity such as that required for typing, playing a musical instrument, or operating a video game? Answers to these questions await a more sophisticated understanding of the brain's molecular and cellular constituents and of the complex intercellular communication that underlies the functioning of neural circuits.

NORMAL CONTROL OF MOVEMENT

The intention to perform a particular voluntary movement originates in cortical association areas. These areas act in cooperation with cerebellar hemispheres and the basal ganglia during the planning phase of movement. Commands to move are continually devised and initiated by the motor cortex, and portions of the cerebellum and basal ganglia are updated constantly by collateral connections and by peripheral sensory receptors that indicate the body's position.

Motor control is subserved by multiple, highly interconnected circuits. The corticospinal pathway consists of upper motor neurons with cell bodies in the cerebral cortex whose axons synapse on lower motor neurons in the spinal cord (Figure 14–1). This pathway is often termed the pyramidal tract because the axons of upper motor neurons form a pyramid-shaped bundle as they traverse the brain stem. Other pathways that ultimately influence lower motor neurons have been collectively referred to as extrapyramidal motor systems. These diverse pathways involve the basal ganglia, the cerebellum, and several brain stem nuclei that influence cerebellar and spinal function.

ANATOMY OF THE CORTICOSPINAL PATHWAY

The cell bodies of upper motor neurons are located in frontal (motor) areas of the cortex. These neurons descend through the internal capsule and brain stem pyramids and synapse onto lower motor neurons in the anterior horn of the spinal cord, which in turn directly synapse onto their specific muscle targets (see Figure 14–1). Upper motor neurons are glutamatergic, and lower motor neurons are cholinergic. The actions of acetylcholine at postsynaptic specializations on muscle fibers, termed *muscle end plates*, are mediated by nicotinic cholinergic receptors (see Chapter 9).

Because the axons of upper motor neurons must travel a considerable distance to synapse onto lower motor neurons, they are among the longest in the body; indeed, they can be as long as a meter in some individuals. Both upper and lower motor neurons are topographically organized. Upper motor neurons that control the activities of certain muscle groups are grouped in corresponding regions of the cortex; these neurons synapse onto closely spaced lower motor neurons located at a given level of the spinal cord, which in turn innervate the appropriate muscle fibers.

The corticobulbar tract comprises upper motor neurons of the cortex that synapse onto lower motor neurons in the brain stem; thus this area is functionally and anatomically related to the corticospinal tract. Axons from lower motor neurons of the corticobulbar tract exit the brain stem through various cranial nerves and control muscles for facial expressions, eye movements, and various other motor functions of the head and neck. Cranial nerves involved in the coticobulbar tract include cranial nerve VII, which innervates facial muscles; cranial nerve V, the trigeminal nerve that innervates jaw muscles; and cranial nerve XII, the hypoglossal nerve that innervates the tongue.

ANATOMY OF THE EXTRAPYRAMIDAL SYSTEM

Basal ganglia　The basal ganglia are a collection of bilateral subcortical nuclei that are so named because they lie at the base of the forebrain in primates. The major components of this region of the brain are the caudate nucleus, the putamen, and the globus pallidus. The cau-

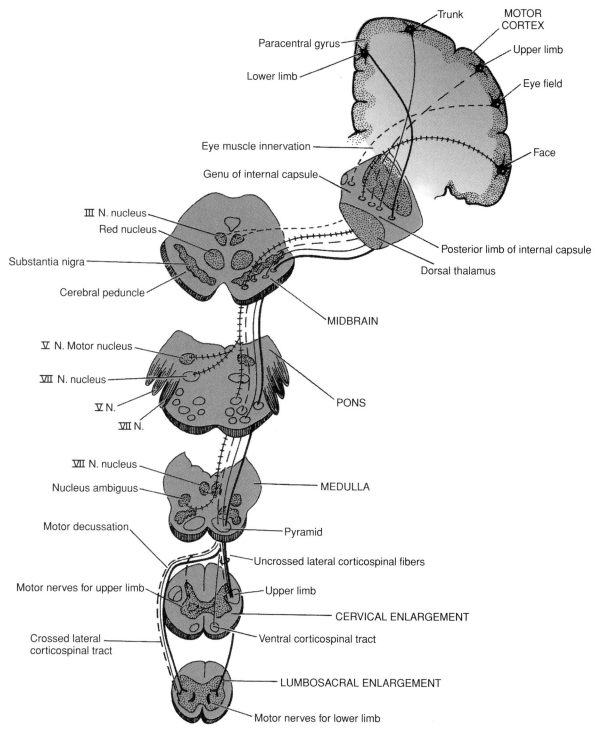

Figure 14-1. Corticospinal and corticobulbar tracts. Upper motor neurons in the cerebral cortex project to lower motor neurons in the brain stem (corticobulbar tract) or in the spinal cord (corticospinal tract). Note the topographic organization of upper motor neurons in the cortex. The roman numerals and N. refer to the numbers of cranial nerve. (Adapted with permission from Adams RD, Victor M. 1993. *Principles of Neurology,* 5th ed, p. 43. New York: McGraw-Hill.)

date and putamen are collectively known as the neostriatum because of striations apparent in tissue dissected from this region. The term *striatum* is often used to encompass both the neostriatum (also called the dorsal striatum) and more ventral extensions referred to as the ventral striatum, the principal component of which is the nucleus accumbens. Two other subcortical nuclei, the subthalamic nucleus and the substantia nigra, are interconnected with the neostriatum functionally and anatomically. The substantia nigra is located in the midbrain and has two main parts: the pars compacta, which contains dopaminergic neurons, and the pars reticulata, which contains γ-aminobutyric acid (GABA)ergic neurons. It was given its name because it contains black melanin pigment in its dopaminergic neurons.

The basal ganglia and associated nuclei, together with the mediodorsal nucleus of the thalamus, form a large-scale neural circuit that receives and processes input from the cerebral cortex, and subsequently provides feedback to the cortex. In this way, the basal ganglia are involved in the integration of complex information that underlies the generation and initiation of voluntary movement; moreover, these regions most likely are involved in selecting responses to certain stimuli. The basal ganglia also assist in forming certain types of implicit memory, especially habit-related memories that permit automatization of motor programs. Accordingly, diseases that affect the basal ganglia may result in serious motor disturbances ranging from a paucity of movement to abnormal involuntary movements.

The striatum receives excitatory, glutamatergic input from all cortical areas. Neocortical areas project mainly to dorsal parts of striatum, whereas other regions of the cortex, such as the hippocampus and amygdala, project mainly to ventral parts of striatum. The ultimate feedback from the striatum to the cortex, which is delivered by means of the mediodorsal thalamus, is directed primarily to the frontal cortex, which comprises areas involved in motor planning.

Circuitry   More than 90% of striatal neurons are medium-sized GABAergic neurons that project out of the striatum and have dense dendritic spines arranged in distinctive patterns; thus they are termed *medium spiny neurons*. A simplified model of basal ganglia circuitry that has been useful in understanding the symptoms of **Parkinson disease** is based on two major loops that process cortical information and feed the processed information back to the cortex (Figure 14–2). One loop, often called the direct pathway, involves

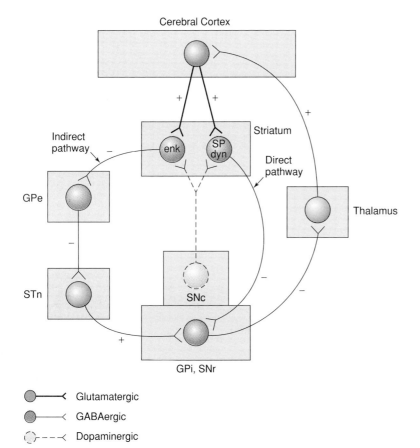

Figure 14–2. Simplified representation of neural circuitry in the basal ganglia. Glutamatergic neurons from the cortex innervate two major types of GABAergic neurons in the striatum. One type, which coexpresses the neuropeptides dynorphin (dyn) and substance P (SP), projects directly to the globus pallidus pars interna (GPi) and substantia nigra pars reticulata (SNr). The other type of GABAergic neuron, which coexpresses enkephalin (enk), projects indirectly to the GPi and SNr by means of the globus pallidus pars externa (GPe) and subthalamus nucleus (STn). Dopaminergic neurons in the substantia nigra pars compacta (SNc) modulate these striatal outputs. The activity of these dopamine neurons is controlled by GABAergic projections from the striatum and by GABAergic neurons in the SNr (not shown). The major output neurons of the basal ganglia are GABAergic neurons in the GPi and SNr, which project to the thalamus and to the brain stem (not shown).

approximately half of the medium spiny neurons in the striatum (those that express substance P and dynorphin). The neurons in this loop project to the internal segment of the globus pallidus and to the substantia nigra pars reticulata; these closely related output structures of the basal ganglia subsequently extend to the thalamus, which projects back to the cortex. The second loop, called the indirect pathway, involves the other half of the medium spiny neurons in the striatum, which express enkephalin. This pathway is described as indirect because it entails additional processing of information before it reaches the output structures of the basal ganglia. Accordingly, medium spiny neurons of the indirect pathway project to the external segment of the globus pallidus, which extends to the subthalamic nucleus, which in turn continues to the internal segment of the globus pallidus and to the substantia nigra pars reticulata. These output structures send feedback to the thalamus and ultimately to the cortex as they do in the first loop described. The medium spiny neurons of both pathways, as well as interneurons in the striatum, are densely innervated by dopaminergic afferent fibers from the substantia nigra pars compacta. Degeneration of these dopaminergic neurons causes Parkinson disease.

The ventral striatum is characterized by an analogous circuitry; however, these circuits receive dopaminergic input from the ventral tegmental area (VTA) instead of from the nearby substantia nigra pars compacta. Neurons from the VTA also innervate the amygdala, the hippocampus, and especially in primates, large portions of the cerebral cortex. The neurons that project from the ventral striatum, like those that project from the dorsal striatum, are GABAergic medium spiny neurons. One subset of these neurons projects to the ventral pallidum by a route analogous to the indirect pathway described for the dorsal striatum; the other subset projects back to the VTA by a route analogous to the direct pathway previously described. Ventral striatal neurons are believed to be involved in the regulation of motivational states and motor activity. As discussed in Chapter 16, the dopaminergic pathway (mesoaccumbens) that extends from the VTA to the nucleus accumbens is a critical substrate for the reinforcing properties of natural rewards (e.g., food and sex) and of **drugs of abuse**. Dopaminergic projections (mesocortical) from the VTA to the frontal cortex have been implicated in working memory (see Chapter 17); those from the VTA to the hippocampus play a role in spatial memory in rodents and may regulate explicit memory in humans (see Chapter 20). Regulation of dopamine in mesocorticolimbic circuits most likely underlies some of the actions of **antipsychotic** drugs and may be involved in the formation of psychotic symptoms in **schizophrenia** (see Chapter 17).

Cellular organization of the striatum Each medium spiny neuron may receive excitatory synapses from thousands of cortical neurons. This anatomic organization enables the integration of information from many sources. Medium spiny neurons are deeply hyperpolarized at rest and thus are silent most of the time, until simultaneous activity in many glutamatergic afferent neurons propels them into an active mode. After they have entered this mode, small changes in input can trigger action potentials, and in turn can cause the cells to fire in bursts. The operation of striatal neurons is complex and interesting; for example, the firing of these neurons sometimes is context-dependent. A striatal neuron may fire in conjunction with a movement when it is associated with a particular behavioral task, but may not be activated when the same movement occurs as part of a different task.

All other neurons in the striatum are interneurons; these include small GABAergic interneurons and very large cholinergic interneurons. Such neurons modulate the activity of GABAergic medium spiny projection neurons and of the glutamatergic and dopaminergic nerve terminals that innervate the striatum. The striatum can be subdivided into patch (striosome) and matrix compartments, based on the selective localization of various proteins; such compartments are interspersed throughout striatal tissue (Figure 14–3). The Ca^{2+}-binding protein calbindin, for example, is localized to a subset of GABAergic interneurons, and its

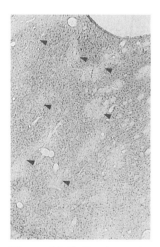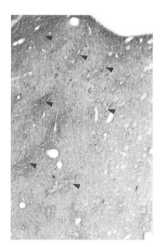

Figure 14–3. Patch–matrix compartments of the striatum. Compartments in sections of rat caudate–putamen are delineated by the immunoreactivity of calbindin (*left*) and calretinin (*right*). Patches (striosomes) are calbindin-poor and calretinin-rich areas (*arrowheads*) surrounded by calbindin-rich calretinin-poor matrix. The blank area in the upper right corner represents the lateral ventricle. (Borrowed with permission from N. Hiroi, Albert Einstein College of Medicine, Bronx, NY.)

presence or absence can be used as a marker of the patch–matrix organization of the striatum; calbindin-rich regions define matrix, whereas calbindin-poor regions define patches. In some species, patches are also marked by μ opioid receptors.

As previously discussed, the two subtypes of GABAergic medium spiny neurons in the striatum can be distinguished by the neuropeptides they express: striatonigral neurons, which project by means of the direct pathway, express substance P and dynorphin, whereas striatopallidal neurons, which project by means of the indirect pathway, express enkephalin. However, it is important to emphasize that these distinctions are not absolute; a small number of medium spiny neurons express both substance P and enkephalin. Moreover, the localization of dopamine receptor subtypes within these medium spiny neuron populations has been a subject of considerable debate. Investigators initially proposed a sharp delineation in receptor expression; accordingly it was believed that D_1-like receptors are expressed only by dynorphin- and substance P-positive cells and that D_2-like receptors are expressed only by enkephalin-positive cells. Other investigators argued that most medium spiny neurons express both D_1- and D_2-like receptors. Currently the prevailing view is somewhere in between: a majority of striatonigral medium spiny neurons express predominantly D_1-like receptors and also are dynorphin- and substance P-positive, and a majority of striatopallidal neurons express predominantly D_2-like receptors and are enkephalin-positive. However, considerable overlap most likely exists, and many neurons that predominantly express one type of receptor also may express small amounts of other receptor subtypes.

Considerable debate also surrounds the net functional effect of dopamine in the striatum. It is generally believed that dopamine's activation of either D_1-like or D_2-like dopamine receptors inhibits the firing of GABAergic projection neurons. However, as with many classes of G protein-coupled receptors, it appears that dopamine receptors cannot be characterized as simply inhibitory or excitatory. The ionic basis of dopamine's actions at either receptor remains unclear, and the circumstances under which the activation of either receptor results in antagonistic or synergistic functional effects also have not been determined with certainty. Some of the complexity of dopamine's effects may be traced to cellular heterogeneity in the striatum and the related difficulty associated with isolating effects experimentally and attributing them to interaction with one type of neuron or synapse. Moreover, dopamine's effects vary depending on the physiologic state of the medium spiny neuron.

Yet dopaminergic transmission in the striatum undoubtedly serves to increase locomotor activity. Indeed, psychomotor stimulants such as **cocaine** and **amphetamine** cause locomotor activity by increasing such transmission. Agonists that act directly at D_1-like or D_2-like dopamine receptors also activate locomotion. It appears that the ventral striatum, or nucleus accumbens, mediates ambulatory locomotor activity induced by a psychomotor stimulant and that the dorsal striatum (the caudate nucleus and putamen) mediates more complicated activity—at higher doses producing stereotypy, or repetitive movements without purpose such as rearing. However, considerable overlap in the behavioral output of these systems most likely exists.

Adenosine receptor antagonists such as **caffeine** represent another class of stimulants whose effects are believed to be mediated at least in part at the level of the striatum (see Chapter 10); adenosine A_{2A} receptors are co-localized with D_2 receptors in the striatum, and significant dopamine–adenosine interactions have been reported. Substantial serotonin innervation of the basal ganglia by means of the midbrain raphe nuclei also occurs (see Chapter 9). Such serotonergic input is gaining attention because antagonism of 5-HT$_{2A}$ and other serotonin receptors appears to be a critical property of second-generation antipsychotic drugs such as **clozapine, risperidone,** and **olanzapine,** which are less likely than older antipsychotic agents to cause extrapyramidal (Parkinson disease-like) motor symptoms.

The anatomic and chemical complexity of striatal neurons have made it difficult to understand how specific behaviors are mediated by striatal circuitry. Yet modulation of the striatum by dopamine and other neurotransmitters remains a topic of intense interest because such modulation has been implicated in a wide range of neuropsychiatric disorders discussed here and in subsequent chapters, including **Parkinson disease, Huntington disease, drug addiction, schizophrenia, obsessive–compulsive disorder,** and **Tourette syndrome.**

CEREBELLAR CONTROL OF MOVEMENT

The cerebellum plays an important role in the execution of a variety of voluntary movements by helping to maintain proper posture, initiate sequential movements, and control properties of movement such as speed and trajectory. Disorders of the cerebellum typically interfere with movements involving rapidly alternating motoric functions and also disturb the balance necessary for walking and running. Such impairment typically results in movements that are slow, clumsy, and poorly organized.

Located in the posterior fossa, the cerebellum is a bilaterally symmetrical structure divided into two large lateral masses called cerebellar hemispheres, which fuse near the midline along a narrow portion called the

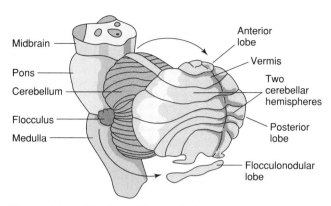

Figure 14-4. Structure of the cerebellum.

Midbrain

Pons

Cerebellum

Flocculus

Medulla

Anterior lobe

Vermis

Two cerebellar hemispheres

Posterior lobe

Flocculonodular lobe

vermis. Cerebellar peduncles are large collections of axons that connect the cerebellum to the pons and medulla and serve to reciprocally link the cerebellum with several brain stem nuclei; such connections provide a constant account of motor activity as determined by signals from various inputs. The vermis and the intermediate zones of the anterior and posterior lobes of the cerebellar hemispheres receive input from the spinal cord; the flocculonodular lobe and the cerebellar hemispheres receive input from the vestibular nuclei and the cerebral hemispheres, respectively (Figure 14–4). Additional sensory information from the skin, joints, and muscles reaches the cerebellum through spinocerebellar tracts.

DISORDERS OF MOVEMENT

Some movement disorders primarily involve motor weakness, whereas many others are characterized by abnormal involuntary movements or impaired regulation of voluntary movement. The abnormal movements that are hallmarks of the latter disorders are not caused by weakness or sensory deficits; rather they result from a dysfunction of brain areas that control normal movement. Hypokinetic disorders are characterized by a paucity of movement, and hyperkinetic disorders are characterized by an increase in abnormal, involuntary movements. Table 14–1 lists the types of abnormal movements that are associated with various movement disorders.

Many abnormal movements can be traced to specific lesions in the brain. Lesions or neoplasms in or near the basal ganglia interrupt the normal flow of impulses to the globus pallidus, and consequently disrupt flow to the thalamus and cerebral cortex. Lesions in the subthalamic and caudate nuclei, for example, result in hemiballism and hemichorea. In adults, such lesions are often the result of **strokes**. The degeneration of

Table 14-1 Types of Abnormal Movements Associated With Movement Disorders

Type of Movement	Description
Akathisia	Subjective feeling of inner restlessness that is relieved by stereotypic and complex movements (e.g., squirming, crossing/uncrossing legs, rocking and pacing)
Asterixis	Periods of sudden cessation of muscle contraction, most easily observed when patient's arms are extended in front; considered a form of myoclonus
Athetosis	Sinuous, slow, writhing or wormlike movements involving the extremities, trunk, and neck
Ballismus	Wild flinging, flailing movements of the arm and leg that represent proximal choreiform movements; often unilateral (hemiballismus)
Bradykinesia	Movements that are slow or of diminished frequency or amplitude
Catalepsy	Maintenance of abnormal positions; passive movement of limbs, often characterized by waxy flexibility
Chorea	Rapid irregular muscle jerks that occur involuntarily and unpredictably in alternating parts of the body in a continuous and non-purposeful pattern; disappear during sleep
Dyskinesia	Any excessive movement
Dystonia	Twisting movements sustained for variable periods of time
Freezing	Brief episodes during which a motor act is temporarily blocked or halted; most often affect walking
Myokymia	Quivering or rippling of muscle
Rigidity	Increased muscle tone during passive motion in all directions (i.e., affects flexors and extensors equally)
Tachykinesia	Movements of speech that are characterized by continuous acceleration or loss of amplitude
Tics	Sudden, quick, coordinated, repetitive movements or sounds that are voluntarily suppressible for short periods; diminish during voluntary activity and disappear during sleep
Tremor	Regular, rhythmic, oscillatory movements that may be present at rest or during action

specific neuronal cell types, such as upper or lower motor neurons or basal ganglion neurons, can lead to a vast array of motor abnormalities. Drugs also can produce abnormal movement. The precise genetic loci of some inherited movement disorders caused by single gene mutations have been determined (Table 14–2).

Table 14–2 Inheritable Movement Disorders

Disorder	Mode of Inheritance	Site of Genetic Defect	Gene Product
Huntington disease	AD	4p16.3	Huntingtin
Idiopathic torsion dystonia	AD	9q32-34	Not known
	AR	Unknown	
	XL	Xq21.3	
Wilson disease	AR	13q14.1	Copper transporter
Benign (essential) familial tremor	AD	Unknown	Not known
X-linked dystonia/parkinsonism	XL	Xq11.2	Not known
Dopa-responsive dystonia	AD	14q	GTP-cyclohydrolase I
Parkinson disease			
• familial adult onset	AD	4q21-q23	α-Synuclein
• familial juvenile onset	AR	6	Parkin
Benign hereditary chorea	AD, AR	Unknown	Not known
Familial chorea/acanthocytosis	AR	Unknown	Not known
Paroxysmal choreoathetosis	AD	2q	Not known
Familial amyotrophic lateral sclerosis	AD	21q	CuZn-SOD
Spinobulbar muscular atrophy[1]	XL	Xq13	Androgen receptor

[1]Also known as Kennedy disease.
AD, autosomal dominant; AR, autosomal recessive; XL, X-linked; SOD, superoxide dismutase; GTP, guanosine 5′-triphosphate.

DISORDERS OF THE PYRAMIDAL TRACT AND CEREBELLUM

Motor function can be disturbed by the dysfunction of many parts of the central or peripheral nervous system, including that of upper or lower motor neurons, the cerebellum, basal ganglia, peripheral nerves, or neuromuscular junctions. Any disease that directly affects muscles also can perturb motor function.

Various clinical criteria are used to determine whether upper or lower motor neurons are affected by a particular disease (Table 14–3). Diseases that affect lower motor neurons are characterized by weakness and wasting of affected muscles. If muscles involved in locomotion are affected, gait also may be altered. Diseases that affect upper motor neurons are characterized by loss of voluntary control of motor function as well as motor weakness. In contrast, cerebellar dysfunction typically results in abnormal balance and coordination.

Amyotrophic lateral sclerosis Also known as Lou Gehrig's disease in the United States, amyotrophic lateral sclerosis (ALS) is a motor neuron disease that generally occurs in individuals between 30 and 60 years of age. It is characterized by the degeneration of upper and lower motor neurons in both the corticospinal and corticobulbar tracts. The distribution of resulting deficits in movement can be traced to predominant involvement of either the limbs or cranial nerves, and the predominant involvement of either upper or lower motor neurons, and can be used to distinguish the clinical variations of this disorder. In approximately 20% of patients, for example, the disease is limited to weakness of the bulbar muscles; bulbar involvement is characterized by difficulty in swallowing, chewing, coughing, breathing, and speaking. ALS is progressive and typically results in a fatal outcome within three to five years.

Table 14–3 Comparison of Motor Neuron and Cerebellar Dysfunction

Upper Motor Neuron Lesions
- Weakness or paralysis
- Spasticity
- Increased tendon reflexes
- Abnormal Babinski response
- Loss of abdominal reflexes
- Little or no muscle atrophy

Lower Motor Neuron Lesions
- Weakness or paralysis
- Hypotonia
- Loss of tendon reflexes
- Normal Babinski response
- Normal abdominal reflexes
- Wasting of involved muscles
- Muscle fasciculations

Cerebellar Dysfunction
- Ataxia
- Hypotonia
- Decreased tendon reflexes
- Gait abnormalities
- Abnormal eye movements
- Dysarthric speech

Box 14–1 Intracellular Inclusions and Gain-of-Function Mutations

An important lesson that has evolved from the study of movement disorders is that genetic mutations may cause disease not by affecting the normal function of a particular protein but by producing a new and toxic function of the protein. Many mutant proteins, for example, induce the formation of intracellular inclusion bodies, which exert toxic effects on cells by disrupting basic cellular processes (see table). Diseases caused by such gain-of-function mutations often exhibit dominant transmission because only one copy of the responsible gene is required for pathogenesis.

Movement Disorder	Cellular Site of Inclusions	Possible Effect of Inclusions
Parkinson[1] disease	Cytoplasm (Lewy bodies)	Disruption of proteasomes
Huntington disease	Nucleus	Disruption of RNA processing
Amyotrophic lateral sclerosis	Cytoplasm; cellular processes	Disruption of transport Impaired control of glutamate
Myotonic dystrophy	Unknown	Disruption of RNA processing

[1]Familial forms.

Patients with bulbar involvement generally are given a poorer prognosis because of breathing and swallowing difficulties and associated aspiration and pulmonary infections. Motor neuron disease in children, such as **Werdnig-Hoffmann disease (infantile spinal muscular atrophy)**, typically presents early in life and is characterized by impaired swallowing or sucking and muscle wasting of the limbs.

Most cases of ALS are sporadic; only 10–20% are characterized by familial transmission. In approximately 20% of familial cases (a very small percentage of all cases), the disease is caused by a mutation in the gene for the enyme Cu/Zn superoxide dismutase (SOD), which is involved in removing oxygen-reactive species from cells (see Chapter 11). This finding initially suggested an excitotoxic mechanism of neuronal damage. Accordingly it was believed that mutations in SOD lead to a loss of its function, which in turn increases oxidative stress on cells. However, further investigation suggested a more complicated situation. First, SOD is involved in only a small percentage of cases of ALS. Second, knockout mice that lack SOD do not develop signs of ALS. Third, some disease-causing mutations in the protein do not result in reduced enzyme activity. Yet despite such data, transgenic mice that overexpress a mutant form of SOD have exhibited a loss of motor neurons.

Currently it is believed that mutant forms of SOD associated with ALS may reflect a gain of function (Box 14–1); such mutant proteins cause the development of inclusions in the cytoplasm and cellular processes that in turn cause damage to cells. Details regarding this process remain controversial; for example, some researchers argue that these inclusions initially form in astrocytes of the spinal cord, reducing their ability to transport glutamate and thereby interfering with the termination of synaptic glutamate signals (see Chapter 7). Such interference might result in excitotoxicity. Others argue that inclusions initially form in motor neurons and thereby directly disrupt aspects of neuronal function; such disruption most likely would not depend on excitotoxicity. In one small family lineage, ALS is caused by a mutation in a gene that encodes a neurofilament subunit; although this mutation is associated with intracellular inclusions, little else is known about its role in motor neuron death. Other aspects of the association between SOD and ALS also remain puzzling. Because the expression of SOD is ubiquitous, researchers have yet to determine why the mutation of its gene results in the selective degeneration of upper and lower motor neurons, and why this degeneration occurs relatively late in life, in a relatively synchronized fashion.

Until recently, treatment of ALS has been symptomatic. However, two medications currently in use may be effective in slowing the progression of the disease. **Riluzole** is believed to exert ameliorative effects by decreasing synaptic levels of glutamate. Such activity is consistent with the hypothesis that ALS may be caused by glutamate-mediated excitotoxicity. **Gabapentin** is an anticonvulsant that potentiates GABAergic transmission at the synapse, perhaps by reducing GABA reuptake (see Chapter 21). Because GABA inhibits excitatory neurons, its usefulness in the treatment of ALS is also consistent with an excitotoxic model of the disease.

Experimental therapies for ALS currently are focused on the use of various **neurotrophic factors,** based on evidence that these factors can protect motor neurons from degeneration in cell culture and in some animal models of the disease (see Chapter 11). However, most patients cannot tolerate the weight loss and other side effects associated with such treatment approaches; thus their implementation must await further research. Nevertheless, the evolving understanding of the pathophysiology of the disease, particularly that of its familial forms, raises hope that future treatment of the disorder might be directed at its underlying cause.

Cerebellar dysfunction   Disorders that affect the cerebellum typically alter muscle tone and the smooth execution of movements (see Table 14–3). Alteration of motor skill resulting from cerebellar malfunction is called *cerebellar ataxia.* Involvement of midline cerebellar structures, especially the vermis, leads to truncal ataxia, which is characterized by a gait that is clumsy, irregular, unsteady, and broad-based; in extreme cases, the affected individual cannot stand without falling. A lesion of one of the cerebellar hemispheres results in an unsteady gait and causes a patient to consistently fall to one side. Cerebellar dysfunction also may cause tremors and difficulty in controlling the trajectory or placement of body parts during active movements. If such dysfunction occurs gradually, defects may be compensated for by other brain circuits. Accordingly, disease that progresses slowly results in defects that are more subtle than those caused by acute injury to the cerebellum.

One of the most common causes of cerebellar dysfunction is **acute alcohol intoxication**. Alcohol produces this effect by facilitating $GABA_A$ receptor function (see Chapter 7), particularly that of receptors that contain the α_6 subunit, which is concentrated in cerebellar neurons. This finding enabled the development of **RO15–4513,** a drug that selectively antagonizes the effects of alcohol at the α_6 subunit (see Chapters 7 and 15). Although this drug reverses the ataxic effects of alcohol, it has no effect on other actions attributed to alcohol, such as cognitive impairment and sedation, which are mediated by other α subunits outside the cerebellum. Consequently, RO15–4513 remains unsuitable for use as a sobering agent. Yet its effectiveness in reversing some of the deleterious effects of alcohol demonstrates how knowledge of molecular mechanisms can lead to the development of highly specific drugs with selective behavioral effects.

PARKINSON DISEASE

Parkinson disease is characterized by tremor at rest, bradykinesia, and cogwheel rigidity. The characteristic resting tremor is typified by a pill-rolling motion at a frequency of 3–5 Hz. Bradykinesia refers to a slowness of movements—in particular, a difficulty in initiating movements—which interferes with the performance of daily tasks. Rigidity and impaired reflexes are partly responsible for the parkinsonian gait, which is traditionally described as festinating, or characterized by short rapid steps. Patients with Parkinson disease also may experience micrography, or small handwriting; weight loss; and alterations in autonomic function; masked facies, or a blank facial expression caused by less frequent eye blinking, and bradykinesia of the facial muscles also is common among affected individuals.

Pathophysiology   Parkinson disease is caused by the death of dopamine neurons in the substantia nigra pars compacta, with consequent dopamine depletion in the caudate nucleus and putamen. Pathologic manifestations include degenerative changes, such as neuronal deterioration and depigmentation in the substantia nigra, and the appearance of intracellular inclusions called *Lewy bodies* in dopamine neurons. Death of dopaminergic neurons in the VTA and that of other monoaminergic neurons (e.g., noradrenergic and serotonergic neurons in the brain stem) also may occur on a much smaller scale.

The functional effects of the loss of dopamine in patients with Parkinson disease can be understood, to some degree, based on our knowledge of striatal circuits (see Figures 14–2 and 14–5). Normally, dopamine exerts an inhibitory influence on GABAergic projection neurons of the striatum. Consequently, the loss of dopamine causes increased activity among these neurons, and in turn causes increased inhibitory output from the basal ganglia to the thalamus (see Figure 14–2). Increased activity among striatal GABAergic neurons decreases the activity of GABAergic neurons in the globus pallidus. These events lead to increased activity among glutamatergic neurons in the subthalamic nucleus, which in turn leads to increased activity among GABAergic neurons of the substantia nigra pars reticulata. Such activity causes increased inhibition of the thalamic ventral tier nuclei. Because these nuclei are responsible for the activation of cortical areas involved in the initiation of movements, the ultimate effect of dopamine deficiency is paucity of movement.

Healthy individuals possess a large reserve of nigrostriatal dopaminergic neurons; consequently, overt parkinsonian symptoms do not occur until approximately 80% of these neurons have been lost. Compensatory responses in remaining neurons, such as the up-regulation of tyrosine hydroxylase (see Chapter 8), enable these cells to make more dopamine. The functional reserve provided by these adaptations causes most cases of Parkinson disease to be characterized by a slow, progressive loss of dopamine cells. Rapidly evolving lesions, such as those produced by neurotoxins, can produce parkinsonian symptoms in response to the loss of many fewer dopaminergic neurons. Interestingly, a very slow, progressive loss of dopamine neurons occurs—even in the absence of Parkinson disease—in normal individuals throughout adult life.

Genetic factors   Increasing evidence suggests that there may be a genetic contribution to the etiology of Parkinson disease, but the exact nature of this contribution remains unclear. In most cases, the disease appears to be sporadic; that is, it occurs in individuals who do not appear to have a family history of the disease. However, this pattern of disease may reflect genetic susceptibility that only gives rise to illness when certain environmental factors, such as exposure to dopaminergic neurotoxins, are also present.

In addition to the sporadic, common forms of Parkinson disease, there are rare familial forms that are characterized by Mendelian transmission. Two specific genes responsible for such transmission have been identified by genetic linkage analysis. One gene encodes a previously unknown protein, called *parkin;* the other encodes a protein of unknown function termed α-*synuclein.* How mutations in these genes cause the death of dopaminergic neurons remains unknown, but ubiquitin–mediated protein degradation pathways have been implicated. Ubiquitin is a small protein that is added covalently to other cellular proteins targeted for proteolytic degradation by cellular organelles called *proteasomes* (see Chapter 6). Lewy bodies, the pathognomonic feature of Parkinson disease, are heavily stained with antibodies to ubiquitin and related proteins, and with anti-α-synuclein antibodies, even in sporadic cases that lack α-synuclein mutations. Interestingly, parkin is highly homologous to ubiquitin; consequently it has been hypothesized that mutations in parkin or α-synuclein may lead to abnormalities in proteasome pathways. Further evidence for this hypothesis is drawn from a form of Parkinson disease in a single German lineage; this variation is caused by a mutation in *UCHL1,* a gene that encodes a thiol protease that also is involved in the ubiquitin pathway. Whether disease-causing mutations in these various proteins reflect loss-of-function or gain-of-function mutations remains unknown, although most investigators currently believe that the latter type of mutation occurs. Why mutations in proteins expressed widely in the brain result in the selective death of dopamine neurons is a question that also remains unanswered.

Environmental factors   The belief that environmental factors may be a cause of common idiopathic forms of Parkinson disease was prompted by the discovery of a severe form of parkinsonism that developed in a group of young adults after intravenous use of a preparation of **meperidine,** a synthetic opiate, which contained

Normal

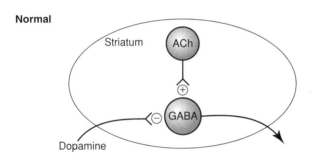

Parkinson disease

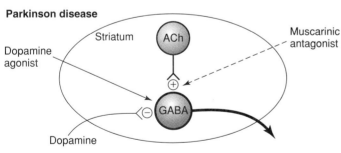

Huntington disease

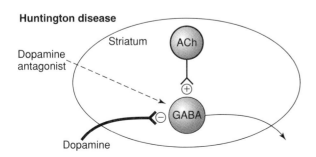

Figure 14–5. Dopamine-acetylcholine (Ach) interactions in the striatum. According to a simplified scheme, the net activity of striatal γ-aminobutyric acid (GABA)ergic projection neurons is determined by the relative activity of inhibitory dopaminergic input (mediated by D_1 and D_2 receptors) and of excitatory cholinergic input (mediated by muscarinic receptors). In individuals with Parkinson disease, the degeneration of dopaminergic neurons leads to increased excitation of GABAergic projection neurons and to motor symptoms associated with parkinsonism. Such symptoms can be reduced by L-dopa, which partially restores the inhibitory influence of dopamine, or by muscarinic cholinergic antagonists. Huntington disease is characterized by the degeneration of the GABAergic projection neurons, which leads to motor symptoms such as choreoathetoid dyskinesias. GABAergic function in affected individuals can be partially restored by dopamine receptor antagonists; theoretically, GABAergic function also should be restored by muscarinic cholinergic agonists, but the use of these agents has not resulted in clinical improvement.

the harmful by-product **1-methyl-4-phenyl-1,2,3,6-tetra-hydropyridine** (**MPTP**). Such patients exhibited rapid and extensive loss of dopamine neurons, resulting in severe parkinsonism. Investigators have since learned that MPTP is directly toxic to dopaminergic neurons (see Chapter 8).

The possibility that environmental neurotoxins may cause sporadic cases of Parkinson disease—albeit with less dramatic effects than MPTP—has been further supported by epidemiologic evidence that the disease is more common in people who reside in rural areas, drink well water, and have regular exposure to herbicides and pesticides. Potential disease-causing toxins have been identified. The pesticide rotenone can reproduce features of Parkinson disease in animal models. In Guam a very high incidence of Parkinson disease and other neurodegenerative syndromes, such as **ALS** and **dementia,** has been explained by reliance on the **cycad plant** as a dietary staple; it is believed that the seeds of this plant contain one or more neurotoxins that kill dopaminergic and other neurons. Heavy metal poisoning, particularly from exposure to Mn^{2+} or Al^-, also has been associated with Parkinson disease. Moreover, a high incidence of the disease has been noted after certain viral epidemics; thus a viral contribution to the disease is conceivable. However, specific toxins and viruses that cause common forms of Parkinson disease have yet to be identified with certainty.

Rodent and nonhuman primate models of Parkinson disease are achieved surgically or pharmacologically. Surgical lesions of either the substantia nigra or the median forebrain bundle, which carries dopaminergic axons from the midbrain to the striatum, lead to behavioral effects shortly after such lesions are placed. A model that more closely reflects the slow, progressive degeneration of nigrostriatal dopamine neurons that occurs in humans is achieved with the direct delivery of a neurotoxin into the striatum by means of slow infusion. Delivery of **MPTP** or **6-hydroxydopamine** (another selective dopaminergic neurotoxin) by means of osmotic minipumps has resulted in a 50–60% loss of dopaminergic neurons over days or weeks. Unilateral destruction of dopamine cells in rodents has been used to produce one of the most widely used behavioral assays of dopaminergic systems (Box 14–2).

DRUG-INDUCED PARKINSONISM

Certain drugs are common causes of a reversible parkinsonian-like syndrome. Patients with drug-induced parkinsonism can be symptomatically indistinguishable from those with idiopathic Parkinson disease. A large percentage of patients treated with typical **antipsychotic** medications, or **neuroleptic** agents, including various **phenothiazines** and **butyrophenones** develop drug-induced parkinsonism (see Chapter 17). Dopamine-depleting agents such as **reserpine,** previously used to treat hypertension but now rarely used (see Chapters 8 and 12), also result in a parkinsonian-like syndrome.

Drug-induced parkinsonism is most common among elderly patients, presumably because they have a smaller reserve of dopamine neurons. Symptoms develop within days to months after use of the offending drug commences (Table 14–4), and disappear over weeks or months after cessation of the drug. Resting tremor, cogwheel rigidity, and akinesia or bradykinesia are common symptoms. Akathisia also occurs and appears to be more strongly associated with drug-induced parkinsonism than with Parkinson disease.

Parkinsonian-like symptoms caused by typical antipsychotic medications are among a large number of so-called extrapyramidal side effects produced by these drugs (see Table 14–4). Such side effects are caused by the D_2-like dopamine receptor antagonist properties of these agents. Blockade of these receptors produces functional effects that mimic those of increased activity of GABAergic projection neurons, such as occurs with the loss of dopaminergic neurons (see Figure 14–5). In animals, typical extrapyramidal side effects include catalepsy and a waxy rigidity of the tail and extremities. As mentioned in Chapter 8, there are three D_2-like receptors: D_2, D_3, and D_4 receptors. Animal research suggests that antagonism of the D_2 receptor is the most likely cause of neuroleptic-induced parkinsonism because selective antagonists of the D_3 and D_4 receptors do not produce catalepsy. In addition, knockout mice lacking D_2 receptors, but not those lacking D_3 or D_4 receptors, exhibit catalepsy.

The fact that antipsychotic drugs reduce psychosis, presumably through D_2 antagonism in the mesocorticolimbic dopamine system, and cause extrapyramidal side effects, presumably through D_2 antagonism in the nigrostriatal dopamine system, has provided clinicians with a dilemma. Agents that tend to reduce psychosis also have tended to increase the severity of motoric side effects, and agents that tend to reduce motoric side effects also have tended to aggravate psychosis. A similar dilemma is encountered in the treatment of Parkinson disease: although L-dopa is effective in replacing lost dopamine, it can cause dyskinetic side effects and psychotic symptoms after prolonged use. Likewise, agents that are used to reduce the dyskinetic side effects associated with L-dopa tend to increase the severity of parkinsonian symptoms. As discussed in a subsequent section of this chapter, the introduction of newer antipsychotic medications has helped to reduce some of these complications.

Box 14–2 Rotating Rodents

A classic procedure designed to test the impact of striatal function on behavior in rodents involves the placement of lesions on one side of the nigrostriatal pathway. Various types of dopamine-promoting drugs are subsequently administered to such animals to induce rotational behavior—the tendency to turn to a particular side (see figure). This rotation is caused by asymmetry in the dopamine pathways in the two hemispheres of the brain and is produced by the unilateral lesion; the direction of the rotation depends on the mechanism of action of the drug. Dopamine receptor agonists, such as **apomorphine,** cause rotation away from the side in which the lesion is placed because they produce a greater effect on the side of the lesion, where striatal dopamine receptors are hypersensitive, most likely in response to the loss of dopamine. In contrast, indirect dopamine agonists, such as **amphetamine,** cause rotation toward the side that contains the lesion; because these drugs cause the release of dopamine from striatal nerve terminals, they produce a lesser effect on the lesioned side, where many dopaminergic terminals have been destroyed.

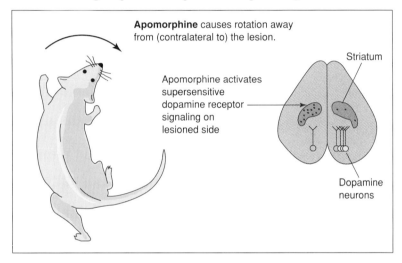

Apomorphine causes rotation away from (contralateral to) the lesion.

Striatum

Apomorphine activates supersensitive dopamine receptor signaling on lesioned side

Dopamine neurons

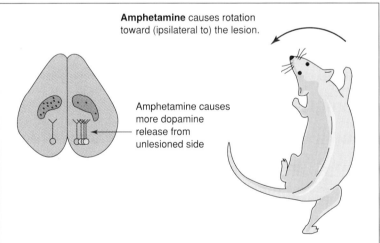

Amphetamine causes rotation toward (ipsilateral to) the lesion.

Amphetamine causes more dopamine release from unlesioned side

Why does increased dopaminergic function on one side of the striatum cause rotation away from that side? Although this question remains unanswered, it is known that drugs that activate the dopamine pathway, such as cocaine and amphetamine, also activate locomotion. This phenomenon can be understood based on interactions represented in Figures 14–2 and 14–5. These figures indicate that increased dopaminergic function decreases GABAergic output from the striatum. In the indirect striatal pathway, such reduction in output leads to reduced GABAergic output from the substantia nigra pars reticulata and, in turn, to reduced inhibition of afferent signals from the thalamus to the cortex. Although this series of events represents an oversimplified view of basal ganglia circuitry, it helps to provide a functional context for dopamine-related alterations in movement.

Table 14–4 Extrapyramidal Side Effects of Antipsychotic Drugs

Side Effect	Features	Period of Maximal Risk	Treatment
Acute dystonia	Spasms of muscles in tongue, face, neck, and back	First 5 days of treatment	Antiparkinsonian agents
Akathisia	Motor restlessness	5 to 60 days after treatment begins	Reduction of dose or change to different drug; antiparkinsonian agents, benzodiazepines, or propranolol may help
Parkinsonism	Bradykinesia, rigidity, variable tremor, mask-like facies, shuffling gait	5 to 30 days after treatment begins	Antiparkinsonian agents
Neuroleptic malignant syndrome	Catatonia, stupor, fever, unstable blood pressure, myoglobinemia; can be fatal	Weeks after treatment begins; can persist for days after neuroleptic is discontinued	Immediate discontinuation of neuroleptic; dantrolene or bromocriptine may help; antiparkinsonian agents not effective
Tardive dyskinesia	Oral-facial dyskinesia; widespread choreoathetosis or dystonia	After months or years of treatment; is exacerbated by withdrawal	Prevention is crucial; treatment is unsatisfactory

Tardive dyskinesia   Antagonism of D_2 receptors has been implicated in a particularly severe extrapyramidal side effect of traditional antipsychotic medications known as tardive dyskinesia (TD). TD is unlike other extrapyramidal side effects in that it requires prolonged exposure to the offending drug; indeed, the longer the exposure, the greater the likelihood of developing this syndrome. Moreover, unlike other extrapyramidal side effects, it can persist for long periods, even for a lifetime, after the precipitating medication has been discontinued. TD involves excessive, abnormal movements, particularly choreoathetoid movements that are reminiscent of **Huntington disease**. These abnormal movements, which predominate in the head and neck and typically involve the mouth and tongue, can be debilitating. TD must be distinguished from withdrawal dyskinesias that occur in many individuals after the cessation of antipsychotic treatment and gradually subside over weeks or months.

The Huntington disease-like features of TD symptoms have led to the proposal that TD represents a state of supersensitivity to dopamine in the striatum that develops as an adaptation to persistent D_2 receptor antagonism. Indeed, one treatment for TD symptoms involves raising the dose of the precipitating D_2 antagonist, a practice that is not ultimately beneficial because it leads to a vicious cycle of TD symptoms followed by increasing doses of medication, which in turn cause a worsening of TD symptoms. Despite a great deal of research, the drug-induced changes in the striatum or elsewhere in the brain that cause TD are not yet

known. Increased expression of specific dopamine receptor subtypes or of specific post-receptor signaling proteins, and neurodegenerative changes of striatal medium spiny neurons, have been proposed as underlying mechanisms of TD but remain conjectural. TD also has been traced to disruptions in neural circuitry; accordingly it has been proposed that facilitation of pallidal–subthalamic GABAergic projections may lead to inhibition of the subthalamic nucleus (see Figure 14–2).

Side effects of atypical antipsychotic drugs   A major advance in the treatment of psychosis occurred with the introduction of **clozapine,** which has been termed an atypical antipsychotic based on its superior clinical efficacy and on the absence of related extrapyramidal side effects such as parkinsonism and TD (see Chapter 17). However, clozapine can produce life-threatening agranulocytosis (most likely through an immune mechanism), a side effect that has limited its use and has led to an intense search for medications that share clozapine's superior clinical profile but do not produce deleterious effects on white blood cells. Unfortunately, the property of clozapine that is responsible for its atypical profile is not known. Clozapine has a relatively weak affinity for D_2 receptors and a higher affinity for D_3 and D_4 receptors than many other antipsychotic drugs. In addition, it has a relatively high affinity for 5-HT_{2A} receptors, at which it also acts as an antagonist. Consequently, investigators have hypothesized that a high 5-HT_{2A} to D_2 ratio is critical for an atypical profile. Several newer antipsychotic medications have been developed based on this theory, including **risperidone, olanzapine, quetiapine,** and **ziprasidone**. These drugs are associated with a lower risk for extrapyramidal side effects—including both parkinsonism and TD—compared with most other antipsychotic medications, but a higher risk compared with clozapine. It also appears that they lack the superior efficacy of clozapine.

TREATMENT OF PARKINSON DISEASE

As mentioned in Chapter 8, tyrosine is the starting point in the biosynthesis of dopamine; it is taken up into the brain by means of a low-affinity amino acid transport system, and is taken up from the extracellular space into dopaminergic neurons by means of amino acid transporters. After tyrosine has entered a neuron, it is converted to L-dopa by the cytosolic enzyme tyrosine hydroxylase, through a reaction that is the rate-limiting step in dopamine biosynthesis. Aromatic amino acid decarboxylase subsequently converts L-dopa to dopamine. Dopamine is taken up into synaptic storage vesicles and released in response to the arrival of an action potential. Dopaminergic terminals contain reuptake transporters that help to terminate neurotransmitter action and maintain homeostasis.

Currently the treatment of Parkinson disease and parkinsonism typically consists of the administration of medications that enhance dopaminergic function in the basal ganglia. Such agents may act at any of the aforementioned sites. Oral administration of **L-dopa** is the most effective symptomatic treatment available for Parkinson disease (Figure 14–6). L-dopa is transported

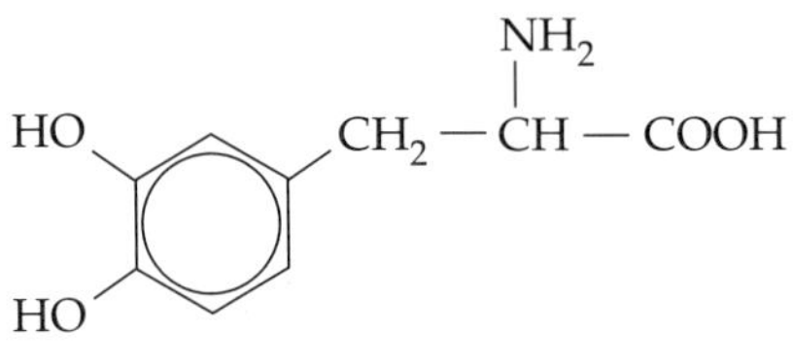

L-Dopa

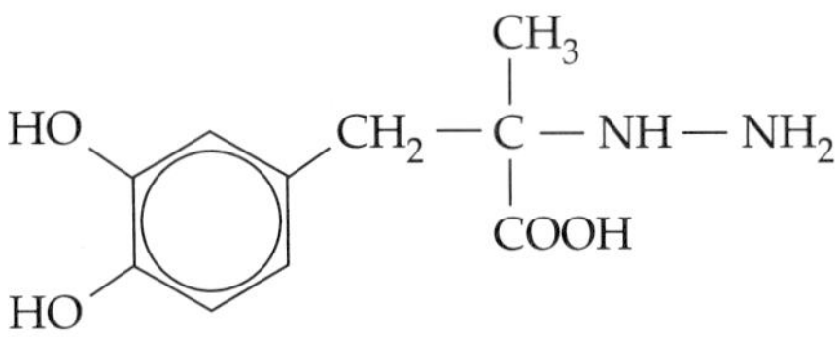

α-Methyldopa-hydrazine
(Carbidopa)

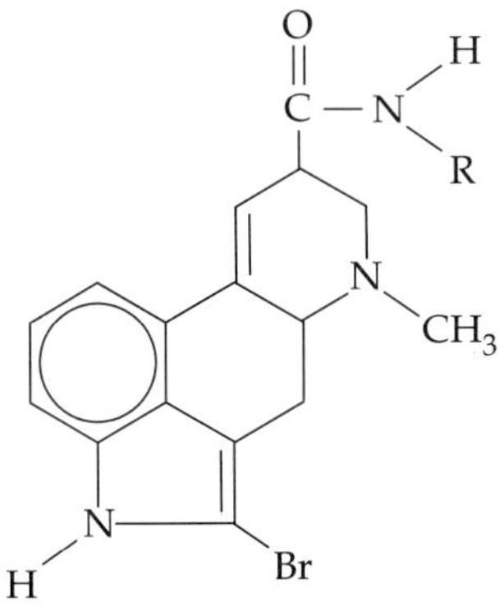

Bromocriptine

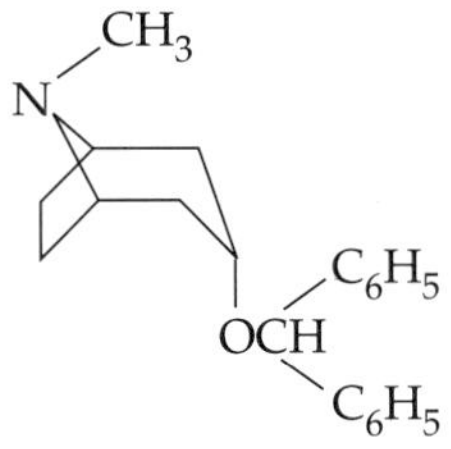

Benztropine

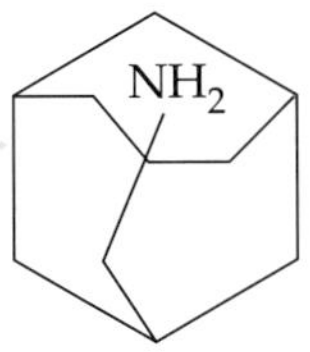

Amantadine

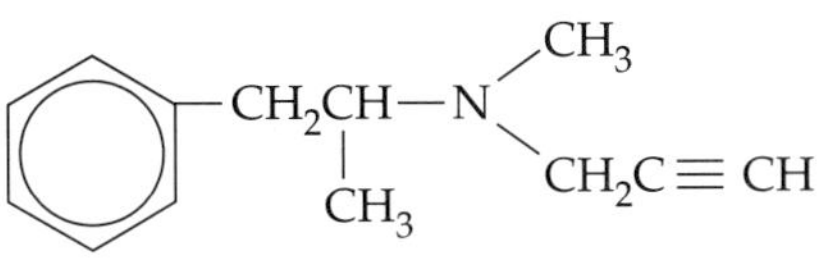

(–)-Selegiline (Deprenyl)

Figure 14–6. Chemical structures of drugs commonly used in the treatment of Parkinson disease.

across the blood–brain barrier and is converted to dopamine; thus it substitutes for missing neurotransmitter. In contrast, tyrosine itself cannot be used as a treatment for two reasons: circulating tyrosine levels normally saturate the amino acid transporter at the blood–brain barrier, and brain levels of tyrosine normally saturate tyrosine hydroxylase expressed in dopamine neurons.

L-dopa efficiently restores neurologic function, particularly during the early stages of Parkinson disease. Yet systemically administered L-dopa cannot possibly replicate dopaminergic innervation of the striatum, either spatially or temporally. Moreover, the efficacy of L-dopa decreases after 5 to 6 years and, as previously mentioned, side effects in addition to dyskinesias begin to appear, including visual hallucinations and other psychotic symptoms, sleep disturbances, and confusion. A late complication of L-dopa therapy, referred to as the on–off phenomenon, involves abrupt and transient fluctuations in the severity of parkinsonism at different intervals of the day; such fluctuations are unrelated to drug dosage. To minimize this phenomenon, individuals often restrict their use of L-dopa to times of the day when therapeutic relief is required.

Peripheral side effects caused by the conversion of L-dopa into dopamine by aromatic amino acid decarboxylase expressed in liver and other peripheral tissues may include severe hypotension and nausea. Such problems with L-dopa have been controlled by aromatic amino acid decarboxylase inhibitors such as **carbidopa** and **benserazide** (see Figure 14–6). When administered with L-dopa, such agents, which cannot cross the blood–brain barrier, inhibit peripheral aromatic amino acid decarboxylase and reduce the peripheral conversion of L-dopa into dopamine. Such actions reduce the peripheral side effects of L-dopa and enable the drug to be administered in much smaller doses. L-dopa and carbidopa are available in a fixed-ratio preparation called **Sinemet. Entacapone,** an inhibitor of catechol-O-methyltransferase (COMT), is also used in conjunction with L-dopa in the treatment of Parkinson disease. Since L-dopa is metabolized peripherally by COMT (see Chapter 8) as well as by aromatic amino acid decarboxylase, entacapone can prolong the efficacy of a dose of L-dopa.

Dopamine agonists, which theoretically should be effective during later stages of Parkinson disease, mimic endogenous dopamine by directly stimulating dopamine receptors and, unlike L-dopa, do not require enzymatic transformation. Many dopamine agonists also are not metabolized by L-dopa oxidative pathways and thus do not produce the potentially toxic metabolites of this agent. **Bromocriptine** is an ergot derivative that directly stimulates dopamine D_2-like receptors. It is believed to be slightly less effective than L-dopa in providing symptom relief, but produces less dyskinesia and less of the on–off phenomenon, possibly because of its direct receptor activation. Like bromocriptine, **pergolide** is an ergot derivative and dopamine receptor agonist, but it acts on both D_1-like and D_2-like receptors. These medications are used most commonly as an adjunct to L-dopa and, by reducing the amount of L-dopa needed, can decrease the long-term complications of L-dopa therapy. Not surprisingly, the pharmaceutical industry has expressed considerable interest in developing more selective D_1 and D_2 dopamine receptor agonists for the treatment of Parkinson disease.

Muscarinic cholinergic antagonists are helpful in alleviating tremor and rigidity but are generally less effective than dopaminergic drugs. However, they are the mainstay of treatment for parkinsonism induced by D_2 antagonists because dopaminergic therapy increases the severity of associated psychiatric symptoms. The mechanism by which muscarinic anticholinergic agents reduce parkinsonism can be understood based on the actions represented in Figure 14–5. Normally, cholinergic interneurons provide an excitatory influence on striatal medium spiny neurons; consequently, the loss of dopaminergic inhibition of these medium spiny neurons can be compensated for by a decrease in cholinergic excitation. Muscarinic antagonists commonly used to treat parkinsonism include **benztropine, trihexyphenidyl,** and **diphenhydramine** (see Figure 14–6).

Amantadine, introduced originally as an anti-influenza medication, has more recently proven to be useful in the treatment of Parkinson disease. It may be given alone or in combination with anticholinergic medications and is believed to potentiate the release of dopamine. It appears to exert this effect by acting as a weak antagonist at N-methyl-D-aspartate (NMDA) glutamate receptors, although precisely how this action leads to enhanced dopamine release is not yet known. Amantadine improves all of the clinical features of parkinsonism, and associated side effects are uncommon. However, the benefits of this drug are relatively modest and short-lived.

Selegiline (deprenyl) is a selective inhibitor of monoamine oxidase B (MAOB). It was introduced into clinical use because MAOB converts MPTP into its active neurotoxic form, MPP^+. It was hypothesized that the progression of idiopathic Parkinson disease may involve neurotoxins that act like MPTP but are as yet unidentified; accordingly, it was speculated that selegiline might retard the progression of Parkinson disease. Large multicenter studies indicate that although selegiline may offer benefits during early stages of the illness, its efficacy wanes as the disease progresses. In addition, selegiline may not provide a neuroprotective effect but may simply increase dopamine levels by inhibiting monoamine oxidase.

Drugs that act at various types of adenosine receptors are currently under evaluation for use in the treatment of Parkinson disease. These compounds, which are discussed in Chapter 10, may act by means of interactions at dopaminergic synapses in the striatum, as previously discussed.

New approaches to treatment   Because patients treated pharmacologically soon become refractory to L-dopa and related therapies, other treatment strategies have been explored. Excess output from the subthalamic nucleus is postulated to play a critical role in the pathophysiology of Parkinson disease (see Figure 14–2). Surgical lesions of this nucleus, or of the internal segment of the globus pallidus (called a pallidotomy) have reduced major motor disturbances such as akinesia, rigidity, and tremor. However, because such treatment involves an irreversible lesion, it is reserved for the most severe and medication-refractory cases. More recently, deep brain stimulation with a stimulating electrode in the subthalamic nucleus has shown promise as a reversible alternative to placing a lesion. At appropriate stimulation frequencies, the subthalamic nucleus is inactivated and symptoms are relieved, at least temporarily.

Cell transplantation—for example, the administration of fetal mesencephalic dopaminergic neurons into the striatum—also has been evaluated as a treatment for Parkinson disease. This approach is based on the expectation that fetal cells will proliferate, establish synaptic connections, and synthesize and release dopamine in the striatum. The use of fetal neurons as a source of dopamine has some advantages; for example, such neurons express normal dopamine release mechanisms, which provide potential sites of regulation. However, clinical trials have been disappointing. Some patients experience minor improvement, but most patients remained severely disabled. Moreover, transplantation procedures require immunosuppression, and multiple donors of fetal tissue of the appropriate age are needed for each patient. Furthermore, it appears that only a small number of fetal neurons survive transplantation. More recently, the hope of reprogramming stem cells to become dopaminergic neurons has reinvigorated this area of research.

Gene therapy refers to the transfer of a therapeutic gene into a target tissue and the maintenance of its function for a sufficient length of time. Gene therapy for neurologic disorders can be achieved when genes are delivered into the brain either by transplantation of genetically modified cells or by direct injection of genes (e.g., by means of viral vectors) into the striatum. Because tyrosine hydroxylase is the rate-limiting enzyme for dopamine biosynthesis, it has been proposed that expression of the gene for this enzyme in the striatum

could be of use in Parkinson disease treatment. Such expression would be functionally equivalent to L-dopa administration, yet it would restrict treatment to the striatum, avoid certain side effects, and better maintain stable L-dopa levels in the striatum. Tyrosine hydroxylase also might be subject to endogenous control mechanisms such as phosphorylation (see Chapter 8). However, although expression of tyrosine hydroxylase might achieve symptomatic palliation, it would not interfere with the disease progression that ultimately leads to abnormal involuntary movement. Transplantation of tyrosine hydroxylase-expressing cells, or injection of viral vectors that encode the enzyme, have shown some promise in animal models but remain unproven in humans.

Yet another approach to the treatment of Parkinson disease involves the use of neurotrophic factors, which support the survival of neurons. An active search for neurotrophic factors that support dopaminergic neurons (see Chapter 11) is underway. Thus far most therapeutic efforts have focused on brain-derived neurotrophic factor (**BDNF**) and on glial cell line-derived neurotrophic factor (**GDNF**). Local infusion of either factor into the substantia nigra reduces the death of these neurons and associated behavioral sequelae in animal models of Parkinson disease—for example, in animals with 6-hydroxydopamine or MPTP lesions. The delivery of neurotrophic factors to humans may prove to be a major challenge. Delivery by direct striatal injections would require such factors to act on surviving dopaminergic nerve terminals in the striatum or be transported retrogradely or anterogradely to the midbrain, where they might act on dopaminergic cell bodies. An alternative method of delivery might involve viral vectors; for example, a recombinant adeno-associated virus vector expressing GDNF has been proven to significantly improve cell survival in animal models of Parkinson disease and has led to the reversal of some behavioral abnormalities. Yet such approaches remain in the early stages of development.

ESSENTIAL TREMOR

Benign essential tremor is a postural tremor that may be prominent in otherwise normal individuals and that often has a familial basis. The most prevalent of movement disorders, it occurs in approximately 1–2% of individuals 65 years of age or older. Symptoms typically include a tremor in one or both hands and may affect the legs, jaw, tongue, head, or voice; such symptoms may appear in teenagers or young adults but often do not emerge until patients are older.

In some families, essential tremor appears to be inherited as an autosomal dominant trait; the genetic locus for this disorder, *FET1*, has been mapped to chromosome 3q13 by linkage analysis in 16 Icelandic families, but the specific gene responsible has not yet been found. Although essential tremor is not associated with characteristic histopathologic patterns, positron emission tomography (PET) studies have demonstrated increased cerebral blood flow during tremor and at rest in affected individuals. Patients report that a small amount of **alcohol** can provide transient relief; the mechanism responsible for such relief is unknown but may involve enhanced $GABA_A$ receptor function (see Chapter 7).

Treatment with **propranolol** or other β-adrenergic receptor antagonists (see Chapter 8) is effective in reducing the amplitude of disabling tremors, and can be used in anticipation of precipitating circumstances. The anticonvulsant medication **primidone** also has been effective in the treatment of essential tremor. Primidone is a congener of **phenobarbital** and presumably acts by facilitating $GABA_A$ receptor function (see Chapters 7 and 15).

Lithium-induced tremor   One of the most common side effects of **lithium** therapy, which is used in the treatment of bipolar disorder and depression (see Chapter 15), is a 7-Hz action tremor. Associated side effects can include hyperexcitability of skeletal muscle and fasciculations. The mechanism by which exposure to lithium causes tremor is not known. Lithium-induced tremor responds symptomatically to β-adrenergic receptor antagonists.

HUNTINGTON DISEASE

Huntington disease is an autosomal dominant disorder caused by a mutation of the huntingtin gene on the short arm of chromosome 4. The clinical manifestations of the disease typically begin in midlife, with a mean age of onset of 40 years. Initially, the symptoms are subtle and include minor coordination problems, jerky eye movements, and occasional movements of the fingers, limbs, or trunk. Such symptoms may be accompanied by depression, psychotic symptoms, irritability, impulsiveness, and cognitive changes. Deterioration leads to progressive dementia, emotional lability and personality changes, and choreiform movements. Progressive cognitive decline causes disruption of memory and difficulty with complicated tasks; in addition, mood swings, depression, and apathy become more pronounced. During late stages of the disorder choreiform movements regress and dystonia and rigidity are typical symptoms.

In approximately 10% of cases of Huntington disease, symptoms occur before age 20. Individuals with juvenile-onset disease exhibit a more rapidly progressive course and are more likely to experience dystonia

with seizures and cerebellar ataxia than chorea. As discussed in the next section, genetic factors are an important determinant of early onset of disease.

Pathophysiology   Huntington disease is associated with degenerative changes that are most apparent in the caudate nucleus and putamen. Such destruction is selective and is restricted to populations of GABAergic medium spiny projection neurons, particularly those that form the previously described indirect pathway and project to the globus pallidus. Neuronal loss also occurs in the thalamus and cerebral cortex. Striatal cholinergic interneurons, as well as midbrain dopaminergic neurons, are largely unaffected. Indeed, choreiform activity is believed to result from excessive activity of preserved nigrostriatal dopaminergic neurons in conjunction with decreased activity of striatal GABAergic neurons (see Figures 14–2 and 14–5). However, the connection between a loss of GABAergic output from the striatum and choreiform movements is not yet understood.

Genetics and pathogenesis   Huntington disease is a Mendelian dominant genetic disorder; individuals who inherit only one mutated copy of the gene do not differ clinically from individuals who possess two defective copies. The molecular basis of Huntington disease is an expansion of a trinucleotide repeat sequence $(CAG)_n$ within the coding region of a gene on chromosome 4p16.3. This gene, identified in a linkage study of a large lineage with the disease, encodes a protein that has been named *huntingtin*. On chromosomes of normal individuals, the repeated CAG triplet encodes an average of 5 to 30 copies of the amino acid glutamine within the normal huntingtin protein. Huntington disease results from an expansion of these triplet repeats that yields 37 to 86 or more glutamines. Such expansion of nucleotide repeats is common to several inherited neuropsychiatric diseases (Table 14–5). Longer repeats in individuals with Huntington disease

Table 14–5 Examples of Diseases Caused by Trinucleotide Repeats

Disease	Repeat
Fragile X	$(GGC)_n$ on *FMR1* gene
Myotonic dystrophy	$(CTG)_n$ on myotonin protein kinase gene
Spinobulbar muscular atrophy	$(CAG)_n$ on coding sequence of the androgen receptor gene
Huntington Disease	$(CAG)_n$ on huntingtin gene

FMR1, Fragile X mental retardation gene.

are associated with an earlier age of onset and, in some cases, with more severe symptoms. Moreover, repeat lengths are unstable and tend to increase from one generation to the next through transmission from both sexes. This expansion most likely occurs during spermatogenesis, and is believed to be characterized by average increases of 0.4 and 9 repeat units in female and male transmissions, respectively. Such changes result in the clinical phenomenon of *anticipation*—an earlier age of onset or an increase in the severity of disease across successive generations.

As previously mentioned, the increased length of the trinucleotide repeat in huntingtin is associated with a younger age of onset of Huntington disease; juvenile onset occurs in individuals with the highest number of trinucleotide repeats. Although the age of onset is most dependent on repeat length, it also is influenced by modifying genes and environmental factors; for example, two individuals with the same number of repeats can exhibit very different courses of the disease when they are members of different families. There is great interest in identifying genetic and environmental factors that lead to such modifications because such knowledge might improve management or prevention of the disease and shed light on its pathogenesis. The expanded repeats in huntingtin can be detected in gene carriers by a simple polymerase chain reaction (PCR)-based assay. Consequently family members can be tested before they are symptomatic to determine whether they carry the defective gene, and the gene also can be detected in fetuses through prenatal testing.

The mechanism underlying Huntington disease represents a classic example of a gain-of-function mutation. The disease is caused by a single copy of a mutant gene that leads to a new biologic effect, rather than a simple increase or decrease in the normal effect of the gene (see Box 14–1). The new function of mutant huntingtin remains incompletely understood. However, according to an emerging hypothesis, the longer the glutamine repeat is, the more likely the huntingtin protein is to accumulate within vulnerable neurons as intranuclear inclusion bodies, which have been identified during pathologic examination of striatum from patients with Huntington disease. Such inclusion bodies lead to disruptions in critical cellular functions, including RNA processing, and eventually cause cell death. It has been hypothesized that the gain of function in mutant huntingtin is the neural toxicity of the expanded polyglutamine domain of the mutant protein. Consistent with this theory are recent findings from mice that overexpress a mutant huntingtin gene; these animals exhibit nuclear inclusion bodies and morphologic changes in vulnerable neurons—early signs of apoptosis that parallel the patterns of cell death associated with Huntington

disease. Such mice represent models that can be used to develop new therapies. Interestingly, the huntingtin gene is widely expressed throughout the brain and most other organs; therefore, why mutant huntingtin leads to a relatively selective pathologic process within striatal GABAergic neurons remains a mystery.

The normal function of huntingtin is also something of a mystery. Knockout mice that lack huntingtin die early during embryonic development, exhibiting features of apoptotic cell death. Such findings indicate that huntingtin plays a critical role in many cell types, yet investigators have yet to uncover clues to its function.

Treatment of Huntington disease   Unfortunately, no specific treatment is available for Huntington disease. The drugs most commonly used for controlling associated dyskinesias are dopamine receptor antagonists, including antipsychotic agents such as **haloperidol** and **chlorpromazine**. These drugs are effective because the blockade of dopamine action relieves dopamine's inhibitory influence on dying GABAergic neurons, thereby increasing net GABAergic output from the striatum (see Figure 14–5). The use of antipsychotic drugs also has the beneficial effect of reducing psychosis in patients who experience such symptoms. Other pharmacologic treatment of Huntington disease targets specific symptoms, such as depression and impulsive behavior, for which **antidepressants** and **propranolol** have been used, respectively. However, the therapeutic efficacy of the latter agent, a β-adrenergic antagonist, is limited.

The interactions represented in Figure 14–5 suggest that drugs that increase GABAergic or cholinergic function in the striatum should ameliorate the symptoms of Huntington disease. However, attempts to alleviate chorea and other dyskinesias with drugs that exert such effects have not yielded consistent clinical responses.

Lessons from Huntington disease   Experience with Huntington disease has raised several points that are essential to remember as we strive to identify the causes of other neuropsychiatric disorders. First, the gene that causes Huntington disease was previously unknown; its discovery illustrates the power of "reverse genetics"—that is, approaches to finding a disease-related gene that can proceed without prior knowledge of the disease's pathophysiology. Second, the discovery of a disease-related gene provides essential tools for investigating pathogenesis. Indeed, classic approaches to understanding disease pathophysiology did not succeed in explaining Huntington disease. Moreover, classic neuropharmacologic approaches would have been based on the assumption that GABAergic and dopaminergic mechanisms were central to the disease. Yet the culprit is a protein that is expressed throughout the body, is not even enriched in the striatum, and is not directly involved in neurotransmission.

Third, the path that leads from the identification of a disease-related gene to definitive treatment can be long and arduous. Five years after identification of the gene, little is known about the normal product of the gene and we are just beginning to understand how the mutant product generates disease. Definitive treatment of Huntington disease and preventive measures await our ability to discover and exploit such information.

It should be emphasized that this section describes a disease caused by a single genetic mutation and characterized by a straightforward diagnosis, uncomplicated familial transmission, and definitive pathologic findings. The process of determining the mechanisms that underlie other neuropsychiatric disorders, particularly those that represent heterogeneous, genetically complex syndromes, is likely to be much more arduous.

DYSTONIA

The dystonias are a heterogeneous group of disorders that result in sustained involuntary contractions of the agonist and antagonist muscles of the face, neck, limbs, or trunk. Dystonia can be generalized, segmental, or focal and can be triggered by specific motor acts such as playing a piano or by voluntary movements. It is exacerbated by stress and fatigue and improved by sleep and relaxation. Types of dystonia are distinguished based on clinical or pharmacologic features. Dystonia can be very painful as well as disfiguring.

Torsion dystonia   Dystonic movements and postures characterize torsion dystonia in the absence of other neurologic signs. These dystonias may be inherited as autosomal dominant, autosomal recessive, or X-linked recessive disorders. The genetic loci for some types have been determined; other types may occur on a sporadic basis. Such disorders also can be classified in terms of age of onset or according to the physical distribution of symptoms. The precise pathogenesis of these disorders is unknown.

Generalized dystonia is most prevalent among members of the Ashkenazi Jewish population, and in these individuals apparently can be traced to a founder mutation in DYT1, a dystonia gene located on chromosome 9q. However, a mutation in the same gene has been found in a large non-Jewish family. The protein encoded by this gene has not yet been characterized extensively. Symptoms typically begin in one limb at approximately 12 years of age and spread to other limbs within 5 years.

Another subtype of torsion dystonia is hereditary dystonia, an autosomal dominant disorder of abnormal movements that is responsive to **alcohol**. This disease is characterized by early onset and relatively insignificant progression during life, and is not associated with degenerative changes. Alcohol is believed to exert its palliative effects by facilitating GABA$_A$ receptor function (see Chapter 7).

Dystonia musculorum deformans is a rare disorder whose onset, which typically occurs between the ages of 5 and 15, is often benign yet insidious. It consists of mild dystonic movements of an extremity or the neck, which result in conditions such as writer's cramp or torticollis (a contraction of muscles that turns the neck to one side). Such symptoms slowly progress to involve the trunk and other extremities. Ultimately children with this disease are physically twisted and deformed and experience multiple secondary contractures. An incorrect psychiatric diagnosis often is made initially because of the bizarre postures and positions assumed by affected children.

Dopa-responsive dystonia   The majority of patients with dopa-responsive dystonia (DRD) exhibit autosomal dominant inheritance. The disease appears to be caused by mutations in the gene for GTP cyclohydrolase I (GTPCH), which has been mapped to chromosome 14. GTPCH is an enzyme involved in the formation of tetrahydrobiopterin, a cofactor of dopamine synthesis. As discussed in Chapter 8, tetrahydrobiopterin is a cofactor for tyrosine hydroxylase, phenylalanine hydroxylase, and tryptophan hydroxylase, thus patients with DRD show reduced activities of these enzymes.

The clinical spectrum of DRD is wide, but the disease most often presents with posturing or a gait disorder in a previously normal child at 6 years of age. Symptoms typically intensify throughout the day or after exercise. Parkinsonism, including postural instability, bradykinesia, and rigidity, may occur in some patients.

Patients with DRD exhibit a dramatic and sustained response to low-dose therapy with L-dopa. Fluorodopa PET studies, which provide a measure of striatal aromatic amino acid decarboxylase activity, indicate that such activity is normal in patients with DRD and suggest an intact nigrostriatal pathway and a lack of dopaminergic cell loss. Nevertheless, patients can exhibit a profound decrease in dopamine in the striatum because of impairment in tyrosine hydroxylase activity caused by mutations in GTPCH.

Treatment   L-dopa therapy often is an effective treatment for primary dystonias or DRDs. Muscarinic cholinergic receptor antagonists such as **trihexyphenidyl** also are effective. **Baclofen**, a GABA$_B$ receptor agonist, and **carbamazepine**, an anticonvulsant agent (see Chapter 21), can be of benefit for some patients. Hemiballism, hemichorea, and segmental dystonia have been successfully treated with **clonazepam,** a benzodiazepine that suppresses GABA-mediated inhibition in thalamic relay neurons through its effects (i.e., facilitation of GABA$_A$ receptor function) on nucleus reticularis neurons in the brain stem. Focal dystonias dramatically improve in response to treatment with **botulinum toxin type A,** which inhibits the release of acetylcholine from presynaptic cholinergic terminals (see Chapters 4 and 9). An injection placed directly into the spasmodic muscle can be effective for as many as 3–6 months, at which time sprouting and regrowth of nerve terminals is believed to occur. Stereotactic thalamotomy is sometimes helpful in cases of unilateral dystonia that predominantly involve the limbs.

Drug-induced dystonia   Perhaps the most common cause of dystonia, including manifestations such as lock-jaw, blepharospasm, torticollis, and facial grimacing, is the use of typical **antipsychotic** medications. Like the previously mentioned extrapyramidal side effects of these drugs, dystonia is caused by the blockade of D$_2$ dopamine receptors, presumably in the striatum. It is one of the first extrapyramidal side effects elicited by such drugs, and often appears within an hour of drug administration. Why, based on neural circuitry, the blockade of D$_2$ receptors causes this abnormal movement is not understood. Acute dystonic reactions often require immediate medical attention; in such cases, the treatment of choice is administration of muscarinic cholinergic antagonists, by systemic injection if necessary.

TOURETTE SYNDROME

Gilles de la Tourette syndrome is a disorder of unknown etiology that usually develops during early adolescence. Onset of the syndrome is marked by one or more poorly controlled symptoms, which consist of intermittent facial grimacing, multiple motor tics that can involve the head or extremities, and the spasmodic production of vocalizations or vocal tics, including barks and coughs. The disorder is notoriously associated with coprolalia (involuntary uttering of obscenities); however, this feature of the disease is rare. Characteristic tics can be voluntarily suppressed, but only for brief periods; in severe cases, they can cause marked distress and impairment in social and occupational functioning. Milder cases of tics are not classified as Tourette syndrome per se but may be related pathophysiologically or etiologically.

Tourette syndrome typically is characterized by familial transmission. In many families, a sex-influenced, possibly autosomal dominant mode of inheritance with variable expressivity is seen. However, specific genes related to the disorder have not been identified despite extensive investigation. Tourette syndrome is associated with obsessive–compulsive disorder and with attention deficit–hyperactivity disorder, each of which occurs in 25% to 50% of patients with the syndrome. Consequently, obsessions have been speculatively conceptualized as cognitive tics, and compulsions as complex motor performance tics.

The pathogenesis of Tourette syndrome is unknown. It is believed to be caused by an abnormality in striatal function that has yet to be specified. Because dopamine-blocking drugs have beneficial effects on associated tics, dopaminergic hyperactivity in the brains of patients with Tourette syndrome has been postulated; however, no direct evidence supports this theory. Some evidence does support pathologic changes in the striatum as a cause of the disease. Elevated levels of the dopamine transporter—the protein responsible for termination of the dopamine signal at the synapse (see Chapter 8)—are reported in the caudate and putamen of a limited number of individuals with Tourette syndrome (Figure 14–7). Although these findings offer important clues, much remains to be learned about this disorder.

Tics can be socially embarrassing and severe enough to interfere with daily functioning. **Antipsychotic** drugs (D$_2$ dopamine receptor antagonists) are very effective at reducing tics, but typically are avoided except in extreme cases because of their troubling extrapyramidal side effects, which can include tardive dyskinesia. Consequently, α_2-adrenergic agonists such as **clonidine** and **guanfacine** are the first line of treatment for patients

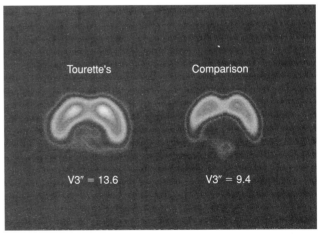

Figure 14–7. SPECT images of striatal [^{123}I]β-CIT (2 β-carbomethoxy-3 β-4-iodophenyltropane) binding in a patient with Tourette syndrome and in an age- and gender-matched healthy control. (Adapted with permission from Malison RT, McDougle CJ, van Dyck CH, et al. 1995. *Am J Psychiatry* 152:1359.)

with Tourette syndrome. These agents are reported to improve motor and vocal tics in approximately 50% of children. It has been speculated that these drugs inhibit central noradrenergic neurons through the activation of inhibitory autoreceptors (see Chapters 8 and 12), but how this action leads to symptom reduction remains unknown. In patients with concomitant obsessive–compulsive disorder, which is discussed further in a subsequent section of this chapter, treatment with a selective serotonin reuptake inhibitor (SSRI) (e.g., **fluoxetine, sertraline,** or **fluvoxamine**) or with a serotonergic tricyclic antidepressant (e.g., **clomipramine**) can improve tics and obsessive–compulsive symptoms. In patients with concomitant attention deficit–hyperactivity disorder, stimulant drugs such as **methylphenidate,** which relieve symptoms of inattention and hyperactivity (see Chapter 18), may be used but can be problematic because they can exacerbate tics in some cases.

SYDENHAM CHOREA

A movement disorder that occurs primarily as a complication of group-A β-hemolytic streptococcal infection in children, Sydenham chorea most commonly occurs between the ages of 5 and 15. The onset of symptoms may occur before, in association with, or after other manifestations of rheumatic fever or polyarthritis; however, some patients have no recent history of sore throat or fever. Approximately one third of affected children develop valvular heart disease.

Clinical symptoms often are dramatic; choreiform movements may be observed in the fingers, hands, extremities, face, and even in the diaphragm. The movements often intensify during periods of agitation or activity and usually disappear during sleep. Psychiatric symptoms may be noted before the onset of other abnormalities, and may range from mild personality changes and emotional lability to psychotic features. Saint Vitus's dance, an obsolete name for this syndrome, may be explained by such symptoms: affected children were at one time believed to be possessed by demons.

Increasing evidence indicates that Sydenham chorea results from autoantibodies that cross-react with epitopes of the streptococcus organism and with the neuronal surface of basal ganglia neurons. The disease is often diagnosed based on associated signs, such as arthritis, carditis, a history of rheumatic fever, and streptococcal tonsillitis. Serum studies may not indicate an elevation of acute-phase reactants, including antistreptolysin O (ASLO), because a latency period often occurs between streptococcal infection and the onset of chorea. The chorea usually lasts 1 to 3 months, and

haloperidol or other D_2 antagonists can be effective in reducing associated movements. Traditional treatment includes bed rest, sedation, and prophylactic antibiotic therapy, even when no other signs of acute rheumatic fever are present. Long-term prognoses are primarily based on the severity of cardiac abnormalities.

A subgroup of patients that exhibit **obsessive–compulsive disorder** or **Tourette syndrome** in the context of group-A β-hemolytic streptococcal infection are affected by pediatric autoimmune neuropsychiatric disorders associated with streptococcal infections (**PANDAS**). Such patients typically are distinguished from those with Sydenham chorea because they do not exhibit signs of rheumatic fever or chorea; however, patients with a particular histocompatibility marker—human leukocyte antigen (HLA) type D8/17—may have both rheumatic fever and PANDAS. The antibodies that recognize cross-reacting epitopes on bacteria and on striatal neurons in patients with PANDAS may recognize a different subpopulation of neurons in Sydenham chorea. In preliminary trials, patients with PANDAS have exhibited good clinical responses to antibiotic therapy, including resolution of tics and obsessive–compulsive symptoms.

OBSESSIVE–COMPULSIVE DISORDER

Obsessive–compulsive disorder (OCD) is characterized by stereotyped, repetitive, and intrusive thoughts and fears that can be relieved temporarily by the performance of compulsive behaviors. Obsessions are ideas, impulses, and images that repeatedly intrude upon a patient—often without relief. Most patients develop compulsions such as counting, touching, checking, or cleaning in an attempt to ward off unwanted events or to satisfy an obsession. OCD is a relatively common disorder; it affects approximately 2% of the population, presents with varying degrees of severity, and is chronic. The onset of the disorder can be acute or gradual; first symptoms typically appear when patients are in their early 20s.

Although the cause of OCD is unknown, it is believed to involve abnormal functioning of the basal ganglia. It has been speculated that the disorder affects perseverative functioning in cortical–striatal–thalamic–cortical loops, but this theory is not yet supported by evidence. A well-conducted morphometric MRI study revealed that individuals with OCD have a reduced caudate volume compared with control subjects. This finding represents the first piece of evidence that directly links OCD with pathology in striatal regions of the brain.

Familial patterns of transmission of OCD have not yet been fully established. Based on observed patterns of transmission, the risk for OCD appears to be genetically complex, and most likely involves multiple interacting loci. The gene that encodes the serotonin transporter was evaluated as a cause of OCD but proved to have no bearing on the disorder. The results of such evaluation underscore the limitations of creating pathophysiologic hypotheses based on the efficacy of agents used in treatment (see Chapter 1).

SSRIs and clomipramine (a serotonin-selective tricyclic compound) are the only agents that have been used successfully in the treatment of OCD (see Chapter 15). Interestingly, the treatment of OCD requires doses of these agents that are higher than those used to treat depression. Moreover, the latency period before the onset of therapeutic effect is longer when such agents are used to treat OCD; patients may take these drugs for as long as 10 weeks before a reduction in obsessive–compulsive symptoms becomes apparent. Most patients with OCD exhibit only partial improvement with the use of these drugs, yet such limited improvement can be dramatic in terms of restoring an individual's ability to function socially and occupationally. However, because of the limited value of these drugs, a need for therapies with greater efficacy persists.

WILSON DISEASE

Wilson disease, also known as hepatolenticular degeneration, is an autosomal recessive disorder of copper metabolism that produces abnormal copper deposition, particularly in the liver, cornea, and brain. In the brain, depositions in the striatum, cerebral cortex, and cerebellum predominate. This disease typically appears during childhood or young adulthood, and is characterized by progressive hepatic and neurologic dysfunction that involves various combinations of symptoms, which may include dysarthria, tremor, dystonia, choreiform movements, parkinsonism, or ataxia. Personality changes also may occur. Bilateral brown rings on the cornea that result from copper deposition, known as Kayser–Fleischer rings, are the most common ocular finding.

The pathogenesis of Wilson disease involves a reduction in the binding of copper to ceruloplasmin, a transport protein. This reduction results in large amounts of unbound copper that enter the circulation and are deposited in the tissues previously mentioned. All cases of the disease are caused by mutations in a single gene (*ATP7B*) that encodes a membrane-bound, copper-binding, adenosine triphosphatase involved in transmembrane copper transport. However, distinct mutations in the protein occur in different families and lead to different functional effects, which explain the clinical variability of the disease. Laboratory investigations reveal abnormal liver function, a low serum level of ceruloplasmin, and increased urinary excretion of copper. Brain imaging may reveal basal ganglia abnormalities or cerebrocortical atrophy.

Treatment is aimed at the removal of excess copper and subsequent maintenance of copper balance. The mainstay of treatment is **penicillamine,** a copper-chelating agent that promotes both extraction of copper from tissue sites and its urinary excretion. **Trientine,** a chelator that increases urinary excretion of copper, is also used. **Zinc** salts are used to induce intestinal cell metallothionein, which has a high affinity for copper and forms a mucosal barrier to copper absorption. **Tetrathiomolybdate** forms a complex with proteins and copper and is used to block the absorption of copper from the gut. Some evidence suggests that L-dopa may help to reverse neurologic symptoms that are not improved by chelation therapy.

SELECTED READING

Adams RD, Victor M. 1993. *Principles of Neurology,* 5th ed. New York: McGraw-Hill.

Albin RL, Young AB, Penney JB. 1990. The functional anatomy of basal ganglia disorders. *Trends Neurosci* 12:366.

Bartholome K, Ludecke B. 1998. Mutations in the tyrosine hydroxylase gene cause various forms of L-dopa-responsive dystonia. *Adv Pharm* 42:48–49.

Betarbet R, Sherer TB, MacKenzie G, et al. 2000. Chronic systemic pesticide exposure reproduces features of Parkinson's disease. *Nature Neurosci* 3:1301–1306.

Cleveland DW. 1999. From Charcot to SOD1: Mechanisms of selective motor neuron death in ALS. *Neuron* 24:515–520.

Davies SW, Turmaine M, Cozens BA, et al. 1997. Formation of neuronal intranuclear inclusions underlies the neurological dysfunction in mice transgenic for the HD mutation. *Cell* 90:537–548.

Dunnett SB, Bjorklund A. 1999. Prospects for new restorative and neuroprotective treatments in Parkinson disease. *Nature* 399(suppl):A32–A39.

Elsworth JD, Roth RH. 1997. Dopamine synthesis, uptake, metabolism, and receptors: Relevance to gene therapy of Parkinson disease. *Exp Neurol* 144:4–9.

Ferrigno P, Silver PA. 2000. Polyglutamine expansions: Proteolysis, chaperones, and the dangers of promiscuity. *Neuron* 26:9–12.

Freeman TB. 1997. From transplants to gene therapy for Parkinson's disease. *Exp Neurol* 144:47–50.

Galvin JE, Lee VM, Schmidt ML, et al. 1999. Pathobiology of the Lewy body. *Adv Neurol* 80:313–324.

Gasser T, Bereznai B, Muller B, et al. 1996. Linkage studies in alcohol-responsive myoclonic dystonia. *Mov Disord* 11:363–370.

Gerfen CR, Wilson DJ. 1996. The basal ganglia. In Swanson LW, Bjorklund A, Hokfelt T (eds): *Handbook of Chemical Neuroanatomy*, vol 12. Amsterdam: Elsevier.

Graybiel AM. 1995. Building action repertoires: Memory and learning functions of the basal ganglia. *Curr Opin Neurobiol* 5:733–741.

Graybiel AM, Rauch SL. 2000. Toward a neurobiology of obsessive-compulsive disorder. *Neuron* 28:343–347.

Gulcher JR, Jonsson P, Kong A, et al. 1997. Mapping of a familial essential tremor gene, *FET1*, to chromosome 3q13. *Nature Genetics* 17:84–87.

Gusella JF, MacDonald ME. 2000. Molecular genetics; unmasking polyglutamine triggers in neurodegenerative disease. *Nature Rev Neurosci* 1:109–115.

Huntington's Disease Collaborative Research Group. 1993. A novel gene containing a trinucleotide repeat that is expanded and unstable on Huntington's disease chromosomes. *Cell* 72:971–983.

Ichinose H, Nagatsu T. 1997. Molecular genetics of hereditary dystonia: Mutations in the GTP cyclohydrolase I gene. *Brain Res Bull* 43:35–38.

Jankovic J, Beach J, Pandolfo M, Patel PI. 1997. Familial essential tremor in 4 kindreds: Prospects for genetic mapping. *Arch Neurol* 54:289–294.

Lang AE, Lozano AM. 1998. Parkinson's disease. *New Engl J Med* 339:1130–1143.

Leckman JF, Riddle MA. 2000. Tourette's syndrome: when habit-forming systems form habits of their own? *Neuron* 28:349–354.

Malison RT, McDougle CJ, van Dyck CH, et al. 1995. [^{123}I]β-CIT SPECT imaging of striatal dopamine transporter binding in Tourette's disorder. *Am J Psychiatry* 152: 1359–1361.

Miller GW, Gainetdinov RR, Levey AI, Caron MG. 1999. Dopamine transporters and neuronal injury. *Trends Pharmacol Sci* 20:424–429.

Neiman J, Lang AE, Fornazzari L, Carlen PL. 1990. Movement disorders in alcoholism: A review. *Neurology* 40:741–746.

Nygaard TG. 1995. Dopa-responsive dystonia. *Curr Opin Neurol* 8:310–313.

Onn SP, West AR, Grace AA. 2000. Dopamine-mediated regulation of striatal neuronal and network interactions. *Trends Neurosci* 23(suppl):S48–S56.

Ozelius LJ, Hewett JW, Page CE, et al. 1997. The early-onset torsion dystonia gene (*DYT1*) encodes an ATP-binding protein. *Nature Genetics* 17:40–48.

Palumbo D, Maughan A, Kurlan R. 1997. Hypothesis III: Tourette's syndrome is only one of several causes of a developmental basal ganglia syndrome. *Arch Neurol* 54: 475–483.

Robinson D, Wu H, Munne RA. 1995. Reduced caudate nucleus volume in obsessive–compulsive disorder. *Arch Gen Psychiatry* 52:393–398.

Swedo SE, Leonard JL, Mittleman BB, et al. 1997. Identification of children with pediatric autoimmune neuropsychiatric disorders associated with streptococcal infections by a marker associated with rheumatic fever. *Am J Psychiatry* 154:110–112.

Zoghbi HY, Orr HT. 2000. Glutamine repeats and neurodegeneration. *Annu Rev Neurosci* 23:217–247.

Chapter 15
Mood and Emotion

KEY CONCEPTS

- Emotions activate behavioral repertoires and physiologic outputs that represent adaptive responses to external and internal stimuli.

- Emotion refers to transient responses to environmental, internal, and cognitive stimuli, while mood refers to the predominant emotional state over time.

- The neural circuitry of fear is well understood in part because fear responses are well conserved across evolution, permitting the development of good animal models.

- Information about threatening stimuli is transmitted from the thalamus and cerebral cortex to the amygdala where it is processed; fear-related efferent signals are sent from the central nucleus of the amygdala to multiple effector sites in the brain responsible for adaptive responses.

- Anxiety, a state characterized by arousal, vigilance, physiologic preparedness, and negative subjective states, may share certain critical circuits with fear.

- Mood disorders are divided into unipolar disorders, which are characterized by depression only, and bipolar disorders, which are diagnosed if the person has ever had an episode of mania.

- Mood disorders are highly influenced by both genes and environment, but the circuitry in the brain underlying mood disorders is not yet well understood.

- Individuals with major depression often exhibit abnormal excessive activation of the hypothalamic–pituitary–adrenal axis.

- Most of the effective treatments for depression interact with proteins at monoamine synapses, generally enhancing neurotransmission by norepinephrine, serotonin, or both.

- The tricyclic antidepressants inhibit reuptake of norepinephrine or serotonin by binding to their respective transporters; the selective serotonin reuptake inhibitors (SSRIs) bind only to the serotonin transporter; and the monoamine oxidase inhibitors (MAOIs) inhibit the metabolism of norepinephrine, serotonin, and dopamine.

- Although the initial molecular targets of antidepressants are well characterized, the actual mechanism of action is not understood. The 2- to 4-week latency of onset of therapeutic effects suggests that slowly developing adaptive responses to initial enhancement of monoamine neurotransmission are required for efficacy.

- Therapies for bipolar disorder include lithium and several drugs, including valproic acid, that were originally developed as anticonvulsants.

- Although the mechanism of action of lithium is not well understood, the two leading candidate mechanisms are inhibition of the inositol phosphate second messenger pathway and inhibition of Wnt signaling via inhibition of the glycogen synthase kinase 3β pathway.

Emotions represent far more than subjective feelings; indeed they are critical to survival. They activate behavioral repertoires and physiologic outputs that constitute adaptive responses to environmental or interoceptive (internal) stimuli and often are necessary to sustain life. A distinction typically is made between emotion (also called *affect*) and mood. The term *emotion* generally refers to transient responses to environmental, interoceptive, or cognitive stimuli. In contrast, the term *mood* typically is used to characterize the predominant emotional state of an individual over time. Although there are many subtle forms of emotion, they may be divided into two broad categories. Negative emotions, such as fear, are elicited under normal circumstances by stimuli that connote danger, pain, or other noxious conditions and generally lead to avoidance, escape, or protective responses. Positive emotions are elicited by stimuli that connote food, safety, comfort, or other rewarding situations and lead to approach behaviors.

Almost everything that is known about mood regulation and much that is known about emotion has been gleaned from pathology. Many common human diseases produce pathologic emotional states that may be transient or enduring. Although most of these emotional disorders can be treated successfully with pharmacologic agents, in many cases the mechanisms of action that underlie the efficacy of such agents are not well understood. For example, the initial molecular targets of **anxiolytic** (anti-anxiety) and **antidepressant** drugs have for the most part been determined; however, the mechanisms by which antidepressants and mood-stabilizing

drugs ultimately produce their therapeutic effects have yet to be adequately characterized. Most commonly used antidepressant drugs block serotonin or norepinephrine reuptake after initial exposure, but only alleviate the symptoms of depression after several weeks of administration. Thus the antidepressant response is not caused by the blockade of monoamine reuptake per se; rather, such blockade causes other changes in the brain that underlie the relief from depression. The pharmacology of agents used to alleviate anxiety and treat mood disorders is the focus of this chapter. The pharmacology of addictive drugs, which similarly tap into systems that regulate emotion (especially positive emotion) and motivation, is discussed in Chapter 16.

REPRESENTATION OF EMOTION IN THE BRAIN

The neural underpinnings of emotion were initially explored in relation to a hypothetical general processing system composed of evolutionarily old brain regions lying deep to the neocortex called the *limbic system* (Figure 15–1). Classic components of the limbic system include the amygdala and hippocampus. These limbic structures, in conjunction with paralimbic regions of the cerebral cortex such as the orbital and medial prefrontal cortex, play critical roles in the processing of emotion. However, recent research on the physiology and pharmacology of emotion has led to the recognition of neural circuits in the brain that are relevant to specific emotions. As with other complex brain functions, improvements in our understanding of the neural

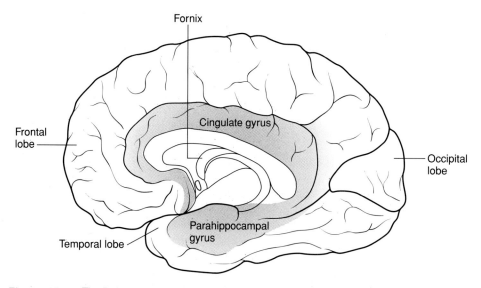

Figure 15–1. The limbic lobe. This ring of tissue (limbus) encircles the upper brain stem and consists of evolutionarily older forms of cortex. It comprises the cingulate and parahippocampal gyri as well as deeper structures such as the hippocampus and amygdala.

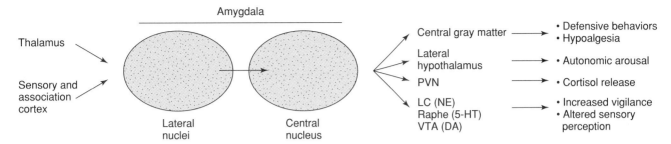

Figure 15-2. Flow of information into and out of the amygdala. Fear-related information enters the amygdala by means of its lateral nuclei. These nuclei project to the central nucleus, which projects to structures that produce the diverse physiologic and behavioral responses characteristic of fear, including the central or periaqueductal gray matter, lateral hypothalamus, paraventricular nucleus of the hypothalamus (PVN), monoaminergic nuclei such as locus ceruleus (LC), raphe nuclei, ventral tegmental area (VTA), and many regions not shown. NE, norepinephrine; 5-HT, serotonin; DA, dopamine.

basis of emotion will require that the functional anatomy of emotion be viewed in terms of distributed circuits rather than in terms of a general purpose system. Such a perspective also will be necessary to facilitate the identification of new sites of action for psychotropic drugs designed to influence emotion.

Emotion-processing circuits produce adaptive responses to salient stimuli. Accordingly, these circuits must appraise the significance of a stimulus and subsequently activate output systems that prepare an organism to respond appropriately. Appraisal of a stimulus (e.g., as dangerous, novel, or desirable), except in the first few hundred milliseconds that elapse during an emergency, requires that highly processed sensory and cognitive information from the association cortex gain access to these circuits and that relevant new experiences be encoded in memory to provide appropriate warnings in the future. Circuits that process emotion may suppress ongoing behavior to activate automatic defensive or approach repertoires. They also may regulate arousal and attention, in part by activating monoamine and cholinergic systems in the brain (see Chapters 8 and 9), and may control the internal milieu by means of neuroendocrine systems (see Chapter 13) and the autonomic nervous system (see Chapter 12).

FEAR

During the past decade, the greatest progress in emotion research has resulted from analysis of the circuitry underlying fear. Such research has been facilitated by apparent evolutionary conservation in the fear circuitry and fear-related behavior ascribed to animals and humans. Experiments involving animals have indicated that information about threatening stimuli is transmitted to the lateral nuclei, the major input nuclei of the amygdala, which in turn project both directly and indi-

rectly to the central nucleus, the major output nucleus of the amygdala (Box 15–1). Efferent projections from the central nucleus activate numerous effector sites for physiologic and behavioral fear responses (Figure 15–2). Projections to the lateral hypothalamus mediate activation of the sympathetic nervous system, and projections to the paraventricular nucleus (PVN) of the hypothalamus induce the synthesis and release of corticotropin-releasing factor (CRF) (see Chapters 10 and 13). The release of CRF activates a cascade that ultimately leads to the release of glucocorticoids from the adrenal cortex. Glucocorticoids cause the body to enter a catabolic state; they also suppress inflammatory responses and may heighten alertness. The CRF-activated hypothalamic–pituitary–adrenal (HPA) axis often is chronically hyperactive in individuals with **depression,** as discussed in subsequent sections of this chapter. Because CRF also serves as a neurotransmitter for neurons in the central nucleus of the amygdala, through which it may mediate certain aspects of the fear response and other negative emotional responses, **CRF antagonists** are being tested as antidepressants and anxiolytics.

Projections from the amygdala to the periaqueductal gray matter (PAG) in the core of the brain stem activate descending analgesic responses that involve endogenous opioid peptides, which can suppress pain in response to intense fear and stress (see Chapter 19). Projections to a different region of the PAG activate species-specific defensive responses, such as behavioral freezing in rats and mice. Projections to the noradrenergic locus ceruleus, the serotonergic raphe nuclei, and the dopaminergic ventral tegmental area increase arousal and vigilance and enhance the formation of explicit and implicit memories of circumstances under which danger has occurred.

Under normal circumstances, these various physiologic and behavioral responses are adaptive and enhance

Box 15–1 Studying Fear Circuitry

Studies of fear circuitry have exploited the discovery that emotionally salient stimuli are strong inducers of memory formation. Accordingly, simple classical conditioning experiments, similar to those first described by Pavlov, have been used to analyze the mechanisms by which animals learn about and then predict danger. In such experiments, a neutral stimulus such as a tone or a light consistently precedes a strongly aversive stimulus, or unconditioned stimulus (US), such as foot shock. (Pavlov used a bell to signal the arrival of food, a rewarding rather than an aversive stimulus.) After a period of learning, known as conditioning, the animal regards the previously neutral stimulus, now the conditioned stimulus (CS), as a predictor of the arrival and magnitude of the aversive event. Thus after an animal has undergone associative learning, a tone previously paired with foot shock is capable of producing fear-related behaviors, or a conditioned response (CR), such as freezing or enhanced acoustic startle. With the use of precise lesions and anatomic methods, investigators have been able to trace the pathways between areas in the brain that receive auditory input (the tone) and the areas responsible for behavioral output (the response to fear). Such mapping studies have identified the amygdala, a complex nucleus in the temporal lobes, as a critical node in fear-processing circuits. When a tone signals danger, the information reaches the amygdala by means of two pathways. Rapidly processed but only approximate information arrives from the medial geniculate nucleus of the thalamus, a way station in auditory processing. More highly processed information arrives, after a brief lag, from the auditory cortex and other cortical regions. The rapid pathway from the thalamus permits an organism to get ready to respond to danger even before the sensory and cognitive processing that distinguishes a real danger from a false alarm has been completed.

survival. Indeed, fear helps ensure that we avoid and escape from dangerous environments. However, it has been hypothesized that symptoms of anxiety disorders occur in response to the abnormal function of such fear circuitry.

ANXIETY

The anticipation of danger that is characteristic of anxiety results in arousal, vigilance, physiologic preparedness, and negative subjective states that are qualitatively similar to those associated with fear. Yet anxiety differs from fear in that it is triggered in the absence of an immediately threatening stimulus. Moreover, anxiety often is elicited by generalized cues, whereas fear is elicited by discrete, explicit cues.

The amygdala appears to play a critical role in the processing of fearful stimuli and in the encoding of fearful memories in humans as well as in animals. This hypothesis is supported by observations of patients who have had lesions of the amygdala that resulted from stroke, infection, or head injury. Patients with amygdala lesions, for example, often lack autonomic and other conditioned responses to a fearful stimulus, even though their declarative memory (their ability to remember a specific stimulus) is intact. Moreover, neuroimaging studies of responses to fearful stimuli have suggested that the processing of such stimuli occurs in the amygdala, although these studies have not revealed the precise circuitry involved.

Despite these findings, lesions of the central nucleus of the amygdala do not abolish behavioral outputs in certain animal models of anxiety; thus it is believed that other regions of the brain must be involved in the anxiety response. In a rodent model of anxiety, for example, lesions of the central nucleus of the amygdala do not reduce anxiety-like behavior triggered by the elevated plus maze (Box 15–2). Such experiments have indicated that neural circuits responsible for mediating output related to anxiety may be distinct from those that mediate output related to fear. Moreover, research has suggested that the bed nucleus of the stria terminalis (BNST) rather than the central nucleus of the amygdala may give rise to projections involved in physiologic and behavioral expressions of anxiety; in particular, CRF may act in this region to induce anxiety-like behaviors. The BNST is considered an extended region of the amygdala, and indeed resembles the central nucleus of the amygdala with regard to its cellular organization; yet it is hypothesized that this area may respond to less specific stimuli than the central nucleus and thus may mediate the more generalized symptoms of anxiety. If this hypothesis is confirmed, sites in the BNST may become targets of anxiolytic agents that have yet to be discovered.

ANXIETY AND EMOTIONAL MEMORY

The memories produced by fearful situations have both a cognitive and an affective component. The cognitive component, which depends at least in part on the hippocampus, records the precise setting in which danger is experienced and details of the experience. The affective component, which appears to involve the amygdala, is capable of reinitiating the physiologic and behavioral cascade of the fear response. Under normal circumstances affective, or emotional, memories are

Box 15–2 Elevated Plus Maze

One of the best-established devices for observing anxiety-like behavior in rodents is the elevated plus maze (see figure). This apparatus is elevated above a table and consists of two arms that intersect to form the shape of a plus sign. The sides of one arm are closed, and the sides of the other arm are open. An animal is placed at the intersection of the arms, and the amount of time it chooses to spend in each arm is measured. Rodents normally prefer the closed arm; this preference has led investigators to hypothesize that rodents experience an aversive state akin to anxiety in the open arm. Behavior exhibited by these animals in response to the administration of a variety of drugs appears to confirm this hypothesis. **Benzodiazepines** such as **diazepam** serve to dramatically increase the amount of time an animal spends in the open arm, as indicated on the hypothetical bar graph. In contrast, **β-carboline (β-CCE)**, an inverse agonist at the benzodiazepine site that is anxiogenic in humans, reduces the amount of time an animal spends in the open arm. Drugs that do not produce anxiolytic or anxiogenic responses in humans are without effect when administered to animals placed in the elevated plus maze.

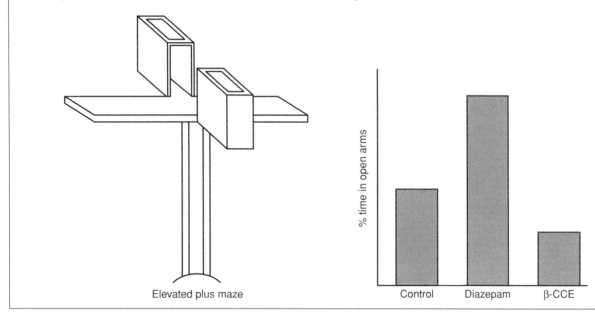

Elevated plus maze

adaptive; they enable us to avoid putting ourselves in harm's way a second time after we have been burned, bitten, or chased. Such memories enable us to identify cues that predict danger so that when we encounter them we are physiologically and behaviorally ready to fight or flee.

However, the strength and persistence of memories encoded in the presence of intense fear may underlie the pathophysiology of certain anxiety disorders such as **agoraphobia** and **posttraumatic stress disorder** (**PTSD**). Agoraphobia, or a fear of public places, often results from the association of an extremely frightening experience known as a **panic attack** with previously neutral contexts in which panic attacks have occurred. PTSD has been hypothesized to involve strong stimulation of amygdala-based fear pathways, which leads to the development of powerful, maladaptive associative emotional memories. In individuals with PTSD, cues reminiscent of an original trauma elicit both explicit (conscious) memories of the experience and emotional memories, or the repertoire of physiologic and behavioral responses to fear that characterized the original traumatic situation.

Evidence has suggested that the exceptional sharpness of explicit (cognitive) memories encoded in the presence of strong negative emotional experiences can be partly attributed to peripheral adrenergic stimulation. Moreover, such enhanced encoding can be blocked by β-adrenergic receptor antagonists such as **propranolol;** indeed, studies involving rodents have suggested that these drugs may be used clinically to dampen memories in human trauma victims when administered within 2 hours after a traumatic event is experienced.

Positive experiences also are believed to elicit emotional memories. Memories resulting from positive experiences most likely result from activity in the nucleus accumbens, the major structure of the ventral striatum, as well as activity in the amygdala. Involvement of the nucleus accumbens is postulated based on evidence that it is a critical neural substrate for reinforcing responses to drugs of abuse and for responses to natural reinforcers such as food, sex, and drink (see Chapter 16). Interestingly, a region of the nucleus accumbens, called the shell, has such significant anatomic and neurochemical similarities to the amygdala that the former is considered by some to be part of an "extended amygdala." Together, amygdala- and nucleus accumbens-based circuitry determine the emotional valence of an experience and assist in encoding that valence in memory.

MOOD REGULATION

Compared with the neural mechanisms that underlie emotions such as fear and anxiety, those that underlie mood regulation are less well understood. Experimental models of fear and anxiety in animals do not have obvious counterparts that might facilitate the investigation of an animal's emotional state over time. Yet considerable overlap appears to exist among the neural systems that regulate fear, anxiety, and mood, and anxiety and mood disorders often occur in the same patients. Because of the lack of suitable animal models of mood, much of the investigation of mood regulation has required the use of noninvasive neuroimaging techniques such as positron emission tomography (PET) and magnetic resonance imaging (MRI) in studies of human subjects. Based on research conducted thus far, structures that are likely to be involved in mood regulation and mood disorders include the orbital and medial prefrontal cortex, amygdala, ventral striatum, hippocampus, and hypothalamus.

PHARMACOLOGY OF ANXIETY AND ANXIETY DISORDERS

Anxiety disorders refer to a heterogeneous group of conditions, each of which features some type of anxiety as its most prominent symptom (Table 15–1). It is important to emphasize that the categorization of these disorders currently is based exclusively on syndromal groupings of subjective and behavioral symptoms; thus any one of these putative disorders may represent a heterogeneous collection of diseases of disparate etiology. Growing evidence, drawn in part from studies of monozygotic and dizygotic twins, suggests that genetic factors contribute to some anxiety disorders; however, despite persistent research efforts during the past two decades, investigators have not yet identified a specific gene that might predispose an individual to any one of these disorders. Barriers to the identification of anxiety

disorder-related genes include inaccurate diagnoses of anxiety disorders, limited knowledge of the pathophysiology of these disorders, and the likelihood that illness results from the interaction of multiple genetic and nongenetic factors. Thus, the discovery of such genes may have to await significant improvements in phenotyping and in genetic technologies, which are developing rapidly.

Despite gaps in our understanding of the pathophysiology of anxiety disorders, several highly effective treatments are available. **Acute anxiety,** for example, has been successfully treated with **benzodiazepines, generalized anxiety disorder** with antidepressants or

Table 15–1 Anxiety Disorders

Panic Disorder

Panic attacks are discrete episodes of intense anxiety accompanied by somatic symptoms such as tachycardia, tachypnea, and dizziness. Panic disorder is diagnosed when multiple panic attacks occur or when one or a few attacks are followed by persistent fear of having another attack.

Generalized Anxiety Disorder (GAD)

GAD is characterized by unrealistic and excessive worry for more than six months accompanied by specific anxiety-related symptoms, such as motor tension, sympathetic hyperactivity, and excessive vigilance.

Posttraumatic Stress Disorder (PTSD)

PTSD occurs after serious trauma and is characterized by numbing, cue-elicited reliving of the traumatic experience, increased startle, and nightmares.

Simple Phobias

Simple phobias are characterized by intense fear of and avoidance of specific stimuli, such as snakes, dogs, airplane travel, and exposure to heights.

Social Phobia (Social Anxiety Disorder)

Social phobia is a persistent fear of one or more social situations involving possible exposure to scrutiny by others, and associated fear of humiliation. An example of a specific social phobia is stage fright. A social phobia may generalize, in which case it may lead to avoidance of all social situations, resulting in substantial social and occupational disability. The boundary between shyness and this type of social phobia has not been well clarified.

The anxiety disorders listed here are described in the American Psychiatric Association's *Diagnostic and Statistical Manual of Mental Disorders*, 4th ed. (American Psychiatric Association, 1993). Obsessive–compulsive disorder also is listed in the manual as an anxiety disorder but appears to be pathophysiologically distinct. The disorders listed in this table have, as their primary symptom, dysregulation of fear, whereas the primary symptom of obsessive-compulsive disorder appears to be intrusive, unwanted thoughts, which most likely are the products of different neural circuits.

benzodiazepines, **panic disorder** with long-term administration of certain **antidepressant drugs** or with high-potency benzodiazepines (often in combination with behavioral therapies), and obsessive–compulsive disorder with long-term administration of **selective serotonin reuptake inhibitor (SSRI) antidepressants** or **clomipramine** together with behavioral therapies. Treatment of **PTSD** remains problematic, although various antidepressants provide modest relief. For some patients, **cognitive–behavioral therapies** are highly effective adjuncts or alternatives to medication therapy; the efficacy of these therapies emphasizes the importance of learning and memory in anxiety.

Although neurobiologic causes of anxiety are not well understood, much is known about the mechanisms by which anxiolytic medications (Figure 15–3) act to reduce anxiety. Therefore the discussion that follows approaches the topic of anxiety disorders from a treatment perspective.

MOLECULAR PHARMACOLOGY OF THE GABA$_A$ RECEPTOR

As discussed in Chapter 7, the GABA$_A$ receptor, like many other ligand-gated channels, is a heteropentamer whose subunits are arranged like staves around a barrel. Three major types of GABA$_A$ receptor subunits, termed α, β, and γ, are known, and multiple subtypes of each have been identified. Several binding sites on the GABA$_A$ receptor complex are summarized in Table 15–2. **Benzodiazepines** bind to a site on the α subunit of the GABA$_A$ receptor complex and thereby increase the affinity of the β subunit for GABA; the presence of a γ subunit is required for such binding. Thus benzodiazepines facilitate the ability of GABA to activate the GABA$_A$ receptor's intrinsic Cl$^-$ channel and in turn facilitate inhibitory neurotransmission. In the absence of GABA, benzodiazepines exert little effect on GABA$_A$ receptors.

Competitive antagonists of anxiolytic benzodiazepines have been discovered and include agents such as **flumazenil**. These antagonists do not exert independent effects on GABA$_A$ receptor function but competitively reverse effects on the receptor produced by benzodiazepine agonists such as **diazepam**. Clinically, flumazenil is useful in the treatment of benzodiazepine overdoses; however, this drug can precipitate withdrawal in benzodiazepine-dependent patients in much the same way that opiate antagonists such as **naloxone** produce withdrawal symptoms in opiate-dependent patients (see Chapter 16).

Inverse agonists, which decrease GABA-activated Cl$^-$ conductance, bind at or near the benzodiazepine binding site on the GABA$_A$ receptor α subunit but

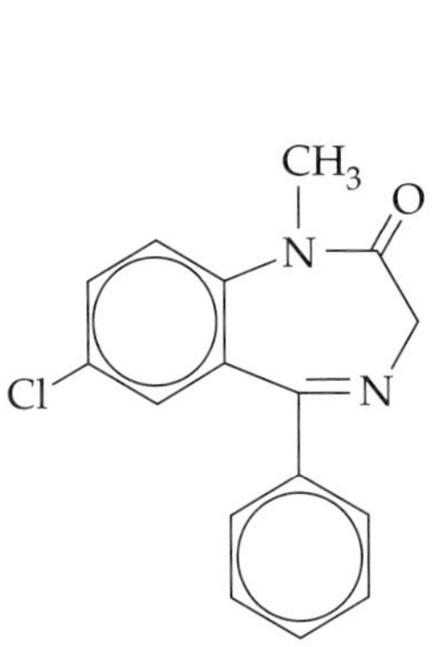

Diazepam

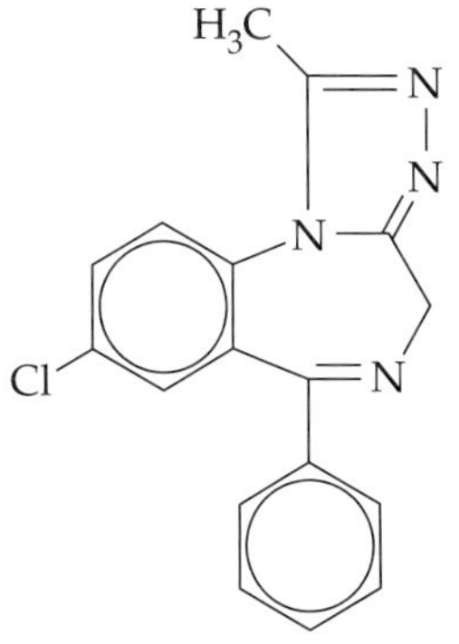

Alprazolam

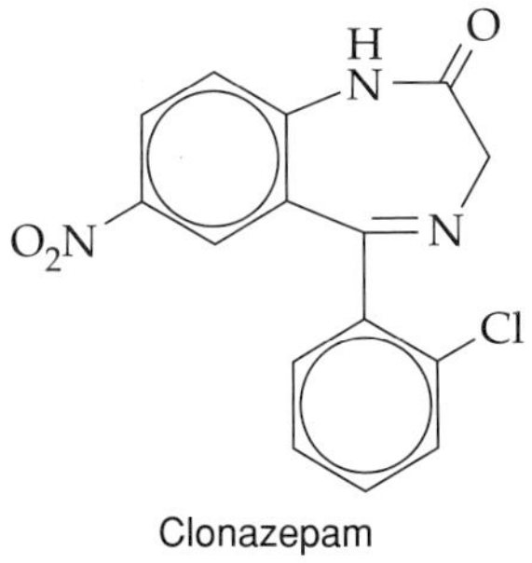

Clonazepam

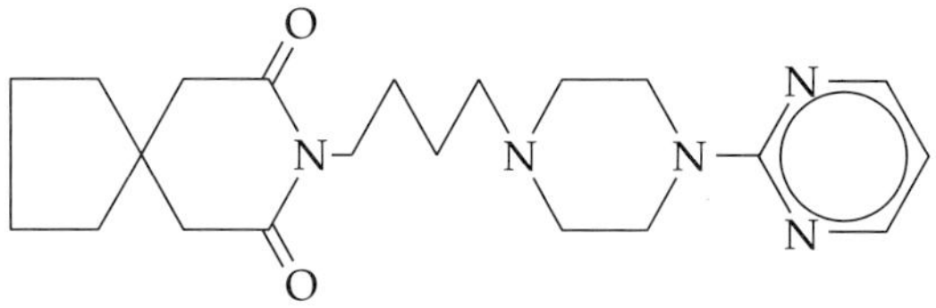

Buspirone

Figure 15–3. Chemical structures of representative anxiolytics. (See Chapter 18 for the structures of benzodiazepines and related compounds that are used primarily in the treatment of insomnia.)

Table 15–2 Pharmacologically Significant Binding Sites on GABA$_A$ Receptors

Site	Agonists	Antagonists	Inverse Agonists
GABA	GABA Muscimol	Bicuculline	
Benzodiazepine	Diazepam	Flumazenil	β-carbolines RO-15-4513
Barbiturate	Pentobarbital		
Convulsant[1]	Picrotoxin Pentylenetetrazole		
Neuroactive steroid[2] (site uncertain)	3α and 5α-THP	DHEA-S	

[1]The categorization of picrotoxin and pentylenetetrazole as agonists at this site may seem paradoxical because these agents antagonize GABA$_A$ receptor function. The term *agonist* is used to indicate that the drugs bind to an allosteric site in the receptor complex that exerts an effect (albeit an inhibitory one) on the receptor.
[2] See Chapter 13 for a more in-depth discussion of neuroactive steroids.
3α and 5α-THP, tetrahydroprogesterone; DHEA-S, dehydroepiandrosterone sulfate.

exert opposite effects on receptor function compared with those produced by benzodiazepines (see Table 15–2). The prototypical inverse agonist is β-carboline-3-carboxylic acid ethyl ester (**β-CCE** or **β-carboline**), which is characterized as proconvulsant and proconflict when administered to animals undergoing the conflict test. During the conflict test, which is used to screen for benzodiazepine effects in animals, a rat presses a lever for food or water and simultaneously receives a shock, which tends to inhibit further pressing of the lever. The pairing of these events is believed to create a state of conflict in the animal, which is faced with both the desire for food and the expectation of punishment. Benzodiazepines administered to such animals are characterized as anticonflict: they release behaviors inhibited by conflict. Thus under the influence of a benzodiazepine, the rat continues to eat or drink despite the threat of punishment. β-CCE exerts the opposite effect in this assay. In non-human primates, β-CCE produces dose-related increases in behavioral agitation, plasma cortisol, blood pressure, and heart rate. Likewise, inverse agonists have produced sympathetic arousal and intense feelings of inner tension and impending doom in human volunteers. The pharmacodynamics and clinical effects of benzodiazepines, together with those of the competitive antagonists and inverse agonists described here, clearly indicate that central GABAergic transmission is involved in the modulation of anxiety symptoms. Yet no direct evidence has suggested that GABAergic systems are abnormal in humans with anxiety disorders.

The discovery of benzodiazepine binding sites in the brain led investigators to hypothesize that, analogous to the endogenous opioids found in the brain (see Chapter 10), there might be an endogenous diazepam-like substance. However, such an entity has yet to be identified. Some reports allege that benzodiazepine molecules have been extracted from mammalian brain, but these assertions lack corroborating evidence such as a corresponding enzyme cascade for synthesis or a release mechanism.

EFFECTS OF GABAERGIC DRUGS ON ANXIETY

Benzodiazepines   Benzodiazepines are a class of drugs with anxiolytic, sedative, muscle relaxant, and anticonvulsant properties (Table 15–3). Benzodiazepines also produce anterograde amnesia, a property that is exploited when high-potency, short-acting benzodiazepines are used as preoperative anxiolytics, but that otherwise represents an unwanted side effect. All benzodiazepines exert their pharmacologic effects by facilitating GABA$_A$ receptor function, as previously mentioned. A related drug, **zolpidem,** which is chemically distinct from the benzodiazepines, nonetheless binds to the same site on the GABA$_A$ receptor and exerts similar pharmacologic effects. Many benzodiazepines are available for clinical use; the major distinguishing features of these agents are their pharmacokinetic properties. Some of these drugs exhibit particularly short half-lives, and thus are desirable for use as **hypnotics,** or **sleeping pills;** examples include **triazolam, zolpidem,** and **lorazepam.** Drugs with longer half-lives are preferable for **generalized anxiety,** or for the treatment of drug withdrawal, as discussed in a subsequent section of this chapter; examples include **diazepam** and **chlordiazepoxide. Alprazolam** and **clonazepam** are widely prescribed for the treatment of **panic disorder** because they are high-potency drugs that produce less sedation (sleepiness) at equipotent doses than many other benzodiazepines. The chemical structures of representative benzodiazepines used in the treatment

Table 15–3 Commonly Used Benzodiazepines

Agonists		
Alprazolam	Flurazepam	Prazepam
Chlordiazepoxide	Halazepam	Quazepam
Clonazepam	Lorazepam	Temazepam
Clorazepate	Midazolam	Triazolam
Diazepam	Nitrazepam	Zolpidem[1]
Estazolam	Oxazepam	

Antagonist
Flumazeni

[1]The nonbenzodiazepine, zolpidem, is an imidazopyridine that acts on the same site of the $GABA_A$ receptor as do benzodiazepines.

of anxiety disorders appear in Figure 15–3; the structures of related agents that are more commonly used to treat insomnia are provided in Chapter 18.

The various clinical effects of benzodiazepines are likely mediated by $GABA_A$ receptors expressed in different regions of the brain. Based on data derived from animal models it has been hypothesized that the anxiolytic properties of benzodiazepines reflect actions on neurons in the amygdala and other components of the fear–anxiety circuitry. GABAergic inhibition of serotonergic, noradrenergic, and many other types of neurons that project to brain structures involved in emotional processing also may contribute to anxiolysis. Depending on the focus of a seizure, the anticonvulsant actions of benzodiazepines may take place in the cerebral cortex, hippocampus, or amygdala. Sedative effects of benzodiazepines have been ascribed to interaction with receptors in brain stem nuclei and in the cerebral cortex; however, this mechanism of action remains conjectural.

The binding site for benzodiazepines was first identified by means of radioreceptor binding assays. Originally called the benzodiazepine receptor, a misnomer because the receptor has no known endogenous ligand, the site is best described as an allosteric regulatory binding site on the $GABA_A$ receptor. Evidence that this site is related to the clinical efficacy of benzodiazepines was drawn from classic pharmacologic investigations, which demonstrated that the affinities of various benzodiazepine drugs for this site neatly corresponded to their clinical potencies (e.g., clonazepam > lorazepam > diazepam > oxazepam). However, these early studies were carried out before the molecular cloning of multiple subtypes of benzodiazepine binding sites (i.e., multiple α subunits of the $GABA_A$ receptor). Such cloning has raised the theoretical possibility of generating benzodiazepines with selective effects on these various subunits.

The benzodiazepines in clinical use today do not exploit such subunit diversity. A major goal of current research is to identify the particular α subunit that is most closely linked to each clinical action produced by benzodiazepines and in turn to develop more selective compounds. The α_1 subunit has been associated with the hypnotic effects of these drugs, the α_5 subunit with some of their cognitive effects, and the α_2 subunit with anxiolysis. A benzodiazepine-like drug designed to be selective for an anxiety-specific subunit like α_2 might be capable of producing anxiolysis without the sedative and amnestic effects of most of the benzodiazepines in current use.

Barbiturates Like benzodiazepines, barbiturates interact with the $GABA_A$ receptor; however, they bind to a physically different site on the receptor, which is believed to be in close proximity to the Cl^- channel (see Table 15–2; also see Chapter 7). Whereas benzodiazepines increase the likelihood that Cl^- channels will open in a GABA-dependent manner, barbiturates increase not only the probability that they will open but also the duration of their opening. Moreover, at high doses barbiturates can act independently of GABA; consequently they can lead to far greater inhibition of the nervous system than can benzodiazepines. Accordingly, a much greater risk of serious respiratory depression and death are associated with barbiturate overdose. Overdoses of benzodiazepines can result in coma but very rarely cause death unless combined with the use of a cross-reactive substance such as a barbiturate or alcohol. Many barbiturate-like drugs, including **methaqualone** (quaaludes), **ethchlorvynol, meprobamate,** and **chloral hydrate,** have been introduced into clinical practice with the hope that their use might result in fewer side effects and less abuse compared with barbiturates. None have withstood the test of time; today barbiturates and related compounds are rarely used for sedation or anxiolysis. Such agents not only produce unwanted side effects, such as induction of hepatic microsomal enzymes, they are more likely to cause dependence and addiction and are not as effective as benzodiazepines in the treatment of anxiety. Short-acting barbiturates currently are used primarily for anesthesia. A prototypical agent used for this purpose is **pentobarbital.** A long-acting barbiturate, **phenobarbital,** is still used for certain seizure disorders (see Chapter 21).

Neuroactive steroids represent yet another class of molecules that modulate the function of $GABA_A$ receptors; however, their precise mechanisms of action remain unknown. These molecules are discussed in greater detail in Chapter 13.

Alcohol Concentrations of ethyl alcohol produced in humans from the consumption of alcoholic beverages facilitate the GABA-mediated opening of $GABA_A$ receptor Cl^- channels. Thus it should not be surprising that a reduction in anxiety is among the most prominent effects of alcohol, at least at low doses and while blood levels continue to rise (see Chapter 16). This characteristic helps to explain why alcohol is widely self-administered to enhance social interaction. Indeed, **social anxiety disorder** is a risk factor for alcoholism. When alcohol is taken with benzodiazepines or barbiturates its effects are greatly intensified because each of these agents alters $GABA_A$ receptor conformation to increase the efficacy of the others. Because of this cross-reactivity, which is synergistic, mixtures of these drugs can be lethal. Such cross-reactivity is exploited in alcohol detoxification regimens, which typically replace alcohol with a benzodiazepine which is then slowly tapered. Benzodiazepines, such as **chlordiazepoxide,** are used for detoxification because they have a longer half-life than alcohol; thus they permit a smoother detoxification process (i.e., less risk of withdrawal symptoms), cause fewer side effects, and may reduce the likelihood of relapse.

As discussed in Chapter 7, an inverse agonist compound designated **RO15–4513** has been demonstrated to inhibit ethanol-induced Cl^- conductance of $GABA_A$ receptors. It also is capable of reversing some behavioral effects (e.g., staggering gait and impaired righting reflex) of ethanol-induced intoxication in rats. Only $GABA_A$ receptors that contain the α_6 subunit can bind RO15–4513; moreover, this receptor subtype does not bind other benzodiazepines or inverse agonists. The selective antagonism of ethanol-induced motor incoordination and ataxia by this novel compound may be explained by the relatively selective expression of the α_6 subunit in cerebellar granule cells. However, the selective expression of this subunit also has limited the clinical utility of RO15–4513, which is unable to antagonize noncerebellar actions of alcohol.

TOLERANCE AND DEPENDENCE ASSOCIATED WITH BENZODIAZEPINES

Benzodiazepines differ significantly from many other psychotropic drugs with regard to their latency of action. In contrast to antidepressants, lithium and other mood-stabilizing agents, and antipsychotic drugs, which take weeks to achieve maximal therapeutic effects, the therapeutic effects of benzodiazepines are directly related to current serum levels. Although the short-term effects of these medications can be clinically desirable, the long-term actions of benzodiazepines and barbiturates on the nervous system can be deleterious. These agents can produce tolerance and dependence and, in a small per-

centage of individuals, can trigger addictive behaviors (see Chapter 16).

Chronic administration of a benzodiazepine generally causes tolerance to its sedating and anticonvulsant effects. This characteristic has severely limited the utility of these agents; for example, in the treatment of seizure disorders, benzodiazepines are—with few exceptions—used only in acute settings. This property also has complicated the use of these drugs as hypnotics in the long-term treatment of chronic insomnia. In contrast, appreciable tolerance to the anxiolytic effects of benzodiazepines does not develop in most patients. Indeed, many individuals maintain a daily low dose of a benzodiazepine to reduce anxiety over a period of years and in some cases for most of their lifetimes.

Dependence produced by the long-term administration of a benzodiazepine is marked by a characteristic withdrawal syndrome, which features both psychological and physical symptoms in response to the discontinuation of drug treatment. The intensity of this withdrawal syndrome appears to be greater with the discontinuation of high-potency short half-life compounds such as **alprazolam**. Symptoms of benzodiazepine withdrawal include rebound symptoms, or a worsening of the symptoms (e.g., insomnia or anxiety) for which the drugs were originally administered, and the onset of new symptoms such as tremulousness, anxiety, paresthesias, and, in some cases, seizures.

It is important to distinguish tolerance and dependence from addiction, which is marked by inappropriate drug-seeking behavior and the compulsive nonmedical use of a drug despite adverse consequences (see Chapter 16). Benzodiazepines commonly produce dependence but are much less likely to produce addiction, which tends to occur most commonly in individuals with a prior history of drug abuse. Barbiturates and related compounds and alcohol are far more likely to cause addictive behaviors. Nevertheless, concerns about benzodiazepine addiction, and confusion regarding tolerance, dependence, and addiction, have caused physicians and patients alike to be wary of the use of these drugs. This is unfortunate because, when prescribed appropriately, benzodiazepines remain among the safest and most effective psychotropic medications.

The molecular mechanisms that underlie benzodiazepine tolerance and dependence continue to be investigated. Some researchers have proposed that a covalent modification of the $GABA_A$ receptor, such as phosphorylation, may explain the occurrence of such phenomena. Accordingly, phosphorylation of a receptor subunit may reduce the sensitivity of the receptor complex to GABA and benzodiazepines. Alternatively, tolerance and dependence may be explained by altered expression of GABA$_A$ receptor subtypes with different functional properties. Chronic administration of alcohol to laboratory animals, for example, causes region-specific alterations in the patterns of expression of several GABA$_A$ receptor subunits in the brain; however, such changes have not been definitively linked to the development of tolerance and dependence.

NONBENZODIAZEPINE ANXIOLYTICS

Considerable effort has been devoted to the development of anxiolytic agents with novel mechanisms of action. Examples under consideration include previously mentioned CRF$_1$R receptor antagonists, Substance P NK$_1$ receptor antagonists, and NPY Y$_1$ receptor agonists (see Chapter 10), but the viability of such agents will require a great deal of additional preclinical and clinical research. However, the development and use of two types of agents with mechanisms of action other than GABA$_A$ receptor facilitation deserve further comment.

Buspirone   Buspirone, an azaspirodecanedione partial agonist at 5-HT$_{1A}$ serotonin receptors, is marketed as an anxiolytic. 5-HT$_{1A}$ receptors serve as autoreceptors on serotonin neurons and also as postsynaptic receptors (see Chapter 9). When administered to animals, buspirone has a taming effect on rhesus monkeys, inhibits conditioned avoidance responses in rats, and reduces shock-elicited fighting in mice. However, it is generally ineffective as an anticonflict agent in rats and monkeys. Buspirone is approved for use in the treatment of **generalized anxiety disorder,** although it is less effective than benzodiazepines or certain antidepressants when used for this or related purposes. The major advantage of buspirone and SSRIs compared with benzodiazepines is that they are less likely to give rise to dependence, and they are virtually without abuse liability. Clinical experience with buspirone and related 5-HT$_{1A}$ agonists has been disappointing because the 5-HT$_{1A}$ receptor had been strongly implicated in anxiolytic and antidepressant actions in some animal models. Such experience highlights the continuing difficulty of predicting with certainty the clinical efficacy of a new psychotropic drug based on its activity in available animal models and in vitro receptor assays.

One feature that dramatically distinguishes buspirone from the benzodiazepines is that its clinical efficacy, albeit weak, requires repeated drug administration for several weeks. This characteristic suggests that initial actions at the 5-HT$_{1A}$ receptor are not anxiolytic per se, but induce long-term adaptations in brain function—perhaps involving altered expression of receptors or intracellular messenger proteins—that ultimately are

anxiolytic. However, the adaptations that mediate buspirone's actions have yet to be determined.

Adenosine receptor agonists   Another target for anxiolytic drugs may prove to be the adenosine A$_1$ receptor (see Chapter 10). Adenosine is a purine neuromodulator that inhibits the release of other neurotransmitters, including acetylcholine, norepinephrine, glutamate, dopamine, 5-HT, and GABA, in specific regions of the brain through actions at its A$_1$ receptor. This action is mediated through the opening of K$^+$ channels, the inhibition of Ca^{2+} channel opening, and the inhibition of adenylyl cyclase—all by means of the G$_{i/o}$ family of G proteins. Adenosine is sedative, anticonvulsant, analgesic, and anxiolytic. Adenosine receptor antagonists, including **methylxanthines** such as **caffeine** and **theophylline,** produce stimulant effects. Large doses of caffeine are anxiogenic, and high doses administered into the brain may produce seizures.

Benzodiazepines, acting through their binding sites on GABA$_A$ receptors, have important interactions with adenosine. Adenosine and diazepam, for example, have synergistic actions; moreover, caffeine can antagonize many of the behavioral effects of benzodiazepines. Although the role of adenosine in human anxiety is unclear, A$_1$ adenosine receptor agonists may prove to be useful in the treatment of various types of anxiety disorders.

TREATMENT OF ANXIETY DISORDERS

As previously suggested, both benzodiazepines and some types of antidepressants have been effective in the treatment of anxiety (see Table 15–1). The preferred treatment for **panic disorder** is the use of an antidepressant. An **SSRI** typically is selected, but among the currently approved antidepressants only **bupropion** and **trazodone** have proven to be ineffective for this indication. The most common alternative is the use of a high-potency benzodiazepine such as **alprazolam** or **clonazepam.** Generally, **cognitive-behavior therapies** can be used as adjuncts to medication and sometimes may be used in place of medication. For specific phobias (e.g., animal phobias), cognitive-behavioral therapies aimed at desensitization are the treatment of choice. **Social phobia,** also called **social anxiety disorder,** is characterized by a persistent fear of experiencing humiliation in one or more social situations in which an individual may be exposed to scrutiny by others. Affected individuals may experience stage fright or find that they are unable to speak out in class or during social gatherings. The anxiety experienced may be characterized as low-grade or tolerable, or may reach the intensity of a panic attack.

Social phobia is distinguished from normal anxiety in part by the extent of avoidance or social and occupational limitation that occurs. Alcoholism appears to be a common complication of social phobia, most likely because alcohol has temporary anxiolytic effects. Specific performance anxiety, such as stage fright, is a highly circumscribed form of social anxiety disorder and is associated primarily with autonomic symptoms such as pounding heart, dry mouth, and tremor. Because benzodiazepines can adversely affect mental acuity, the treatment of choice for this disorder typically is a β-adrenergic receptor antagonist such as **propranolol** or **atenolol,** which is likely to have fewer cognitive side effects. Individuals with generalized social phobia appear more likely to benefit from the use of an SSRI antidepressant in conjunction with cognitive behavioral therapy; alternatively, the use of high-potency benzodiazepines may be considered.

PTSD initially was identified in veterans exposed to intense combat situations. Symptoms include cue-induced reexperiencing of a traumatic event accompanied by autonomic and other physiologic aspects of the fear response. Nightmares and general feelings of emotional numbness are also common. During the past few decades PTSD has been identified as a common response to many types of trauma, including rape, sexual abuse, child abuse, and motor vehicle accidents. Although these clinical syndromes are becoming increasingly well-defined in terms of characteristic symptoms, much remains to be learned about their underlying neurobiology. Investigators have proposed that abnormalities in amygdala circuitry contribute to the development of such disorders, but this hypothesis remains unproven. PTSD is not adequately treated by available medications. The use of an **SSRI** or **monoamine oxidase inhibitor (MAOI)** in conjunction with psychotherapy leads to modest improvement in many patients. It is currently hypothesized that **β-adrenergic receptor antagonists** may reduce the enhanced recall of explicit memories associated with trauma when administered within the first 1–2 hours after trauma. The development of improved treatments for PTSD remains a major goal of current research.

OBSESSIVE–COMPULSIVE DISORDER

Obsessive–compulsive disorder (OCD) involves either 1) recurrent intrusive thoughts that an individual recognizes as products of his or her own mind (obsessions); or 2) repetitive, seemingly purposeful behavior designed to prevent or neutralize a dreaded occurrence, often as a consequence of the obsession (compulsions); or both. Although it traditionally has been classified as an anxiety disorder, growing evidence suggests that OCD differs from other anxiety disorders with regard to its neurobiologic substrates. As described in Chapter 14, current hypotheses associate OCD with a disruption in the neural circuit that extends from the frontal cortex to the striatum, continues to the thalamus, and returns to the cortex. Other neuropsychiatric diseases that are believed to affect the striatum, including **Tourette syndrome** and child-onset movement disorders such as **Sydenham chorea,** also may feature obsessive–compulsive symptoms (see Chapter 14).

OCD currently is treated with **SSRIs,** or with the tricyclic drug **clomipramine,** which also preferentially inhibits the 5-HT transporter (Table 15–4). However, higher doses of these drugs are generally required compared with doses used for the treatment of depression. Interestingly, therapeutic action also tends to occur after a longer latency period than that associated with the treatment of depression; indeed, delays in the onset of drug action may be as great as 10–12 weeks. Pharmacologic treatment of OCD is hypothesized to take place within the striatum, although little direct evidence supports this theory. Investigators also have yet to determine why SSRI antidepressants and clomipramine are uniquely effective in the treatment of this disorder. Cognitive-behavior therapy has proven to be useful in the treatment of some patients, especially with regard to reducing or eliminating compulsive rituals.

PHARMACOLOGY OF MOOD DISORDERS

Throughout the world mood disorders are among the most prevalent causes of morbidity and disability and are the leading cause of suicide. Based on symptoms and patterns of familial transmission, these disorders can be assigned to one of two broad categories. Individuals with **unipolar depression** experience episodes of depression only; those with **bipolar disorder** experience at least one episode of mania, and most commonly experience alternating episodes of depression and mania (Table 15–5). Yet it must be emphasized that these clinical entities, much like anxiety disorders, most likely represent a heterogeneous group of disparate pathophysiologic processes. Moreover, considerable overlap exists among anxiety and mood disorders.

Mood disorders generally are characterized by an episodic course, although they can become chronic. A striking feature of mood disorders is that their symptoms appear to reflect abnormal functioning in many different regions of the brain. Sleep disturbances may be traced to alterations in brain stem monoamine or cholinergic nuclei or, based on the stereotypical diurnal pattern of common sleep disturbances, to disruptions of the circa-

Table 15-4 Effects of Tricyclic and Related Tetracyclic Antidepressants on Receptors and Transporters[1]

Drug	Transporters		Receptors		
	NE	5-HT	Muscarinic Acetylcholine	H₁ Histamine	α₁ Adrenergic
Amitriptyline	+/−	+ +	+ + + +	+ + + +	+ + +
Amoxapine	+ +	0	0	+/−	+ +
Clomipramine	+	+ + +	+ +	+	+ +
Desipramine	+ + +	0	+	0	+
Doxepin	+ +	+	+ +	+ + +	+ +
Imipramine	+	+	+ +	+	+ +
Maprotiline	+ +	0	+	+ +	+
Nortriptyline	+ +	+/−	+ +	+	+
Protriptyline	+ +	0	+ + +	+	+
Trimipramine	+	0	+ +	+ + +	+ +

[1]Number of plus (+) signs indicates binding affinity. 0, undetectable. All effects listed are antagonistic. Desipramine is the desmethyl metabolite of imipramine, and nortriptyline is the desmethyl metabolite of amitriptyline.

dian pacemaker in the suprachiasmatic nucleus of the hypothalamus (see Chapter 18). Changes in appetite and energy may reflect abnormalities in various hypothalamic nuclei. Depressed mood and anhedonia (lack of interest in pleasurable activities) in depressed individuals, and euphoria and increased involvement in goal-directed

Table 15-5 Mood Disorders[1]

Major Depression

Characterized by sad mood or loss of interest in usual pursuits, accompanied by abnormalities of sleep, appetite, energy, sex drive, and motivation. Other features may include psychomotor retardation or agitation, and abnormal thoughts, such as guilt, hopelessness, and suicidal ideas.

Dysthymia

Represents chronic milder depression. Its course is often punctuated by episodes of major depression.

Bipolar Disorder (Manic-Depressive Illness)

Characterized by episodes of mania, with or without distinct episodes of depression. The symptoms and signs of depression are the same whether the disorder is unipolar or bipolar. Mania is characterized by euphoria or irritability, increased energy, and a decreased need for sleep. Patients often are intrusive, hypersexual, and impulsive; they have inflated self-esteem, which may be delusional. Cognitively, they are distractible; their speech is often rapid and pressured. Psychotic symptoms are common.

[1]Based on the American Psychiatric Association's *Diagnostic and Statistical Manual of Mental Disorders*, 4th ed. (American Psychiatric Association, 1993).

activities in patients who experience mania, may reflect opposing abnormalities in the ventral striatum, medial prefrontal cortex, amygdala, or other structures. Anxiety, which is a common symptom of depression, may reflect abnormalities in the functioning of the amygdala and BNST, as previously mentioned. The excessive release of stress hormones, such as cortisol, that occurs in many individuals with mood disorders may result from hyperfunctioning of the PVN of the hypothalamus, hyperfunctioning of the amygdala (which activates the PVN), or hypofunctioning of the hippocampus (which exerts a potent inhibitory influence on the PVN). Alterations in the content of thought, which are a cardinal feature of depression and mania, most likely reflect abnormal functioning of the cerebral cortex. A neurobiologic explanation of mood disorders must be able to demonstrate how diverse brain regions are affected, why associated abnormalities are episodic, and how both genes and environment can affect the pathogenesis of these disorders. Circuits that can directly or indirectly influence all of the structures affected by these disorders are currently a focus of research. Because of their widespread projections, and because of their role in antidepressant action, monoamine systems in the brain historically have been thought to play an important role in the pathophysiology of mood disorders. Even if they are not the primary cause of mood disorders, monoamine systems may serve to generalize an abnormality initiated elsewhere so that it affects much of the rest of the brain.

One obstacle to research in depression has been a lack of good animal models. Several well-characterized

Box 15–3 The Search for Animal Models of Depression

A major obstacle to research on depression has been the lack of good animal models. Two tests that are commonly used to predict the efficacy of antidepressant drugs illustrate the weaknesses in current models. The Porsolt test, or *forced swim test*, involves placing a rodent in a bucket of water. Most rodents struggle for a time before adopting a floating position without further struggle. The administration of an antidepressant, regardless of the type, increases the amount of time the animal spends struggling. Consequently it has been hypothesized that such drugs cause these animals to work harder and refuse to give up. This interpretation is not at all obvious. Moreover, the effects of the antidepressants administered during this test are observed immediately, even though their clinical effects in humans require long-term administration. In addition, cocaine and other stimulants increase struggling in these animals but do not produce antidepressant effects in humans.

Another test used to investigate the effects of antidepressant drugs is referred to as *learned helplessness*. Animals that undergo this test are repeatedly given a mild foot shock but are not permitted to escape from the environment in which they receive the shock. After a suitable training period, these animals are permitted to escape after receiving a shock. Under these circumstances, a subpopulation of rodents typically fails to attempt escape. It has been hypothesized that these animals shows signs of having "given up"; in other words, such animals exhibit learned helplessness. The administration of an antidepressant facilitates escape behavior. This test has greater face validity than the forced swim test; however, unlike antidepressants administered to humans, the drugs given to these animals are effective after several doses.

All available antidepressants are active in both of the tests described here. This should not be surprising because

only compounds that have been active in these tests have been pursued as antidepressants for human use. This has created a catch-22. Although these tests are good predictors of available antidepressants, it is not at all clear that they are likely to detect the effectiveness of agents with truly novel mechanisms of action. A non-monoamine-based agent, for example, might be effective in humans despite its failure to produce expected results in these tests.

Recent research has focused on developing models of depression that have greater validity and that can be reversed only with long-term antidepressant administration. Various types of chronic stress models have been proposed, some of which involve animals subjected to low levels of stress for relatively long periods of time (weeks to months). In some laboratories, stress is created by exposing animals to highly aggressive dominant males. Other models subject young pups to maternal separation and study the animals as adults. Animals used in each of these cases exhibit some of the signs that are characteristic of depression in humans; for example, they develop sleep disorders, exhibit reduced feeding and sexual behavior, and show abnormalities in the HPA axis. These models are being used to identify neurobiologic and genetic substrates of mood disorders.

A related approach involves the use of different genetic strains of rodents in chronic stress models. It has long been known that inbred strains vary greatly in their responses to stress and in their performance in stress-related tests. A particularly vulnerable strain subjected to chronic stress might represent a viable model of a particular type of depression, or might at least reproduce certain symptoms of depression. Of course, a better model of depression might involve the placement of mutant (depression-causing) human genes in mice. However, this type of model must await the identification of such genes.

---

tests (e.g., forced swim or learned helplessness) are used to predict antidepressant responses in rodents, but are limited in terms of their ability to produce models of depression (Box 15–3). Rodent models used to explore various types of chronic stress have more accurately exhibited certain aspects of depression. Limitations associated with animal models have required the use of human subjects for much of the research that has been devoted to mood disorders.

A substantial focus of research has been the documentation of abnormalities in monoamine systems because of the efficacy of antidepressant drugs that target norepinephrine, serotonin, and less commonly, dopamine systems. Although it is widely recognized that such pharmacologic treatments may act on synapses that are unrelated to the pathophysiology of depression or mania, a large number of studies have examined

monoamine turnover, monoamine receptors on accessible peripheral blood cells, and the neuroendocrine and behavioral effects of various pharmacologic challenges such as the depletion of monoamine systems. Many of these active challenges can provoke symptoms or alter physiologic responses, but they have yielded little specific information about disease pathophysiology or even mechanisms of drug action. Certain antidepressant drugs have proved efficacious for a wide range of emotional and other disorders, including depression, panic disorder, obsessive–compulsive disorder, PTSD, eating disorders, enuresis (bed wetting), and chronic pain syndromes. Thus serotonin and norepinephrine are not exclusively related to depression. Rather, it appears that modulation of the brain's serotonergic or noradrenergic systems can result in palliative effects on many pathophysiologic mechanisms.

GENETICS OF MOOD DISORDERS

The lifetime prevalence of serious major depression in the United States is 5%; thus among serious diseases of the brain depression is arguably the most common. Less severe forms of depression may affect an additional 10% of the population. The risk of developing unipolar depression is approximately twice as great among women as among men in almost all cultures studied. The prevalence of bipolar disorder, which tends to affect men and women equally, is approximately 1% throughout the world. Both bipolar disorder and depression are characterized by familial transmission, but the familial nature of bipolar disorder is especially pronounced; the incidence of bipolar disorder among first-degree relatives of affected individuals is 8–25%, compared with 1% in the general population. Evidence drawn from twin and adoption studies strongly supports a genetic contribution to mood disorders. Yet molecular analyses have thus far failed to identify specific genetic mutations (or polymorphisms) that cause these disorders. As with many complex genetic disorders, most efforts to trace the heritability of depression and bipolar disorder have led to the view that multiple genetic loci and nongenetic factors are involved. Moreover, the critical nongenetic factors that influence the occurrence of these disorders and their course in some cases may not be shared by members of a family, and thus have been difficult to analyze. Stress, for example, has been implicated as a factor in the onset of depression; however, each individual tends to interpret particular events as stressors in a relatively unique way.

Several rare genetic diseases are characterized by disorders of mood in addition to a variety of other manifestations. An example is **Wolfram syndrome,** which is caused by a microdeletion of chromosome 4. The critical gene responsible for this disease appears to encode wolframin, a protein whose function is not yet known. Homozygotes with this mutation exhibit diabetes mellitus and optic deformities, but heterozygotes commonly exhibit depression. Another example is **velocardiofacial syndrome,** which is caused by a microdeletion of chromosome 22. The relevant gene(s) associated with this disorder remain unknown. Patients typically present with deformities of the palate, heart, and face, as the name of the syndrome implies, and also exhibit prominent behavioral abnormalities that include mania-like symptoms. The relationship between these diseases and common mood disorders has yet to be determined, but such disorders may provide clues to the types of genetic abnormalities and pathophysiologic mechanisms that can cause mood disorders.

NEUROENDOCRINE ABNORMALITIES ASSOCIATED WITH DEPRESSION

Abnormal, excessive activation of the HPA axis (see Chapter 13, Figure 13–3) occurs in approximately half of all individuals who experience an episode of major depression. These individuals may exhibit increased cortisol production, as measured by increases in free cortisol in urine, and a reduced ability to suppress plasma cortisol, adrenocorticotropic hormone (ACTH), and β-endorphin after administration of dexamethasone, a potent synthetic glucocorticoid. Direct and indirect evidence suggests that these individuals also exhibit hypersecretion of CRF. Moreover, ACTH responses to intravenously administered CRF are blunted, and concentrations of CRF in cerebrospinal fluid (CSF) tend to be increased. A postmortem study of depressed individuals has revealed increases in CRF in the PVN of the hypothalamus. This finding has suggested that the primary source of hypercortisolism is located at or above the level of the hypothalamus.

As previously indicated, increases in cortisol induce catabolism, suppress the immune system, and may have temporary elevating effects on mood, energy, and cognition. Although short-term administration of glucocorticoids often produces euphoria and increased energy, the impact of long-lasting increases in endogenous glucocorticoids produced during depression can involve complex adaptations such as those that occur in **Cushing syndrome** (see Chapter 13). For example, evidence indicates that prolonged increases in cortisol can be toxic to hippocampal neurons in animals and humans. Because the hippocampus is required for feedback inhibition of CRF neurons (Figure 15–4), episodes of depression marked by severe hypercortisolemia may produce further impairment in feedback regulation of the HPA axis and predispose affected individuals to chronic depression or to future recurrences.

Striking parallels exist among melancholic depression, the stress response, and behavioral and physiologic effects produced by CRF injected into cerebral ventricles. These include increased arousal and vigilance, decreased appetite, decreased sexual behavior, and increased heart rate and blood pressure. Thus whether hypothalamic abnormalities are a primary cause of depression or secondary to the initial cause of the disease, they undoubtedly contribute to the generation of serious symptoms and have an impact on the course of depression and its somatic sequelae. Accordingly new pharmacologic agents currently under investigation have been designed to correct some of these abnormalities. CRF receptor antagonists, particularly **CRF$_1$R antagonists,** that are now being evaluated in clinical trials for the treatment of depression may act in the PVN to limit hypercortisolism. Inhibition of CRF$_1$ receptors in the amygdala and its projection areas also may contribute to a reduction in symptoms of depression and anxiety. Thus far it appears that CRF$_1$ receptor antagonists do not cause adrenal insufficiency, a side effect that would severely limit their utility, because ACTH synthesis and release is controlled by multiple mechanisms, including the actions of vasopressin (see Chapter 13). Also undergoing evaluation is the feasibility of designing a drug that might influence central CRF function by interfering with CRF-binding protein (CBP). The physiologic function of this protein is incompletely understood, but it appears to regulate levels of free active CRF.

ANXIETY DISORDERS AND DEPRESSION

Many individuals with **panic disorder, PTSD,** or other **anxiety** disorders develop major depression, and many individuals with **major depression** also experience severe anxiety. Moreover, there appears to be an overlapping genetic risk for panic disorder and depression in some families. Interestingly, both depression and panic disorder have been effectively treated with **tricyclic antidepressants, SSRIs,** and **MAOIs,** and SSRIs and MAOIs appear to provide some benefit in the treatment of PTSD. Together these observations have raised the question of whether overlapping neural circuitry is involved in the pathophysiology of depression and of certain anxiety disorders. The answer to this question must await a better understanding of the neural circuits underlying emotion and mood, and of the specific genes that predispose families to these illnesses. Meanwhile, evidence for common pathophysiologic mechanisms in anxiety and depression continues to accumulate. Preliminary findings suggest, for example, that small-molecule antagonists of the receptors for substance P and CRF may exhibit both antidepressant and anxiolytic properties in animal models and in humans.

ANTIDEPRESSANT DRUGS

Antidepressant drugs are a heterogeneous group of compounds that are effective in the treatment of major depression (Table 15–6). As previously mentioned, most are also effective in the treatment of some anxiety disorders, including **panic disorder**. A number of these agents, including **clomipramine** and the **SSRIs,** also are effective in the treatment of **obsessive–compulsive disorder**. Based on structural and neurochemical properties, antidepressant drugs often are subdivided into groups that include **tricyclic** and related cyclic antidepressants; **SSRIs;** norepinephrine selective reuptake inhibitors (**NRIs**); serotonin and norepinephrine reuptake inhibitors (**SNRIs**); **MAOIs;** and miscellaneous antidepressants. The chemical structures of representative antidepressants are shown in Figure 15–5.

Tricyclic antidepressants inhibit serotonin and/or norepinephrine reuptake to varying extents (see Tables 15–4 and 15–6). They also antagonize several neurotransmitter receptors, particularly muscarinic cholinergic, H$_1$ histaminergic, and α_1 adrenergic receptors (see Table 15–4); such antagonism explains their many side

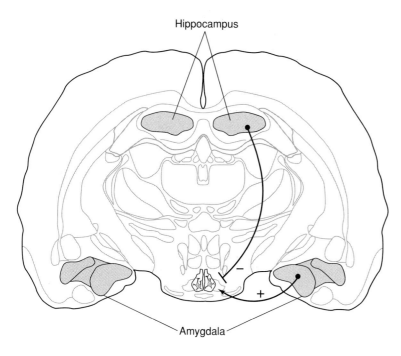

Figure 15–4. Regulation of the hypothalamic–pituitary–adrenal (HPA) axis. Neurons of the paraventricular nucleus (PVN) of the hypothalamus containing corticotropin-releasing factor integrate information relevant to stress. Prominent neural inputs include excitatory afferent signals from the amygdala and inhibitory afferent signals from the hippocampus. Other important inputs are received from ascending monoamine pathways and from the periphery, the latter of which include inhibitory inputs from circulating endogenous glucocorticoids such as cortisol (see Chapter 13).

Table 15–6 Commonly Used Antidepressant Medications

Tricyclics[1]	
5-HT-selective reuptake blockers	
Amitriptyline[2]	
Imipramine[2]	
Clomipramine	
NE-selective reuptake blockers	
Nortriptyline	
Desipramine	
SSRIs	
Citalopram	
Fluoxetine	
Fluvoxamine	
Paroxetine	
Sertraline	
NE-selective reuptake inhibitors (NRIs)	
Reboxetine	
Mixed 5-HT/NE reuptake inhibitors (SNRIs)	
Venlafaxine	
MAOIs	
Tranylcypromine	
Phenelzine	
Antidepressants with other mechanisms	
Bupropion	
Mirtazepine	
Nefazodone	
Trazodone	

[1]See Table 15–4 for additional examples of tricyclic and related tetracyclic antidepressants.
[2]Although these compounds predominantly inhibit 5-HT reuptake, they are metabolized into nortriptyline and desipramine, antidepressants in their own right that are NE reuptake inhibitors.
5-HT, serotonin; NE, norepinephrine; MAOI, monoamine oxidase inhibitors.

effects, including sedation, dry mouth, and constipation. SSRIs were developed to selectively inhibit the serotonin transporter, without activity at cholinergic, histaminergic, or adrenergic receptors; their use has represented a rational means of avoiding side effects associated with tricyclic agents. Likewise, **reboxetine** is an NRI that lacks many side effects associated with tricyclic agents because it lacks activity at the same receptors. **Venlafaxine** inhibits both serotonin and norepinephrine reuptake and also lacks many of the side effects of tricyclic antidepressants because of selective actions at the serotonin and norepinephrine trans-

porters. MAOIs were developed as selective inhibitors of MAO enzymes. Their development was based on the serendipitous discovery five decades ago that the antitubercular drug iproniazid alleviates depression, and the subsequent discovery that such alleviation stems from MAO inhibition (see Chapter 8).

In contrast to these antidepressants, the mechanisms of action of most other antidepressant agents, which often are described as atypical, remain poorly understood. **Bupropion,** an aminoketone, is an effective antidepressant that does not produce appreciable effects on the serotonin or norepinephrine systems. Its effectiveness has been attributed to its inhibition of dopamine reuptake; however, this is unlikely to be a sole mechanism of action, because cocaine also inhibits dopamine reuptake but does not serve as an effective antidepressant. **Mirtazepine,** an antidepressant recently introduced into clinical practice, is reported to be an antagonist at α_2-adrenergic and 5-HT_{2A} and 5-HT_3 serotonin receptors; however, the relationship between these actions and its antidepressant effects has not been ascertained. **Trazodone** and **nefazodone,** both triazoloperidine derivatives, influence serotonin systems in several ways; however, it appears that trazodone is not as effective as other available agents.

Antidepressants with novel mechanisms of action are in great demand. Some mechanisms by which new agents might act (e.g., antagonism of CRF_1R and glucocorticoid receptors) already have been discussed in this chapter, and several are mentioned in subsequent sections. Another type of agent, an **NK_1 (substance P) receptor antagonist,** deserves comment. One such antagonist, **MK-869,** is reportedly effective in animal models of depression, and one study has indicated that it is useful in the treatment of depression, although the results of another study failed to confirm efficacy. Other NK_1 antagonists also are currently being tested in humans. How an NK_1 receptor antagonist might treat depression is unknown but has been related to the high density of these receptors in the amygdala. If such a connection is confirmed, it may provide important new leads in antidepressant research.

There has been considerable popular interest in the use of so-called natural remedies, or **herbal products,** to treat depression. However, the safety and efficacy of these preparations have not yet been established. **St. John's Wort,** an herbal product available over the counter, has been used by many individuals as an antidepressant, yet the component in St. John's Wort that might be responsible for its putative effectiveness has not been identified. Interestingly, it has been determined that St. John's Wort induces the metabolism of, and therefore diminishes the effectiveness of, oral contraceptives, certain immunosuppressants, and some of

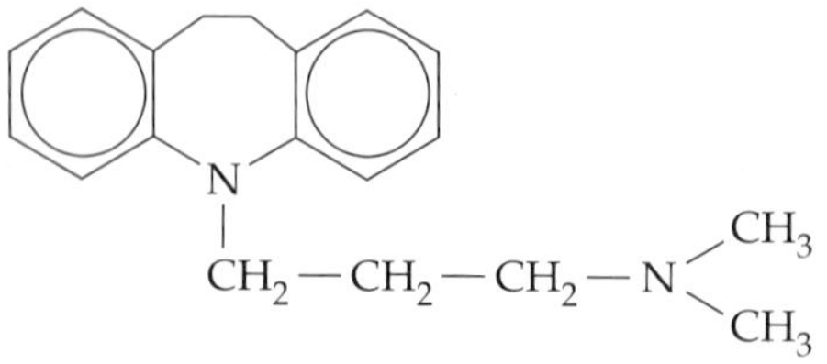

Imipramine

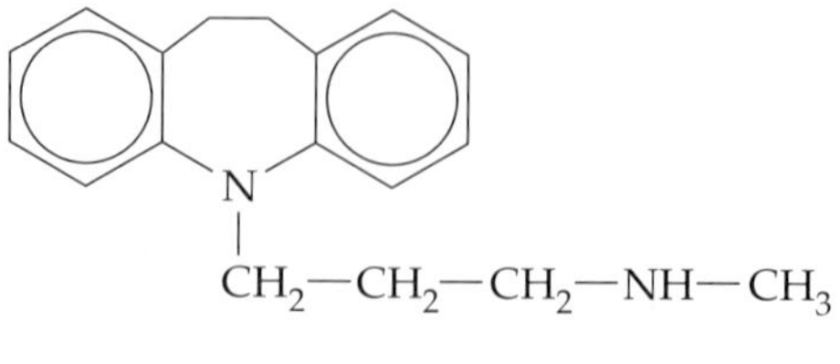

Desipramine

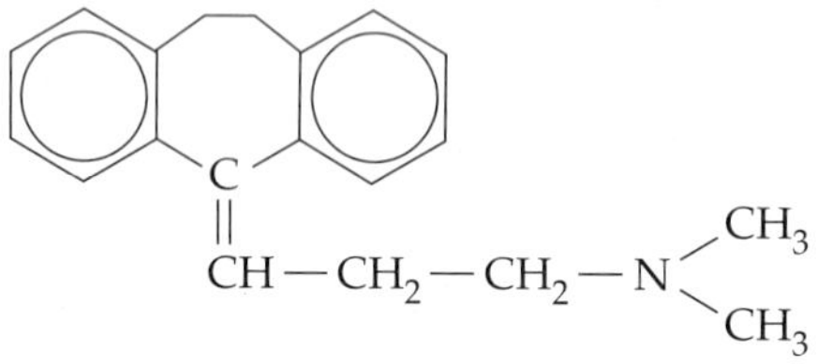

Amitriptyline

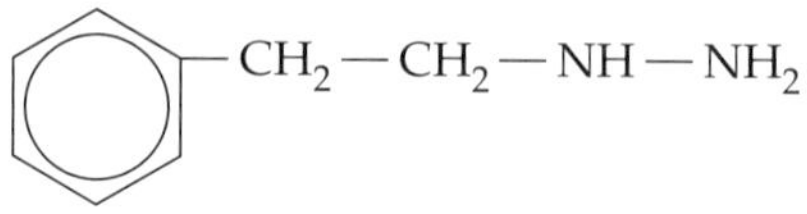

Phenelzine

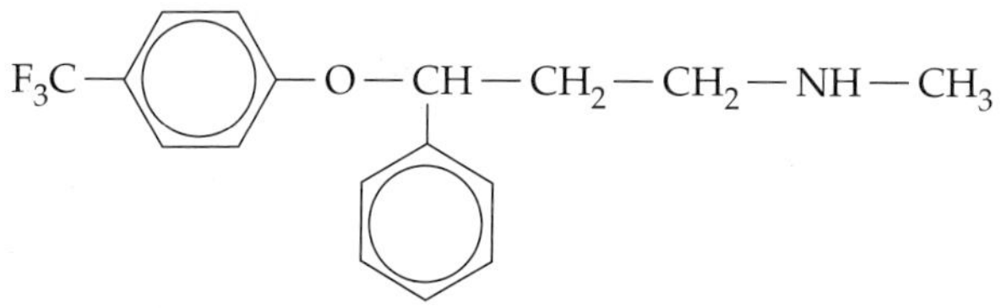

Fluoxetine

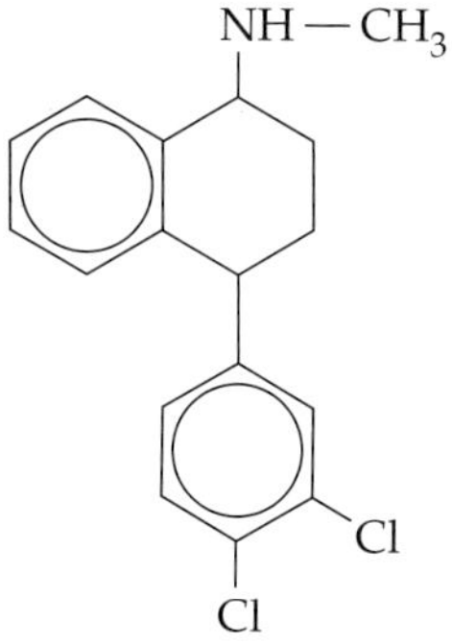

Sertraline

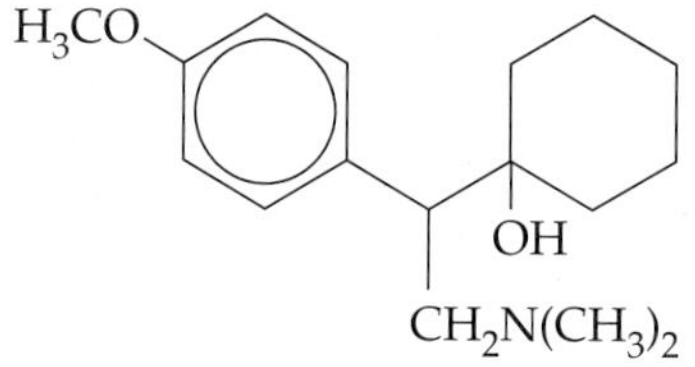

Venlafaxine

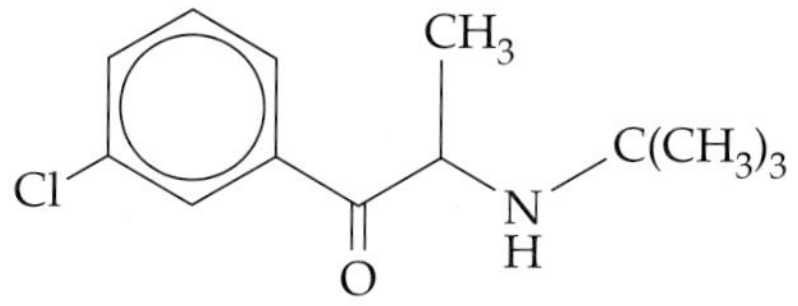

Bupropion

Figure 15–5. Chemical structures of representative antidepressants.

the drugs used to treat HIV infection. (See Chapter 18 for further discussion of herbal products.)

With the exception of **amoxapine,** a rarely prescribed tetracyclic drug with tricyclic antidepressant-like effects, antidepressants have not been determined to cause cumulative or long-term deleterious effects in patients with unipolar depression. Amoxapine, like many antipsychotic medications, is a D_2 dopamine receptor antagonist and is potentially capable of causing tardive dyskinesia (see Chapters 14 and 17). In patients with bipolar disorder, antidepressants may shorten the length of cycles and thereby lead to more rapid cycling for reasons that are unknown. Long-term treatment with SSRIs has produced apathy in a small number of patients, a side effect that responds to a decrease rather than an increase in drug dosage. With all classes of antidepressants, there may be a loss of efficacy in a small percentage of patients over time.

No objective test can predict whether a patient with depression will respond to a particular antidepressant treatment. An SSRI or NRI may be prescribed first, and the other of these two types of agents may be tried if the first is ineffective. If both of these agents produce disappointing results, a medication that inhibits reuptake of both neurotransmitters, such as a tricyclic antidepressant or the SNRI venlafaxine, might be considered. Continued treatment failure may require treatment with an MAOI or an atypical drug. The use of MAO inhibitors has been limited because of adverse interactions with sympathomimetic agents and certain foods (see Chapter 8), but such interactions can be avoided when dietary restrictions are observed. When treatment with one antidepressant is ineffective, **lithium** can be added to augment therapy; this is an often effective approach in many treatment-refractory patients. **Electroconvulsive therapy** (**ECT**), which typically involves a series of 6–8 generalized seizures under light anesthesia over 2 to 3 weeks, remains one of the most effective treatments for depression, but its therapeutic effects often are short-lived; for this reason, ECT is often combined with a chemical antidepressant. ECT no longer induces a motor seizure because of the current use of muscle paralyzing agents such as **succinylcholine** (see Chapter 9); to be effective, however, it must produce electroencephalographic evidence of a seizure. The mechanism by which ECT treats depression is unknown.

Monoamine systems and antidepressant action

Altered synaptic levels of modulatory neurotransmitters, such as serotonin or the catecholamines, have a marked influence on behavior, which they regulate through their effects on information processing in multiple circuits that underlie sensation, cognition, emotion, and motor and neuroendocrine outputs. However, their actions must be understood in the proper context. Historically, hypotheses linking mood disorders to norepinephrine and serotonin systems in the brain were oversimplistic, based not on the structure and physiology of these systems but on pharmacologic observations alone. It was observed, for example, that approximately 15% of patients who received long-term treatment with the antihypertensive drug **reserpine** developed a syndrome indistinguishable from naturally occurring depression; concomitantly it was discovered that reserpine depletes neurons of norepinephrine, serotonin, and dopamine (see Chapters 8 and 9). Likewise, studies of the first antidepressants revealed that they influence monoamines; for example, it was discovered that MAOIs inhibit the enzyme that metabolizes monoamine neurotransmitters, as mentioned earlier. Furthermore, it was proposed that because this enzyme is located in presynaptic terminals, its inhibition prolongs the life of monoamine neurotransmitters in the presynaptic cyto-

plasm and in turn increases the amount of these transmitters available for packaging into vesicles and subsequent release. Similarly, it was discovered that **imipramine** and other tricyclic antidepressants inhibit the reuptake of norepinephrine and serotonin in varying ratios. Because reuptake was known to be the primary mechanism by which the synaptic actions of monoamines are terminated, it was posited that tricyclic antidepressants act by dramatically increasing the amount of these neurotransmitters in synapses.

Pharmacologic observations such as these led to a simple hypothesis: depression is the result of inadequate monoamine neurotransmission and clinically effective antidepressants work by increasing the availability of monoamines. Yet this hypothesis has failed to explain the observation that weeks of treatment with antidepressants are required before clinical efficacy becomes apparent, despite the fact that the inhibitory actions of these agents—whether in relation to reuptake or monoamine oxidase—are immediate. This delay in therapeutic effect eventually led investigators to theorize that long-term adaptations in brain function, rather than increases in synaptic norepinephrine and serotonin per se, most likely underlie the therapeutic effects of antidepressant drugs. Consequently, the focus of research on antidepressants has shifted from the study of their immediate effects to the investigation of effects that develop more slowly.

The anatomic focus of research on antidepressants also has shifted. Although monoamine synapses are believed to be the immediate targets of antidepressant drugs, more attention is focused on the target neurons of monoamines, wherein chronic alterations in monoaminergic inputs caused by antidepressant drugs lead to longlasting adaptations that underlie effective treatment of depression. The identification of molecular and cellular adaptations that occur in response to antidepressants, and the location of the cells and circuits in which they occur, are the chief goals that guide current research.

Although the remainder of this section is devoted to a discussion of antidepressant-induced neuroadaptations, a series of clinical studies conducted during the past 10 years that support a role for serotonergic and noradrenergic systems in antidepressant action deserve comment. According to these studies, patients with depression who respond to treatment with an SSRI exhibit a brief relapse when their body stores of tryptophan, the precursor of serotonin, are depleted (see Chapter 9). In contrast, such tryptophan depletion does not cause relapse in patients treated with NRIs. Moreover, patients treated with NRIs experience relapse in response to inhibition of catecholamine synthesis with **α-methylparatyrosine** (**AMPT**), an inhibitor of tyrosine hydroxylase (see Chapter 8), whereas patients treated with SSRIs do not. Overall, these findings indicate that monoamine systems are important substrates for the clinical efficacy of antidepressants. In addition, the brief relapses described here may represent withdrawal phenomena akin to those associated with benzodiazepine antagonists. However, the studies that produced these findings do not reveal the specific changes in the brain that mediate such clinical responses and do not offer information about the pathophysiology of depression.

Long-term adaptations in monoamine systems

The long-term effects of antidepressant drugs that have received the most attention until recently are those that involve alterations in the turnover of monoamine neurotransmitters and in the levels of monoamine receptors in monoaminergic neurons (where they serve as autoreceptors) and their targets neurons. The wealth of studies in this area during the past 20 years, largely performed in rats or mice, has given rise to a new set of hypotheses that attempt to account for antidepressant action. All of these hypotheses correlate the delay in antidepressant efficacy in humans with one or more of the slow-onset adaptive changes in neurotransmitter turnover or receptor sensitivity that have been observed in laboratory animals. However, antidepressant-induced adaptive changes in monoamines and their receptors have not per se proven to be convincing mechanisms of antidepressant action. The first part of the discussion that follows considers some of the technical obstacles that have been encountered during research related to this topic. The second part provides an overview of the best-established long-term adaptive changes that antidepressants induce in the brain and highlights the need to identify alternative mechanisms that might be applied to new neuropharmacologic efforts to alleviate the symptoms of depression.

Obstacles to research

Whether experimental findings in laboratory animals can be generalized to humans is often difficult to determine, and this issue represents a major difficulty associated with antidepressant research. Changes in the levels of most neurotransmitters and neurotransmitter receptors currently cannot be measured in specific brain regions of living human patients. Changes in postreceptor messenger systems are even more difficult to trace. Although advances in PET, single-photon emission computed tomography (SPECT), and MRS technology may eventually enable us to assess some of these changes, human studies have thus far relied on indirect methods of assessment. One such method involves the measurement of monoamine metabolite levels in CSF, blood, or urine—an approach that is compromised by many confounding variables, including peripheral sources of monoamines. The amount of a monoamine metabolite detected in one of these fluids, for example, is not a dependable indicator of the functioning of monoaminergic neurons in the brain. Even metabolite levels measured in CSF reflect a complicated integration of monoaminergic function throughout the brain; they reveal very little about the functioning of specific monoaminergic pathways and nothing about their target neurons.

Another common indirect method previously used in human studies involved the measurement of neurotransmitter receptors in peripheral blood elements such as platelets or white blood cells. This approach was severely limited because receptors and other signaling molecules on blood elements are regulated independently of similar molecules on neurons. Consequently, the state of neurotransmitters and receptors in peripheral cells—which are exposed to a host of peripheral autonomic, hormonal, and metabolic influences—does not provide information relevant to the state of such molecules on small subpopulations of dysfunctional neurons in the brain.

The pharmacologic challenge paradigm, which is analogous to methods used in endocrinology, was also enlisted in an attempt to understand the pathophysiology of mood disorders. This approach allowed the sensitivity of a receptor system to be measured based on altered responses to a challenge drug in ill versus unaffected subjects. Neuroendocrine, autonomic, and subjective responses to the administration of **yohimbine** (an α_2-adrenergic antagonist), for example, were used to estimate the sensitivity of central α_2-adrenergic receptors in depression and anxiety disorders. However, compared with a glucose tolerance test, which provides accurate information about a peripheral metabolic state, challenges related to brain function, such as yohimbine challenges, are not able to provide mechanistic insights into the functioning of neurons in the brain and thus have not yielded robust pathophysiologic data.

A significant obstacle to interpreting the significance of drug-induced changes in neurotransmitter turnover and receptor sensitivity in rat brain stems from the fact that most related research has involved the use of normal laboratory rats. The brain of a depressed human being is unlikely to respond to a drug treatment in the same way that the brain of an unaffected human or laboratory rat might. Indeed, antidepressants administered to humans without depression produce no discernible responses other than typical side effects. Thus we do not know whether regulation of monoamine turnover or receptors in the rat correlates with responses to antidepressants in depressed patients. If neurotransmitter or receptor regulation were the actual mechanism by which antidepressants produce their therapeutic effects, the predicted regulation would be expected to occur in depressed patients who respond to drug treatment, but not in nonresponders. Our ability to investigate this question most likely must await improvements in imaging technologies.

Regulation of noradrenergic systems   Among the most consistently observed effects of long-term antidepressant administration in animals has been the down-regulation of postsynaptic β-adrenergic receptors. Most types of antidepressant treatment, including repeated ECT, produce this effect in the cerebral cortex and other regions of rat brain. Down-regulation of β-adrenergic receptors can be viewed as a homeostatic response to the immediate actions of antidepressant drugs (Figure 15–6). Accordingly, short-term increases in synaptic levels of norepinephrine produced by antidepressants may prompt homeostatic mechanisms to decrease β-adrenergic receptor levels over time and thereby restore noradrenergic signal transduction within the postsynaptic neuron to baseline levels. There are serious problems with the hypothesis that β-adrenergic receptor down-regulation mediates antidepressant effects.

Some antidepressants, such as bupropion, are clinically effective but do not down-regulate β-adrenergic receptors in rat brain. Furthermore, some compounds that modify β-adrenergic receptors exert effects that are inconsistent with a direct correlation between down-regulation of β-adrenergic receptors and mood elevation. **Thyroid hormone** can be helpful as an adjunct therapy for depression despite the fact that it augments rather than diminishes β-adrenergic receptor function; **propranolol,** a β-adrenergic receptor antagonist, is not an antidepressant and indeed can exacerbate depression in a small percentage of vulnerable individuals; and **yohimbine,** an α_2-adrenergic antagonist that facilitates down-regulation of β-adrenergic receptors in response to tricyclic drugs, does not augment the clinical efficacy of these compounds.

Long-term treatment with some antidepressants also appears to influence α_2-adrenergic receptors in the brain, although less reproducibly compared with its effects on β-adrenergic receptors. α_2-Adrenergic receptors primarily function as autoreceptors on presynaptic noradrenergic nerve terminals; activation of these receptors by norepinephrine decreases the amount of the transmitter released in response to subsequent nerve impulses (see Chapter 8). Some evidence, both preclinical and clinical, suggests that long-term admin-

istration of tricyclics and certain other antidepressants leads to down-regulation of α_2-adrenergic receptors, possibly as a homeostatic response to drug-induced increases in synaptic levels of norepinephrine. Down-regulation of these receptors reduces negative feedback on presynaptic cells by norepinephrine and can lead to an increase in overall norepinephrine release. The involvement of antidepressant-induced down-regulation of both α_2- and β-adrenergic receptors in the therapeutic mechanisms that underlie antidepressant drug action seems unlikely because these forms of regulation appear to have opposing effects on noradrenergic signal transduction. When both α_2- and β-adrenergic receptors are down-regulated after long-term treatment with antidepressants, it is not clear whether the postsynaptic neuron is exposed to more or less norepinephrine-induced signaling compared with such signaling before drug administration, if indeed a change occurs at all. Similar uncertainties complicate the interpretation of other drug-induced changes in neurotransmitter receptors. Currently it seems likely that down-regulation of α_2- and β-adrenergic receptors will prove to be markers of increased synaptic norepinephrine rather than critical mechanisms of antidepressant action.

Long-term antidepressant treatments not only regulate adrenergic receptors, they also alter the synthesis of norepinephrine in the brain. All major antidepressant treatments, including long-term ECT, decrease levels of tyrosine hydroxylase in the locus ceruleus, and in turn decrease the capacity of noradrenergic neurons to synthesize norepinephrine. Indeed elevated levels of tyrosine hydroxylase in the locus ceruleus of autopsy specimens taken from depressed patients who committed suicide have been reported. This finding suggests that noradrenergic hyperactivity may occur in at least some depressed patients. Yet further research will be required to determine the precise relationship between altered levels of tyrosine hydroxylase and the pathophysiology and treatment of depression.

Regulation of serotonergic systems   Changes in serotonergic neurotransmission in the brain also occur in response to long-term antidepressant treatment. Ligand-binding assays have indicated that most types of antidepressant drugs down-regulate 5-HT$_{2A}$ receptors. Like the down-regulation of adrenergic receptors, down-regulation of 5-HT$_{2A}$ receptors can be viewed as a homeostatic response to increased synaptic levels of serotonin. However, a direct correlation between 5-HT$_{2A}$ receptor down-regulation and the clinical effects of antidepressants must be questioned because repeated ECT up-regulates 5-HT$_{2A}$ receptors, and some drugs

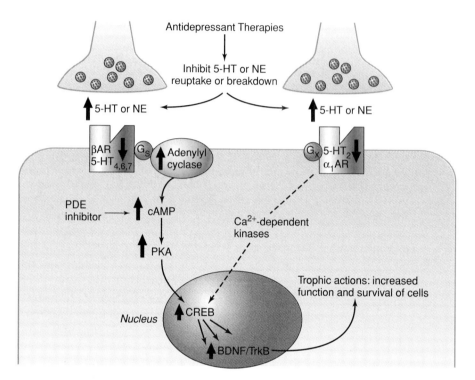

Figure 15–6. Long-term adaptations to antidepressant treatment. Antidepressants acutely increase levels of serotonin (5-HT) and norepinephrine (NE) by inhibiting the reuptake or breakdown of these monoamines. Such increases activate several 5-HT and NE receptors, including those coupled to cAMP and Ca^{2+} pathways. (G_x refers to a variety of G proteins that can influence Ca^{2+} pathways.) Long-term antidepressant administration decreases the function and expression of certain 5-HT and NE receptors, such as βAR and $5-HT_2$. In contrast, the cAMP pathway is up-regulated in the hippocampus and frontal cortex by long-term treatment, resulting in increased levels of adenylyl cyclase and cAMP-dependent protein kinase A (PKA), as well as increased expression and function of the transcription factor CREB. The observation that the cAMP cascade is enhanced after long-term antidepressant treatment indicates that the functional output of 5-HT and NE may be up-regulated, even though levels of certain 5-HT and NE receptors are down-regulated. Brain-derived neurotrophic factor (BDNF) and TrkB represent two of many potential targets of CREB. Antidepressant-induced up-regulation of BDNF and TrkB may influence the function and survival of vulnerable hippocampal and cortical neurons (see Figure 15–7). (Adapted with permission from Duman RS, Heninger GR, Nestler EJ. 1997. *Arch Gen Psychiatry* 54:597.)

that down-regulate $5-HT_{2A}$ receptors do not have antidepressant effects.

Electrophysiologic recordings indicate that antidepressants facilitate serotonergic synaptic transmission at certain cortical and hippocampal synapses. The mechanism that underlies this augmentation of serotonergic neurotransmission remains unknown but appears to be mediated by postsynaptic $5-HT_{1A}$ receptors. This hypothesis provides the conceptual basis for the use of newly developed $5-HT_{1A}$ agonists such as **gepirone** to treat depression, although the clinical efficacy of such compounds has been disappointing. As with the noradrenergic system, the complexity of changes in the serotonergic system has interfered with our ability to determine whether long-term antidepressant treatments increase or decrease or in any way alter overall serotonergic function in the brain.

Regulation of intracellular messenger pathways
Based on our knowledge of the importance of postreceptor events in the brain, it now appears likely that such events assist in mediating the clinical actions of antidepressant treatments. Our inability to fully account for antidepressant action based on neurotransmitter turnover and receptor regulation further supports the involvement of postreceptor mechanisms. Moreover, the

adaptations in monoamines and monoamine receptors previously discussed, whether or not they are therapeutically relevant, are mediated by postreceptor mechanisms. Thus a growing number of investigations have begun to focus on antidepressant-induced regulation of intracellular messengers and neuronal gene expression. Such studies have resulted in promising early findings and should lead to a more comprehensive view of the effects on brain function exerted by antidepressant drugs.

A simplified process by which antidepressants may induce long-term adaptations in neuronal function is represented in Figure 15–6. According to this scheme, antidepressants induce initial changes in the brain by increasing synaptic levels of monoamine neurotransmitters. As previously discussed, antidepressants most likely trigger such changes by inhibiting monoamine reuptake or degradation; however, other contributing actions may be identified in the future. Such initial changes in monoamine function lead to numerous changes in the functional state of target neurons related to the perturbation of intracellular signal transduction pathways (see Chapter 5). These changes in turn are likely to result in alterations in gene expression that develop slowly and become increasingly prominent with continued drug administration; for example, increased levels of the transcription factor CREB (see Chapter 6) have been produced in some regions of the brain by several major classes of antidepressants. Changes in gene expression result in altered levels of specific neuronal proteins, which subsequently underlie long-term changes in the functional properties of target neurons. Currently the critical proteins targeted by antidepressant action remain unknown. However, hypotheses regarding these targets and related mechanisms of action are presented in subsequent sections of this chapter.

If intracellular signaling proteins are indeed targets of long-term administration of antidepressant agents, drugs that directly target such proteins might serve as novel antidepressants. Potential candidates for such agents may include **phosphodiesterase inhibitors**. Several reports have indicated that long-term antidepressant treatment may up-regulate the functioning of the cAMP pathway in the hippocampus and cerebral cortex; the drug-induced increases in CREB previously mentioned may be an example of such up-regulation. This has led to the proposal that increased activity of the cAMP pathway may contribute to the clinical efficacy of these treatments. Consistent with this possibility is the clinical observation that **rolipram,** a type-4 phosphodiesterase inhibitor that increases cAMP levels by decreasing its degradation, reduces the symptoms of depression. Unfortunately, rolipram is poorly tolerated by humans because of its many side effects; however, the recent cloning of num-

erous subtypes of type-4 phosphodiesterase, and the demonstration of their region-specific expression in the brain (see Chapter 5), offers promise for the development of more selective agents that may effectively relieve depression with fewer side effects.

Neurotrophic hypothesis of depression and antidepressant treatments   As discussed earlier in this chapter, the brain reacts to both acute and chronic stress in part by activating the HPA axis. As described in Chapter 6, glucocorticoids such as cortisol, which are the end product of this pathway, act by binding to their cytoplasmic receptors. Such binding induces the translocation of these receptors to the nucleus, where they bind to specific DNA response elements to activate or repress the expression of multiple genes, or interfere with other signaling pathways by binding other transcription factors. The activity of the HPA axis is controlled by numerous brain regions, including the amygdala, which exerts an excitatory influence on hypothalamic CRF-containing neurons in the PVN, and the hippocampus, which exerts an inhibitory influence (see Figure 15–4). Glucocorticoids, by potently affecting the activity of hippocampal neurons, can provide powerful feedback to the HPA axis. Under normal physiologic circumstances, glucocorticoids appear to enhance hippocampal inhibition of HPA activity. However, sustained elevation of glucocorticoids, which occurs in response to prolonged and severe stress, may damage hippocampal neurons. Such damage initially may be manifested by a loss of the highly specialized dendritic spines that enable hippocampal neurons to receive their synaptic inputs (Figure 15–7). The loss of these spines may in turn reduce the inhibitory control that the hippocampus exerts on the HPA axis, further increasing the levels of circulating glucocorticoids and resulting in additional damage to the hippocampus. The pathologic consequences of such a positive feedback process may contribute to the hypercortisolemic state and other abnormalities in the regulation of the HPA axis that are characteristic of some patients with depression.

Stress also may damage hippocampal neurons by a variety of other means. It may injure these neurons by activating particular neurotransmitter systems; for example, the sustained glutamatergic activation of hippocampal neurons that occurs in response to stress is potentially capable of triggering excitotoxic mechanisms of neuronal injury. Indeed, stress increases the vulnerability of hippocampal pyramidal neurons to several forms of excitotoxicity. Moreover, stress has been shown to reduce the expression of brain-derived neurotrophic factor (BDNF; see Chapter 11) in vulnerable hippocampal neurons.

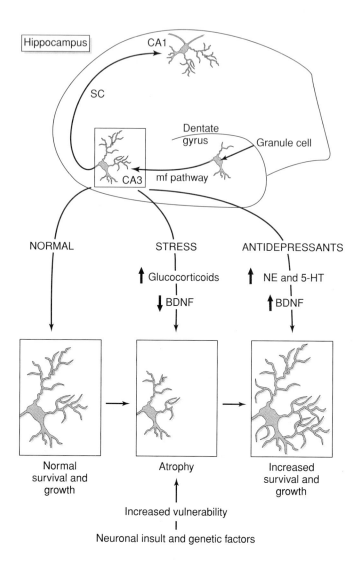

Figure 15–7. Model of the neurotrophic hypothesis of antidepressant treatments and stress-related disorders. The major cell types in the hippocampus and the effects of stress and antidepressant treatments on CA3 pyramidal cells are shown. The three major subfields of the hippocampus—CA3 and CA1 pyramidal cells and dentate gyrus granule cells—are connected by the mossy fiber (mf) and Schaffer collateral (SC) pathways. Chronic stress decreases the expression of brain-derived neurotrophic factor (BDNF) in the hippocampus, which in turn may contribute to the atrophy of CA3 neurons and their increased vulnerability to a variety of neuronal insults. Chronic elevation of glucocorticoid levels is also known to decrease the survival of these neurons. In contrast, antidepressant treatments increase the expression of BDNF, as well as that of TrkB, and prevent the down-regulation of BDNF elicited by stress. Such activity may increase the dendritic arborizations and survival of the neurons, or help repair or protect the neurons from further damage. (Adapted with permission from Duman RS, Heninger GR, Nestler EJ. 1997. *Arch Gen Psychiatry* 54:597.)

In contrast, long-term administration of virtually any type of antidepressant increases BDNF expression in the hippocampus. Antidepressant administration also prevents the down-regulation of BDNF that occurs in response to stress; indeed, antidepressant treatments can enhance the dendritic sprouting of certain hippocampal neurons, in contrast to the effects of stress. Such antidepressant effects are not observed in BDNF knock-out mice. These findings suggest that antidepressant-induced up-regulation of BDNF may help repair stress-induced damage to hippocampal neurons and may protect vulnerable neurons from further damage (see Figure 15–7). Such findings also may help to explain why responses to antidepressants are delayed: antidepressant efficacy may require sufficient time for levels of BDNF to gradually increase and exert their neurotrophic effects. Accordingly, other agents that promote BDNF function may

prove to be clinically effective antidepressants. Currently, no such compounds are available, but the development of small molecules that regulate neurotrophic factors is a major focus of drug development (see Chapter 11). Finally, stress appears to inhibit the birth of new neurons in the hippocampus, and in preliminary findings (see Chapter 11) antidepressants have been shown to increase such neurogenesis. The biologic significance of such findings is not yet clear.

LITHIUM AND OTHER MOOD-STABILIZING DRUGS

Lithium is effective in the treatment of acute mania and is used prophylactically to prevent the recurrence of manic and depressive episodes in individuals with bipolar disorder. As with antidepressants, the clinical effects of this agent require long-term administration. The lightest solid element in the periodic table, lithium circulates as a monovalent cation. Although it has been in use for decades, its mechanism of action remains unknown; however, research has revealed many effects of lithium on the nervous system at concentrations that approximate the therapeutic serum levels of 1 mM. Lithium has immediate and long-term effects, for example, on the release of serotonin and norepinephrine from nerve terminals. At higher concentrations it influences transmembrane ion pumps.

It is believed that lithium's therapeutic benefits may be attributed to its effects on postreceptor intracellular signaling proteins. Long-term lithium administration has been shown to alter 1) the coupling of some neurotransmitter receptors to G proteins, 2) the expression of $G_{\alpha i}$ and subtypes of adenylyl cyclase, 3) the modification of G proteins by ADP-ribosylation, and 4) cAMP-dependent and Ca^{2+}-dependent protein phosphorylation in specific brain regions. Despite these numerous actions, it has been hypothesized that lithium's beneficial effects in the treatment of manic-depressive illness are related to its effects on the phosphatidylinositol and Wnt signaling pathways. A major obstacle to testing these hypotheses has been the lack of a credible animal model of bipolar disorder. However, after the genes responsible for this disorder have been identified, it is anticipated that their placement in mice may yield animal models that are useful for preclinical studies.

Inositol depletion hypothesis Although this explanation of lithium's therapeutic value is more than a decade old, its validity has yet to be determined. Many neurotransmitter receptors, including α_1-adrenergic, 5-HT_2-serotonergic, and muscarinic cholinergic receptors, are linked to the enzyme phospholipase C by means of the G protein G_q. Phospholipase C hydrolyzes phosphatidylinositol bisphosphate (PIP_2), a membrane phospholipid, to yield two second messengers: diacylglycerol and inositol triphosphate (IP_3). Diacylglycerol activates protein kinase C, and IP_3 binds its receptor on the endoplasmic reticulum to release intracellular Ca^{2+}. These pathways are described in detail in Chapter 5.

Phosphatidylinositol is synthesized from free inositol and a lipid moiety. Most cells can obtain free inositol directly from plasma, but neurons cannot because inositol does not cross the blood–brain barrier. Consequently, neurons must either recycle inositol by dephosphorylating inositol phosphates after they are generated from the hydrolysis of phosphatidylinositols, or synthesize it de novo from glucose-6-phosphate, a product of glycolysis. At therapeutic concentrations, lithium inhibits several inositol phosphatases, most significantly inositol

monophosphatase (IMPase). Such inhibition blocks the ability of neurons to generate free inositol from recycled inositol phosphates or glucose-6-phosphate. Thus lithium-exposed neurons have a diminished ability to resynthesize PIP_2 after it is hydrolyzed in response to neurotransmitter receptor activation. Accordingly, it has been hypothesized that when firing rates of neurons are abnormally high, lithium-treated neurons are depleted of PIP_2, and neurotransmission dependent on this second messenger system is dampened.

This hypothesis is intriguing because it suggests that the effects of lithium may be evident only in cells with abnormally high firing rates and that lithium may be capable of treating both manic and depressive states because of its effects on multiple neurotransmitter systems. However, the story is more complex. Chronic inhibition of inositol phosphatases may lead to a buildup of active inositol phosphates, including IP_3, and thus may facilitate rather than dampen the actions of neurotransmitters on this pathway. Indeed, whether long-term lithium administration dampens or facilitates phosphatidylinositol-dependent signal transduction in the brain is not clear. Moreover, the critical cells in the brain that are targets of lithium's therapeutic action remain unknown, and it is unclear which of the many phosphatidylinositol-dependent neurotransmitter systems must be dampened (or facilitated) to produce lithium's effects. More importantly, this hypothesis does not explain why several weeks must elapse before lithium exhibits a therapeutic effect.

Regulation of the Wnt pathway and glycogen synthase kinase 3β In addition to the antimanic properties previously discussed, several teratogenic effects have been attributed to the use of lithium. Studies have revealed, for example, that lithium has teratogenic effects on embryos of *Xenopus laevis,* an African clawed toad, that lead to dorsalization of the embryo (i.e., the production of two spines). Initially it was speculated that lithium's inhibition of IMPase was responsible not only for mood stabilization, as previously discussed, but also for lithium's dramatic developmental effects. However, an important series of investigations led to the discovery that the teratogenic effects of lithium are instead related to its inhibition of glycogen synthase kinase 3β (GSK-3β). Highly selective bisphosphonate blockers of IMPase do not produce teratogenic effects in *Xenopus,* and lithium is capable of altering cell fate in mutants of the yeast *Dictyostelium discoideum* that lack phospholipase C and thus cannot generate inositol triphosphate.

The glycogen synthase kinase 3β pathway is a negative regulator of the Wnt signaling pathway (Box 15–4),

Box 15–4 Wnt Signaling Pathway

The Wnt genes encode a large family of secreted proteins that regulate cell proliferation and differentiation in species as divergent as nematodes, flies, frogs, and humans. In mammals, Wnt genes have been implicated in brain development. The initial gene discovery in mammals was of Int-1, a gene that became activated to produce tumors when the mouse mammary tumor virus integrated next to it in the mouse genome. Int-1 was found to be the mouse version of *wingless* (Wg), a developmental control gene first discovered in *Drosophila*. The contraction of Int-1 with Wg resulted in the term Wnt, of which many members are now known.

Wnt ligands bind to receptor molecules of the Frizzled family to initiate a signal transduction cascade involving a cytosolic protein Dishevelled (Dsh). It is of interest that Dsh knockout mice are defective in social behavior and grooming and have subtle neurologic abnormalities reminiscent of those seen in **schizophrenia** (see Chapter 17). Wnt signaling through Frizzled and Dsh inhibits the serine–threonine kinase known as glycogen synthase kinase 3β (GSK-3β) (see figure). GSK-3β is believed to inhibit the function of β-catenin constitutively by phosphorylation of this protein that leads to its degradation. By inhibiting GSK-3β activity, Wnt signaling (and lithium) leads to stabilization of β-catenin, which in turn translocates to the nucleus, where it interacts with the transcription factor dTCF/LEF-1 to activate expression of Wnt-responsive genes. Potentially relevant genes that might be affected in the brain by lithium inhibition of GSK-3β are currently unknown. GSK-3β is also implicated in **Alzheimer disease;** indeed, the kinase may be partly responsible for the hyperphosphorylation of tau (a microtubule-associated protein), which is believed to be a cause of neurofibrillary tangles (see Chapter 20).

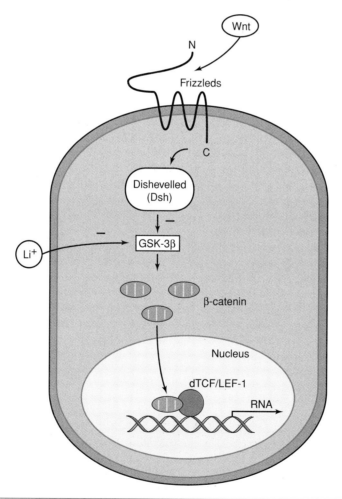

whose inhibition reproduces the teratogenic effects of lithium in several species. Because inhibition of glycogen synthase kinase 3β occurs at lithium concentrations similar to those used therapeutically, questions have been raised as to whether the antimanic properties of lithium also may be mediated at least partly by the inhibition of glycogen synthase kinase 3β. Selective inhibitors of this enzyme must be generated before this hypothesis can be tested in humans.

Lithium regulation of adenylyl cyclase   As previously indicated, lithium directly inhibits adenylyl cyclase in most tissues, including those that comprise the brain. Although the concentrations required to exert this effect in the brain appear to be higher than those required for lithium's clinical effectiveness, such inhibition does appear to account for some of lithium's peripheral side effects. Lithium inhibits the normal activation of adenylyl cyclase by thyroid stimulating hormone (TSH) and antidiuretic hormone (vasopressin), a property that may partly explain its widely observed antithyroid effects and tendency to interfere with the concentration of urine.

Actions of other antimanic agents   Other mood stabilizers are increasingly used as substitutes for lithium in the treatment of mania. Strikingly, most of these drugs initially were developed for use as anticonvulsants (see Chapter 21). **Valproic acid,** for example, appears to act by facilitating GABAergic neurotransmission, possibly by increasing GABA release through mechanisms that thus far have been poorly described. Valproic acid has been established as an effective treatment for mania and is better tolerated than lithium by some patients. Why valproic acid reduces mania is not yet understood. It has been proposed that this agent's effectiveness is consistent with the hypothesis that mania is characterized by excessive neural activity, at least in certain circuits of the brain that have yet to be identified. Other anticonvulsants, such as **carbamazepine, lamotrigine** (an inhibitor of the release of excitatory amino acids), **gabapentin** (which may increase GABA levels through interaction with the GABA transporter), and **topiramate** (which blocks glutamate receptors, inhibits carbonic anhydrase, and modulates Na^+ conductance), also have been used to treat bipolar disorder, and have exhibited varying degrees of clinical efficacy. The introduction of anticonvulsants as agents for the treatment of mania represents one of the few true therapeutic advances in the treatment of psychiatric disorders during the past several decades. Despite this achievement, investigators remain frustrated in their attempts to determine how these agents exert their beneficial effects.

SELECTED READING

Altar CA. 1999. Neurotrophins and depression. *Trends Pharmacol Sci* 20:59–61.

American Psychiatric Association. 1993. *Diagnostic and Statistical Manual of Mental Disorders,* 4th ed. Washington: American Psychiatric Press.

Arborelius L, Owens MJ, Plotsky PM, Nemeroff CB. 1999. The role of corticotropin-releasing factor in depression and anxiety disorders. *J Endocrinol* 160:1–12.

Bale TL, Contarino A, Smith GW, et al. 2000. Mice deficient for corticotropin-releasing hormone receptor-2 display anxiety-like behavior and are hypersensitive to stress. *Nature Gene* 24:410–414.

Bechara A, Damasio H, Damasio AR. 2000. Emotion, decision making and the orbitofrontal cortex. *Cerebral Cortex* 10: 295–307.

Berridge MJ, Downes CP, Hanley MR. 1989. Neural and developmental actions of lithium: A unifying hypothesis. *Cell* 59:411–419.

Breiter HC, Etcoff NL, Whalen PJ, et al. 1996. Response and habituation of the human amygdala during visual processing of facial expression. *Neuron* 17:875–887.

Brown ES, Rush AJ, McEwen BS. 1999. Hippocampal remodeling and damage by corticosteroids: Implications for mood disorders. *Neuropsychopharmacology* 21:474–484.

Buchel C, Morris J, Dolan RJ, Friston KJ. 1998. Brain systems mediating aversive conditioning: An event-related MRI study. *Neuron* 20:947–957.

Cahill L, McGaugh JL. 1998. Mechanisms of emotional arousal and lasting declarative memory. *Trends Neurosci* 21:294–299.

Charney DS. 1998. Monoamine dysfunction and the pathophysiology and treatment of depression. *J Clin Psychiatry* 59(suppl) 14:11–14.

Davis M. 1997. Neurobiology of fear responses: The role of the amygdala. *J Neuropsychiatr Clin Neurosci* 9:382–402.

De Blas AL. 1996. Brain $GABA_A$ receptors studied with subunit-specific antibodies. *Mol Neurobiol* 12:55–71.

Dildy-Mayfield JE, Mihic SJ, Liu Y, et al. 1996. Actions of long chain alcohols on $GABA_A$ and glutamate receptors: Relation to in vivo effects. *Br J Pharmacol* 118:378–384.

Duman RS, Heninger GR, Nestler EJ. 1997. A molecular and cellular hypothesis of depression. *Arch Gen Psychiatry* 54:597–606.

Fanselow MS, LeDoux JE. 1999. Why we think plasticity underlying pavlovian fear conditioning occurs in the basolateral amygdala. *Neuron* 23:229–232.

Fellous J-M. 1999. Neuromodulatory basis of emotion. *The Neuroscientist* 5:283–294.

Hedgepeth CM, Conrad LJ, Zhang J, et al. 1997. Activation of the Wnt signaling pathway: A molecular mechanism for lithium action. *Dev Biol* 185:82–91.

Hyman SE, Nestler EJ. 1996. Initiation and adaptation: A paradigm for understanding psychotropic drug action. *Am J Psychiatry* 153:151–162.

Klein PS, Melton DA. 1996. A molecular mechanism for the effect of lithium on development. *Proc Natl Acad Sci USA* 93:8455–8459.

Kuhl M, Sheldahl LC, Park M, et al. 2000. The Wnt/Ca^{2+} pathway. *Trends Genet* 16:279–283.

LeDoux JE. 2000. Emotion circuits in the brain. *Annu Rev Neurosci* 23:155–184.

Low K, Crestani F, Keist R, et al. 2000. Molecular and neuronal substrate for the selective attenuation of anxiety. *Science* 290:131–134

Manji HK, Bowden CL, Belmaker RH. 1999. *Bipolar Medications: Mechanisms of Action.* American Psychiatric Press.

Mayberg HS. 1997. Limbic-cortical dysregulation: A proposed model of depression. *J Neuropsychiatr Clin Neurosci* 9:471–481.

Newport DJ, Nemeroff CB. 2000. Neurobiology of posttraumatic stress disorder. *Curr Opin Neurobiol* 10:211–218.

Raadsheer FC, van Heerikhuize JJ, Lucassen PJ, et al. 1995. Corticotropin-releasing hormone mRNA levels in the paraventricular nucleus of patients with Alzheimer's disease and depression. *Am J Psychiatry* 152:1372–1376.

Rajkowska G. 2000. Postmortem studies in mood disorders indicate altered numbers of neurons and glial cells. *Biol Psychiatry,* in press.

Rogan MT, Staubli UV, LeDoux JE. 1997. Fear conditioning induces associative long-term potentiation in the amygdala. *Nature* 390:604–607.

Rolls ET. 1998. *The Brain and Emotion.* New York: Oxford University Press.

Roth BL. 1994. Multiple serotonin receptors: Clinical and experimental aspects. *Ann Clin Psychiatry* 6:67–78.

Sapolsky RM. 2000. Glucocorticoids and hippocampal atrophy in neuropsychiatric disorders. *Arch Gen Psychiatry* 57:925–935.

Sapolsky RM, Romero LM, Munck AU. 2000. How do glucocorticoids influence stress responses? Integrating permissive, suppressive, stimulatory, and preparative actions. *Endocrine Rev* 21:55–89.

Shelton RC, Mainer DH, Sulser F. 1996. cAMP-dependent protein kinase activity in major depression. *Am J Psychiatry* 153:1037–1042.

Southwick SM, Paige S, Morgan CA III, et al. 1999. Neurotransmitter alterations in PTSD: catecholamines and serotonin. *Sem Clin Neuropsychiatry* 4:242–248.

Stein MB. 1998. Neurobiological perspectives on social phobia: from affiliation to zoology. *Biol Psychiatry* 44:1277–1285.

Thome J, Sakai N, Shin KH, et al. 2000. cAMP response element-mediated gene transcription is upregulated by chronic antidepressant treatment. *J Neurosci* 20:4030–4036.

Chapter 16

Reinforcement and Addictive Disorders

KEY CONCEPTS

- The defining feature of addiction is compulsive, out-of-control drug use, despite negative consequences.

- Addictive drugs induce pleasurable states or relief from distress, thus motivating repeated drug use.

- Drugs of abuse are both rewarding and reinforcing. Rewards are stimuli that the brain interprets as intrinsically positive, and reinforcing stimuli are those that increase the probability that behaviors paired with them will be repeated.

- The brain reward circuitry targeted by addictive drugs, which normally responds to natural reinforcers, such as food, water, and sex, includes the dopaminergic projections from the ventral tegmental area (VTA) of the midbrain to the nucleus accumbens (NAc) and other forebrain structures.

- Repeated use of addictive drugs produces multiple unwanted changes in the brain that may lead to tolerance, sensitization, dependence, and addiction.

- Dependence is an adaptive state that develops in response to repeated drug administration; when unmasked by cessation of drug use, this adapted state may lead to withdrawal symptoms.

- Tolerance refers to the diminished effect of a drug after repeated administration at the same dose, or to the need for an increase in dose to produce the same effect; sensitization describes the opposite response to repeated drug administration.

- Cocaine and amphetamines produce their psychoactive effects by potentiating monoaminergic transmission through actions on the dopamine transporter, together with actions on the serotonin and norepinephrine transporters.

- The reinforcing effects of opiate drugs result from their binding to endogenous opioid receptors, most importantly μ-opioid receptors in both the VTA and NAc.

- The immediate effects of ethanol are believed to result primarily from facilitation of $GABA_A$ receptors and inhibition of NMDA glutamate receptors. At higher doses, ethanol inhibits the functioning of most voltage-gated ion channels as well.

- Nicotine differs from cocaine and opiates in that it is powerfully reinforcing in the absence of subjective euphoria.

- The effects of nicotine are caused by its activation of nicotinic acetylcholine (nACh) receptors; its reinforcing effects may depend on nACh receptors located on VTA dopamine neurons.

- Delta-9-tetrahydrocannabinol, the active psychotropic ingredient in marijuana, exerts its primary pharmacologic effects by binding to a G protein-coupled receptor in the brain known as the CB_1 receptor.

- The psychotomimetic drugs of abuse, phencyclidine (angel dust, PCP) and ketamine, bind specific sites in the channel of the NMDA glutamate receptor, where they act as noncompetitive NMDA antagonists.

Drug addiction is a progressive and often fatal behavioral syndrome characterized by compulsive drug seeking and consumption despite serious negative consequences. The drug-centered existence of addicts can cost them their jobs, personal relationships, financial standing, happiness, and, in some cases, their lives. Drug-addicted individuals often appear to have lost the ability to make choices that promote their own happiness and survival. Many drug addicts who seek treatment report that they realize the destructive nature of their addiction but are *unable* to alter their addictive behavior.

In laboratory settings in which social and environmental variables are controlled, normal animals with access to addictive drugs typically engage in self-administration of these substances. Such behavior indicates that addiction is the result of a conserved neurobiologic substrate in animal and human brains that is vulnerable to regulation by addictive drugs. The actions of such drugs on this neural substrate tend to promote continued drug-taking behavior in a way that becomes increasingly involuntary.

The biologic determinants of addiction, and the biologic factors responsible for individual vulnerability to addiction, must be thoroughly understood before truly effective treatment and prevention strategies can be developed. Thus it is necessary to determine: 1) the neurochemical and anatomic basis, and naturally intended function, of reward circuitry in the healthy brain; and 2) the changes in this circuitry produced by addictive drugs that cause the addicted brain to be fundamentally different from a drug-free brain.

BRAIN REWARD PATHWAYS

Addictive drugs are both *rewarding* and *reinforcing*. A reward is a stimulus that the brain interprets as intrinsically positive, or as something to be approached. A reinforcing stimulus is one that increases the probability that behaviors paired with it will be repeated. Not all reinforcers are rewarding; for example, a negative or punishing stimulus might reinforce avoidance behaviors. The neural substrates that underlie the perception of reward and the phenomenon of positive reinforcement are a set of interconnected forebrain structures often called brain reward pathways; these include the nucleus accumbens (NAc; the major component of the ventral striatum), the basal forebrain (components of which have been termed the extended amygdala, as discussed in this chapter), and regions of the medial prefrontal cortex. These structures receive rich dopaminergic innervation from the ventral tegmental area (VTA) of the midbrain. It appears that addictive drugs are reward-ing and reinforcing because they act in brain reward pathways to enhance either dopamine release or the effects of dopamine in the NAc or related structures, or because they produce effects similar to dopamine.

Drug-induced pleasurable states are important motivators of initial drug use. Drug actions that produce these states also produce associated, but ultimately undesirable, changes in brain reward circuitry that promote future drug use. Another form of positive reinforcement involves the alleviation of unpleasant symptoms—either from preexisting states or caused by drug withdrawal—by means of drug use. Conditioned reinforcement, which occurs when previously neutral stimuli become associated with the pleasurable effects of drugs, is yet another type of positive reinforcement. All of these mechanisms contribute to repetitive drug taking that, in vulnerable individuals, may result in an addicted state.

The reinforcing effects of drugs can be demonstrated in experiments in which drug acquisition is contingent upon a specific behavioral response; for example, an animal may learn that it will receive an injection of drug every time it presses a particular lever in its cage. The drug acts as a reinforcer if it increases the occurrence of the behavior (pressing the lever) that leads to acquisition of the drug. In this *self-administration* paradigm, the amount of work an animal does to gain access to a given amount of drug indicates the strength of reinforcement induced by the drug. The strength with which different drugs reinforce behavior in animals correlates well with their tendency to reinforce drug-seeking behavior in humans. Cocaine, for example, is highly reinforcing when injected intravenously. Laboratory animals readily learn behaviors necessary to self-administer this drug, and some of them will give up survival necessities, such as food and water, or work excessively, even to the point of death, in order to gain access to cocaine. Such evidence of the power of cocaine's reinforcing properties helps to explain its addictiveness in humans. In general, drugs that are less addictive in humans (such as marijuana) are not as likely to be self-administered by animals, and drugs that are not addictive in humans are not reinforcing in or self-administered by animals. Nicotine appears to represent an exception to this rule; although it does not strongly reinforce drug-seeking behavior in animals, it produces strong addiction in some humans.

Another paradigm used to investigate drug reward in animal research is known as *conditioned place preference*. In this type of experiment, animals learn to associate a particular environment with passive drug exposure; for example, a rodent will learn to spend more time on the side of a box where it was previously given cocaine. This paradigm is believed to demonstrate the strong cue-conditioned effects of addictive drugs and to provide an indirect measure of drug reward. In the *conditioned reinforcement* paradigm, animals learn to associate a neutral cue, such as light, with a natural reinforcer, such as water. With sufficient training, the neutral cue becomes a conditioned reinforcer, or a desirable phenomenon that animals will exhibit appropriate behavior, such as pressing a lever, to obtain. Addictive drugs dramatically potentiate the degree to which animals will work for conditioned reinforcers.

A COMPARISON BETWEEN ADDICTIVE DRUGS AND NATURAL REINFORCERS

The brain reward circuitry that is targeted by addictive drugs is believed to mediate the pleasure and strengthening of behaviors associated with natural reinforcers, such as food, water, and sexual contact. Thus drugs tap into neural networks that apparently evolved to reinforce behaviors that are necessary for survival and reproduction. These systems can be viewed as complementary to survival networks in the brain that mediate learning about dangerous and harmful stimuli (see Chapter 15).

Sensory cues produced by natural reinforcers activate reward pathways under normal circumstances, whereas addictive drugs directly activate the same neural circuitry by chemical means, bypassing the need for evolutionarily useful behaviors. Thus the powerful control over behavior exerted by addictive drugs may stem from the brain's inability to distinguish between the activation of reward circuitry by drugs and natural activation of the same circuitry by useful behaviors. Any activity, whether related to drug-taking or survival, that activates this circuitry is regarded as one that should be repeated. Moreover, chemical activation of reward circuitry by addictive drugs can be much more reliable and powerful than activation triggered by natural reinforcers. Exposure to addictive chemicals not only produces extreme euphoric states that may initially motivate drug use, but also causes equally extreme adaptations in reinforcement mechanisms and motivated behavior that eventually lead to compulsive use. Accordingly, the evolutionary design of human and animal brains that has helped to promote our survival also has made us vulnerable to addiction.

Repeated exposure to an addictive drug induces profound cellular and molecular changes within neurons of the brain reward circuitry, which in turn are believed to cause the alterations in reinforcement mechanisms that contribute to addiction. Drug-induced adaptations reflect both homeostatic compensations for excessive stimulation by drugs and alterations in multiple memory systems in the brain that serve to sustain addiction over long periods of time. These adaptations gradually alter normal control of motivated behavior, and eventually produce the compulsive and increasingly involuntary drug-seeking behavior that characterizes addiction. Thus compared with the normal brain, the addicted brain programs behavior in a fundamentally different way that can be long-lasting and perhaps even permanent.

FUNCTIONAL CONSEQUENCES OF LONG-TERM DRUG EXPOSURE

Familiar pharmacologic terms such as tolerance, dependence, and sensitization are useful in describing some of the time-dependent processes believed to underlie addiction. *Tolerance* refers to the diminishing effect of a drug after repeated administration at the same dose, or to the need for an increase in dose to produce the same effect. Tolerance may develop to some of the effects of a drug but not to others; for example, tolerance frequently develops to the analgesic, euphoric, and respiratory depressant effects of opiates, but not to the pupillary constriction produced by these drugs. *Pharmacokinetic* tolerance is caused by increased drug metabolism or clearance, whereas *pharmacodynamic* tolerance is a result of adaptations in the neural elements that respond to drugs initially. Pharmacodynamic tolerance is the more important mechanism in terms of its contribution to behavior, including addiction. *Sensitization,* which may be referred to as reverse tolerance, occurs when repeated administration of the same drug dose elicits escalating effects. *Dependence,* which is defined as an adaptive state that develops in response to repeated drug administration, typically is unmasked during *withdrawal,* which occurs when drug-taking stops. Dependence resulting from long-term drug use may have both a somatic component, manifested by physical symptoms that develop when drug use ceases, and an emotional–motivational component, manifested by dysphoria and anhedonic symptoms that occur when a drug is discontinued.

According to modern definitions, *drug addiction* is characterized by compulsive, out-of-control drug use, despite adverse consequences; thus current definitions emphasize emotional–motivational aspects of dependence (Box 16–1). Older definitions of addiction required the presence of physical dependence as a necessary component; however, this criterion is not relevant to the use of certain highly addictive drugs, such as cocaine and amphetamines, which are associated with emotional and motivational aspects of withdrawal despite the absence of prominent physical withdrawal symptoms. Compulsive users of cocaine, for example, often do not exhibit physical withdrawal signs upon termination of drug use, but may complain of depression-like

Box 16–1 Criteria for Substance Dependence and Substance Abuse According to the Diagnostic and Statistical Manual of Mental Disorders, Fourth Edition

Substance Dependence[1]

A maladaptive pattern of substance use, leading to clinically significant impairment or distress, as manifested by the occurrence of three (or more) of the following during the same 12-month period:

(1) Tolerance, as defined by either of the following:
  (a) a need for markedly increased amounts of a substance to achieve intoxication or a desired effect,
  (b) markedly diminished effect with continued use of the same amount of a substance
(2) Withdrawal, as manifested by either of the following:
  (a) symptoms characteristic of withdrawal from a substance,
  (b) the ability to take a substance or one closely related to it, to relieve or avoid withdrawal symptoms
(3) A need to take a substance in larger amounts or over a longer period than intended.
(4) A persistent desire or unsuccessful efforts to cut down or control substance use
(5) A great deal of time spent in activities necessary to obtain a substance (e.g., visits to multiple doctors or driving long distances), to use a substance (e.g., chain-smoking), or to recover from its effects.
(6) Abandonment of or absence from important social, occupational, or recreational activities because of substance use.
(7) Continued substance use despite knowledge of having a persistent or recurrent physical or psychological problem that is likely to have been caused or exacerbated by the substance (e.g., continued cocaine use despite recognition of cocaine-induced depression, or continued drinking despite recognition that an ulcer is made worse by alcohol consumption).

Substance Abuse[2]

A maladaptive pattern of substance use leading to clinically significant impairment or distress, as manifested by occurrence of one or more of the following during a 12-month period:

(1) Recurrent substance use resulting in a failure to fulfill major role obligations at work, school, or home (e.g., repeated absences or poor work performance related to substance use; substance-related absences, suspensions, or expulsions from school; neglect of children or household).
(2) Recurrent substance use in situations in which it is physically hazardous (e.g., driving an automobile or operating a machine when impaired by substance use).
(3) Recurrent substance-related legal problems (e.g., arrests for substance-related disorderly conduct).
(4) Continued substance use despite having persistent or recurrent social or interpersonal problems caused or exacerbated by the effects of the substance (e.g., arguments with spouse about consequences of intoxication, or physical fights).

Reprinted with permission from American Pyschiatric Association. 1994. *Diagnostic and Statistical Manual of Mental Disorders*, 4th ed. Washington, DC: American Psychiatric Association pp. 181–183.

[1]DSM uses the term *dependence* to mean addiction. As discussed in the text, dependence is just one type of molecular and cellular process that contributes to addiction.
[2]According to DSM, substance abuse is diagnosed when an individual meets the conditions listed, but does not meet the criteria for substance dependence (i.e., addiction). Thus, the distinction between abuse and addiction is arbitrary.

symptoms and, more importantly, may experience an intense craving for the drug. Moreover, signs of physical dependence can subside over the course of weeks, whereas the risk of relapse associated with addiction can last for years. Furthermore, the presence of physical dependence alone is not sufficient evidence of addiction because many drugs that are nonaddictive (eg, β-adrenergic antagonists, tricyclic antidepressants, and antipsychotics) produce physical dependence and withdrawal symptoms but do not lead to compulsive use.

REWARD PATHWAYS: ANATOMY AND NEUROCHEMISTRY

Olds and Milner observed that electrical stimulation of discrete brain regions in rats could produce rein-

forcement of operant responses that were contingently paired with such stimulation, and thereby discovered that specific neural substrates in the brain are capable of mediating reinforcement. Such *intracranial self-stimulation* paradigms allow experimental animals to receive electrical stimulation in specific brain regions (containing implanted electrodes) in response to a particular behavior, such as pressing a lever. Although electrical stimulation of several brain structures is reinforcing, stimulation of the medial forebrain bundle and closely associated areas results in the strongest reinforcement of paired behavior. The medial forebrain bundle consists of ascending and descending fiber tracts that connect rostral basal forebrain and midbrain structures, and includes dopaminergic, noradrenergic, and serotonergic fibers derived from monoamine nuclei of the brain stem (see Chapters 8 and 9).

Addictive drugs and reinforcing electrical brain stimulation activate the same brain reward circuitry, as suggested by the synergistic effect that addictive drugs have on brain stimulation reward (BSR) thresholds; in the presence of drugs, less stimulation is needed to produce a particular response. Virtually all addictive drugs enhance BSR, including amphetamines, cocaine, opiates, nicotine, phencyclidine (PCP) and ketamine, cannabinoids, benzodiazepines, barbiturates, and ethanol.

Reinforcement produced by stimulation of the medial forebrain bundle appears to be caused primarily by activation of the mesocorticolimbic dopamine system; this system is also a critical substrate for the reinforcing effects of drugs and natural stimuli, as previously mentioned (Figure 16–1). Mesocorticolimbic dopaminergic projections originate in the VTA of the ventral midbrain and project through the medial forebrain bundle to limbic and forebrain structures. The dopaminergic projection that extends from the VTA to the NAc is the best-established substrate for reinforce-

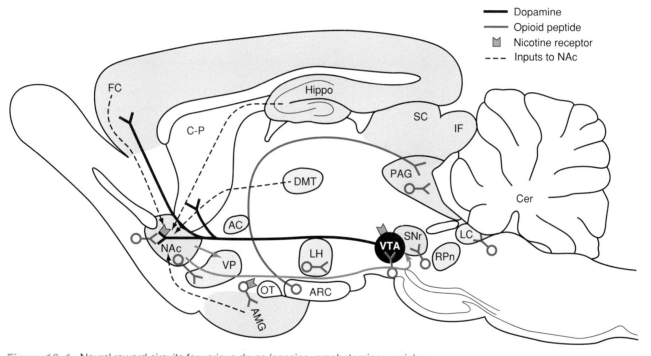

Figure 16-1. Neural reward circuits for various drugs (cocaine, amphetamines, opiates, nicotine, and alcohol) in a sagittal section of rat brain. A limbic–extrapyramidal motor interface is apparent. Dashed lines indicate limbic afferent inputs to the nucleus accumbens (NAc). A solid gray line represents efferent signals from the NAc believed to be involved in drug reward. Solid black lines indicate projections of the mesocorticolimbic dopamine system, which are believed to be critical substrates for drug reward. This dopamine system originates in the ventral tegmental area (VTA) and projects to the NAc, olfactory tubercle, ventral striatal domains of the caudate–putamen (C–P), and amygdala (AMG). Blue lines indicate opioid peptide-containing neurons, which comprise systems that may be involved in opiate, ethanol, and possibly nicotine reward; these systems include local enkephalinergic circuits (*short segments*) and the hypothalamic β-endorphin circuit of the midbrain (*long segment*). Blue areas indicate the approximate distribution of GABA$_A$ receptor complexes, some of which may mediate sedative/hypnotic (ethanol) reward. Gray solid structures indicate nicotinic acetylcholine receptors, which are hypothesized to be located among dopaminergic and opioid peptidergic systems. AC, anterior commissure; ARC, arcuate nucleus; Cer, cerebellum; DMT, dorsomedial thalamus; FC, frontal cortex; Hippo, hippocampus; IF, inferior colliculus; LC, locus coeruleus; LH, lateral hypothalamus; OT, olfactory tract; PAG, periaqueductal gray; RPn, raphe pontis nucleus; SC, superior colliculus; SNr, substantia nigra pars reticulata; VP, ventral pallidum. (Adapted with permission from Koob GF, Nestler EJ. 1997. In Salloway S, Malloy P, Cummings JL (eds): *The Neuropsychiatry of Limbic and Subcortical Disorders,* p. 179. Washington, DC: American Psychiatric Press.)

Table 16-1 Examples of Acute Pharmacologic Actions of Drugs of Abuse

Drug	Action
Opiates	Agonist at μ, δ, and κ opioid receptors[1]
Cocaine	Inhibits monoamine reuptake transporters
Amphetamine	Stimulates monoamine release[2]
Ethanol	Facilitates $GABA_A$ receptor function and inhibits NMDA glutamate receptor function[3]
Nicotine	Agonist at nicotinic acetylcholine receptors
Cannabinoids	Agonist at cannabinoid (CB_1 and CB_2) receptors[4]
Hallucinogens	Partial agonist at $5-HT_{2A}$ serotonin receptors
Phencyclidine (PCP)	Antagonist at NMDA glutamate receptors
Inhalants	Unknown

[1]μ and γ receptors mediate the reinforcing actions of opiates.
[2]Amphetamine produces this effect via actions at monoamine transporters.
[3]It is not known whether ethanol produces these effects by direct binding to these targets or by indirect mechanisms.
[4]CB_1 receptors mediate the reinforcing actions of cannabinoids.

ment. In vivo microdialysis studies have indicated that most if not all addictive drugs, including cocaine, amphetamines, opiates, nicotine, and ethanol, unlike nonaddictive drugs, cause selective elevation of extra-cellular dopamine levels in the medial subdivision of the NAc, known as the shell. Although the mesolimbic dopamine system is a site of convergence for the rewarding effects of virtually all major classes of addictive drugs, these drugs act by very different mechanisms, which are described in the section that follows (Table 16-1; Figure 16-2).

INITIAL ACTIONS OF DRUGS OF ABUSE AND NATURAL REINFORCERS

PSYCHOSTIMULANTS

Cocaine, amphetamines, and **methamphetamine** are the major psychostimulants of abuse. The related drug **methylphenidate** is also abused, although it is far less potent. These drugs elicit similar initial subjective effects (Table 16-2); differences generally reflect the route of administration and other pharmacokinetic factors. Such agents also have important therapeutic uses; cocaine, for example, is used as a **local anesthetic** (see Chapter 3), and amphetamines and methylphenidate are used in low doses to treat **attention deficit–hyperactivity** disorder and in higher doses to treat **narcolepsy** (see Chapter 18). Despite their clinical uses, these drugs are strongly reinforcing, and their long-term use at high doses is linked with potential addiction, espe-

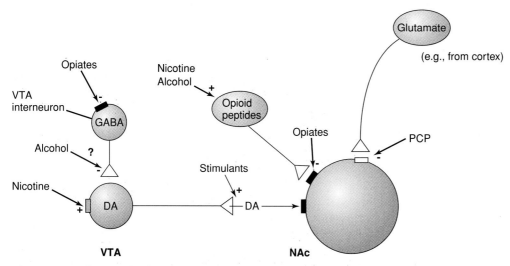

Figure 16-2. Proposed sites at which drugs of abuse act in the mesolimbic dopamine system. Opiates increase the firing of dopaminergic (DA) neurons in the VTA by inhibiting γ-aminobutyric acid (GABA) neurons. The inhibition of GABA neurons reduces the tonic inhibition of DA neurons, and in turn increases their firing. Opiates also have a direct impact on neurons in the nucleus accumbens (NAc). Cocaine and amphetamine act on dopaminergic terminals in the NAc to potentiate dopaminergic transmission, by blocking dopamine uptake and by increasing dopamine release, respectively. Nicotine and ethanol activate dopaminergic neurons of the VTA and also may activate opioid peptidergic neurons afferent to the NAc. Phencyclidine (PCP) blocks excitatory glutamatergic input to the NAc.

Table 16–2 Acute Effects of Psychostimulants and Withdrawal Symptoms

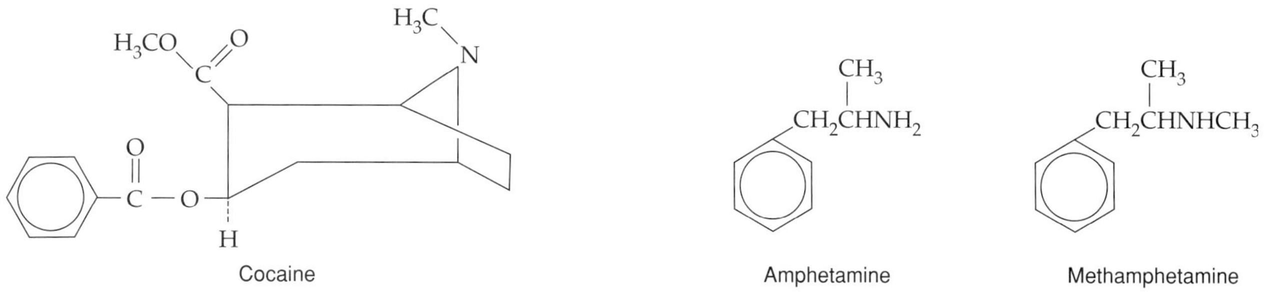

Cocaine

Amphetamine

Methamphetamine

Short-Term Effects	Withdrawal Symptoms
Euphoria	Dysphoria
Increased arousal	Depression
Suppression of fatigue	Fatigue/exhaustion
Increased sense of confidence	Anxiety
Appetite suppression	Hyperphagia

cially when they are rapidly administered or when high-potency forms are given. Moreover, amphetamines and their derivatives can be toxic to monoaminergic neurons when given at high doses.

Addictive use of psychostimulants often consists of intermittent binges and escalating intake, compared with the patterns of continual or daily administration most often associated with the use of opiates, nicotine, and alcohol. As previously mentioned, long-term psychostimulant use is more strongly associated with emotional and motivational dependence than with physical dependence (see Table 16–2).

Cocaine and amphetamines produce their psychoactive effects by potentiating monoaminergic transmission through actions on dopamine, serotonin, and norepinephrine transporters (Figure 16–3). These proteins normally transport synaptically released neurotransmitter back into the presynaptic nerve terminal and thereby terminate transmitter action (see Chapters 4, 8, and 9). Actions at the dopamine transporter are believed to be most important for the reinforcing effects of these drugs; for example, mice with a null mutation in the dopamine transporter (DAT) gene are much less sensitive than normal mice to the behavioral effects of cocaine or amphetamines. Yet mice with this mutation retain some responsiveness to these drugs; thus it is likely that actions at other transporters, particularly serotonergic transporters, may contribute to reinforcement.

Cocaine and amphetamines affect monoamine transporters in different ways, although the net effect of these drugs—an increase in monoaminergic neurotransmission—is similar. Cocaine binds to and competi-

tively inhibits the functioning of the dopamine transporter, thereby increasing the duration of action of dopamine that is released into the synaptic cleft. Cocaine similarly affects serotonin and norepinephrine transporters. In contrast, amphetamines and related drugs are believed to potentiate dopaminergic or other types of monoaminergic neurotransmission by acting as a substrate for monoamine transporters. These drugs are transported into dopamine, serotonin, and norepinephrine nerve terminals, where they act to cause reverse transport of dopamine, serotonin, and norepinephrine from the terminals. These drugs may produce this effect by disrupting the ability of synaptic vesicles to concentrate these neurotransmitters, perhaps by impairing H^+ transport in the vesicles; however, this theory remains conjectural. The result is increased cytoplasmic levels of the neurotransmitters, which appears to lead to their release from the terminals by means of the transporters.

The reinforcing effects of cocaine and amphetamines require an intact mesolimbic dopamine system. Systemic administration of dopamine antagonists, or of the dopamine synthesis inhibitor **α-methylparatyrosine** (AMPT), decreases self-administration; in contrast, antagonists of various adrenergic receptors have little or no effect on such behavior. Selective antagonists for multiple dopamine receptor subtypes (D_1, D_2, and D_3) are effective in decreasing the reinforcing actions of cocaine. Dopamine release is increased in the NAc during self-administration of amphetamine or cocaine, as mentioned previously, and blockade of dopaminergic transmission in the NAc—for example, in response to

A   Cocaine inhibits
monoamine reuptake

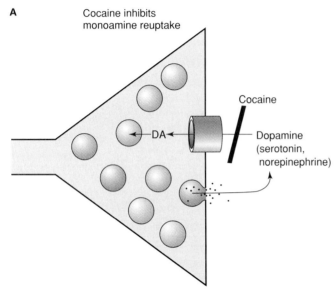

B   Amphetamine and methamphetamine
increase monoamine release

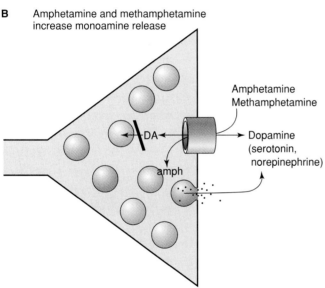

Figure 16–3. Mechanism of action of cocaine and amphetamine on monoamine nerve terminals. **A.** Cocaine potentiates the actions of monoamines at the synapse by inhibiting monoamine transporter proteins, which normally carry previously released transmitter back into the nerve terminal. **B.** Amphetamine serves as a substrate for monoamine transporter proteins and is transported into the nerve terminal. In the nerve terminal, amphetamine disrupts the vesicular storage of monoamine transmitters, which leads to an increase in their extravesicular levels; consequently these transmitters are pumped out of the nerve terminal by a reverse action of the transporters.

intra-NAc injections of dopamine receptor antagonists or of the toxin **6-hydroxydopamine** (see Chapter 8)—dramatically reduces drug reinforcement. The predominant effect of dopamine in the NAc is the inhibition of γ-aminobutyric acid (GABA)ergic medium spiny projection neurons; however, why inhibition of these neurons contributes to drug reinforcement remains unknown.

OPIATES

The opiates and their synthetic analogs are the most effective analgesic agents known (see Chapter 19), yet they are widely abused because of their effects on brain reward circuitry (Table 16–3). **Morphine** and **heroin** are among the most commonly abused opiates. Abuse of these drugs may be driven by a variety of factors, including their reinforcing effects, their ability to relieve both preexisting dysphoria and unpleasant symptoms related to drug withdrawal, and the intense craving they produce after long-term use. Physical dependence on opiates can occur independently of addiction; for example, patients with cancer pain may become physically dependent on these drugs but do not compulsively abuse them. Termination of opiate use is accompanied by emotional–motivational symptoms as well as somatic withdrawal symptoms (see Table 16–3).

Immediate effects of opiate drugs result from their binding to endogenous opioid receptors. As discussed in Chapter 10, the three types of opioid receptors—μ, δ, and κ—are distinguished by their pharmacologic profiles and anatomic distributions. These receptors

Table 16-3 Acute Effects of Opiates and Withdrawal Symptoms

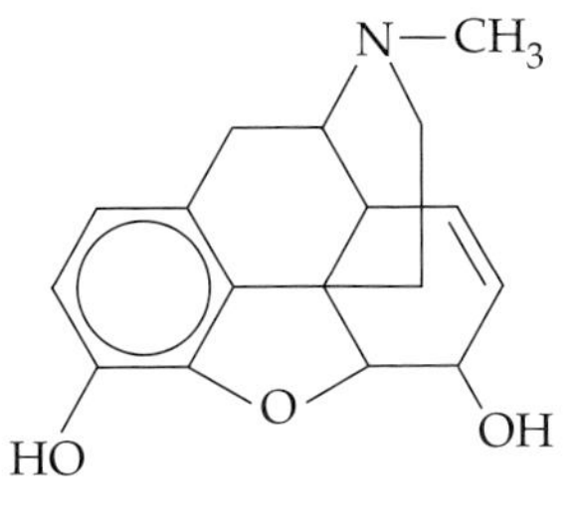

Morphine

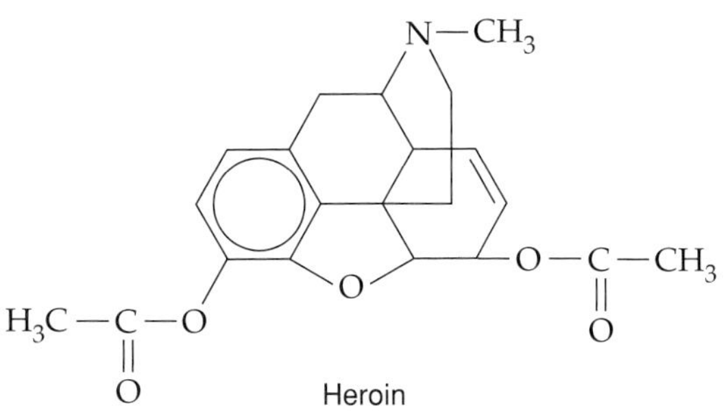

Heroin

Short-Term Effects	Withdrawal Symptoms
Analgesia	Increased pain sensitivity
Euphoria	Dysphoria; irritability
Sedation	Restlessness; insomnia
Constipation	Diarrhea
Respiratory depression	Hyperventilation

belong to the G protein-coupled receptor superfamily and exhibit significant homology, particularly in transmembrane and intracellular regions. Opioid receptors couple with $G_{i/o}$ proteins to inhibit adenylyl cyclase, to activate inwardly rectifying K^+ channels, and to inhibit voltage-gated Ca^{2+} channels. They typically mediate inhibitory responses that involve a reduction in excitability and cell firing, and inhibition of neurotransmitter release. Examples of neural and behavioral actions mediated by μ, δ, and κ opioid receptors are listed in Table 16–4.

Opiates are hypothesized to activate brain reward circuitry by means of at least two mechanisms: 1) disinhibition of the VTA, which results in dopamine release in the NAc, and 2) dopamine-independent activity in the NAc. Although the injection of morphine, selective μ or δ opioid receptor agonists, or enkephalin analogs into several areas of the brain can be reinforcing, the VTA is particularly sensitive. Moreover, reinforcing effects of intravenous heroin can be partly attenuated by administration of an opioid receptor antagonist

directly into the VTA or by lesions in dopaminergic neurons of the VTA. Opiate activation of such neurons results from opiate inhibition of the GABAergic interneurons in the VTA that normally inhibit principal dopamine neurons (see Figure 16–2).

Opiates also produce reinforcement through direct dopamine-independent actions on μ, and perhaps δ, receptors expressed in NAc neurons. These receptors are normally targets of the enkephalinergic (and possibly endorphinergic) neurons that innervate this brain region. Animals will work to self-administer morphine directly into the NAc, even in the presence of dopamine receptor blockade or 6-hydroxydopamine lesions of dopaminergic terminals in this region of the brain. Within the NAc, opiates appear to directly inhibit the same populations of medium spiny projection neurons that are inhibited by dopamine. Thus opioid and dopaminergic systems appear to converge on a common efferent reward pathway in the NAc (see Figure 16–2).

μ and δ opioid receptor subtypes, both of which are present in the NAc and VTA, are important factors in

Table 16-4 Receptor Subtypes Implicated in Actions of Opiates

	Receptor Subtype	Effect of Agonists	Effect of Antagonists
Analgesia	μ, δ, κ	Analgesia	No effect[1]
Respiratory function	μ	Respiratory depression	No effect[2]
Gastrointestinal tract function	μ, δ	Decreased motility	No effect
Sedation	μ, κ	Sedation	No effect
Reward function	μ, δ	Reinforcement	Possibly mild aversion
	κ	Aversion	Unknown

[1]Can block stress-induced analgesia.
[2]Can reverse respiratory depression caused by μ receptor agonist.

opiate reinforcement. In contrast, κ opioid receptor activation is not reinforcing; indeed, it is aversive in both animals and humans. Activation of κ receptors can decrease dopamine release in the NAc; thus the mesolimbic dopamine system may mediate aversive effects of opiates as well as their reinforcing properties. Tonic activation of the different opioid receptors in the reward circuitry by endogenous opioid peptides may modulate responses to natural reinforcers and influence an individual's motivational state.

ETHANOL

Ethanol is a CNS depressant that shares some behavioral effects with sedative–hypnotic drugs such as barbiturates and benzodiazepines (Table 16–5; see Chapters 7, 15, and 18). In humans it is clearly reinforcing and addictive, as evidenced by its widespread compulsive use. Ethanol reinforcement can be demonstrated in animal studies involving oral and other routes of self-administration. The many serious health problems associated with long-term ethanol use, such as gastritis, cirrhosis, and malnutrition, most likely are related to the extremely large amounts of ethanol that are necessary for its psychoactive effects (as much as 100 mM in tolerant users), and also to the ability of this small molecule to interact with numerous physiologic systems.

Two to three decades ago it was hypothesized that ethanol produces its behavioral effects by dissolving into neuronal plasma membranes in a nonspecific manner, and subsequently by altering the liquidity of membrane lipids and disrupting membrane function. More recently it has become clear that ethanol exerts more specific effects in the brain, particularly at moderate concentrations. Accordingly, the initial effects of ethanol currently are believed to result primarily from facilitation of $GABA_A$ receptors and inhibition of NMDA glutamate receptors. At higher doses, ethanol also inhibits the functioning of most ligand- and voltage-gated ion channels. The mechanisms by which ethanol causes these effects are unknown but may be related to generalized effects on cell membranes; that is, various ligand-gated and voltage-gated channels may be preferentially affected by ethanol because, as highly complex multimeric proteins, they may be particularly vulnerable to changes in their lipid surroundings. Alternatively, direct interactions with particular intramembranous regions of these proteins have been postulated.

Regardless of its precise mechanisms of action, ethanol allosterically regulates the $GABA_A$ receptor to enhance GABA-activated Cl^- flux. The anxiolytic and sedative effects of ethanol, as well as those of **barbiturates** and **benzodiazepines,** are believed to result from this enhancement of GABAergic function. Not all $GABA_A$ receptors are ethanol sensitive. As mentioned in Chapters 7 and 15, $GABA_A$ receptor complexes comprise combinations of five distinct subunit families. The regional distribution and relative abundance of these subunit combinations vary, and thus may explain differences in the sensitivity of $GABA_A$ receptors to ethanol in different brain regions. As with other sedative–hypnotics, such as barbiturates, facilitation of $GABA_A$ receptor function is believed to contribute to ethanol's reinforcing effects.

Ethanol also acts as an NMDA antagonist and allosterically inhibits the passage of glutamate-activated Na^+ and Ca^{2+} currents through the NMDA receptor. The sensitivity of NMDA receptors to ethanol, like that of $GABA_A$ receptors, may depend on receptor subunit composition. Other NMDA antagonists, such as **phencyclidine,** produce profound cognitive deficits and psychotic symptoms; thus the dissociative and psychotomimetic effects of ethanol (at higher doses) may be mediated by means of such antagonism. Because other NMDA antagonists are reinforcing, it is believed that some of ethanol's addicting properties also are mediated by this mechanism; however, this possibility is only beginning to be explored.

Other immediate actions of ethanol include potentiation of the action of serotonin at $5-HT_3$ receptors, which, like NMDA receptors, are excitatory, cation-selective ion channels. These receptors are located primarily on inhibitory interneurons; consequently ethanol potentiation at $5-HT_3$ receptors most likely increases the inhibitory influence of these interneurons. Ethanol also inhibits L-type voltage-gated Ca^{2+} channels, which are believed to be important in regulating second messenger functions of calcium. Moreover, as previously mentioned, ethanol inhibits most voltage-gated ion channels at very high concentrations; such inhibition most likely explains the profound CNS-depressant effects of high concentrations of ethanol, which can lead to coma and death.

Table 16–5 Acute Effects of Ethanol and Withdrawal Symptoms

$$CH_3-CH_2-OH$$

Ethanol

Short-Term Effects	Withdrawal Symptoms
Loss of inhibition	Irritability; tremor
Anxiolysis	Anxiety
Sedation	Sleep disturbance
Decreased motor coordination	Seizures

The primary neurochemical mechanism through which ethanol influences reinforcement systems is not yet known but evidence suggests the involvement of several neurotransmitter systems (see Figure 16–2). The reinforcing effects of ethanol are partly explained by its ability to activate mesocorticolimbic dopamine circuitry, although it is not known whether this effect is mediated at the level of the VTA or the NAc. It also is not known whether this activation of dopamine systems is caused primarily by facilitation of $GABA_A$ receptors or inhibition of NMDA receptors, or both. Serotonin also appears to be involved in ethanol consumption and reinforcement; ethanol consumption is generally curbed by experimental manipulations that increase serotonergic function, and experiments with rats selectively bred for ethanol preference suggest that strong ethanol preference is associated with reduced serotonergic function. $5-HT_3$ antagonists such as **odansetron** can block both ethanol-induced dopamine release in the NAc and ethanol consumption in rats, suggesting that this receptor subtype is involved in ethanol reinforcement as well. Ethanol reinforcement also is mediated in part by ethanol-induced release of endogenous opioid peptides within the mesolimbic dopamine system, although whether the VTA or NAc is the predominant site of such action is not yet known. The opioid receptor antagonist **naltrexone** reduces ethanol self-administration in animals; moreover, it reduces ethanol consumption, relapse, and craving, and has been reported to diminish ethanol-induced euphoria in humans addicted to ethanol. Conversely, drugs that block the degradation of endogenous opioids increase voluntary ethanol consumption in rats.

NICOTINE

Nicotine is the main psychoactive ingredient of tobacco and is responsible for the stimulant effects, reinforcement, dependence, and addiction that result from tobacco use (Table 16–6). Cigarette smoking rapidly delivers pulses of nicotine into the bloodstream. Nicotine differs from cocaine and opiates in that it is powerfully reinforcing in the absence of subjective euphoria. The high incidence of carcinogenicity associated with long-term tobacco use is related to compounds other than nicotine that are either contained in tobacco or generated by its combustion.

The initial effects of nicotine are caused by its activation of nicotinic acetylcholine (nACh) receptors. nACh receptors are ligand-gated cation channels (see Chapters 9 and 12); in the CNS, they are located postsynaptically and also on presynaptic terminals, where they facilitate transmitter release. The reinforcing effects of nicotine, like those of other addictive drugs,

Table 16–6 Acute Effects of Nicotine and Withdrawal Symptoms

Nicotine

Short-Term Effects	Withdrawal Symptoms
Increased alertness	Difficulty concentrating
Mild Euphoria	Dysphoria; irritability
Muscle relaxation	Restlessness; anxiety
Nausea	Increased appetite
Increased psychomotor activity	Hyperventilation

depend on an intact mesolimbic dopamine system. nACh receptors located on VTA dopamine neurons are implicated in nicotine reinforcement. Systemic nicotine self-administration is disrupted when antagonists are administered directly into the VTA but not when they are administered into the NAc; moreover, nicotine is rewarding when injected directly into the VTA. nACh receptors on VTA dopamine neurons are normally activated by cholinergic innervation from the laterodorsal tegmental nucleus or the pedunculopontine nucleus. In addition, nicotine may stimulate dopamine release in the NAc through actions on presynaptic nACh receptors located on dopamine terminals within the NAc. Nicotine self-administration also can be blocked by opioid receptor antagonists, such as naltrexone. These findings indicate the involvement of endogenous opioid systems in the reinforcing effects of nicotine, and raise the possibility that such antagonists may be of use in the treatment of nicotine addiction.

CANNABINOIDS

Delta-9-tetrahydrocannabinol (THC) is one of several cannabinoid compounds contained in **marijuana,** and is primarily responsible for the psychoactive effects of cannabis preparations (Table 16–7). The addictive potential of THC has been a matter of debate, but reinforcing effects of cannabinoids comparable to those of other addictive drugs have not been demonstrated in animals. Nonetheless, there are many compulsive users of marijuana. Withdrawal symptoms typically do not occur with termination of long-term marijuana use, probably because of the persistence of accumulated THC in the tissues of long-term users. However, cannabinoid dependence can be demonstrated experimentally with the use of cannabinoid receptor antago-

Table 16–7 Acute Effects of Cannabinoids and Withdrawal Symptoms

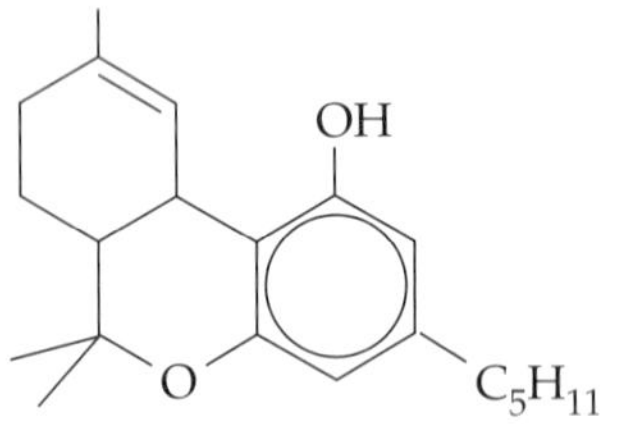

Delta-9-tetrahydrocannabinol

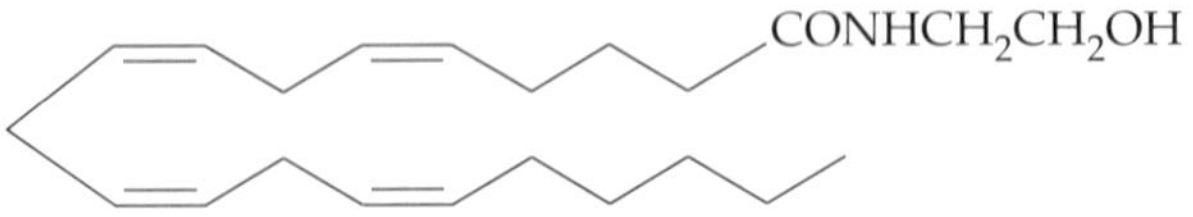

CONHCH$_2$CH$_2$OH

Anandamide [1]

Short-Term Effects	Withdrawal Symptoms
Euphoria	Irritability
Disinhibition	Restlessness
Cognitive deficits	Sleep disturbance
Increased hunger	Nausea
Altered sensory perception	

[1]Arachidonyl ethanolamide (for the structure of arachidonic acid, see Chapter 5).

nists, which precipitate profound withdrawal symptoms that are both physical and emotional–motivational.

THC exerts its primary pharmacologic effects by binding to a G protein-coupled receptor in the brain known as the CB$_1$ receptor—a misnomer because cannabinoids are not natural ligands for this receptor. Most evidence suggests that the endogenous ligand for this receptor is an arachadonic acid derivative termed anandamide; however, the nature of anandamide's function in the brain remains unclear. Evidence indicates that other endogenous ligands also may bind at this receptor. Although THC does not measurably alter overall dopamine release in the NAc, it does appear to selectively induce dopamine release in the shell of the NAc through a specific action on CB$_1$ receptors. This effect may be indirect and mediated in part by cannabinoid regulation of endogenous opioid systems in the VTA. The pharmacology and psychoactive effects of cannabinoids are discussed in greater detail in Chapter 17.

PHENCYCLIDINE

Phencyclidine (**PCP** or **angel dust**) and **ketamine** (also known as special K) are structurally related drugs (Figure 16–4) that are classified as dissociative anesthetics. These drugs are distinguished from other psychotomimetic agents, such as hallucinogens, by their distinct spectrum of pharmacologic effects, including their reinforcing properties and risks related to compulsive abuse (see Chapter 17).

The reinforcing properties of PCP and ketamine are mediated by the binding of these drugs to specific sites in the channel of the NMDA glutamate receptor, where they act as noncompetitive antagonists. PCP is self-admin-

istered directly into the NAc, where its reinforcing effects are believed to result from the blockade of excitatory glutamatergic input to the same medium spiny NAc neurons inhibited by opioids and dopamine (see Figure 16–2).

OTHER DRUGS OF ABUSE

Several other classes of drugs are categorized as drugs of abuse (see Figure 16–4) but rarely produce compulsive use. These include psychedelic agents, such as **lysergic acid diethylamide (LSD)**, which are used for their ability to produce perceptual distortions at low and moderate doses. The use of LSD and other indolealkylamine psychedelics typically does not lead to compulsive abuse; rather, these drugs are associated with the rapid development of tolerance and the absence of positive reinforcement (see Chapter 17). Partial agonist effects at 5-HT$_{2A}$ receptors are implicated in the psychedelic actions of LSD and related hallucinogens.

3,4-methylenedioxymethamphetamine (**MDMA**), commonly called **ecstacy,** is a methoxylated amphetamine derivative. Categorized as a phenethylamine psychedelic, it produces a combination of psychostimulant-like and weak LSD-like effects at low doses. Unlike LSD, MDMA is reinforcing—most likely because of its interactions with dopamine systems—and accordingly is subject to compulsive abuse. The weak psychedelic effects of MDMA appear to result from its amphetamine-like actions on the serotonin reuptake transporter, by means of which it causes transporter-dependent serotonin efflux. MDMA has been proven to produce lesions in the terminals of serotonin neurons in animals. There is preliminary evidence of neurotoxic effects on humans as well (see Chapter 9).

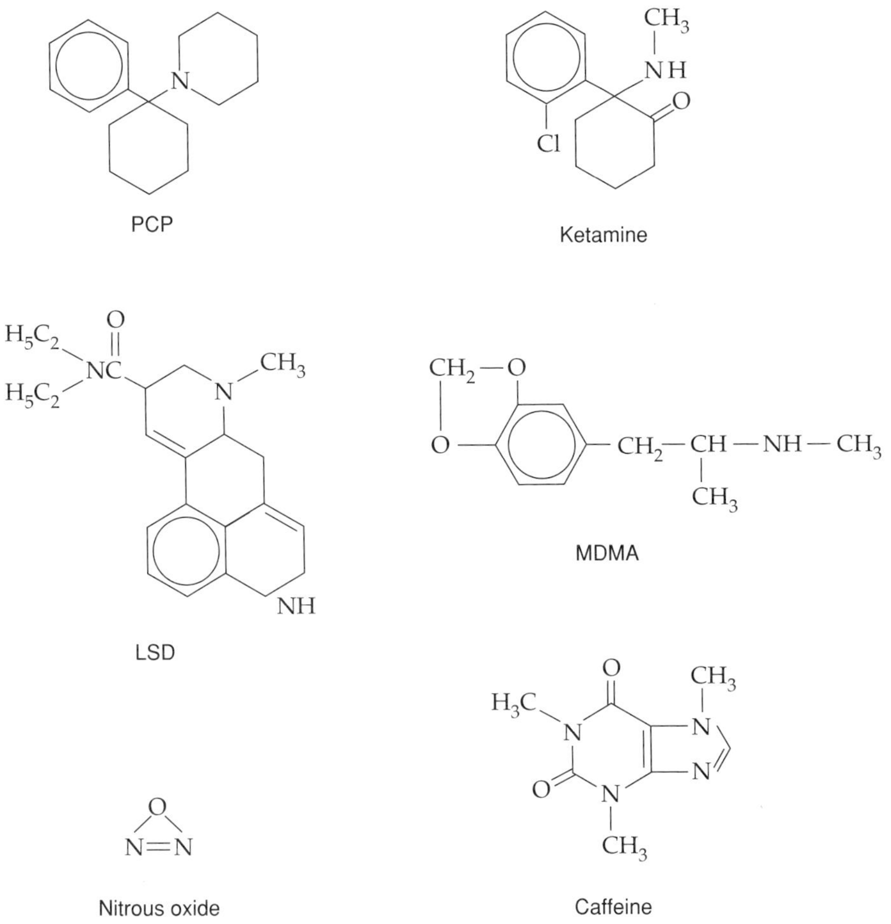

PCP

Ketamine

LSD

MDMA

Nitrous oxide

Caffeine

Figure 16–4. Chemical structures of some miscellaneous drugs that are self-administered for psychotropic effects.

A variety of volatile chemicals are abused as **inhalants** because of their ability to produce rapid and brief intoxication, which generally consists of some degree of euphoria and light-headedness. Abused inhalants include commercial products that are readily obtained by minors and that consist of diverse chemical classes—for example, aerosol products, household solvents, adhesives, gasoline, and **nitrous oxide**. Their pharmacologic effects and toxicity vary, depending on their constituent chemicals; however, their mechanisms of action remain obscure. Compulsive use of inhalants can be severe.

Caffeine, theophylline, and **theobromine** are methylxanthines that stimulate the CNS, produce increased alertness, improve psychomotor performance, and decrease fatigue. Long-term caffeine use can lead to mild physical dependence. A withdrawal syndrome characterized by drowsiness, irritability, and headache typically lasts no longer than a day. True compulsive use of caffeine has not been documented. The main mechanism responsible for the pharmacologic effects of caffeine and other methylxanthines appears to be competitive antagonism of G protein-coupled adenosine A_1

and A_{2A} receptors (see Chapter 10). An interesting finding from a study that must be replicated is that regular caffeine consumption appears to protect dopamine neurons and thereby may have a preventive effect on **Parkinson disease**.

ACTIVATION OF REWARD CIRCUITRY BY NATURAL REINFORCERS

As previously indicated, the neural circuitry activated by reinforcing brain stimulation and by addictive drugs is believed to be part of an endogenous reward mechanism that motivates individuals to pursue natural reinforcers such as food and sex. This reward mechanism involves activation of the mesolimbic dopamine system. Dopamine neurons in the VTA, and in the pars compacta of the substantia nigra, are activated by food and water, and dopamine release in the NAc is stimulated by the presence of natural reinforcers, such as food, water, or a sexual partner.

The mechanisms by which natural reinforcers activate reward circuitry differ somewhat from those involved in drug use. The complex reinforcing effects of food rewards, for example, are maintained after lesions are placed in the mesolimbic dopamine system. Both endogenous opioid pathways and complex hypothalamic peptidergic circuitry are known to be involved in feeding (see Chapter 13). In a study of individual NAc neurons in monkeys working for rewards, differences between neuronal responses to cocaine and neuronal responses to juice were detected; the results of this study suggest that responses to cocaine and natural reinforcers are separable at the neuronal level. Accordingly, it is possible that cocaine reinforcement can be altered without disrupting natural reward pathways, and consequently that current efforts to develop medications for cocaine addiction may be successful.

Can compulsive eating, shopping, gambling, and sex be related to the abnormal regulation of endogenous reward mechanisms in certain individuals? Just as addictive drugs can powerfully activate reward pathways and consequently modify motivated behavior, it is possible that these pleasurable behaviors may excessively activate reward-reinforcement mechanisms in susceptible individuals. As with drugs, such activation may result in profound alterations in motivation that promote the repetition of initially rewarding behavior, despite the impact of negative consequences associated with the resulting compulsion. Indeed, addictions to both drugs and behavioral rewards may arise from similar dysregulation of the mesolimbic dopamine system. Because such behaviors as shopping and gambling cannot be easily examined in animals, confirmation of neurophysiologic links between drug use and other compulsive behaviors may have to await improvements in human neuroimaging technologies.

DOPAMINERGIC NEURONS AND REWARD-DEPENDENT LEARNING

How does increased dopaminergic transmission in the NAc, elicited by natural reinforcers, drugs, or rewarding brain stimulation, strengthen the motivated behavior produced by these stimuli? Dopamine's precise role in reinforcement has been recently reevaluated. Instead of simply mediating subjective pleasure, dopamine may affect motivation and attention to salient stimuli, including rewarding stimuli. Indeed, several experimental findings suggest that the pleasure associated with food does not necessarily depend on dopamine; rather, it appears to be more affected by drugs that influence opioid and GABA systems. Dopaminergic lesions of the NAc and caudate nucleus, as well as dopamine receptor antagonists, can alter the *motivation* to eat, but do not affect the hedonic value assigned to taste. It is important to mention that such lesions and antagonists also do not involve the impair-

ment of motor capabilities (see Chapter 14) . If motivational drive is described in terms of *wanting*, and hedonic evaluation in terms of *liking*, it appears that wanting can be dissociated from liking and that dopamine may influence these phenomena differently. Differences between wanting and liking are confirmed in reports by human addicts, who state that their desire for drugs (wanting) increases with continued use even when pleasure (liking) decreases because of tolerance. Moreover, during withdrawal the desire for drugs can be more strongly associated with dysphoria than with pleasure. Imaging studies of human cocaine users have demonstrated dynamic changes in neural networks in response to cocaine-induced euphoria and cocaine-induced craving; such studies further support the idea that liking and wanting are separate phenomena mediated by somewhat distinct neural substrates.

The involvement of dopaminergic neurons in the regulation of attention and motivation is suggested by electrophysiologic studies of dopaminergic neurons in the midbrain of the monkey. These neurons respond to reward-predicting stimuli as well as to unexpected—but not expected—rewards. Thus they appear to signal not a reward per se but salient events that warrant attention. Therefore, it is predictors of reward and *unexpected* rewarding stimuli that elicit significant responses in dopaminergic neurons of the midbrain; indeed, these neurons do not respond to rewards that have become predictable based on previous experience. When predicted rewards fail to occur, dopaminergic neurons signal this deviation from expected events by a decrease in activity at the time the reward was predicted to have occurred. Based on such findings, it appears that these neurons can signal positive and negative outcomes in relation to predicted rewards. It has been suggested that the dopamine signal may constitute a mechanism of learning relevant to rewards. Dopaminergic innervation of the prefrontal cortex has been strongly associated with regulation of executive functions such as working memory (see Chapter 17), a finding that further demonstrates the potent effects of dopamine—and of drugs that affect dopaminergic transmission—on attention and planning.

EXTENDED REWARD CIRCUITRY

Dopaminergic neurons of the midbrain are believed to function in reward and reinforcement as part of a neural circuit at the interface between limbic emotional–motivational information and extrapyramidal regulation of motor behavior (see Chapter 14). The major components of this circuit and the critical substrates for drug reward are represented in Figure 16–1. A macrostructure postulated to integrate many of the functions of this circuit is described by some investigators as the *extended amygdala*. The extended amygdala is said to comprise several basal forebrain structures that share similar morphology, immunocytochemical features, and connectivity and that are well-suited to mediating aspects of reward function; these include the bed nucleus of the stria terminalis, the central medial amygdala, the shell of the NAc, and the sublenticular substantia innominata.

The NAc and VTA are central components of the circuitry underlying reward and memory of reward. As previously mentioned, the activity of dopaminergic neurons in the VTA appears to be linked to reward prediction. The NAc is involved in learning associated with reinforcement and the modulation of motoric responses to stimuli that satisfy internal homeostatic needs. The shell of the NAc appears to be particularly important to initial drug actions within reward circuitry; addictive drugs appear to have a greater effect on dopamine release in the shell than in the core of the NAc.

As mentioned earlier, the anatomic connections among GABAergic medium spiny neurons of the NAc are believed to be a critical component of the postulated limbic–extrapyramidal interface involved in reward and reinforcement. As they do in the dorsal striatum (see Chapter 14), these neurons integrate glutamatergic inputs from the cerebral cortex with dopamine inputs from the midbrain. In contrast to activity in the dorsal striatum, however, cortical inputs to the NAc arise from frontal association cortex (rather than from motor cortex and many other areas) and dopamine inputs originate in the VTA (rather than in the substantia nigra). In both the NAc and dorsal striatum, the interactions between dopamine and glutamate may underlie learning and presumably involve plasticity at synapses formed between cortical pyramidal neurons and neurons of the NAc and dorsal striatum. The actions of addictive drugs in these circuits may underlie the acquisition of learned drug-seeking behaviors, in accord with dopamine's postulated involvement in the prediction of reward in animals.

Of the two main subtypes of GABAergic medium spiny neurons in the NAc (see Chapter 14), the type that forms the striatopallidal pathway may be most strongly linked to reward-related behaviors. These neurons, which coexpress enkephalin and, to some extent, D_2 receptors, project from the NAc to the ventral pallidum. This pathway appears to be activated by rewarding stimulation of the VTA, and lesions placed in this pathway reduce cocaine and opiate reinforcement. Activation of the pathway also powerfully stimulates cocaine-seeking behavior, as described later in this chapter. However, it is important to emphasize that the other major subpopulation of GABAergic medium spiny neurons appears to

assist in the regulation of reinforcement and motivation. These neurons project directly to the VTA and coexpress dynorphin, substance P, and predominantly D_1 receptors. A major goal of current research is to more clearly define the role of D_1 and D_2 receptors in dopamine's complex actions on neural systems and the behaviors they mediate. Another critical challenge is to determine precisely why decreased firing of NAc neurons—a common response to the actions of addictive drugs and presumably also a response to natural reinforcers—leads to reinforcement.

The reinforcing function of the amygdala is postulated to involve its role in an individual's orientation to and memory of emotionally salient stimuli. In addition, the amygdala is implicated in the modulation of perception by attention. Projections between the NAc and the amygdala are believed to be important to the formation of stimulus–reward associations. Neurons in the amygdala fire in response to food-related stimuli. Lesions of the amygdala disrupt the ability of experimental animals to remember the pairing of a stimulus with a reward (without disrupting recognition of the stimulus) and can lessen the response to a conditioned reinforcer previously paired with a natural reward. The central nucleus of the amygdala also has been implicated in aversive aspects of drug withdrawal, as described in a subsequent section of this chapter, and is associated with fear, as discussed in Chapter 15.

The hypothalamus assists in the regulation of many homeostatic functions (see Chapter 13). Neurons of the lateral hypothalamus appear to signal the motivational value of a reward in relation to internal drive states. Indeed, the lateral hypothalamus was one of the original structures identified as able to support self-stimulation in early brain stimulation experiments. Important reciprocal projections between the lateral hypothalamus and the extended amygdala may regulate reward mechanisms.

MOLECULAR AND CELLULAR MECHANISMS OF ADDICTION

The loss of control over drug use that characterizes addiction develops progressively as a consequence of time-dependent, drug-induced processes in the brain, which eventually usurp normal volitional control of motivated behavior. Tolerance, dependence, and sensitization are believed to represent time-dependent adaptive processes induced in neurons as a result of repeated drug exposure; when induced by drugs within reinforcement systems, such processes become critical components of addiction. These adaptations can be viewed as examples of drug-induced neural plasticity and may consist of experience-dependent changes in several molecular and cellular processes, including the regulation of receptors, ion channels, intracellular signaling proteins, and gene expression. Multiple neural circuits may undergo adaptive changes in response to a single drug; the functional consequences of the changes in each circuit are related to: 1) the nature of the adaptations, and 2) the normal function of the neurons that undergo adaptations.

Time-dependent adaptations accompany long-term exposure to many psychotropic drugs, regardless of their addictive properties, and indeed are believed to be critical to the therapeutic actions of **antidepressant** (see Chapter 15) and **antipsychotic** (see Chapter 17) medications. Moreover, adaptations that occur in response to long-term drug exposure are not restricted to the nervous system. Other tissues of the body undergo progressive functional alterations in response to the continued presence of a drug. Such adaptations often are homeostatic; they serve to counteract the effects of initial drug exposure and thereby return the system to equilibrium. One example of a drug-induced homeostatic adaptation in peripheral tissues is the generation of metabolic enzymes in the liver in response to long-term ethanol exposure. Such enzymes increase the metabolism and lower blood levels of ethanol and diminish behavioral effects that result from a given dose of the drug.

A current challenge in addiction research is to determine how each adaptation contributes to long-term aspects of the addictive process, and to ascertain the cellular and molecular actions of drugs that lead to such adaptations. The sections that follow summarize some of the adaptive processes induced in neurons by long-term drug administration, many of which may underlie the alterations in reinforcement systems that cause addiction.

ADAPTATIONS THAT PRODUCE TOLERANCE AND PHYSICAL DEPENDENCE

Withdrawal symptoms associated with physical dependence vary depending on the type of drug that has triggered dependence. Such symptoms are mediated by adaptations in neural substrates that are uniquely affected by the presence of different drugs. More is known about adaptations that produce tolerance and physical dependence than about adaptations related to emotional and motivational aspects of dependence. Tolerance and physical dependence are believed to result from homeostatic regulatory processes in the body, which, in the continued presence of a drug, are initiated to counteract the effects of drug presence and to return the system to a normal level of function.

The emergence of withdrawal signs in response to cessation of drug use in a physically dependent individual indicates that the body has adapted to the presence of the drug and, by virtue of the adaptation, requires it for normal function. During withdrawal, the overcompensated system is suddenly unopposed by the drug. Consequently, withdrawal symptoms appear that generally are opposite to the immediate effects produced by drug exposure.

OPIATE TOLERANCE AND DEPENDENCE

The molecular adaptations that underlie tolerance and physical dependence are best established for repeated opiate administration. Opiate tolerance and dependence cannot be adequately explained by changes in endogenous opioid peptides or in opioid receptor affinity or number. Rather, changes in intracellular signaling proteins have been implicated as important contributors to physical dependence on, and possibly tolerance to, opiates (Figure 16–5).

The locus ceruleus (LC), located in the dorsal pons, is the major noradrenergic nucleus of the brain and is important for the regulation of attentional states and autonomic nervous system activity (see Chapters 12 and 18). The LC also has been implicated in the autonomic and stress-like effects of opiate withdrawal. The activity of LC neurons is inhibited by opiates, but continued exposure to these drugs results in tolerance and dependence: depressed firing rates gradually return to normal and the administration of an opioid receptor antagonist causes a dramatic increase in firing rates. The excitation of LC neurons during opiate withdrawal is sufficient to produce many of the signs and symptoms of physical withdrawal.

Alterations in the cAMP signaling pathway in LC neurons contribute to the changes in excitability that these neurons undergo (see Figure 16–5). Opiates initially inhibit the cAMP pathway in many types of neurons, including LC neurons, through actions on G protein-coupled opioid receptors. In the LC, μ opioid receptor activation also results in the activation of inwardly rectifying K^+ channels, by means of direct G protein $\beta\gamma$ binding, and in the inhibition of Na^+ current, caused by the inhibition of protein kinase A. Both actions of μ receptor activation lead to the initial inhibition of LC neurons. After long-term opiate treatment, cAMP pathways are up-regulated in the LC, resulting in increased concentrations of adenylyl cyclase and protein kinase A. This up-regulation can be viewed as a homeostatic response of LC neurons to persistent opiate inhibition of the cAMP pathway. Accordingly, the up-regulated cAMP pathway increases the electrical excitability of LC neurons, by activating

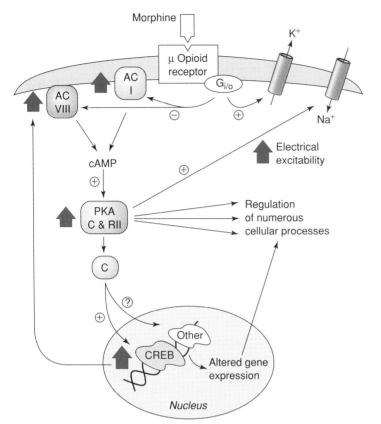

Figure 16-5. Opiate actions in the locus ceruleus. Opiates inhibit neurons of the locus ceruleus (LC) by increasing the conductance of an inwardly rectifying K^+ channel through coupling with subtypes of $G_{i/o}$, and by decreasing a Na^+-dependent inward current through coupling with $G_{i/o}$ and the consequent inhibition of adenylyl cyclase. Reduced levels of cAMP decrease protein kinase A (PKA) activity and the phosphorylation of the responsible channel or pump. Inhibition of the cAMP pathway also decreases the phosphorylation of numerous other proteins and thereby affects many additional processes in the neuron; for example, it reduces the phosphorylation state of CREB, which may initiate some of the longer-term changes in LC function. Upward bold arrows summarize the effects of prolonged exposure to morphine in the LC. Such long-term exposure increases levels of types I and VIII adenylyl cyclase, PKA catalytic (C) and regulatory type II (RII) subunits, and several phosphoproteins, including CREB. These changes contribute to the altered phenotype of the drug-addicted state. For example, the intrinsic excitability of LC neurons is increased by enhanced activity of the cAMP pathway and Na^+-dependent inward current, which contribute to the tolerance, dependence, and withdrawal exhibited by these neurons. Up-regulation of type VIII adenylyl cyclase is mediated by CREB, whereas up-regulation of type I adenylyl cyclase of the PKA subunits appears to occur through CREB-independent mechanisms. (Adapted with permission from Nestler EJ, Aghajanian EK. 1997. *Science* 278:58.)

this Na^+ current, and thereby serves as a mechanism for tolerance and dependence. Such up-regulation helps to return LC firing to normal rates in the continued presence of an opiate (tolerance), and increases LC firing—to rates far higher than normal—in response to removal of the opiate (dependence and withdrawal).

Activation of LC neurons during opiate withdrawal is also partly mediated by a mechanism extrinsic to the LC. This mechanism involves increased glutamatergic activation of these neurons by inputs from the nucleus paragigantocellularis in the rostral ventral medulla. Lesions of the paragigantocellularis, or glutamate receptor antagonists administered locally in the LC, attenuate withdrawal-induced increases in LC firing rates by approximately 50%. An up-regulated cAMP pathway also may mediate this effect on LC neuronal activity because long-term use of opiates causes up-regulation of the cAMP pathway not only in the paragigantocellularis but also in the dorsal root ganglion and dorsal horn of the spinal cord, which provide major afferent input to the paragigantocellularis.

The molecular mechanisms that underlie opiate up-regulation of the cAMP pathway in the LC currently are being determined (see Figure 16–5). Up-regulation of adenylyl cyclase is caused by increased expression of two isoforms of the enzyme: types I and VIII. Up-regulation of protein kinase A can be traced to increased levels of catalytic and type-II regulatory subunits of the kinase. Two general types of mechanisms—transcriptional and posttranslational—appear to mediate these adaptations. The former type involves opiate regulation of the transcription factor CREB, which mediates many of the effects of the cAMP pathway on gene expression (see Chapter 6). Long-term use of opiates increases the expression of CREB in the LC. This increased expression appears to be mediated by a homeostatic autoregulatory mechanism. Opiate inhibition of the cAMP pathway leads to decreased activity of protein kinase A and lower levels of phosphorylated (activated) CREB, which—at a cAMP response element (CRE) site in the CREB gene—results in increased CREB gene transcription. This induction of CREB increases the expression of type-VIII adenylyl cyclase by a CRE site in the gene encoding this enzyme. Mutant mice deficient in CREB are less likely to develop physical dependence on opiates, which supports CREB's involvement in such dependence.

Opiate-induced up-regulation of protein kinase A does not involve CREB and may be mediated posttranslationally. It is known that a free catalytic subunit of the kinase is highly vulnerable to proteolysis, whereas inactive catalytic subunits bound to regulatory subunits are resistant to proteolysis. Thus it currently is speculated that protein kinase A subunits accumulate in the LC during long-term opiate treatment because the enzyme is more stable when it is inhibited by the persistent presence of an opiate. As the number of enzyme molecules increases, more of the molecules are activated by the low levels of cAMP present in LC neurons (cAMP levels also increase gradually as adenylyl cyclase is induced). Although aspects of this scheme remain hypothetical, it can be used to understand mechanisms of tolerance and dependence at the molecular level.

EMOTIONAL AND MOTIVATIONAL ASPECTS OF DEPENDENCE

An emotional and motivational component of drug dependence is indicated by withdrawal symptoms such as anhedonia, depression, anxiety, and negative motivational states. The fact that these symptoms can be characterized as antithetical to the initial effects of addictive drugs suggests that they may result from counteradaptations to prolonged drug exposure. Moreover, just as the reinforcing effects of addictive drugs are believed to be related to actions on brain reward circuitry, emotional and motivational aspects of dependence associated with the long-term use of these drugs may be related to drug-induced adaptations in the same circuitry. The sections that follow illustrate some of the adaptations induced by addictive drugs within reward pathways, which may be potential mediators of drug withdrawal states.

ADAPTATIONS IMPLICATED IN EMOTIONAL–MOTIVATIONAL DEPENDENCE

The VTA and NAc are implicated not only in the immediate reinforcing effects of addictive drugs but also in the emotional and motivational aspects of dependence induced by long-term exposure to these drugs. More specifically, reduced mesolimbic dopaminergic activity is associated with aversive states and with the dysphoria associated with drug withdrawal. Thus these regions of the brain may be sites for common drug-induced adaptations related to the time-dependent changes in drug reinforcement that underlie emotional–motivational dependence.

Up-regulation of the cAMP pathway   Up-regulation of the cAMP pathway in the NAc is a common adaptation to long-term exposure to several types of addictive drugs, including opiates, cocaine, and ethanol, but it is not a feature associated with the use of nonaddictive drugs. Like previously described opiate-induced

adaptations in the cAMP pathway of LC neurons, such up-regulation consists of increased levels of adenylyl cyclase and protein kinase A and decreased levels of $G_{i/o}$ proteins.

Self-administration experiments in which inhibitors or activators of protein kinase A have been injected directly into the NAc have suggested that inhibition of protein kinase A is associated with increased drug reinforcement, whereas activation of this enzyme opposes drug reinforcement. These findings support the hypothesis that up-regulation of the cAMP pathway in the NAc in response to long-term drug administration may contribute to the negative motivational states that characterize withdrawal. The substrate proteins through which protein kinase A exerts these effects have not been identified, but ion channels and glutamate receptor subunits whose phosphorylation would lead to the altered excitability of NAc neurons and, therefore, to altered motivational states are being evaluated. Yet it is important to note that adaptations in the cAMP pathway also have been related to other functional aspects of addiction, such as locomotor sensitization and even enhancement of conditioned reward. The precise functional roles of such molecular adaptations are difficult to determine because the NAc comprises several different cell types with distinct inputs and outputs that may undergo distinct adaptations.

Up-regulation of the cAMP pathway also may occur in the GABA interneurons that innervate dopaminergic neurons of the VTA. Activation of the pathway in these cells during withdrawal may lead to increased GABA release and consequently to reduced firing of the dopaminergic cells that they normally inhibit. Such activity might account at least in part for the reductions in dopaminergic neurotransmission from the VTA to the NAc that have been found to occur during early phases of withdrawal and that are believed to contribute to aversive withdrawal states.

Regulation of CREB   The involvement of CREB in emotional and motivational aspects of dependence might be expected based on our knowledge of drug-induced up-regulation of the cAMP pathway in the NAc. Long-term morphine and cocaine treatment have been found to alter CREB function in the NAc and related striatal regions. Such regulation of CREB may mediate the effects of drug exposure on several neuropeptide genes known to contain CRE sites. Cocaine and amphetamines, for example, can induce the expression of preprotachykinin and prodynorphin mRNA (both of these genes contain CRE sites) and their encoded peptides in striatal neurons. Indeed, cocaine regulation of prodynorphin expression has been shown to depend directly on CREB in vivo.

Drug regulation of dynorphin expression may contribute to the generation of aversive states during withdrawal. Dynorphin acts to decrease dopamine release in the NAc through an action on κ opioid receptors located on presynaptic dopaminergic nerve terminals in this region. Dynorphin most likely is one of many gene products whose expression is regulated by drug-induced changes in CREB function in the NAc. A major goal of current research is to identify other CREB-regulated genes and relate them to specific features of dependence.

Regulation of dopamine transporters   Alterations in dopamine transporter function and expression, which have been reported in humans and in animals after long-term cocaine exposure, may contribute to withdrawal states associated with the termination of cocaine use. However, inconsistencies in the changes reported have made the precise contributions of such adaptations difficult to ascertain.

Regulation of GABA$_A$ and NMDA receptors by ethanol   Changes in ion channel function and altered expression of GABA$_A$ and NMDA receptor subunits are the adaptations most often cited in connection with behavioral consequences of long-term ethanol exposure. Long-term use of ethanol decreases benzodiazepine- and ethanol-induced enhancement of GABA$_A$-mediated responses; such findings suggest that ethanol produces a change in the GABA$_A$ receptor. The nature of this change has remained elusive, despite intensive investigation. It has been hypothesized that long-term ethanol exposure alters the expression of specific GABA$_A$ receptor subunits in discrete brain regions; however, the functional implications of such alterations are not yet clear, and ethanol-induced changes in GABA$_A$ receptor function can occur in the absence of detectable changes in subunit expression. Thus other modifications, such as phosphorylation, may produce relevant changes in the receptor, but none of these has been established with certainty.

Regardless of the underlying mechanism, ethanol-induced decreases in GABA$_A$ receptor sensitivity are believed to contribute to ethanol tolerance. Decreased receptor sensitivity also may mediate some aspects of physical dependence on ethanol (see Chapter 15). However, whether these changes contribute to aversive symptoms that occur during ethanol withdrawal remains unknown.

The NMDA receptor complex also undergoes adaptive changes in response to long-term ethanol exposure, which appear to significantly contribute to physical dependence. Long-term use of ethanol has been reported to increase the number of binding sites for NMDA receptor ligands and also the magnitude of NMDA-mediated Ca^{2+} fluxes in certain brain regions. Increases in protein and mRNA for specific NMDA receptor subunits may mediate some of these ethanol-induced changes. Increased NMDA receptor function parallels the time course for seizure susceptibility in animals during ethanol withdrawal; this phenomenon may also explain the reduction in withdrawal signs that occurs after the administration of NMDA antagonists. Ethanol-induced up-regulation of the NMDA receptor complex also has been speculated to contribute to the changes in mesolimbic dopamine function that are associated with ethanol withdrawal.

Drug regulation of CRF   Corticotropin-releasing factor (CRF) is a neuropeptide that is expressed in neurons of the hypothalamus, central nucleus of the amygdala, and other brain regions (see Chapter 10). It plays an important role in stress responses and has been implicated in anxiety states (see Chapters 13 and 15). Moreover, recent studies have implicated CRF systems in the mediation of many of the anxiogenic and aversive aspects of drug withdrawal. Increased release of CRF, particularly in the central nucleus of the amygdala, occurs during withdrawal from ethanol, opiates, cocaine, and cannabinoids. Accordingly, **CRF antagonists** have successfully reversed the aversive effects of cocaine, ethanol, and opiate withdrawal in laboratory animals, a finding that has led to the current evaluation of these compounds as agents for use in the treatment of withdrawal states.

Glutamatergic regulation of drug-induced adaptations   The development of opiate tolerance and dependence has been reported to depend on glutamatergic transmission. Coadministration of competitive or noncompetitive antagonists of NMDA glutamate receptors, under certain experimental conditions, can block both tolerance to the analgesic effects of opiates and the development of physical dependence on opiates; moreover, by implication they are proposed to block emotional–motivational dependence as well. Such antagonists also can block the locomotor sensitization to psychostimulants and opiates that occurs after repeated drug administration. The effects of NMDA antagonists on opiate tolerance may involve nitric oxide because the inhibition of nitric oxide production—for example, by pharmacologic inhibition of nitric oxide synthase (see Chapter 5)—blocks the development of tolerance.

Interactions between NMDA antagonists and opiates or psychostimulants most likely are quite complex, and the coadministration of these agents may lead to complications. Like other addictive drugs, NMDA antagonists have powerful stimulant and reinforcing effects of their own and can potentiate the stimulant and reinforcing effects of other addictive drugs. Consequently, long-term coadministration of an NMDA antagonist with an opiate or psychostimulant may potentiate the addictiveness of both drugs, regardless of effects on tolerance and dependence per se. Functional interactions between dopaminergic and glutamatergic transmission in striatal and cortical regions of the brain have received a great deal of attention, and related findings should help to explain how NMDA antagonists modify responses to these and other addictive drugs.

OTHER MECHANISMS RELATED TO TOLERANCE

Many of the mechanisms underlying tolerance appear to overlap with those underlying dependence; for example, the up-regulation of the cAMP pathway in the LC in response to long-term use of morphine, which has been implicated in physical dependence, also may contribute to tolerance because this adaptation opposes the inhibitory effects of opiates on adenylyl cyclase in these neurons. However, additional mechanisms appear to underlie tolerance to morphine because opiate effects that are not mediated by the inhibition of adenylyl cyclase—for example, the activation of K^+ channels—also exhibit tolerance. One mechanism that has received a great deal of attention is the functional uncoupling of opioid receptors from their G proteins. Such uncoupling may involve phosphorylation-mediated changes in affinities of the receptors or in their G proteins that may decrease their functional interaction. Such phosphorylation may be mediated by cAMP- or Ca^{2+}-dependent protein kinases or by G protein receptor kinases (GRKs), all of which are known to be regulated by opiate exposure. As explained in Chapter 5, GRKs phosphorylate agonist-bound forms of G protein-coupled receptors, including opioid receptors, and can contribute to receptor internalization and desensitization. The efficacy of opioid receptor transduction also might be reduced by drug-induced alterations in levels of relevant G proteins. Long-term exposure to opiates or cocaine has been demonstrated to decrease the expression of G_i and G_o α subunits in specific brain regions, including the NAc. The $G_{i/o}$ family of G proteins represents the primary coupling mechanisms for opioid, D_2-like dopamine, and CB_1 receptors and may represent an important common substrate for drug-induced alterations in signal transduction in these receptor systems.

Tolerance also may be mediated by a host of other proteins that modulate receptor–G protein interactions. RGS proteins (regulators of G protein signaling), for example, control the functioning of G protein α subunits by regulating the GTPase activity intrinsic to such subunits (see Chapter 5). Opiate-induced increases in levels of these proteins in specific brain regions might be expected to contribute to a state of tolerance. Such mechanisms are currently undergoing investigation.

Tolerance to nicotine is believed to involve yet another receptor-mediated mechanism. Long-term exposure to nicotine increases the number of nACh receptors in most brain regions. This change most likely reflects the stabilization of receptor subunits because no related change in mRNA expression has been detected. Despite this increase in receptor number, most studies indicate that exposure to nicotine decreases the functional responsiveness of the receptors. Thus it appears that tolerance is related to a desensitization of receptors caused by the persistent presence of nicotine (see Chapter 12).

SPECIFICITY OF NEURAL SUBSTRATES THAT UNDERLIE DEPENDENCE

Although the nature and sites of adaptations critical to emotional–motivational dependence have not been determined with certainty, the neural substrates for this type of dependence appear to be at least partly distinct from those that mediate physical aspects of dependence. An examination of the neural substrates that underlie dependence on opiates can be used to illustrate such distinctions. As previously discussed, drug-induced adaptations in the LC mediate some aspects of physical dependence, and opiate antagonists injected into the LC can produce physical withdrawal symptoms. However, the LC appears to be less involved in motivational aspects of opiate withdrawal, and opiate antagonists injected into the LC do not alter reinforcement. Conversely, the mesolimbic dopamine system, which mediates reinforcement, does not significantly mediate physical signs of dependence. Moreover, administration of an opiate antagonist into the NAc interferes with opiate reinforcement but does not produce a marked physical withdrawal syndrome. Further evidence for distinct neural substrates for emotional–motivational versus physical opiate dependence has been drawn from studies of mice that lack D_2 dopamine receptors. These mice develop physical dependence on opiates but exhibit markedly reduced rewarding responses to these drugs.

LINK BETWEEN DRUG CRAVING AND RELAPSE OF ADDICTION

Drug-taking behavior associated with addiction is sustained by: 1) the reinforcement produced by drug exposure, and 2) the motivation to alleviate withdrawal-related distress. However, symptoms of both physical and emotional–motivational dependence subside relatively rapidly after drug use is terminated and cannot account for the high incidence of relapse among users of addictive drugs, particularly after signs of withdrawal have long subsided. Drug craving, which can be defined as the desire to reexperience the effects of a psychoactive substance, has been hypothesized to motivate drug seeking during the development of addiction, and also to trigger relapse in response to stress or conditioned stimuli even after years of abstinence. Accordingly, it has been hypothesized that withdrawal-related distress may reflect the presence of homeostatic adaptations in mesolimbic reward circuits that reverse over weeks or months, whereas late relapse may reflect relatively permanent synaptic remodeling in the same regions of the brain or in different regions. This hypothesis is discussed in greater detail in the section that follows.

SENSITIZATION OF NEURAL PROCESSES MAY UNDERLIE DRUG CRAVING

Drug craving can intensify with repeated drug use and can persist during prolonged periods of drug abstinence. Unlike the homeostatic types of adaptations that are believed to underlie tolerance and dependence, the intensification of drug craving is hypothesized to involve adaptations that augment rather than counteract drug reinforcement. It is proposed that sensitization of neural processes related to drug craving, or to environmental stimuli associated with drugs (known as cues), leads to the progressive increase in drug-seeking behavior that characterizes addiction. Such sensitization appears to increase the attractiveness of drug taking and that of drug-associated stimuli.

Sensitization of some drug-responsive systems has been demonstrated in rodents after repeated exposure to addictive drugs and drug-associated stimuli. Well-characterized behavioral sensitization, involving an increase in locomotor activity and the development of stereotyped movements, has been observed after repeated intermittent administration of psychostimulants. Similar locomotor sensitization also has been observed in rodents after repeated administration of opiates, nicotine, ethanol, and PCP. Moreover, cross-sensitization to many of these agents occurs and is consistent with the involvement of common neurobiologic mechanisms.

Because the precise molecular and cellular mechanisms underlying drug-seeking behavior are unknown, it is difficult to demonstrate the extent to which sensitization contributes to an increase in this behavior. However, the desire for a drug is clearly different from the initial rewarding aspect of drug action; indeed, addiction continues in many cases after drugs have lost some of their associated euphoria as a result of tolerance or illness (e.g., alcoholic gastritis, lung cancer, AIDS).

MECHANISMS OF SENSITIZATION

The reinforcing effects of addictive drugs are subject to sensitization. Repeated systemic or intra-VTA administration of psychostimulants, opiates, or ethanol causes a progressive enhancement of their reinforcing actions. Sensitization resulting from such administration requires persistent activation of the mesolimbic dopamine system. Because activation of this system is implicated in initial drug reinforcement, the sensitization observed with repeated drug administration might be mediated by changes in the mesolimbic dopamine system that enhance its responsiveness to subsequent drug exposure.

Adaptations in the VTA   Effects of drugs on the VTA appear to contribute significantly to the *induction* of behavioral sensitization. Morphine or amphetamine injected locally into the VTA can enhance drug-induced behavioral responses, and intra-VTA injections of dopamine antagonists can block the ability of systemic amphetamine to produce sensitization. In contrast, drugs injected locally into the NAc are ineffective in producing sensitization of behavioral responses. Induction of behavioral sensitization in the VTA may involve D_2 autoreceptor subsensitivity. The receptors themselves do not appear to be down-regulated, but levels of G proteins that transduce the D_2 signal ($G_{i/o}$ α subunits) are decreased transiently in the VTA after long-term drug treatment, a finding that suggests an intracellular mechanism for decreased receptor function. Moreover, experimental inactivation of these G proteins with **pertussis toxin** (see Chapter 5) can cause behavioral sensitization to subsequently administered cocaine. Such sensitization can persist even after G protein levels return to baseline; thus short-lived changes in G proteins may play a role in the induction of but not in the expression of behavioral sensitization to psychostimulants.

Long-term drug treatment also produces adaptations in the VTA's glutamate system that may be relevant to the sensitization of drug responses. Long-term psychostimulant administration increases the responsiveness of VTA dopaminergic neurons to AMPA glutamate receptor stimulation. A mechanism underlying this effect may be drug-induced increases in the expression of certain AMPA subunits, which has been observed after long-term treatment with cocaine, opiates, and ethanol. The selective experimental overexpression of AMPA receptor subunits in VTA neurons has been shown to sensitize animals to locomotor-activating and reinforcing effects of morphine, which further suggests that changes in AMPA receptors contribute to sensitization.

Adaptations in the nucleus accumbens Enhanced drug-induced dopamine release in the NAc, a measure of enhanced mesolimbic dopamine activity, can persist for weeks in association with behavioral sensitization after long-term psychostimulant or opiate treatment. The molecular mechanism that underlies such facilitation of dopamine release is unknown but may be related to the adaptations in dopaminergic cell bodies outlined in this chapter.

The previously mentioned up-regulation of the cAMP pathway in the NAc that commonly occurs after long-term use of psychostimulants, opiates, or ethanol also may underlie associated behavioral sensitization. This possibility is supported by the observation that experimentally induced increases in activity in the cAMP pathway increase locomotor responses to cocaine and amphetamine and enhance the development of locomotor sensitization. Such increases also enhance the rewarding effects of psychostimulants in the conditioned reinforcement paradigm.

An increase in functional D_1 receptor sensitivity has been observed electrophysiologically in the NAc after long-term cocaine or amphetamine treatment and also may be related to drug-induced up-regulation of the cAMP pathway in the NAc. This increase in D_1 sensitivity occurs in the absence of measurable changes in receptor number or affinity. Because stimulation of D_1 receptors activates the cAMP pathway through G_s, an up-regulated cAMP pathway may augment the effects of D_1 stimulation and produce this functional change. However, behavioral sensitization to D_1 receptor activation most likely does not mediate sensitization of drug craving. As explained later in this chapter, cocaine-seeking behavior in animals is not stimulated by D_1 agonists or by experimentally induced enhancement of the cAMP pathway. Instead, cocaine craving is triggered or enhanced by D_2 agonists and also by experimentally induced inhibition of the cAMP pathway.

Sensitization to psychostimulants is associated with a reduction in the excitability of NAc neurons, which is manifested by reduced responses to AMPA glutamate receptor stimulation and by a reduction in the activity of voltage-gated Na^+ channels. Such adaptations may be mediated by altered expression of specific AMPA subunits and by increased phosphorylation of Na^+ channels by protein kinase A, respectively. These findings underscore the association between reinforcement and reduced excitability of NAc medium spiny neurons, and indicate that long-term reductions in such excitability may contribute to sensitization.

Duration and conditioning of sensitization Behavioral sensitization is long-lasting. Sensitization resulting from single injections of amphetamine, cocaine, or morphine can last for months, and sensitization induced with repeated and escalating doses of amphetamines can last as long as 1 year in rodents. The development of sensitization also can be influenced by environmental factors; indeed as previously mentioned, conditioned responses assist in promoting addictive behavior. One of the major challenges in drug abuse research today is to identify the mechanisms that underlie such long-lasting changes. As with other areas of neuroscience research, such as those focused on learning and memory, efforts are directed toward understanding experience-dependent plasticity. It is hoped that current studies of alterations in gene expression and attendant changes in synaptic structure may lead to the discovery of plausible mechanisms by which the brain undergoes stable changes related to sensitization.

IMPACT OF GENE EXPRESSION ON LONG-LASTING ADAPTATIONS

Regulation of gene expression has been pursued as a mechanism that may be responsible for the mediation of long-lasting features of addiction. Accordingly, it has been hypothesized that drug-induced changes in transcriptional regulatory machinery (e.g., transcription factors) may lead to the altered expression of specific target genes, which in turn may underlie the long-lasting behavioral abnormalities that characterize addiction. Although such a scheme might explain the involvement of gene expression in the initiation of the addiction process, it fails to explain how related alterations in gene expression are sustained long after drug use ceases. The previously discussed drug regulation of CREB highlights these issues. Long-term drug exposure causes changes in CREB function in the LC and NAc, among other brain regions. However, the resulting changes in gene expression, like the changes in CREB itself, are relatively short-lived and have been implicated in aspects of dependence that resolve within weeks of drug abstinence.

The discovery that the transcription factor ΔFosB has a long life has provided insight into one cause of sustained drug-induced alterations in gene expression. In contrast to all other members of the Fos family of transcription factors, which are induced rapidly and transiently in response to various perturbations, ΔFosB is induced only slightly by initial stimuli (see Chapter 6). However, with repeated stimulation, ΔFosB begins to accumulate in neurons because of its remarkable stability. This phenomenon occurs with many classes of addictive drugs. Long-term, but not short-term, administration of cocaine, amphetamine, opiates, nicotine, ethanol, or PCP has been proven to induce ΔFosB in the NAc and in related striatal regions. This induction appears to occur selectively within the dynorphin- and substance P-containing subset of GABAergic medium spiny neurons, and only addictive drugs induce ΔFosB in these cells. Long-term exposure to **antipsychotic** drugs, for example, induces ΔFosB in the NAc and in the dorsal striatum but in a different class of medium spiny neurons. Recent studies involving the selective expression of ΔFosB in dynorphin- and substance P-containing medium spiny neurons in adult mice has provided direct evidence that induction of ΔFosB in these neurons per se can cause sensitized behavioral responses to drugs of abuse.

The accumulation of ΔFosB after long-term drug exposure is interesting because it represents a molecular mechanism by which drug-induced changes in gene expression can persist long after drug use has been discontinued; future research is likely to reveal many additional mechanisms underlying such long-lived changes. Despite evidence that supports the involvement of ΔFosB in persistent changes in gene expression, the target genes through which ΔFosB and other stable transcriptional mechanisms exert their effects on neural and behavioral plasticity remain unknown. Among the many gene products targeted by ΔFosB in the NAc appear to be certain AMPA glutamate receptor subunits; indeed, such targets might explain how long-term cocaine use alters AMPA responses in these neurons. It is important to emphasize that ΔFosB, although stable, does undergo proteolysis at a finite rate; thus it cannot mediate the life-long changes in behavior that accompany addiction. Rather, these semipermanent changes, which are perhaps best viewed as memories, may involve alterations in neuronal morphology and synaptic structure initiated by more transient regulation of transcription factors.

ADAPTATIONS IN NEURONAL MORPHOLOGY AND SURVIVAL

Increasing evidence from studies of learning and memory suggests that changes in gene expression can lead to alterations in neuronal function through corresponding changes in neuronal structure. Such changes may affect the shape and size of specific neurons, the number of synaptic connections they form, and their survival.

Of the changes that impact neuronal survival in the context of drug addiction, the best established are neuronal injury and neuronal death. These can be elicited by a single dose of any of several amphetamine derivatives. **Methamphetamine**, for example, is directly toxic to dopaminergic neurons, and **MDMA** is toxic to serotonergic neurons. The mechanisms that underlie such toxicity are unknown, but appear to involve the selective uptake of these drugs (by means of dopamine and serotonin transporters, respectively) into the monoaminergic neurons, which are then vulnerable to oxidative injury caused by drug metabolites.

In contrast to amphetamine derivatives, most other drugs of abuse, including opiates, cocaine, alcohol, cannabinoids, and nicotine do not appear to produce overt damage to specific neurons in the brain, even after long-term administration. Yet evidence suggests that these drugs produce more subtle changes in neuronal structure and morphology. Long-term exposure to opiates or cocaine decreases levels of neuron-specific intermediate filament proteins and increases levels of glial-specific intermediate filament proteins in the VTA. As might be expected, these adaptations are associated with reduced axoplasmic transport from the VTA to the NAc, and with a reduction in the size of dopaminergic neurons in the VTA. Knowledge of the functional consequences of these adaptations is incomplete. Such adaptations might, for example, reflect an impairment of mesolimbic dopamine function, which in turn might contribute to aversive withdrawal states; moreover, these adaptations might serve to compensate for repeated activation of dopamine neurons by a drug. However, it is critical to emphasize that no direct evidence supports these interpretations. Indeed, as discussed further in a subsequent section of this chapter, considerable evidence suggests that long-term administration of **methadone**, an opioid receptor agonist, produces no lasting damage in humans.

A particularly interesting and long-lasting example of a structural change associated with exposure to an addictive drug is the modification in dendritic structure that has been observed in cells of the NAc and prefrontal cortex after repeated psychostimulant administration. These structural changes consist of increases in the length and degree of branching of dendrites and in the density of dendritic spines, and suggest altered synaptic connectivity. Long-term administration of morphine produces opposite changes. Such changes, which may be important mediators of long-term behavioral alterations (e.g., sensitization) after repeated drug exposure, do not represent toxic effects; rather they appear to be identical to changes that are postulated to underlie experience-dependent plasticity (e.g., learning) in brain regions such as the hippocampus (see Chapter 20).

Drug-induced adaptations in neuronal morphology raise the interesting possibility that neurotrophic factors may in some way be involved in drug addiction. Indeed, infusions of certain neurotrophic factors, such as brain-derived neurotrophic factor (BDNF) or glial-derived neurotrophic factor (GDNF), into the VTA prevent and reverse specific molecular adaptations to long-term opiate or cocaine administration. Such infusions also prevent the drug-induced morphologic changes that occur in dopaminergic neurons of the VTA. Accordingly, it is possible that medications designed to target neurotrophic factors or their signaling pathways might be useful in the treatment of addictive disorders.

ADAPTATIONS RELEVANT TO CONDITIONED CRAVING AND RELAPSE OF ADDICTION

A long-term feature of drug addiction that can be quantified in animal models is relapse, or the reinstatement of previously learned drug-seeking behaviors after a period of abstinence. In animals, exposure to a drug of abuse, to stimuli associated with that drug, or to stress can potently reactivate drug-seeking behavior. In fact, animal research and clinical experience have indicated that, under certain circumstances, drug-associated stim-uli and stress can induce drug-seeking behavior even more dramatically than exposure to the drug itself.

Animal models have enabled the identification of some neurobiologic mechanisms responsible for the reinstatement of drug-seeking behavior. Some of the neural pathways that are implicated in mediating responses to drug-associated stimuli and stress, and in mediating relapse of addiction, are represented in Figure 16–6. Not surprisingly, psychostimulants induce drug-seeking behavior by activating the mesolimbic dopamine system, a finding that supports the close relationship between mechanisms relevant to relapse and those related to drug reinforcement. Effects of the mesolimbic dopamine system on drug-seeking behavior appear to be achieved through the activation of D_2 dopamine receptors and the inhibition of protein kinase A in the NAc; the activation of D_1 receptors does not underlie these effects. In fact, D_1 receptor agonists are reported to diminish the drug-seeking behavior induced by psychostimulants. This finding, which is surprising because D_1 agonists themselves can be reinforcing, suggests that D_1 and D_2 receptors may make qualitatively

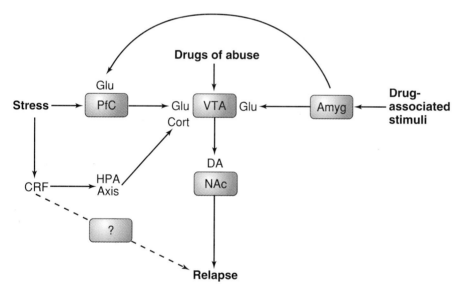

Figure 16–6. Primary pathways through which stress, drugs of abuse, and drug-associated stimuli are hypothesized to trigger relapse of drug-seeking behavior. Stress and drug-associated stimuli activate excitatory glutamate (Glu) projections to the VTA from the prefrontal cortex (PfC) and amygdala (Amyg), respectively. Drugs of abuse stimulate dopamine (DA) release from dopaminergic neurons of the VTA that project to the nucleus accumbens (NAc). Projections from the amygdala to the prefrontal cortex represent a secondary pathway through which drug-associated stimuli may access dopaminergic neurons of the VTA. Stress-induced relapse may involve corticotropin releasing factor (CRF) and the hypothalamic–pituitary–adrenal (HPA) axis, and subsequently, the activation of VTA dopaminergic neurons by means of corticosterone (Cort) secretion. Although dopamine release in the NAc may be the common neurochemical event by which all three stimuli trigger relapse, stress and CRF also may act on unknown brain regions by means of dopamine-independent mechanisms to cause a return to drug-seeking behavior. (From Self DW, Nestler EJ. 1998. *Drug Alcohol Depend* 51:49.)

different contributions to the mechanisms of reinforcement and reward. Such differences may be related to the different cellular locations of these receptor subtypes in the NAc and to their different roles in NAc circuits.

Stimulation of drug-seeking behavior by drug-associated stimuli and stress is believed to be mediated by dopamine-dependent and dopamine-independent mechanisms. The mechanisms that depend on dopamine are becoming increasingly well understood (see Figure 16–6). Drug-associated stimuli are believed to activate circuits of the amygdala, which are implicated in memories of emotionally salient events. The amygdala, in turn, is believed to activate dopaminergic neurons of the VTA directly, by means of glutamatergic or CRF inputs, and indirectly, through the prefrontal cortex. Stress is believed to activate the mesolimbic dopamine system through effects on the prefrontal cortex, amygdala, and hypothalamic–pituitary–adrenal (HPA) axis (see Chapter 13). The effect of stress-induced activation of the HPA axis may be mediated by CRF or by increased levels of circulating glucocorticoids.

TREATMENT OF ADDICTION

The primary goals of addiction treatment are the facilitation of abstinence and the prevention of relapse. Such goals have proven difficult to attain in the treatment of many forms of addiction; indeed, maintenance on long-acting opiates has been accepted as an alternative to abstinence for many opiate-addicted individuals. Pharmacologic treatment often is used to reduce withdrawal symptoms, but thus far has not been effective in preventing relapse. The potential for relapse lasts longer than withdrawal symptoms and involves complex mechanisms that include associative learning. Yet it remains a theoretical possibility that medications that block the reinforcing effects of drugs or drug-induced plasticity might reduce drug craving and the likelihood of relapse. Such medications might prove to be effective if they can act without producing potent reinforcing or anhedonic effects by themselves, and if they can exert their beneficial effects without interfering with the body's responsiveness to natural rewards. Unfortunately, with the exception of naltrexone, which is only partly efficacious in the treatment of alcoholism, no reward-reducing drug treatment has yet been developed for clinical use.

PSYCHOSTIMULANTS

Pharmacologic treatment for psychostimulant addiction is generally unsatisfactory. As previously discussed, cessation of cocaine use and the use of other psycho-

stimulants in dependent individuals does not produce a physical withdrawal syndrome but may produce dysphoria, anhedonia, and an intense desire to reinitiate drug use. In rodents, withdrawal from these drugs is characterized by a greater threshold for brain stimulation reward, which may represent a model of anhedonia. It has been hypothesized that these symptoms result from the decreased responsiveness of the mesolimbic dopamine system that is characteristic of withdrawal from psychostimulants; accordingly it has been postulated that dopamine agonists might ameliorate such symptoms and that these agents might be clinically useful as long as they are not themselves highly reinforcing. Unfortunately, dopamine D_2 agonists such as **bromocriptine** and the weak dopamine indirect agonist **amantadine** have been unimpressive clinically. Dopamine D_1 agonists, which have shown some promise in animal models, have not yet been adequately tested in clinical trials.

Desipramine, a tricyclic antidepressant and a relatively selective inhibitor of norepinephrine reuptake (see Chapter 15), also has been used to ameliorate dysphoric mood and other depression-like symptoms but has not proven to be especially effective. Selective serotonin reuptake inhibitors (SSRIs), such as **fluoxetine** and **sertraline,** have been tested clinically and also have proven to be disappointing. Thus far the 5-$HT_{2A/2C}$ receptor antagonist, **ritanserin,** and several other serotonin-based drugs, including 5-HT_{1A} partial agonists such as **buspirone,** have proven to be ineffective as well.

Attempts also have been made to immunize animals to cocaine, and thereby decrease the bioavailability of subsequently administered drug. Such immunotherapy remains controversial for drugs such as cocaine that already have an extremely short half-life; it also would be selective for one type of drug, such as cocaine, and would not work for a replacement drug such as amphetamine. However, investigators hope to develop a medication that might bind to the cocaine-binding site on the dopamine transporter and thereby block the binding of cocaine, without affecting transporter function. Whether it will be possible to develop such a cocaine antagonist remains unknown. Currently, cognitive–behavioral therapies are the most successful treatment available for preventing the relapse of psychostimulant use.

OPIATES

Treatment of opiate addiction is two-fold. The first and most straightforward step involves the detoxification of an addicted patient, which is undertaken with an effort to minimize physical withdrawal symptoms. The second, and far more difficult, step involves the treatment of emotional–motivational symptoms of withdrawal and efforts that enable the patient to maintain abstinence. One type of detoxification involves the substitution of a safer drug. For example, a long-acting opiate agonist, such as **methadone,** may be substituted for heroin, which has a much shorter half-life (Figure 16–7); subsequently the methadone may be slowly tapered. An alternative approach involves the use of an α_2-adrenergic receptor agonist, such as **clonidine,** which acts in part on autoreceptors of neurons in the LC to counteract the previously discussed rebound hyperactivity implicated in physical withdrawal syndromes. Clonidine permits a relatively comfortable and

rapid withdrawal from methadone and other opiates. Its use also is compatible with the administration of an opioid receptor antagonist, such as **naltrexone,** in rapid detoxification protocols. In the absence of clonidine, naltrexone precipitates a very severe and intolerable withdrawal syndrome.

A long-acting opiate antagonist, naltrexone has been used not only for detoxification but also to prevent relapse in detoxified opiate users. Morning use of naltrexone blocks the euphoria that accompanies heroin or other opiates, in the event that these are administered during the day; thus relapse to active drug use is less likely if a dose of heroin is taken impulsively. Over

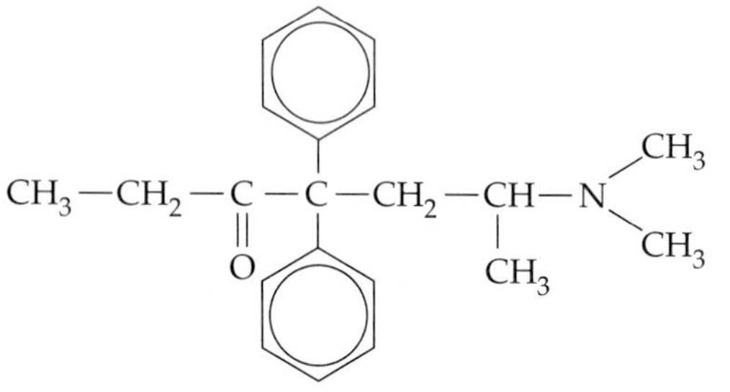

Methadone
(long-acting agonist)

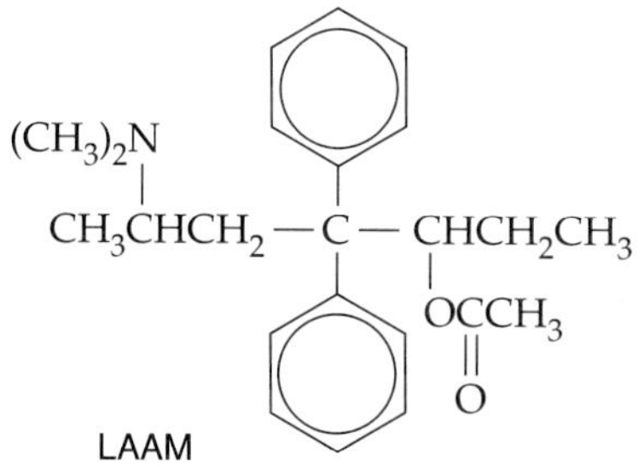

LAAM
(extended-duration agonist)

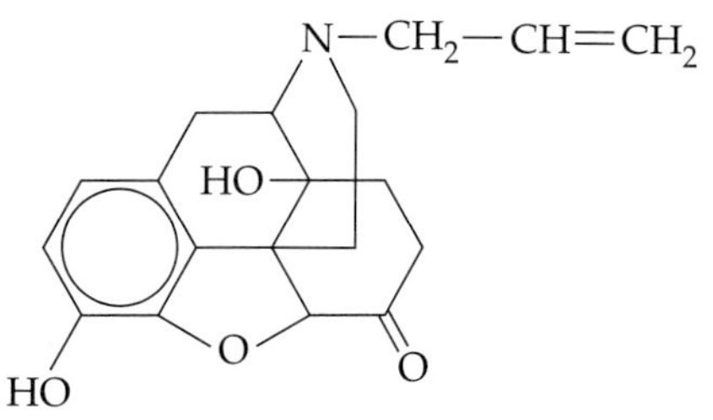

Naloxone
(antagonist)

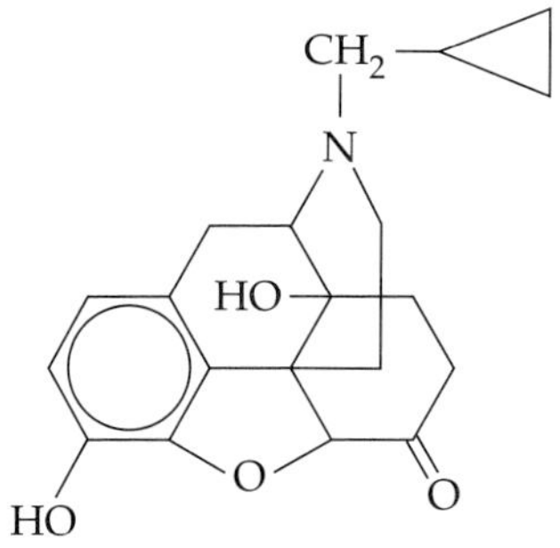

Naltrexone
(antagonist)

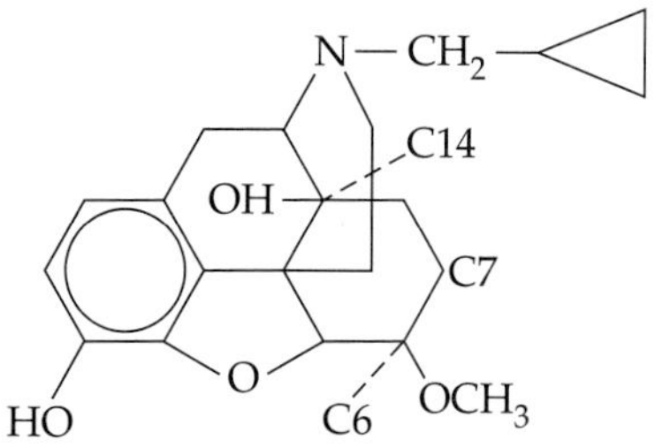

Buprenorphine
(partial agonist)

Figure 16–7. Chemical structures of some clinically useful opioid receptor agonists and antagonists. (See Chapter 19 for structures of opiate agonists used in the treatment of pain.)

time this treatment also may help extinguish the association of drug-taking behaviors with reinforcement. However, the clinical use of naltrexone is limited because it is associated with low rates of compliance, which have been well documented. Moreover, opiate addicts often report that naltrexone induces dysphoria. An alternative agent is **buprenorphine,** a partial μ opioid receptor agonist. This drug, which has only mild reinforcing effects by itself, blocks the effects of heroin by binding to the μ receptor and does not produce dysphoria (see Figure 16–7).

Many opiate addicts cannot achieve abstinence. For these individuals, pharmacologic treatment involves maintenance on a long-acting oral opiate, such as levo-α-acetylmethadol (**LAAM**) or **methadone** (see Figure 16–7). Such treatment has several advantages. It suppresses craving and drug-seeking behavior, and limits intravenous drug use and associated risks of hepatitis and AIDS. Moreover, by smoothing out the peaks and valleys that often characterize heroin use, and blocking the urge to seek heroin during the day, this treatment facilitates rehabilitation and increases an individual's ability to sustain employment and stabilize social relationships. Methadone and LAAM are generally administered in the context of highly structured psychosocial interventions.

ALCOHOL

Detoxification from alcohol typically involves the administration of benzodiazepines such as **chlordiazepoxide,** which exhibit cross-dependence with ethanol at $GABA_A$ receptors (see Chapters 7 and 15). A dose that will prevent the physical symptoms associated with withdrawal from ethanol, including tachycardia, hypertension, tremor, agitation, and seizures, is given and is slowly tapered. Benzodiazepines are used because they are less reinforcing than ethanol among alcoholics. Moreover, the tapered use of a benzodiazepine with a long half-life makes the emergence of withdrawal symptoms less likely than direct withdrawal from ethanol.

Several pharmacologic agents intended for use in conjunction with psychosocial therapies have been examined for their efficacy in the prevention of relapse. Two drugs in particular—**naltrexone** and **acamprosate**—have shown promise in clinical trials and in clinical practice. Animal studies that have linked alcohol reinforcement to endogenous opioid systems have supported the use of naltrexone (and a less well-studied opiate antagonist known as **nalmefene**) to prevent recurring alcohol addiction. In several clinical trials, naltrexone reduced both the risk of a return to heavy drinking and the overall frequency of drinking, compared with placebo. However, its use in these trials was not associated with a higher rate of total abstinence.

European studies suggest that acamprosate decreases both the frequency of drinking and relapse; yet its mechanism of action remains unknown. Acamprosate is a homotaurine derivative that has some structural similarities to GABA but is not associated with significant activity at GABA receptors. It clearly modulates NMDA receptor function in rodents in a complicated manner that involves the facilitation of the receptors in some regions of the brain, and antagonistic effects in other regions.

Other pharmacotherapies have shown less clinical efficacy. **Disulfiram** irreversibly inhibits aldehyde dehydrogenase, and thereby leads to the buildup of the toxic compound acetaldehyde after alcohol consumption. The alcohol–disulfiram reaction is characterized by flushing, dizziness, nausea, and vomiting. The rationale for disulfiram use is that it devalues alcohol consumption by associating alcohol use with a strongly aversive experience. Yet clinical trial data do not support the use of disulfiram in most cases; although the drug may decrease total drinking days for some individuals, it is not effective in preventing a return to heavy drinking. In addition, the alcohol–disulfiram reaction may produce serious morbidity, including severe hypotension. Some clinicians believe that disulfiram may be useful in selected, highly motivated patients. Studies have evaluated the use of **lithium** or **SSRI** antidepressants in the prevention of relapse, but clinical trial data do not support the use of either of these agents.

SELECTED READING

Berke JD, Hyman SE. 2000. Addiction, dopamine, and the molecular mechanisms of memory. *Neuron* 25:515–532.

Bohn LM, Gainetdinov RR, Lin F-T, et al. 2000. μ-Opioid receptor desensitization by β-arrestin-2 determines morphine tolerance but not dependence. *Nature* 408: 720–723.

Bowman EM, Aigner TG, Richmond BJ. 1996. Neural signals in monkey ventral striatum related to motivation for juice and cocaine rewards. *J Neurophysiol* 75:1061–1073.

Breiter HC, Gollub RL, Weisskoff RM, et al. 1997. Acute effects of cocaine on human brain activity and emotion. *Neuron* 19:591–611.

Cadet JL, Ali SF, Rothman RB, Epstein CJ. 1995. Neurotoxicity, drugs and abuse, and the CuZn–superoxide dismutase transgenic mice. *Mol Neurobiol* 11:155–163.

Carlezon WA Jr, Wise RA. 1996. Rewarding actions of phencyclidine and related drugs in nucleus accumbens shell and frontal cortex. *J Neurosci* 16:3112–3122.

Carlezon WA Jr, Thome J, Olson VG, et al. 1998. Regulation of cocaine reward by CREB. *Science* 282:2272–2275.

Crabbe JC, Phillips TJ, Buck KJ, et al. 1999. Identifying genes for alcohol and drug sensitivity: Recent progress and future directions. *Trends Neurosci* 22:173–179.

Everitt BJ, Parkinson JA, Olmstead MC, et al. 1999. Associative processes in addiction and reward. The role of amygdala-ventral striatal subsystems. *Ann NY Acad Sci* 877:412–438.

Gainetdinov RR, Jones SR, Caron MG. 1999. Functional hyperdopaminergia in dopamine transporter knock-out mice. *Biol Psychiatry* 46:303–311.

Garbutt JC, West SL, Carey TS, et al. 1999. Pharmacological treatment of alcohol dependence: A review of the evidence. *JAMA* 28:1318–1325.

Gardner EL. 1997. Brain reward mechanisms. In Lowinson JH, Ruiz P, Millman RB, Langrod JG (editors): *Substance Abuse: A Comprehensive Textbook*, 3rd ed. Baltimore: Williams and Wilkins, pp 51–85.

Giros B, Jaber M, Jones SR, et al. 1996. Hyperlocomotion and indifference to cocaine and amphetamine in mice lacking the dopamine transporter. *Nature* 379:606–612.

Harris RA, Mihic SJ, Valenzuela CF. 1998. Alcohol and benzodiazepines: Recent mechanistic studies. *Drug Alcohol Depend* 51:155–164.

Hyman S. 1996. Addiction to cocaine and amphetamine. *Neuron* 16:901–904.

Kalivas PW, Nakamura M. 1999. Neural systems for behavioral activation and reward. *Curr Opin Neurobiol* 9:223–227.

Kelz MB, Chen JS, Carlezon WA, et al. 1999. Expression of the transcription factor ΔFosB in the brain controls sensitivity to cocaine. *Nature* 401:272–276.

Kolesnikov Y, Pan Y–X, Babey A, et al. 1997. Functionally differentiating two neuronal nitric oxide synthase isoforms through antisense mapping: Evidence for opposing NO actions on morphine analgesia and tolerance. *Proc Natl Acad Sci USA* 94:8220–8225.

Koob GF, Sanna PP, Bloom FE. 1998. Neuroscience of addiction. *Neuron* 21:467–476.

Koob GF, Nestler EJ. 1997. The neurobiology of drug addiction. In Salloway S, Malloy P, Cummings JL (eds): *The Neuropsychiatry of Limbic and Subcortical Disorders*, pp 179–194. Washington, DC: American Psychiatric Press.

Kreek MJ, Koob GF. 1998. Drug dependence: Stress and dysregulation of brain reward pathways. *Drug Alcohol Depend* 51:23–47.

Malonado R, Saiardi A, Valverde L, et al. 1997. Absence of opiate rewarding effects in mice lacking dopamine D$_2$ receptors. *Nature* 388:586–589.

Martin BR, Mechoulam R, Razdan RK. 1999. Discovery and characterization of endogenous cannabinoids. *Life Sci* 65:573–595.

Nesse R, Berridge KC. 1997. Psychoactive drug use in evolutionary perspective. *Science* 278:63–66.

Nestler EJ, Aghajanian GK. 1997. Molecular and cellular basis of addiction. *Science* 278:58–63.

Nestler EJ. 2000. Genes and addiction. *Nature Genet.* 26:277–281.

Nicola SM, Surmeier DJ, Malenka RC. 2000. Dopaminergic modulation of neuronal excitability in the striatum and nucleus accumbens. *Annu Rev Neurosci* 23:185–215.

O'Brien CP. 1997. A range of research-based pharmacotherapies for addiction. *Science* 278:66–70.

Olds J, Milner PM. 1954. Positive reinforcement produced by electrical stimulation of the septal area and other regions of rat brain. *J Comp Physiol* 47:419–427.

Picciotto M. 1998. Common aspects of the action of nicotine and other drugs of abuse. *Drug Alcohol Depend* 51:165–172.

Pontieri FE, Tanda G, DiChiara G. 1995. Intravenous cocaine, morphine, and amphetamine preferentially increase extracellular dopamine in the 'shell' as compared with the 'core' of the rat nucleus accumbens. *Proc Natl Acad Sci USA* 92:12304–12308.

Robinson TE, Berridge KC. 2000. The psychology and neurobiology of addiction: an incentive-sensitization view. *Addiction* 95(suppl):S91–S117

Robinson TE, Kolb B. 1997. Persistent structural modifications in nucleus accumbens and prefrontal cortex neurons produced by previous experience with amphetamine. *J Neurosci* 17:8491–8497.

Schultz W. 1997. Dopamine neurons and their role in reward mechanisms. *Curr Opin Neurobiol* 7:191–197.

Schultz W. 2000. Multiple reward signals in the brain. *Nature Rev Neurosci* 1:199–207.

Self DW, Nestler EJ. 1998. Relapse to drug-seeking: Neural and molecular mechanisms. *Drug Alcohol Depend* 51:49–60.

Spanagel R, Zieglgansberger W. 1997. Anti-craving compounds for ethanol: New pharmacological tools to study addictive processes *Trends Pharmacol Sci* 18:54–59.

Tabakoff BT, Hoffman PL. 1996. Alcohol addiction: An enigma among us. *Neuron* 16:909–912.

White FJ, Kalivas PW. 1998. Neuroadaptations involved in amphetamine and cocaine addiction. *Drug Alcohol Depend* 51:141–153.

Wise RA. 1998. Drug activation of brain reward pathways. *Drug Alcohol Depend* 51:13–22.

Wolf ME. 1998. The role of excitatory amino acids in behavioral sensitization to psychomotor stimulants. *Prog Neurobiol* 54:679–720.

Wolf ME. 1999. Cocaine addiction: Clues from *Drosophila* on drugs. *Curr Biol* 9:R770–R772.

Chapter 17

Higher Cognitive Function and Psychosis

KEY CONCEPTS

- The prefrontal cortex in higher primates (including humans) is particularly important for working memory, which is a cognitive buffer that allows an organism to maintain a representation based on recent sensory information and use it to plan future behavior.

- Schizophrenia, the most common cause of psychosis, is associated with positive symptoms such as hallucinations and delusions, negative symptoms including amotivation and social withdrawal, and cognitive deficits, such as poor working memory.

- The etiology of schizophrenia is unknown but likely involves a genetic predisposition, the manifestation of which depends on a complex set of environmental circumstances.

- High doses of psychostimulants (cocaine and amphetamine), which cause massive release of monoamine neurotransmitters, such as dopamine and serotonin, can induce a transient psychosis that mimics certain features (paranoid delusions) of schizophrenia.

- Dissociative anesthetics such as PCP also can induce a transient psychosis resembling schizophrenia. These drugs act by interfering with the function of the NMDA glutamate receptor.

- Hallucinogens such as LSD cause profound perceptual disturbances by interacting with a particular subtype of serotonin receptor.

- Cannabinoids, the principal active ingredients of marijuana, act on a specific G protein-coupled receptor found throughout the CNS. Anandamide, a derivative of arachidonic acid, may be an endogenous ligand of the cannabinoid receptor.

- The therapeutic action of classic antipsychotic agents, termed *neuroleptics*, correlates with their potency at antagonizing D_2 dopamine receptors, which also causes significant motor side effects (extrapyramidal symptoms). Other side effects of these drugs are due to their interactions with several other neurotransmitter receptor subtypes.

- Atypical antipsychotic drugs such as clozapine are more efficacious. They also have fewer side effects in many patients, possibly because they have high affinity for serotonin as well as dopamine receptors.

- The chronic adaptations of the brain to antipsychotic medications, rather than the immediate actions of these drugs on neurotransmitter receptors, are responsible for their therapeutic efficacy.

Previous chapters have examined neuropharmacology as it relates to the functioning of the brain, from the basic structure and function of individual neurons to the neural circuitry that provides for the basic physiologic integrity and stability of the organism in a changing and uncertain environment. In this chapter, the focus is on what might be considered *the mind.* In humans, the mind is responsible for such intangible areas of mental functioning as identity, meaning, value, and purpose. Such areas might seem impossible to understand in terms of underlying neural substrates; in fact, some have argued that a gap between the data yielded by neuroscience and the experience of consciousness will always exist.

However, as with every aspect of brain function discussed previously, complex functions ascribed to the mind are grounded in the neural circuitry of the brain. The fact that these functions are more complex simply means that the underlying circuitry is more complex and, consequently, more difficult to elucidate. Indeed, as the components of the mind are broken down into specific aspects of higher cognitive functioning, their neuroanatomic, neurophysiologic, and neurochemical bases become apparent.

NEUROANATOMY OF HIGHER COGNITION

The first functional neuroanatomic maps relied on experiments involving stimulation of the cerebral cortex and subsequent observation of motor activity and physiologic changes. Other experiments involved stimulation of sensory modalities and observation of cortical activity. In these types of investigations, areas of so-called *silent cortex,* which did not appear to be implicated in primary sensory or motor processing, were identified. Interestingly, studies of phylogenetically advanced species gradually revealed that such areas occupy a much larger portion of the cortex than originally believed. In humans, these so-called silent areas comprise much of the cortex. Of course, no area of cortex is truly silent and areas of the cortex not devoted to sensory or motor processing have long since been demonstrated to be involved in many forms of higher cognitive function and information processing. Such areas have come to be known as association cortex.

The association cortex comprises three major regions that serve distinct functions (Figure 17–1). Parietal–temporal–occipital association cortex, which receives input from a variety of sensory cortical areas, integrates and coordinates several types of sensory input and processes language. Paralimbic association cortex comprises the ventral surface of the frontal lobe, the medial surface of the parietal lobe, and the anterior portion of the temporal lobe and is involved in the processing of emotions (see Chapter 15). Prefrontal cortex is located in the anterior portion of the frontal lobe and includes the principal sulcus, the superior prefrontal convexity, and the inferior prefrontal convexity (Figure 17–2). The size of this area of the brain increases dramatically when the brains of lower mammals are compared with those of nonhuman primates and subsequently with those of humans (Figure 17–3). A precise understanding of the function of the prefrontal cortex is elusive, largely because the tasks it performs are so complex and thus difficult to study in animals. Human studies of lesions from strokes, tumors, and injury also are difficult to interpret, because such lesions are irregularly shaped and consequently involve different regions of

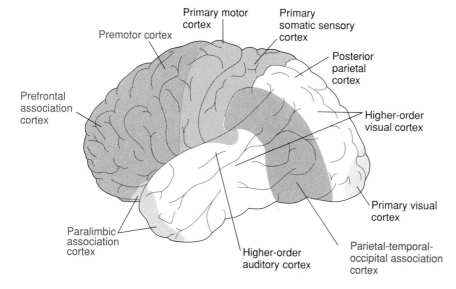

Figure 17–1. Diagram of the human brain showing major areas of association cortex. (Adapted with permission from Kandel ER, Schwartz JH, Jessel TM. 2000. *Principles of Neural Science,* 4th ed, p. 350. New York: McGraw-Hill.)

A Lateral view of monkey brain

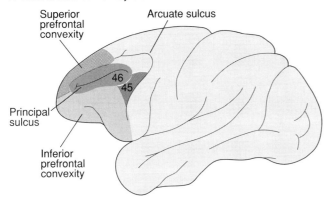

B Ventral view

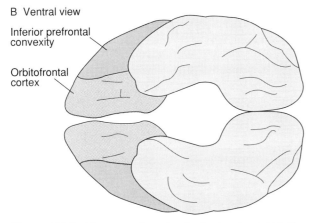

Figure 17–2. Diagrams of monkey brain showing areas of prefrontal cortex (Brodmann areas 45 and 46). **A,** Lateral view. **B,** Inferior view. (Adapted with permission from Kandel ER, Schwartz JH, Jessel TM. 2000. *Principles of Neural Science,* 4th ed, p. 357. New York: McGraw-Hill.)

prefrontal cortex. Nevertheless, based on what is known about this area of the brain, it is reasonable to hypothesize that it is critically important for mediating some of the functions associated with the mind.

WORKING MEMORY
AND COGNITIVE ABSTRACTION

In its most basic sense the nervous system can be thought of as a means by which an organism can sense and respond to its environment. An organism in need of nourishment can perceive food through any of several sensory modalities and respond appropriately with coordinated motor activity to obtain and ingest a meal. This fundamental sense–response relationship is at the core of nervous system functioning. In very simple organisms, this function takes the form of reflex action that occurs without any intermediate processing activity, let alone cognition.

In higher organisms, cognitive processes—many of which depend on memory—can intervene to modulate the response to a stimulus. Organisms learn to recognize that certain organisms are food and others are predators, and their responses to each are dramatically different. Mammals recognize other members of their family and respond with warmth and protection, whereas members of other families may be shunned or attacked. These behaviors are complex and represent a sophisticated integration of stored memories and ongoing sensory stimulation. Although none of these complex responses requires an internalized abstract image of prior sensory stimuli, each does require working memory.

Working memory is a cognitive buffer that allows an organism to maintain an image based on recent sensory

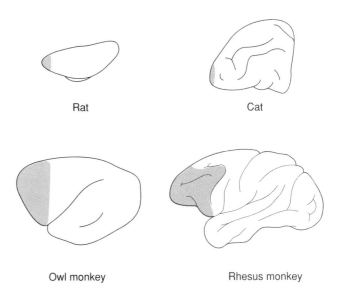

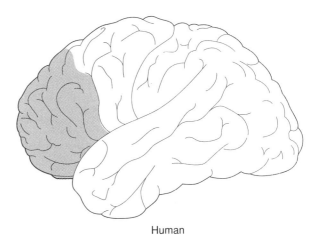

Figure 17–3. Phylogenetic comparison of the proportion of the brain taken up by frontal cortex in five different mammalian species. (Adapted with permission from Kandel ER, Schwartz JH, Jessel TM. 1991. *Principles of Neural Science,* 3rd ed, p. 837. New York: Elsevier.)

information, integrate it with a variety of cognitive and emotional associations, and use it to plan future behavior. Findings drawn from primate research have been used to explain working memory and its central role in higher cognition. A classic experiment involved the placement of bilateral lesions in the frontal association cortex of a chimpanzee and subsequent testing of the animal for delayed spatial responses. The chimpanzee watched as a piece of food was placed under one of several opaque containers. After a brief delay, the animal was allowed to choose a container. Unlesioned control animals uniformly chose the container with food, whereas lesioned animals made random selections. After several additional experiments were performed to determine the types of cognitive deficits involved, it became apparent that the ability to form and maintain a consistent internal image of the food and retain its significance without ongoing sensory stimulation was impaired in the lesioned chimpanzees. Yet the basic sensory and cognitive functions and short-term memory of these animals remained intact.

Our understanding of working memory has expanded considerably since these initial experiments. Subsequent studies, for example, have examined the electrical activity of particular neurons in prefrontal cortex in experimental paradigms that require working memory. In one such study, a monkey was conditioned to fix its eyes on a central point on a video screen. Subsequently a box was displayed briefly in one of eight areas on the screen. After a 3- to 6-second delay, the central fixation point was removed from the screen, and the monkey was trained to shift its gaze to the area where the box previously had been displayed. This study enabled the identification of neurons in prefrontal cortex that are specific for the region of the screen where the box was displayed. Such neurons become more active during the delay phase of the task and return to baseline levels of activity when the gaze returns to the area in which the box appeared. The increased activity of specific neurons during the delay phase appears to be an internal representation of the box, that is, a neural correlate of working memory.

The pharmacologic manipulation of working memory has been the focus of considerable investigation. In particular, investigators have been interested in the effect of dopamine on memory. Mild dopaminergic stimulation of the prefrontal cortex has been shown to enhance working memory; in contrast, higher levels of stimulation profoundly disrupt this function. Current research is aimed at defining the precise dopamine receptor subtypes that are responsible for these effects. Because stress is known to increase dopaminergic transmission to the prefrontal cortex, the actions of dopamine in this brain region may explain why low levels of stress can enhance performance in working memory tasks, whereas higher levels of stress can disrupt performance. Manipulation of the norepinephrine system also has potent effects on working memory; for example, α_2-adrenergic agonists such as **clonidine** and **guanfacine** (see Chapters 8, 12, and 14) appear to increase working memory, a finding that may explain the utility of these agents in the treatment of **attention deficit-related disorders** (see Chapter 18).

Although the studies mentioned thus far involve very simple mental representations, working memory is at the heart of many complex mental tasks in higher mammals. When viewed as a rudimentary form of abstraction, working memory can be seen as crossing from the realm of the brain into that of the mind, where internal representations of the external world are consistent and reliable. The ability to think in abstract terms presumably allows humans to create a sense of identity, to establish aspirations, and to plan for the future. The full importance of these cognitive functions can best be appreciated when they break down.

PSYCHOSIS AND SCHIZOPHRENIA

Psychosis is used to describe a state in which an individual appears to have lost touch with reality. Unlike other neuropsychiatric symptoms, such as depression and anxiety, which involve sensations and thought processes that can be readily understood by an observer, psychosis involves a gross disruption of reality testing—or the ability of a person to understand the external world. Several classic types of psychotic phenomena have been described. *Hallucinations* are perceptions unconnected to external stimuli; individuals who experience these phenomena may report that they hear voices or see things that are not present. *Delusions* are fixed, false beliefs that are not shared by others in an individual's culture, such as the belief that the fillings in one's teeth are radio transmitters. *Illusions* are severely distorted perceptions or misinterpretations of environmental stimuli—for example, the perception that fixed objects are moving or pulsating. *Formal thought disorder* involves a disruption of the logical flow of ideas, such as the loosening of the normal connections between ideas, and many other impairments that are discussed in subsequent sections of this chapter.

Psychosis describes a mental state rather than a specific disorder. It may be associated with a wide range of conditions, including the altered states of consciousness that occur during delirium (see Chapters 18 and 20), the induced perceptual abnormalities caused by drug abuse or endocrine dysfunction, and the gross cognitive impairment caused by advanced cases of **Alzheimer**

Box 17–1 Schizophrenia: A Case History

Martin is a thirty-five-year-old man who is currently homeless and living in shelters or on the street. His childhood was unremarkable until high school, when he began to withdraw from his peers. He tended to eat and play by himself at school and spent much of his time reading science fiction. In college Martin developed a preoccupation with mysticism and religion, often writing lengthy but confusing manifestos that described his beliefs. His parents became concerned at the end of his sophomore year when final exams were approaching and he seemed to become more and more preoccupied with his theories. Finally, Martin broke off contact with his parents, believing that they were sent to prevent him from developing his philosophy, which he believed was sure to revolutionize society. During his junior year, Martin's behavior continued to deteriorate. He began to wear large hats because he believed that people could hear his thoughts and were trying to steal them. When he heard news stories about overseas wars he believed that they were being waged between forces trying to help him and others who were trying to stop him. One night, as Martin was putting aluminum foil around his dorm room to prevent people from using electrical devices to steal his ideas about world communication, he began to hear two voices discussing his work and his philosophy. Their discussion confirmed his fear that his ideas had been stolen. He became more and more infuriated as the voices ridiculed his ideas, until finally he fled his apartment. On the street he saw a policeman he believed was sent to kidnap him. Martin attacked the policeman in what he believed was self-defense.

Martin was brought to a psychiatric hospital where he was sedated and given antipsychotic medication. With treatment, his auditory hallucinations and paranoid delusions subsided over the course of a few weeks, but he remained adamant that he did not want to see his parents. Soon after he was released from the hospital, Martin stopped taking his medications because they made him feel ill. He attempted

to continue his studies but within 6 months dropped out of school because of recurring paranoia about people stealing his ideas and because he was having great difficulty keeping up with his assignments. For the next 6 years he tried to work at a series of jobs but was unable to keep any of them because of unexplained absences and frequent clashes with his bosses and coworkers. During these years he was hospitalized involuntarily six times. Each time he was given an antipsychotic medication that reduced his paranoia and auditory hallucinations; however, he rarely continued to take these drugs for more than a few months because of the many side effects he experienced.

Martin reconciled with his parents and lived with them for several years, but they became increasingly frustrated with his resistance to taking his medications. Because discussions about this issue caused considerable tension, Martin would occasionally leave without a word and live with his one remaining friend or on the street for weeks at a time. He began drinking alcohol and taking drugs, such as marijuana and cocaine, because he was bored or because the drugs would help him ignore the voices that frequently bothered him. Eventually, when he was 29, Martin had a major fight with his parents over his drug use and he moved out of their house, never to return.

During the past 6 years Martin has been living in shelters and on the street. He receives medication from a local public health clinic. Although he continues to take such medication inconsistently, he takes it more frequently because he understands that it helps him stay out of the hospital. He knows some of the other people at the shelters he visits, but in general people make him uncomfortable and he keeps to himself. His parents occasionally send him money but he rarely talks to them more than once a year. Although he still thinks of his philosophy occasionally, it makes less sense to him than it used to. Mostly he spends time alone, making small trinkets out of wire and glass to help him feel safe.

disease or **Huntington disease.** In addition, psychosis is seen in a large number of patients with psychiatric disorders, such as **schizophrenia, mania,** and **depression,** whose diagnoses are based on symptom clusters rather than on known pathophysiologic processes.

Schizophrenia, the most common cause of chronic psychosis, affects approximately 1% of the world's population. Its cardinal signs include active psychosis, such as delusions and hallucinations; the disturbance of logical thought processes; and deterioration of social and occupational function (Box 17–1). The term *schizophrenia* encompasses many different clinical presentations, and very likely many distinct disease states; yet all of these are characterized by chronic disturbances in

perception and in the integration of reality. Most affected individuals also exhibit marked and disabling deficits in cognition and motivation. Although some individuals with mood disorders also exhibit psychotic symptoms, such symptoms generally are episodic and resolve with improvement in mood (see Chapter 15).

Two terms are commonly used to categorize the symptoms of schizophrenia. *Positive symptoms* refer to new mental phenomena, which unaffected people normally do not experience, such as hallucinations and delusions. *Negative symptoms* refer to a loss of normal mental functions such as amotivation and social withdrawal. More recently, impaired cognition has been identified as a third domain of abnormality in schizophrenics. In the past 20 years, the *Diagnostic and Statistical Manual* (*DSM*) of the American Psychiatric Association has provided consensus and consistency in psychiatric diagnosis, based on clinical symptoms and course. The *DSM IV* acknowledges the fundamental importance of positive and negative symptomatology, as well as cognitive deficits, and identifies several subtypes of schizophrenia based on the relative prominence of different symptoms (Box 17–2). However, the current subtypes are not known to be related to different etiologies or pathophysiologic processes, and do not remain consistent across generations of families with schizophrenia.

PATHOPHYSIOLOGY OF SCHIZOPHRENIA

It is currently believed that multiple genetic loci interact to confer vulnerability to schizophrenia and that nongenetic factors convert such vulnerability into illness. However, it has been difficult to identify both risk-conferring genes and nongenetic factors related to schizophrenia. Nongenetic factors may include stochastic, or random, developmental processes. Just as identical twins do not have identical fingerprints, they do not have identical sulcal or gyral patterns in the cerebral cortex, although such patterns are more similar for identical than for nonidentical twins. The fact that genetically identical individuals show differences in these patterns underscores the point that there is a certain amount of chance in the wiring of the hundreds of trillions of synapses that form in the human brain during development. Moreover, epidemiologic findings suggest that environmental insults may confer small increments of risk in some individuals; these include malnutrition and in utero viral infection. The next few sections of this chapter provide a brief overview of the pathophysiology of schizophrenia and conclude with a discussion of the various neurotransmitter systems that influence this disorder.

Neuropsychiatric deficits in schizophrenia   Neuropsychiatric tests, which isolate particular components of mental functioning, have helped to determine specific psychological processing deficits in individuals with schizophrenia. The basic sensorimotor skills and associative abilities of such individuals tend to remain intact, but tasks that require symbolic or verbal representation are undertaken with considerable difficulty. Individuals with schizophrenia also have difficulty integrating novel stimuli with older memories or concepts, and tend to treat familiar associations as though they were unusual and new situations as if they occurred in the recent past. The disorganization of speech, loosening of associations, and word salad speech (a rambling utterance of words that lack obvious sense) that characterize schizophrenia seem to stem from an inability to keep recent thoughts or words in mind.

The internal representation and constancy of ideas that are lacking in individuals with schizophrenia are akin to working memory. In fact, many researchers believe that disturbance of working memory is a primary problem in schizophrenia. Studies that test working memory, similar to previously described studies involving monkeys, have been applied to individuals with schizophrenia to test this hypothesis. In these protocols, a visual target is presented to a human subject for 200 milliseconds, and after a delay of 5 to 30 seconds, the subject is asked to look at the original location of the target. A distracter task is introduced to keep the image from being converted into a verbal representation. People with schizophrenia perform poorly on these tests, compared with normal control subjects, just as monkeys with prefrontal lesions perform poorly in similar paradigms.

Another neuropsychiatric task at which schizophrenic individuals perform poorly is the Wisconsin Card Sorting Test (WCST). Subjects who take this test are asked to sort a deck of cards marked with symbols that vary in number, color, and shape. As each card is dealt, the subject must match the card to a reference deck based on its color, number, or shape. The experimenter indicates whether the subject's match is correct or incorrect, and over time the subject learns the rule of sorting. After a specified number of trials, the experimenter changes the sorting rule without telling the subject, who must realize the test has changed and learn the new rule. Schizophrenics perform well in terms of learning the sorting rule but have a difficult time recognizing and adopting a new sorting rule. Normal subjects appear to learn to associate a card (an external stimulus) with a response (correct or incorrect) until a sorting rule, such as sort by color, is internalized. Schizophrenics appear to be deficient in the working memory component of this task, and thus are over-reliant on the associative component. Lacking normal working memory, the subject with schizophrenia presumably cannot extinguish an initial associative sorting rule and instead exhibits perseveration.

Patients with schizophrenia also demonstrate deficits in working memory when performing the Stroop test. Cards used in this test have the name of a color written on them, but the name is printed in the ink of another color—for example, red is written in blue ink (Figure 17–4). Subjects are asked to give the name of the color in which the word is written, while suppressing the natural tendency to recite the color represented by the word. Patients with schizophrenia have difficulty per-

Box 17–2 Diagnostic Criteria for Schizophrenia and Its Subtypes

Diagnostic Criteria for Schizophrenia

A. Characteristic symptoms: Two (or more) of the following, each present for a significant portion of time during a 1-month period (or less if successfully treated):
  (1) delusions
  (2) hallucinations
  (3) disorganized speech (e.g., frequent derailment or incoherence)
  (4) grossly disorganized or catatonic behavior
  (5) negative symptoms, i.e., affective flattening, alogia, or avolition

  Notes: Only one Criterion A symptom is required if delusions are bizarre or hallucinations consist of a voice keeping up a running commentary on the person's behavior or thoughts, or two or more voices conversing with each other.

B. Social/occupational dysfunction: For a significant portion of the time since the onset of the disturbance, one or more major areas of functioning such as work, interpersonal relations, or self-care are markedly below the level achieved prior to the onset (or when the onset is in childhood or adolescence, failure to achieve expected level of interpersonal, academic, or occupational achievement).

C. Duration: Continuous signs of the disturbance persist for at least 6 months. This 6-month period must include at least 1 month of symptoms (or less if successfully treated) that meet Criterion A (i.e., active-phase symptoms) and may include periods of prodromal or residual symptoms. During these prodromal or residual periods, the signs of the disturbance may be manifested by only negative symptoms or two or more symptoms listed in Criterion A present in an attenuated form (e.g., odd beliefs, unusual perceptual experiences).

D. Schizoaffective and Mood Disorder exclusion: Schizoaffective Disorder and Mood Disorder With Psychotic Features have been ruled out because either (1) no Major Depressive, Manic, or Mixed Episodes have occurred concurrently with the active-phase symptoms; or (2) if mood episodes have occurred during active-phase symptoms, their total duration has been brief relative to the duration of the active and residual periods.

E. Substance/general medical condition exclusion: The disturbance is not due to the direct physiological effects of a substance (e.g., a drug of abuse, a medication) or a general medical condition.

F. Relationship to Pervasive Developmental Disorder: If there is a history of Autistic Disorder or another Pervasive Developmental Disorder, the additional diagnosis of Schizophrenia is made only if prominent delusions or hallucinations are also present for at lease a month (or less if successfully treated).

Diagnostic Criteria for Paranoid Type

A type of schizophrenia in which the following criteria are met:
A. Preoccupation with one or more delusions or frequent auditory hallucinations.
B. None of the following is prominent: disorganized speech, disorganized or catatonic behavior, or flat or inappropriate affect.

Diagnostic Criteria for Disorganized Type

A type of schizophrenia in which the following criteria are met:
A. All of the following are prominent:
  (1) disorganized speech
  (2) disorganized behavior
  (3) flat or inappropriate affect
B. The criteria are not met for Catatonic Type.

Diagnostic Criteria for Catatonic Type

A type of schizophrenia in which the clinical picture is dominated by at least two of the following:
  (1) motoric immobility as evidenced by catalepsy (including waxy flexibility) or stupor
  (2) excessive motor activity (that is apparently purposeless and not influenced by external stimuli)
  (3) extreme negativism (an apparently motiveless resistance to all instructions or maintenance of a rigid posture against attempts to be moved) or mutism
  (4) peculiarities of voluntary movement as evidenced by posturing (voluntary assumption of inappropriate or bizarre postures), stereotyped movements, prominent mannerisms, or prominent grimacing
  (5) echolalia or echopraxia

Diagnostic Criteria for Undifferentiated Type

A type of schizophrenia in which symptoms that meet Criterion A are present, but the criteria are not met for the Paranoid, Disorganized, or Catatonic Type.

Diagnostic Criteria for Residual Type

A type of schizophrenia in which the following criteria are met:
A. Absence of prominent delusions, hallucinations, disorganized speech, and grossly disorganized or catatonic behavior.
B. There is continuing evidence of the disturbance, as indicated by the presence of negative symptoms or two or more symptoms listed in Criterion A for schizophrenia, present in an attenuated form (e.g., odd beliefs, unusual perceptual experiences).

Reprinted with permission from American Psychiatric Association. 1994. *Diagnostic and Statistical Manual of Mental Disorders*, 4th ed. Washington DC: American Psychiatric Association.

forming this task because it requires keeping the rule in working memory and ignoring the immediate stimulus of the content of the word.

Many schizophrenics also exhibit subtle abnormalities that have been referred to as soft neurologic signs. Abnormalities in saccadic eye movements are among the most frequently studied examples. The significance of these minor neurologic impairments remains unknown.

Genetics of schizophrenia Schizophrenia is familial. Although the overall prevalence of schizophrenia in the world is approximately 1%, children of schizophrenic parents exhibit an increased risk, such that approximately 12% of them develop this disorder. This increase in risk appears to result from genetic factors, as indicated by studies of twins. The concordance rate for schizophrenia among monozygotic twins, who share all of their genetic material, is nearly 50%; in contrast, the concordance rate for dizygotic twins, who on average share half of their genetic material, is 7%–12%. Studies of adoptive families indicate that the risk of schizophrenia reflects the status of biologic rather than adoptive parents. Taken as a whole, these studies provide strong evidence for a genetic contribution to schizophrenia. To put this genetic risk in perspective, it would appear that genes play a greater role in schizophrenia than they do for many common diseases that are considered familial, such as type II diabetes mellitus.

The genes responsible for this disorder remain elusive. As discussed in connection with mood disorders in Chapter 15, psychiatric disorders in general, and schizophrenia in particular, are challenging targets for molecular genetic studies for several reasons. First, a biologic test that can be used to define and diagnose a reliable phenotype has yet to be developed. Second, it is possible that many subtypes of schizophrenia exist, which may or may not be related to a common genetic cause. Third, multiple genetic loci most likely contribute to this disorder. Despite these problems, recent studies have identified regions of the human genome that may be related

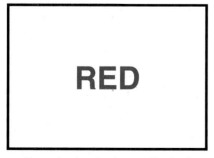

Figure 17–4. Example of a stimulus used in the Stroop test. Individuals are asked to remember the color of the ink rather than the color named by the text.

to schizophrenia. Two studies have linked schizophrenia with 6p22, a region on chromosome 6 (Figure 17–5). This finding has been supported by some studies, but other studies have not identified a linkage in this region. Other chromosomal regions linked to schizophrenia have included 8p21-p22, 22q12-q13.1, and locations on chromosome 13. Chromosome 22 is of particular interest because a microdeletion of this chromosome causes **velocardiofacial syndrome** (see Chapter 15), which in heterozygote form often presents with prominent psychosis. Ultimately, the specific genes in these or other regions of the genome that cause schizophrenia must be identified, and the means by which the products of these genes lead to the neural and behavioral abnormalities associated with schizophrenia must be determined. It is hoped that the increasingly sophisticated tools of molecular genetics will help to accomplish these goals.

Neuroanatomic correlates of schizophrenia Neuroanatomic studies have demonstrated gross differences in the brains of schizophrenic patients compared with the brains of matched controls. The most consistent finding, based on postmortem brain examinations, as well as computerized tomography (CT) and magnetic resonance imaging (MRI) of living patients, is that schizophrenic individuals exhibit decreased brain volumes and enlarged third and lateral ventricles. Worsening abnormalities in brain volume have been documented in the relatively rare syndrome of childhood schizophrenia. In contrast, in adolescent- or adult-onset cases, brain volume abnormalities do not appear to progress after the initial appearance of symptoms. Particularly interesting data from an imaging study of monozygotic twins discordant for schizophrenia revealed that the twin with schizophrenia almost invariably had larger ventricles than the nonschizophrenic twin, even if both had ventricular sizes in the broad normal range. This finding further confirms that nongenetic events affect brain structure.

Abnormalities in particular brain structures also are a feature of schizophrenia. Overall gray matter volume appears to be reduced by 10–15% in schizophrenic individuals, with the most pronounced changes observed in medial and lateral structures in the temporal lobes. Several MRI studies have indicated that the basal ganglia are enlarged in schizophrenia, but these studies have involved patients treated with **antipsychotic** medications, which are known to affect this structure. Accordingly, changes in basal ganglia may be related to the use of these drugs rather than to the presence of schizophrenia.

Functional neuroanatomic studies of schizophrenia have focused on examination of the prefrontal cortex. As previously discussed, this area of brain subserves

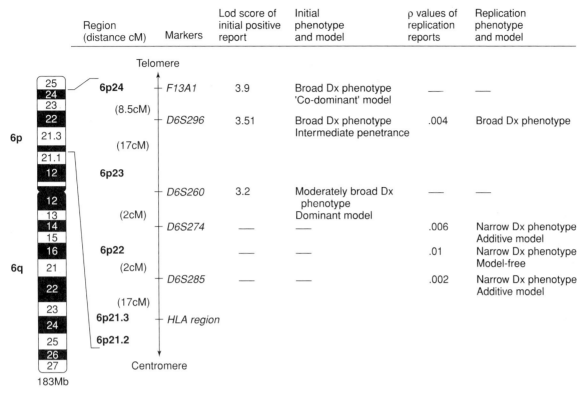

Region (distance cM)	Markers	Lod score of initial positive report	Initial phenotype and model	ρ values of replication reports	Replication phenotype and model
6p24	F13A1	3.9	Broad Dx phenotype 'Co-dominant' model	—	—
(8.5cM)	D6S296	3.51	Broad Dx phenotype Intermediate penetrance	.004	Broad Dx phenotype
(17cM)					
6p23					
	D6S260	3.2	Moderately broad Dx phenotype Dominant model	—	—
(2cM)	D6S274	—	—	.006	Narrow Dx phenotype Additive model
6p22		—	—	.01	Narrow Dx phenotype Model-free
(2cM)	D6S285	—	—	.002	Narrow Dx phenotype Additive model
(17cM)					
6p21.3	HLA region				
6p21.2					

Telomere

Centromere

Figure 17–5. Diagram of chromosome 6 shows specific regions on the chromosome that are reported to be associated with schizophrenia. Such linkage remains to be confirmed. Dx, diagnosis. (Adapted with permission from Egan MF, Weinberger DR. 1997. *Curr Opin Neurobiol* 7:701.)

higher cognitive functioning and working memory, which may be defective in schizophrenia. Studies involving the use of positron emission tomography (PET) or single photon emission computed tomography (SPECT) to measure cerebral blood flow or other evidence of metabolic activity in the brain have revealed decreased basal activity in the dorsolateral prefrontal cortex of schizophrenics and have correlated this pattern with the negative symptoms of schizophrenia. Studies of brain activity during specific tasks also have indicated decreased prefrontal activity in schizophrenia. Healthy individuals exhibit increased brain activity in prefrontal, superior parietal, and medial temporal areas of the cortex during performance of the WCST. In contrast, schizophrenic patients who perform poorly on this test exhibit normal activation of most areas of the cortex but show selective deficits in the activation of dorsolateral areas of the prefrontal cortex.

Some investigators have focused on identifying neuroanatomic changes at the cellular level that may correlate with schizophrenia. This work has relied on analysis of autopsy specimens—an approach fraught with technical challenges, including hour- to day-long delays from death to tissue preservation; the old age at which many patients die (often years or decades after

the time of active pathology); and the patient's prior exposure to antipsychotic drugs. Yet pathologic changes in the brains of schizophrenics have been reported, although the specific brain regions affected and the particular changes identified have varied from study to study. Some reports have indicated decreases in the number of GABAergic interneurons, or in the number of layer 5 pyramidal neurons, in prefrontal or anterior cingulate cortex. Other reports have revealed decreases in the amount of neuropil in these regions, without a change in the total number of neurons. Some researchers have speculated that a deficit in neuronal migration occurs during cortical development, whereas others have observed that pathologic changes occur in the hippocampus. Schizophrenia ultimately must involve molecular and cellular lesions, which may vary with distinct subtypes of the disorder; identification of such lesions may have to await the discovery of specific disease genes.

Electrophysiologic changes in schizophrenia
Several nonspecific EEG abnormalities have been described in schizophrenia, including decreased alpha wave activity, increased theta and delta activity, and increased epileptiform activity, especially after sleep deprivation. However, the significance of these findings

is unclear, especially because many of them have not been universally replicated. In contrast, studies of evoked potentials in schizophrenia have produced more consistent findings. In particular, the P300, a relatively large positive potential that occurs in response to sensory stimulation, is frequently abnormal in schizophrenia; it is smaller and later in response to a given stimulus compared with the same potential in control subjects. The P300 is believed to be the result of a sensory input that has undergone processing at the hippocampus, a major component of the temporal lobes, which, as previously mentioned, may be abnormal in schizophrenia. The significance of an abnormal P300 remains unclear.

The processing of sensory information, often referred to as *sensory gating,* can be manipulated pharmacologically by **nicotinic cholinergic agonists**. Nicotinic receptors composed of homomeric α_7 subunits and concentrated in the hippocampus are believed to mediate this effect (see Chapter 9). Reports suggest that such agonists may improve the gating deficits seen in patients with schizophrenia.

Neurotransmitter systems and schizophrenia

The neurotransmitter most commonly associated with schizophrenia is dopamine. **Antipsychotic** agents, described in subsequent sections of this chapter, are potent antagonists of dopamine receptors and have been shown to disrupt the metabolism of dopamine in the CNS. Moreover, medications used to treat **Parkinson disease,** such as **L-dopa,** act by replacing dopamine in the CNS (see Chapter 14) and can cause psychosis. **Psychostimulants,** which increase synaptic levels of dopamine, also can cause psychosis (see Chapter 16). Furthermore, several neurodegenerative disorders that can cause psychosis, including **Huntington disease,** involve the degeneration of neurons in the striatum, which receives major dopaminergic input (see Chapter 14). The putative involvement of dopamine in schizophrenia and other psychotic syndromes is consistent with the significant dopaminergic innervation of the prefrontal cortex and other limbic regions (see Chapter 8) implicated in psychosis. Despite such supporting evidence, the dopamine hypothesis of schizophrenia is flawed. Antipsychotic drugs block dopamine receptors upon initial drug exposure, but maximal antipsychotic effects are seen only after prolonged drug administration. Conversely, L-dopa and psychostimulants increase dopamine function in the short-term, but generally cause psychosis only after repeated dosing. Indeed, no compelling molecular evidence has suggested that a lesion in the dopamine system is a primary cause of schizophrenia.

Another neurotransmitter implicated in schizophrenia is serotonin, which has received a great deal of attention since the development of second-generation antipsychotic agents. These agents have a relatively low affinity for dopamine receptors compared with older antipsychotic agents, but a higher affinity for 5-HT$_{2A}$ serotonin receptors, where they act as antagonists. **Hallucinogens,** which induce hallucinations and illusions in normal subjects, are partial agonists at this serotonin receptor, as discussed in a subsequent section of this chapter. The neurotransmitter glutamate and the NMDA glutamate receptor also may be factors in schizophrenia because certain psychosis-inducing drugs appear to act on the NMDA receptor, as discussed later in this chapter. Moreover, preliminary research suggests that agents that act at the glycine site on the NMDA receptor complex, and thus would be expected to promote NMDA receptor function, may be of some value in the treatment of schizophrenia.

It must be emphasized that neurotransmitter-related hypotheses that attempt to explain the etiology of schizophrenia are based solely on pharmacologic evidence, and thus are likely to be incomplete or misleading. Although pharmacologic manipulation of neurotransmitter systems may exacerbate or ameliorate psychotic symptoms, aberrations in these systems do not necessarily underlie psychotic disorders. Indeed, it is known that abnormalities in dopamine, serotonin, glutamate, and other neurotransmitter systems are not primary causes of psychotic symptoms associated with many disorders, including Huntington disease and the endocrinopathies.

PHARMACOLOGY OF PERCEPTION AND INTEGRATION

Several classes of pharmacologic agents can affect an individual's ability to perceive his or her environment accurately and integrate multiple perceptions so that they form a consistent reality. High doses of or prolonged exposure to such substances can cause psychosis. In contrast, other agents, known as antipsychotic medications, can reduce psychotic symptoms. Such medications are the agents most commonly used to treat psychotic symptoms associated with schizophrenia, but they are not antischizophrenic agents per se. Antipsychotic medications also are effective in treating psychosis associated with substance intoxication, endocrine dysfunction, mood disorders, delirium, and other conditions.

DRUGS THAT INDUCE PSYCHOSIS

Psychostimulants   **Cocaine** and **amphetamines** are capable of inducing a psychosis that resembles paranoid schizophrenia as well as the psychosis that sometimes accompanies mania. As described in Chapter 16, low doses of both drugs cause an increase in energy and alertness and a subjective sensation of power and euphoria. Higher doses and long-term use of both drugs can lead to psychotic states that are characterized by auditory hallucinations, paranoid delusions, and ideas of reference, such as incorrect beliefs that news reports and other events have personal meaning or reference. These symptoms typically emerge as hypervigilance or vague paranoia and develop gradually over a course of repeated drug use. As paranoia continues, it is magnified by subsequent stimulant use until a severe psychosis develops.

Cocaine and amphetamines increase synaptic levels of all monoamine neurotransmitters (see Chapter 16). The increase in dopamine, in particular, is believed to underlie psychostimulant-induced psychosis because antipsychotic drugs, which block dopamine receptors, decrease this psychosis. Moreover, elevated levels of norepinephrine are associated with increased anxiety and in some cases may cause a panic attack (see Chapter 15). Thus a subjective sense of anxiety coupled with impaired perception and integration may explain the paranoid delusions that often accompany the use of these drugs. The facilitation of serotonergic function may activate 5-HT_{2A} receptors, which also are implicated in psychosis. Yet such speculations do not explain why psychosis typically results from repeated rather than initial psychostimulant exposure. It is more likely that psychostimulant-induced psychosis results from adaptations that occur in response to repeated perturbations of the brain's monoamine systems.

Hallucinogens Hallucinogens encompass numerous drugs that share a unique spectrum of psychological effects. Some of these substances have been used for centuries in folk and religious practices throughout the world. As their name suggests, these compounds have the capacity to induce hallucinations (Box 17–3). Such phenomena are primarily visual but also can be auditory. They can be fully formed images but often tend to be simple distortions, which may involve a brightening of visual sensations or trailers (a stroboscopic effect of moving images). Some hallucinogens cause synesthesia, or a blurring of the boundaries between sensations of different modalities. This sensory distortion can result in a perceived visual representation of sounds and tactile stimuli, or in the perception that visual experiences can amplify or modulate auditory or tactile sensations. Another dramatic effect of hallucinogens is time dilation, or a subjective sense of slowed time that distorts the perceived duration of events. Hallucinogens also can cause an altered sense of self known as ego dissolution. Many of these phenomena are accompanied by a mystical sensation of being united with some larger spiritual phenomenon, often referred to as being at one with the universe.

The hallucinogen **lysergic acid diethylamide (LSD)** helped fuel the countercultural movement that took place during the 1960s, when people were encouraged to "tune in, turn on, and drop out" (Figure 17–6). Initially studied as a potential adjunct to psychotherapy, LSD was subsequently popularized by certain academics

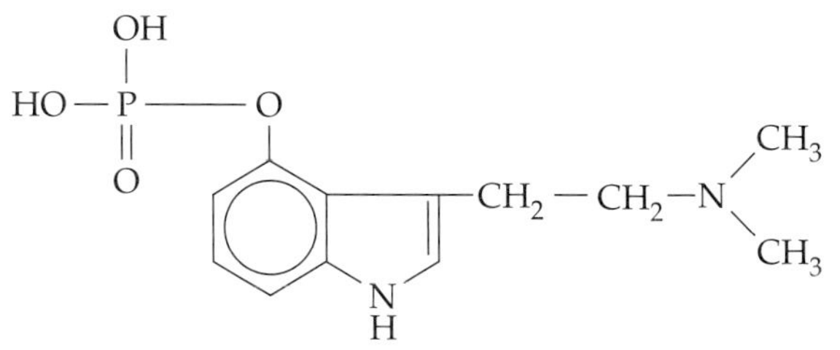

Psilocybin

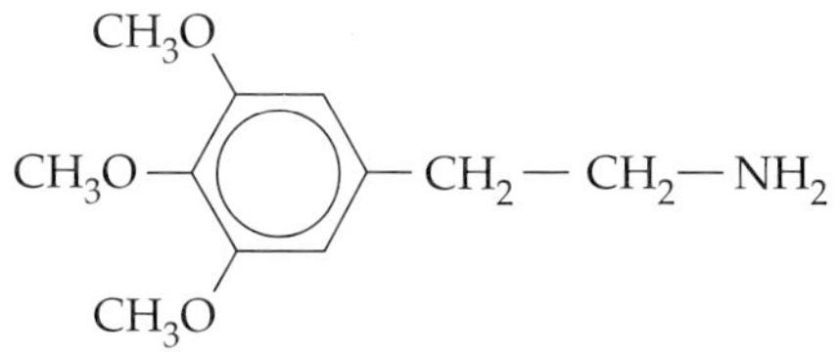

Mescaline

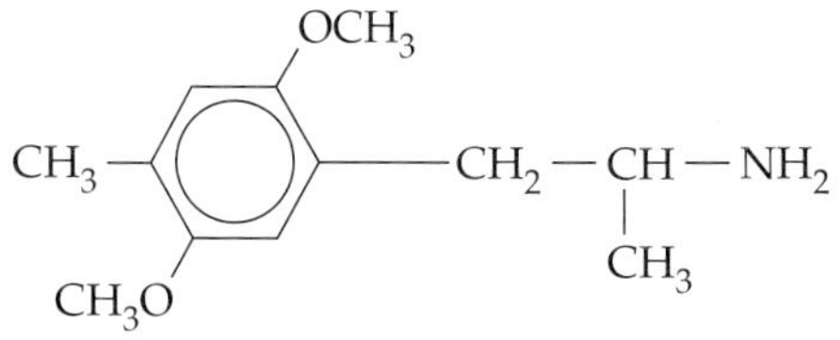

2,5-Dimethoxy-4-methylamphetamine (DOM, STP)

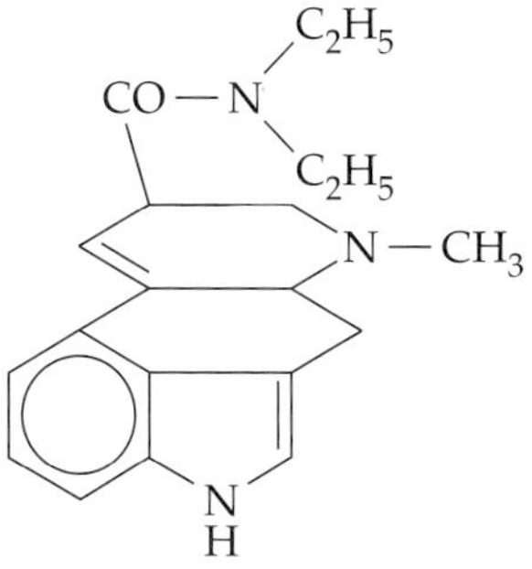

Lysergic acid diethylamide (LSD)

Figure 17–6. Chemical structures of representative hallucinogens.

Box 17–3 The LSD Experience

The first change one is likely to notice after taking a psychedelic drug are changes in sensory perception, especially visual perception. I recall this from my own experimentation with LSD, which took place in a Victorian house on one of the slopes of Twin Peaks, the highest hill in San Francisco. At first, the only notable difference was the appearance of a slight purplish fringe around the objects in my vicinity. Next, every object I focused on began to seem amusingly quaint. The rooftops and facades of houses reminded me of the gingerbread house in Hansel and Gretel, which observation caused me to giggle uncontrollably. As I became more and more entranced by these and other visual sensations, the giggly feeling gradually changed to awe. I looked at the faces of the people around me and noticed details of their physiognomy that had never struck me before. Each pore in my companions' skin was now visible, and every facial expression was laden with significance. As I looked on each person's face I empathized with the exact emotion I thought I saw expressed. At that point, the distortions became more extreme. If I focused upon my forefinger, it would swell. If I concluded that the finger was unimportant, it literally shrank into insignificance. When I gazed at the intricate woodwork that edged the ceiling, the carved designs would undulate back and forth.

About an hour after ingesting the LSD, I clapped my hands and saw sound waves passing before my eyes. When two people clapped their hands at different sound frequencies, I saw two sets of waves that differed in magnitude and seemed to collide with each other. Two hours after taking the drug, I felt I had been under its influence for thousands of years. The remainder of my life on the planet Earth seemed to stretch ahead into infinity—every quarter note seemed to linger for a month. I remember walking from one room to the next with a feeling of having crossed the breadth of the universe. I climbed the stairs to the second floor and looked back down on events that were surely taking place 40,000 miles away.

Boundaries between self and nonself evaporate, giving rise to a serene sense of being at one with the universe. I recall muttering to myself again and again, "All is one, all is one." My wife, who was the sober *observer* for the day, became alarmed and asked me what was going on, to which I could only reply, "What matters? All is one." My ... powerful feeling of oneness with the universe was followed by a loss of awareness of just who I was. I began to call out, "Who am I? Where is the world?" At the height of this disintegration, I was terrified. I tried frantically to remember my name—hoping thus to recapture reality—but it eluded me. In the end, I grasped at the one name I could think of: "San Francisco." I repeated it again and again, "San Francisco, San Francisco, San Francisco." It seemed to be a clue to where I was and who I might be. By this time, eight hours after consuming the LSD, the drug's effects began to wear off. By clinging to the notion that San Francisco was a relevant place, I gradually managed to remember who I was, where I was, and the identities of the people there with me. Very quickly, the world about me coalesced and reality supervened.

Description of a trip on LSD by Solomon Snyder. Reprinted with permission from Snyder SH. 1996. *Drugs and the Brain.* New York: Scientific American Library.

and lay writers. It received attention from the scientific community because the hallucinations and ego dissolution associated with LSD intoxication appeared similar to the phenomena seen in schizophrenia; indeed, the anxiety, agitation, and paranoia that have been reported to accompany a so-called bad trip on LSD are particularly reminiscent of the psychosis that is characteristic of this disorder. For several reasons, most researchers have since abandoned the theory that the hallucinogenic state serves as a useful model of schizophrenia. First, intoxication with hallucinogenic compounds is transient and does not produce residual effects in most individuals. Second, the hallucinogenic experience often elicits euphoria and other positive emotions, which are profoundly different from the dysphoria, anxiety, and paranoia that is common in schizophrenia. Third, unlike the hallucinations that occur with schizophrenia, which often are auditory, the hallucinations produced by LSD typically are visual. Moreover, the use of LSD is not accompanied by the fixed and often elaborate delusions associated with schizophrenia.

Compounds with hallucinogenic properties have very different molecular structures. Hallucinogens initially referred to naturally occurring components of plants, mushrooms, or molds. As pharmacologic methods advanced, these compounds were purified; subsequently new and more potent compounds were synthesized. **Mescaline,** a derivative of the **peyote** cactus *Lophophora williamsii* or *Anhalonium lewinii* (see Figure 17–6), is known in part for its use in religious rituals of native Mexican and American cultures. Although peyote contains many psychoactive compounds, its hallucinogenic properties have been attributed primarily to mescaline. Mescaline itself is a fairly weak drug, but many synthetic congeners, including the methoxyamphetamines, 2,5-dimethoxy-4-methylamphetamine (**DOM**) and **STP,** are quite potent (see Figure 17–6). LSD was identified as a derivative of **ergot** alkaloids from *Claviceps purpurea,* a fungus that grows on rye and other grains. The poisonous effects of ergot alkaloids were described in ancient times, and ergot preparations have been used for centuries to manipulate the sympathetic nervous system (see Chapter 12) for obstetric purposes and in the treatment of migraine headaches.

The ergots and certain other hallucinogenic drugs, such as **psilocybin** and dimethyltryptamine (**DMT**), share basic chemical similarities with serotonin. These similarities help to explain the effectiveness of some of these drugs in the treatment of **migraines** and **uterine bleeding** because serotonin regulates both the cerebral vasculature and uterine smooth muscle contraction. The mechanisms of action that underlie the hallucinogenic properties of these drugs remained obscure until numerous subtypes of serotonin receptors were cloned. Such studies allowed a more precise examination of the effect of hallucinogens on specific serotonin receptors, each of which is expressed in a particular cell type in the brain and in peripheral tissues (see Chapter 9). Different chemical classes of hallucinogens were found to have different affinities for the various serotonin receptors, which likely explains their differential utility in treating migraines and uterine bleeding. The current consensus is that hallucinogens cause perceptual distortions by serving as partial agonists of the 5-HT_{2A} receptor, although the involvement of other serotonin receptor subtypes remains a possibility. Why activation of the 5-HT_{2A} receptor causes these symptoms remains unknown. However, research has shown that this receptor is located in the mid-segments of apical dendrites of deep cortical pyramidal neurons, including those in the prefrontal cortex, where the receptor is ideally situated to influence the sensitivity of these neurons to many synaptic inputs. The study of such cellular mechanisms in the context of working memory and other behavioral paradigms related to higher cognitive function would be of considerable interest.

Certain analogs of the methoxyamphetamines—in particular, 3,4-methylenedioxy-*N*-methylamphetamine (**MDMA**), or **ecstacy** (see Figure 17–6)—are only mildly hallucinogenic but are capable of producing euphoria. MDMA is believed to produce its effect by causing the release of both serotonin and dopamine from nerve terminals (see Chapters 9 and 16).

Phencyclidine and dissociative anesthetics

Phencyclidine, also known as **PCP** or **angel dust,** was originally developed for use as a dissociative anesthetic. Another dissociative anesthetic is **ketamine,** a drug also known as **special K**. These agents produce a sense of dissociation from sensory stimuli. Individuals given these drugs in surgery may experience nociception or the initial perception of pain without the aversive emotional aspects (see Chapter 19). Such agents also induce a replicable and consistent psychotic episode in a dose-dependent manner. As the name angel dust suggests, the use of PCP and related drugs has been associated with depersonalization. Moreover, these drugs can cause visual and auditory hallucinations. Individuals under the influence of these agents have an impaired ability to integrate sensory experiences and are vulnerable to paranoia and panic. The psychosis produced by these drugs resembles that associated with schizophrenia, and the two states can be difficult to differentiate. PCP induces a greater degree of behavioral disinhibition than most other psychotogenic drugs; individuals under its influence do not experience pain or understand the implications of their actions. Psychosis triggered by PCP may represent a medical emergency. The abuse of PCP and ketamine is discussed in greater detail in Chapter 16.

The major actions of PCP initially were believed to occur by means of the sigma receptor, to which the drug binds with a relatively high (200 nM) affinity. This receptor was originally identified as an opioid receptor because it is recognized by benzomorphan opiate drugs such as **pentazocine,** which can induce psychosis. It is now known that this sigma receptor is not a true opioid receptor because it is not antagonized by the opioid receptor antagonist naloxone; rather, it appears to be a mitochondrial protein that remains poorly understood. The sigma site received early interest as a target for antipsychotic drugs. However, interest has waned because stereoisomers of psychosis-inducing opioids that bind to the sigma receptor are behaviorally inactive, and certain stereoisomers that can induce psychosis have lower affinity at the sigma receptor.

PCP has since been shown to have higher affinity for the NMDA glutamate receptor, at which it functions as an open channel blocker (see Chapter 7). This receptor currently is believed to be the primary site of action of PCP, ketamine, and related dissociative anesthetic agents. Such a model of PCP action has suggested that the glutamate system may be exploited in the treatment of schizophrenia. Interestingly, PCP often causes profound retrograde amnesia; it has been hypothesized that this effect can be explained by the drug's interference with NMDA receptor function, which is critically important for certain forms of memory formation (see Chapter 20).

Marijuana and cannabinoids

Marijuana is the most commonly used illicit drug in the United States and in many other countries throughout the world. The term *marijuana,* which is Mexican, refers to a particular form of cannabis that derives mainly from the leaves of the hemp plant. This substance, which typically is smoked, is also commonly referred to as grass, dope, or ganja (a term borrowed from India). Several different formulations are used, including hashish, which consists of the psychoactive resin pressed into blocks, and bhang, a liquid distillate used in India. Throughout much of its history, cannabis has been known more for its analgesic properties than for its psychoactive effects. However, controversy currently surrounds its use as an analgesic and for other medical indications. Although it has been used experimentally to stimulate appetite in patients with AIDS, to reduce intraocular pressure in patients with glaucoma, and to treat the nausea caused by cancer chemotherapy, little formal research has focused on these actions because of concerns about the abuse potential of marijuana (see Chapter 16).

The marijuana intoxication syndrome varies greatly. After exposure to this drug, some individuals become giddy and others become morose and depressed. Use of the drug also may be accompanied by introspection and a sense of time moving slowly. In many ways, marijuana intoxication is similar to intoxication produced by hallucinogens; indeed cannabinoids often are considered "minor hallucinogens". Distortions of sensory perceptions are fairly common during marijuana intoxication and frank hallucinations can be induced, although these are rare. Potential adverse effects include an impairment in short-term and perhaps long-term memory, and impaired motor coordination during the performance of certain tasks.

Significant advances in the pharmacology of cannabinoids, the active constituents of marijuana, have occurred in recent years. It has been determined, for example, that marijuana's mechanism of action is quite different from that of the hallucinogens. The principal psychoactive ingredient of the cannabinoids is $\mathbf{\Delta^9}$-**tetrahydrocannabinol** (**THC**). THC and related cannabinoids have been difficult to study because of their unique lipophilic properties, which make binding studies problematic (see Chapter 16 for the chemical structure of THC). Indeed, these difficulties have caused some researchers to speculate that cannabinoids act directly on membranes rather than through binding to specific receptors. However, in the 1980s relatively water-soluble, potent agents displaying saturable binding and pharmacology consistent with the existence of a so-called cannabinoid receptor in the brain were synthesized (Figure 17–7). These agents were found to cause a GTP-dependent inhibition of adenylyl cyclase, which suggested that the receptor for cannabinoids is a member of the large superfamily of G protein-coupled receptors.

In 1990 the first cannabinoid receptor was identified and cloned in a somewhat serendipitous manner. After the initial cloning and characterization of several G protein-coupled receptors, regions of homology among the receptors were identified, and these were used to isolate novel members of this superfamily of so-called orphan receptors, without knowledge of their ligands. One of these receptors, when localized by in situ hybridization, exhibited a pattern of expression similar to cannabinoid binding sites in the brain. This cannabinoid receptor, now known as CB_1 (Figure 17–8), occurs throughout the CNS and is concentrated in the basal ganglia and cerebellum. Moderate expression of the receptor occurs in the hippocampus and layers I and IV of cerebral cortex, with lower expression seen in the brain stem, medulla, thalamus, and hypothalamus. The anatomic distribution of CB_1 correlates well with the previously mentioned effects of marijuana. A second cannabinoid receptor, CB_2, also has been cloned. It has low overall homology with the CB_1 receptor and is found only in peripheral tissues.

CB_1 and CB_2 receptors couple by means of $G_{i/o}$ proteins. Like other receptors that couple with these G proteins, cannabinoid receptors inhibit adenylyl cyclase and, depending on the cell type, inhibit voltage-gated Ca^{2+} channels or stimulate inwardly rectifying K^+ channels. CB_1 receptors are also reported to increase the transient voltage-dependent K^+ current known as A-type current (see Chapter 3). As with many G_i-coupled receptors, activation of CB_1 inhibits transmitter release and synaptic transmission in a variety of preparations. Moreover, cannabinoids have been shown to impair the generation of long-term potentiation, a cellular model for learning and memory (see Chapter 20). Which cellular actions of cannabinoids account for their profound psychological effects, and in which regions of the brain, are important questions that remain unanswered.

The identification of cannabinoid receptors led to the intriguing speculation that an endogenous cannabinoid-like substance might exist; such speculation was partly based on the discovery of endogenous opioid peptides soon after the detection of opioid receptors (see Chapter 10). Because cannabinoids are highly lipophilic, the search for an endogenous substance focused on membrane extracts from the brain and led to the identification of a derivative of arachidonic acid, called anandamide. This substance fulfills several criteria for an endogenous cannabinoid-like substance: 1) it is located in the brain and can activate cannabinoid receptors, 2) it is released from neurons in response to depolarization, and 3) it appears to undergo rapid inactivation when released. Anandamide is an eicosanoid that consists of arachidonic acid coupled to ethanolamine

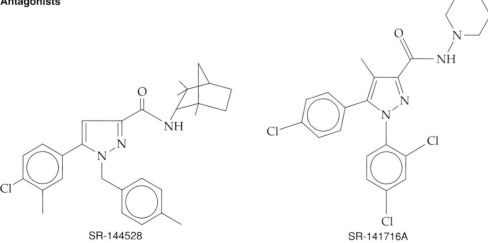

Figure 17–7. Chemical structures of representative agonists and antagonists of cannabinoid receptors.

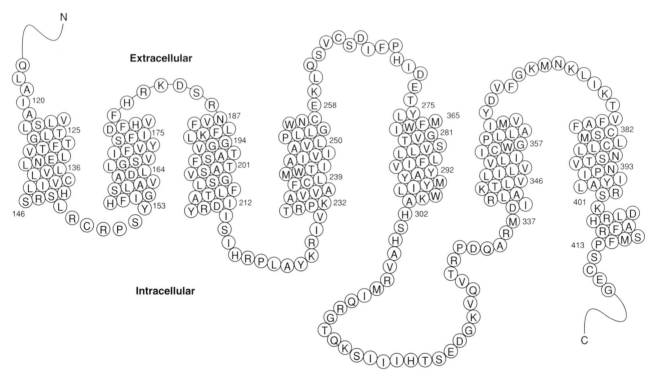

Figure 17–8. Proposed structure of the CB$_1$ receptor. CB$_1$ comprises seven transmembrane domains and is a member of the G protein-coupled receptor superfamily. (Adapted with permission from Julien RM. 1997. *A Primer of Drug Action,* 8th ed. New York: WH Freeman.)

by means of an amide. The route of its biosynthesis is unclear; however, it is possible that increases in intracellular Ca^{2+} activate an *N*-acyl-transferase, which promotes the transfer of arachidonic acid from an *N*-acylphospholipid, such as phosphatidylcholine, to phosphatidylethanolamine (Figure 17–9). Subsequently Ca^{2+}-activated phospholipase D may cleave anandamide from the resulting *N*-acylphosphatidylethanolamine. After its release into the synapse, anandamide may be removed by means of active uptake or may be metabolized.

Although anandamide has been found in many regions of the brain with high levels of CB$_1$ receptors, whether it functions as a neurotransmitter is unclear. It has relatively low affinity for the CB$_1$ and CB$_2$ receptors and, because of its hydrophobicity, it most likely is not stored within synaptic vesicles. Instead, it may be released from a membrane phospholipid precursor in response to activation of the appropriate phospholipase. A second putative endogenous cannabinoid, *sn*-2 arachidonylglycerol (2-AG), has been identified. 2-AG appears to be formed by the Ca^{2+}-stimulated activation of phospholipase C and diacylglycerol lipase. It functions as a full agonist at cannabinoid receptors and, like other cannabinoids, can inhibit hippocampal long-term potentiation.

Some examples of cannabinoid receptor agonists and antagonists are represented in Figure 17–7. Given the potential therapeutic actions of marijuana, the eventual clinical use of these or related compounds appears likely. Anandamide, for example, has potent analgesic actions in animal models of peripheral pain.

The development of cannabinoid antagonists has settled an old question. Years ago it was generally believed that cannabinoids did not induce physical dependence because an obvious withdrawal syndrome was not detectable in animals or humans after the cessation of drug exposure. The absence of a withdrawal syndrome has since been explained by the extremely long half-life of cannabinoids in the brain, which in turn is explained by the drug's strong lipophilic properties. However, when an animal previously exposed to cannabinoids is given a CB$_1$ antagonist, a profound physical withdrawal syndrome ensues (see Chapter 16).

DRUGS THAT REDUCE PSYCHOSIS

Chlorpromazine and **reserpine,** the first antipsychotic drugs, were introduced in the 1950s. These two drugs dramatically improved the treatment of schizophrenia and initiated the first neuropharmacologic studies of the disorder. Chlorpromazine (Figure 17–10) was initially identified as an antihistamine compound and subsequently was credited with improving the safety of surgical anesthesia. Its surgical use led to the discovery of postoperative sedative properties, which in turn led to its use in the reduction of agitation in some patients with schizophrenia. This therapeutic effect could not be attributed to general CNS depression because chlorpromazine reduced agitation in schizophrenic patients without inducing gross sedation. Moreover, this drug appeared to be effective against some of the positive and negative symptoms of schizophrenia. An example of the latter type of effectiveness was the observation that patients with catatonic schizophrenia became more active after treatment with chlorpromazine. Initial studies also revealed that the use of chlorpromazine results in consistent motor side effects. Therapeutic doses caused muscle stiffness and motor slowing similar to that associated with **Parkinson disease.** Because such side effects were believed to be closely related to the therapeutic mechanism of chlorpromazine, related phenothiazine drugs (see Figure 17–10) soon were developed, using motor side effects such as catalepsy (see Chapter 14) as an endpoint in laboratory animals. The term *neuroleptic,* which cur-

rently is used to refer to all first-generation antipsychotic drugs, is Greek for *neuron clasping* and refers to motor side effects of the medications.

Studies of chlorpromazine roughly coincided with the discovery of reserpine's antipsychotic properties. Reserpine, the active component of snakeroot or *Rauwolfia serpentina*, is a medication traditionally used in India to treat psychiatric disorders. However, it was initially used as an antihypertensive agent in the United States (see Chapter 12) until clinical trials demonstrated its effectiveness as an antipsychotic agent. Interestingly, therapeutic doses of reserpine cause motor side effects that are identical to those associated with the use of chlorpromazine. Despite very different molecular structures, these two compounds have a striking number of similar effects. Such similarities provided investigators with important research tools and generated considerable evidence to support the view that schizophrenia can be understood at the neurobiologic level.

Dopamine hypothesis of antipsychotic drug action   In the mid-1950s reserpine administration was shown to reduce the levels of dopamine, norepinephrine, and serotonin in rat brain. The reduction in

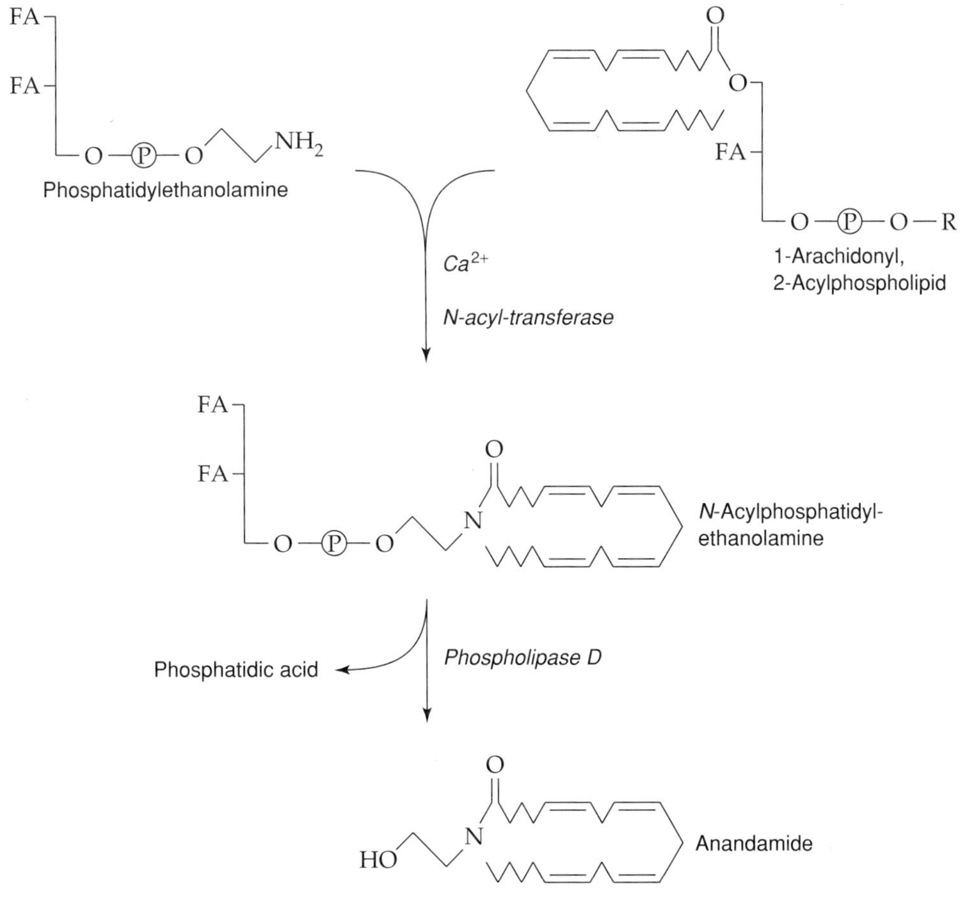

Figure 17–9. Proposed pathway for the biosynthesis of anandamide. FA, fatty acid.

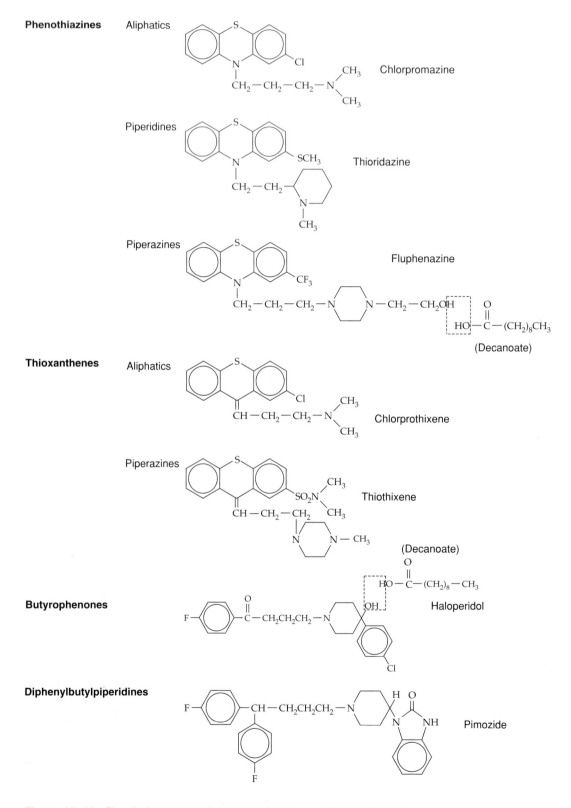

Figure 17–10. Chemical structures of representative classic antipsychotic drugs.

dopamine was a particularly compelling finding because it explained the motor side effects of reserpine; by this time Parkinson disease had been attributed to the death of dopamine neurons in the substantia nigra and the resulting depletion of dopamine from the striatum. Initial studies of chlorpromazine did not support an involvement of dopaminergic systems in its mechanism of action because it had no effect on catecholamine levels in the brain. Instead, Arvid Carlsson and his colleagues observed an increase in the dopamine metabolite homovanillic acid (HVA) in the striatum after administration of chlorpromazine or other neuroleptics (see Chapter 8). They proposed that these drugs worked by blocking dopamine receptors, which leads to a compensatory increase in dopamine release in the striatum and thus to an increase in dopamine breakdown products such as HVA.

Effects of neuroleptics on D_2 dopamine receptors   The dopamine hypothesis of neuroleptic action was bolstered by studies of dopamine receptor binding and function in rat striatum. Such studies identified two major dopamine binding sites, termed D_1 and D_2. Although some older neuroleptics, such as chlorpromazine, are potent antagonists of both receptor types, antagonism of the D_2 receptor is most strongly related to antipsychotic efficacy (Figure 17–11). **Haloperidol,** for example, is a butyrophenone and potent antipsychotic medication with a high affinity for the D_2 but not the D_1 receptor (see Figure 17–10). Molecular cloning studies later revealed that the D_1 binding site consists of D_1 and D_5 receptors and that the D_2 binding site consists of D_2, D_3, and D_4 receptors (see Chapter 8). Although antagonism of the D_2 receptor remains most strongly associated with antipsychotic drug action, the involvement of D_3 and D_4 receptors in such activity has been considered in recent years. The correlation between antipsychotic potency and D_2 antagonism may be flawed because it is supported by circular reasoning: D_2 receptor antagonism has been used to determine dosage ranges of many antipsychotic medications, so it is not surprising that dosage and D_2 receptor affinity correlate. Yet sustained antagonism of D_2 receptors unquestionably decreases psychosis. This finding led to a generation of research regarding a possible role of this receptor or some other component of the dopamine system in the pathophysiology of schizophrenia. As already stated, however, evidence for such a pathophysiologic role is lacking.

How does antagonism of D_2 receptors lead to an antipsychotic effect? The answer to this question, which remains unknown, is likely to be complex for several reasons. First, because it takes neuroleptics several weeks to exert their full antipsychotic effects, it is probably not antagonism of D_2 receptors per se that decreases psychosis; rather this effect is most likely explained by adaptations to sustained D_2 antagonism. Second, the effects of D_2 receptor antagonism must be understood within the context of the neural circuits in which these receptors function, and knowledge of the actions of dopamine in these circuits remains rudimentary. Cortical pyramidal neurons in the prefrontal cortex, for example, receive glutamatergic inputs from other cortical neurons and thalamic neurons. These cortico-cortical and thalamocortical glutamatergic synapses are modulated by local GABAergic interneurons and by numerous afferent projections, including those of distant monoaminergic neurons. A major goal of current research is to delineate how dopamine, acting on D_2 and other dopamine receptors, modifies these various synaptic inputs and pyramidal neuron excitability, and how chronic blockade of D_2 receptors alters the functioning of these circuits to reduce psychosis.

Side effects of neuroleptic drugs   Although neuroleptics have revolutionized the treatment of schizophrenia and have improved the quality of life for millions of individuals, serious drawbacks have limited their clinical use. Their numerous side effects, for example, interfere with adherence to therapy. Pharmacologic studies over the years have revealed that most of these side effects occur because neuroleptics have affinities for multiple receptors in the brain; accordingly, many side effects can be correlated with binding to a particular receptor site (Table 17–1). Sedation, for example, results from the blocking of H_1 histamine receptors in the CNS. Hypotension results from the antagonism of α_1-adrenergic receptors. Dry mouth, blurred vision, and constipation are caused by the antagonism of muscarinic cholinergic receptors. The many neuroleptics available exhibit different affinities at each of these receptors; the degree to which one of these drugs will cause a particular side effect is determined by the drug's potency at the receptor associated with that side effect and the dose of the drug required to achieve therapeutic effects.

The motor side effects caused by neuroleptics are classified as extrapyramidal side effects (EPS) because they relate to drug action that takes place outside of the pyramidal motor system, which controls voluntary movements (see Chapter 14). There are four major categories of EPS. The first consists of a parkinsonian syndrome that resembles true **Parkinson disease**. This syndrome is characterized by rigidity, difficulty in initiating movements, dampened facial expressions, and a resting tremor in the hands and arms. A second and more

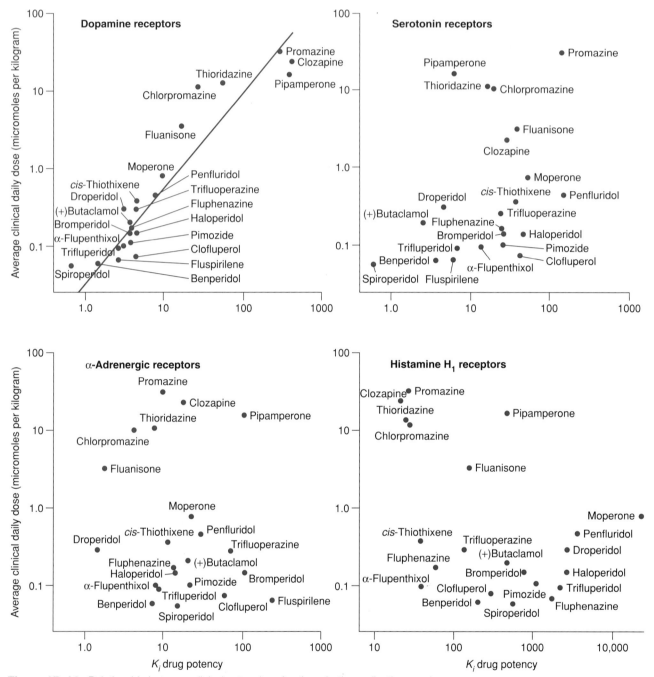

Figure 17–11. Relationship between clinical potencies of antipsychotic medications and their affinities for various receptors. Each graph shows clinical potency as a function of binding to D_2 dopamine, 5-$HT_{2A/C}$ serotonin, α_1-adrenergic, and H_1 histamine receptors. (From Snyder SH. 1996. *Drugs and the Brain.* New York: Scientific American Library.)

severe form of EPS is acute dystonia, which is characterized by a sudden and severe spastic contraction of muscles—most often those of the face and neck. Such dystonic reactions are dramatic and disturbing to individuals who experience them. They also can be dangerous; for example, a related spasm of the tongue can block a patient's airway. A third category of EPS consists of akathisia, a syndrome characterized by a subjective sense of anxiety and restlessness. EPS-related akathisia is commonly mistaken for psychotic agitation. The fourth category of EPS is represented by **tardive dyskinesia,** a syndrome that involves abnormal choreiform movements (see Chapter 14). Unlike other EPS, tardive dyskinesia is more common after repeated drug exposure and is not readily reversible after cessation of drug treatment. A potentially debilitating side effect, tardive dyskinesia has severely limited the use of classic neuroleptics.

Because D_2 receptor antagonism is intimately related to the therapeutic mechanism of neuroleptics and to the emergence of EPS, all neuroleptics cause EPS to some degree. In fact, early studies used EPS to gauge appropriate clinical doses of these medications for various individuals. However, as more antipsychotic drugs became available, it became clear that some caused more frequent and more severe EPS than others. High-potency agents, such as haloperidol, for example, cause more EPS than low-potency agents, such as chlorpromazine. Initially this finding was surprising because high-potency agents were used at much lower doses than low-potency agents. Subsequently, it was appreciated that low-potency neuroleptics tend to have intrinsic anticholinergic activity that ameliorates EPS. This action is believed to be mediated by the antagonism of muscarinic cholinergic receptors in the striatum (see Chapter 14). Currently when high-potency neuroleptics are used, they are often coadministered with a medication, such as **benztropine** or **diphenhydramine,** with antimuscarinic properties (see Chapters 9 and 14).

This practice allows D_2 and muscarinic blocking activities to be titrated independently to reduce EPS.

Atypical antipsychotics   The disadvantages associated with the use of classic neuroleptic antipsychotics have prompted a search for better alternatives. In addition to the complications mentioned in the previous section, classic antipsychotics do not appear to address the primary lesion in schizophrenia. They tend to be relatively ineffective, for example, against the negative symptoms and cognitive deficits that frequently characterize this disorder. Although such clinical problems may be less dramatic than hallucinations and delusions, they can be equally or even more debilitating. The search for better antipsychotics has led to the development of novel agents with pharmacologic properties that appear to be very different from those of the older, conventional neuroleptics; thus these new agents are referred to as atypical antipsychotics.

Atypical antipsychotics can be distinguished from classic neuroleptics by three main characteristics: 1) they are much less likely to induce EPS, 2) they have somewhat better efficacy against the negative symptoms of schizophrenia, and 3) they are able to effectively treat

Table 17-1 Pharmacologic Properties of Classic Neuroleptics

Drug	Approximate Dose Equivalent (mg)	Sedative Effect	Hypotensive Effect	Anticholinergic Effect	Extrapyramidal Effect
Phenothiazines					
Aliphatic					
Chlorpromazine (Thorazine)	100	High	High	Medium	Low
Triflupromazine (Vesprin)	30	High	High	Medium	Medium
Piperidines					
Mesoridazine (Serentil)	50	Medium	Medium	Medium	Medium
Thioridazine (Mellaril)	95	High	High	High	Low
Piperazines					
Acetophenazine (Tindal)	15	Low	Low	Low	Medium
Fluphenazine (Prolixin, Permitil)	2	Medium	Low	Low	High
Perphenazine (Trilafon)	8	Low	Low	Low	High
Trifluoperazine (Stelazine)	5	Medium	Low	Low	High
Thioxanthenes					
Aliphatic					
Chlorprothixene (Taractan)	75	High	High	High	Low
Piperazine					
Thiothixene (Navane)	5	Low	Low	Low	High
Dibenzodiazepines					
Loxapine (Loxitane, Daxolin)	10	Medium	Medium	Medium	High
Clozapine (Clozaril)	100	High	High	High	Very low
Butyrophenones					
Droperidol (Inapsine—injection only)	1	Low	Low	Low	High
Haloperidol (Haldol)	2	Low	Low	Low	High
Indolone					
Molindone (Moban)	10	Medium	Low	Medium	High
Diphenylbutylpiperidine					
Pimozide (Orap)	1	Low	Low	Low	High

Reproduced with permission from Hyman SE, Arana GW, Rosenbaum JF. 1995. *Handbook of Psychiatric Drug Therapy*, 3rd ed. Boston: Little Brown and Co.

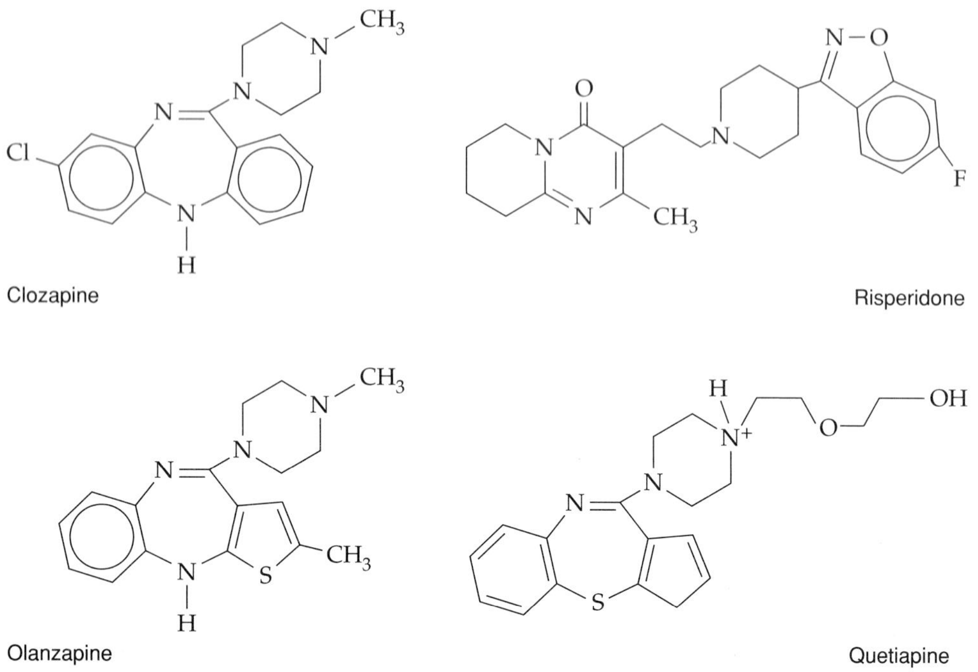

Clozapine

Risperidone

Olanzapine

Quetiapine

Figure 17–12. Chemical structures of clozapine and of several putative atypical antipsychotic drugs that have received approval in the United States.

some patients who are unresponsive to classic neuroleptics. **Clozapine** is the prototype of the atypical antipsychotics (Figure 17–12). It originally was believed to be simply another low-potency antipsychotic because its clinically useful dose is quite high. However, the incidence of EPS associated with its use was far lower than could be explained by its low potency and high anticholinergic activity. Clozapine's introduction into the United States was delayed for many years because its use is associated with a presumed immune-mediated agranulocytosis, or decreased production of white blood cells—a potentially fatal side effect in approximately 1% of patients. Yet clozapine eventually was credited with the effective treatment of many schizophrenic patients who had previously failed to respond to treatment. Large double-blind studies confirmed clozapine's superior efficacy in the treatment of refractory schizophrenia and its effectiveness in reducing negative symptoms. Moreover, studies showed that the use of clozapine resulted in few EPS and virtually no tardive dyskinesia. Clozapine was finally approved in the United States for general use in 1990 and revolutionized the treatment of schizophrenia. Its approval for clinical use stimulated the development of new drugs, discussed in the next section of the chapter, that would mimic clozapine's superior efficacy and minimal EPS without inducing agranulocytosis.

Pharmacology of atypical antipsychotics Detailed examination of clozapine's pharmacologic actions reveals that it antagonizes many known neurotransmitter receptors (Figure 17–13). A primary defining characteristic is its relatively low affinity for the D_2 receptor. This property is believed to partly explain its low incidence of EPS, including tardive dyskinesia. Clozapine exhibits a relatively higher affinity for the D_3 and D_4 dopamine receptors, which are expressed at low levels in the dorsal striatum but at higher levels in the ventral striatum and in limbic regions of cortex (see Chapter 8). Indeed, the D_4 receptor appears to be the predominant D_2-like dopamine receptor in human frontal cortex. These findings have sparked considerable interest in the D_3 and D_4 receptors as the targets for clozapine's unique clinical actions. However, many classic neuroleptics, including haloperidol, exhibit relatively high affinity for the D_3 receptor. Furthermore, several selective D_4 antagonists have thus far failed to exhibit antipsychotic properties in a number of clinical trials. Consequently the role of D_3 and D_4 receptors in atypical antipsychotic drug action remains unclear.

Serotonergic mechanisms also have been hypothesized to underlie the therapeutic actions of atypical antipsychotic medications and their low EPS liability. Such hypotheses initially were based on the previously described serotonergic actions of hallucinogenic drugs such as LSD. Subsequently serotonergic models of psychosis were largely supplanted by the dopamine hypothesis because LSD was determined to be a poor model of schizophrenia and neuroleptics were shown to have high affinities for the D_2 receptor. Yet clozapine's unusual pharmacologic profile rekindled interest in the serotonin receptor actions of antipsychotic agents because it has a high affinity for several serotonin receptors, particularly the 5-HT$_{2A}$ receptor, where the drug appears to act as an antagonist or an inverse agonist. Other putative atypical antipsychotic drugs, which are discussed next, also have a high affinity for 5-HT$_{2A}$ receptors. Consequently, it has been proposed that a low ratio of affinity for the D$_2$ to the 5-HT$_{2A}$ receptor is a defining characteristic of an atypical antipsychotic drug.

This hypothesis sparked the development of several novel antipsychotic drugs that fit this profile and that have been marketed as atypical antipsychotic medications (see Figures 17–12 and 17–13). Examples include **risperidone, olanzapine** (a close chemical analog of clozapine), **quetiapine, ziprasidone,** and **sertindole**. These drugs clearly are effective antipsychotics and cause fewer EPS and other side effects than classic neuroleptics. However, whether they match clozapine and satisfy the three criteria for atypical drugs previously mentioned has been the subject of some controversy. These drugs, which do cause some EPS, including tardive dyskinesia, are generally believed to have less clinical efficacy than clozapine. Yet they represent a major improvement over classic neuroleptics because of their lower incidence of EPS, and are rapidly becoming the drugs of first choice in the treatment of schizophrenia and other psychotic syndromes.

The precise mechanism responsible for clozapine's unique clinical properties has not been defined. Recent clinical studies suggest that antagonism of 5-HT$_{2A}$ receptors per se does not produce an antipsychotic effect, because a highly selective 5-HT$_{2A}$ antagonist (**MDL100907**) has thus far failed to show antipsychotic efficacy in clinical trials. Some attention has been given to other serotonin receptors. Clozapine has relatively high affinity for the 5-HT$_{2C}$, 5-HT$_3$, and 5-HT$_6$ receptors. However, these affinities and other receptor actions of clozapine (see Figure 17–13) appear to provide an imperfect explanation of the clinical actions of this drug; thus further research on this subject is needed.

Long-term effects of neuroleptic treatment Although schizophrenic patients show some clinical improvement shortly after the initiation of antipsychotic drug treatment, weeks of administration often are necessary before maximal therapeutic effects become apparent. This suggests that the prolonged blockade of D$_2$ dopamine receptors and other relevant actions, including perhaps the antagonism of 5-HT$_{2A}$ receptors, cause progressive alterations in particular neuronal populations that eventually lead to a reduction in psychotic symptoms.

Much of the research on long-term effects of neuroleptic treatment has focused on drug-induced alterations in the levels of dopamine receptors. Traditional neuroleptic drugs cause a small but well-replicated up-regulation of D$_2$ dopamine receptors in the striatum and frontal cortex. This change is accompanied by a down-regulation of D$_1$ dopamine receptors. These changes take place days to weeks after the initiation of drug treatment and may continue for several months. Interestingly, clozapine and other putative ayptical drugs also cause changes in dopamine receptor levels in the brain, particularly down-regulation of D$_1$ receptors in the prefrontal cortex. Such findings have led to specu-

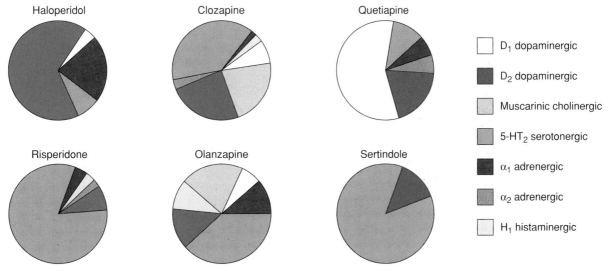

Figure 17–13. Pie graphs comparing pharmacologic profiles of haloperidol, clozapine, and several putative atypical antipsychotic drugs. (From Casey DE. 1997. *J Clin Psychiatry* 58(suppl)10:55.)

lation that alterations in the balance of D_1 and D_2 receptors in certain cortical regions may contribute to the gradual improvement that occurs in response to treatment with antipsychotic agents, and also may provide a common mechanism of typical and atypical antipsychotic drug action.

Yet the therapeutic actions of antipsychotic medications are unlikely to be explained by changes in dopamine receptors alone. Antipsychotic drugs given to laboratory animals also cause significant region-specific changes in the expression of many gene products, including neuropeptides, neurotransmitter receptors, and signal transduction proteins. Some of these changes may be mediated by drug-induced alterations in levels of specific transcription factors, such as the Fos family of proteins described in Chapter 6. Interestingly, classic neuroleptics induce Fos family transcription factors in the dorsal striatum as well as in the ventral striatum and prefrontal cortex, whereas clozapine produces changes only in the latter brain regions. The areas affected by other putative atypical agents, such as risperidone and olanzapine, are somewhere in between those that clozapine and classic neuroleptics affect. However, these data simply recapitulate what we already know: clozapine, and to a lesser extent other putative atypical drugs, somehow target limbic circuits rather than dorsal striatal circuits. Future research is needed to relate molecular and cellular adaptations produced by antipsychotic drugs to both the desirable and unwanted clinical actions of these medications.

Other strategies for treating schizophrenia   The NMDA glutamate receptor has been proposed as a target for antipsychotic drug action primarily because of two discoveries. First, PCP, a well-described psychotomimetic drug, is an NMDA receptor antagonist. Second, clinical studies of schizophrenic patients have produced evidence of decreased glutamate in their cerebral spinal fluid that is independent of drug treatment. However, these findings have not been universally replicated. Postmortem brain studies have led to reports of altered levels of expression of NMDA receptor subunits in the forebrains of schizophrenics compared with normal brains. Together these results offer at least a suggestion—albeit a highly speculative one—that some form of glutamate system dysregulation may be characteristic of schizophrenia.

If indeed NMDA receptor hypofunction contributes to schizophrenia-like psychosis, based on the actions of PCP, it has been reasoned that agents that augment NMDA receptor function might reverse such psychosis. Such reasoning led to clinical trials involving the use of glycine in the treatment of schizophrenia. As discussed in Chapter 7, glycine promotes NMDA receptor function by binding to a positive allosteric regulatory site on the receptor complex. **Milacemide** and **D-cycloserine,** which lead to the in vivo formation of glycine, also have been tried in humans. Some evidence suggests that the drugs might improve negative symptoms in schizophrenic patients when used in combination with neuroleptics or atypical antipsychotics. Trials with inhibitors of the glycine transporter (GLYT1), which may increase synaptic levels of glycine and thereby potentiate NMDA receptor function, are expected to get under way soon.

Dopaminergic neurons in the CNS contain high levels of several neuropeptides, which may act as modulators of dopaminergic neurotransmission. Consequently, these peptide systems have been considered putative targets for the actions of novel antipsychotic drugs. Specific neuropeptides of interest include β-endorphin, neurotensin, and cholecystokinin. This research has been limited by difficulties associated with using peptides as drugs and the general lack of availability of small-molecule drugs that act on neuropeptide receptors (see Chapter 10). As previously indicated, nicotinic cholinergic agonists also have been suggested for use in the treatment of schizophrenia; however, the utility of such agents remains hypothetical.

Despite the extraordinary advances in the treatment of schizophrenia and other psychotic disorders that have occurred during the second half of the past century, much work remains to be done. In particular, it will be important to gain a much more sophisticated understanding of the etiology and pathophysiology of psychotic disorders so that rational drug treatments can be developed.

SELECTED READING

American Psychiatric Association 1994. *Diagnostic and Statistical Manual of Mental Disorders,* 4th ed. Washington, DC: American Psychiatric Association.

Atkins J, Carlezon WA, Chlan J, et al. 1999. Region-specific induction of ΔFosB by repeated administration of typical versus atypical antipsychotic drugs. *Synapse* 33:118–128.

Barondes S. 1993. *Molecules and Mental Illness.* New York: Scientific American Library.

Benes FM. 1999. Evidence for altered trisynaptic circuitry in schizophrenic hippocampus. *Biol Psychiatry* 46:589–599.

Bergeron R, Meyer TM, Coyle JT, Greene RW. 1998 Modulation of *N*-methyl-D-aspartate receptor function by glycine transport. *Proc Natl Acad Sci USA* 95:15730–15734.

Carlsson A, Waters N, Waters S, Carlsson ML. 2000. Network interactions in schizophrenia—therapeutic implications. *Brain Res Rev* 31:342–349.

Casey DE. 1997. The relationship of pharmacology to side effects. *J Clin Psychiatry* 58(10):55–62.

Egan MF, Weinberger DR. 1997. Neurobiology of schizophrenia. *Curr Opin Neurobiol* 7:701–707.

Felder CC, Glass M. 1998. Cannabinoid receptors and their endogenous agonists. *Annu Rev Pharmacol Toxicol* 38:179–200.

Goldman-Rakic PS. 1995. Cellular basis of working memory. *Neuron* 14:477–485.

Goldman–Rakic PS, Muly EC 3rd, Williams GV. 2000. D$_1$ receptors in prefrontal cells and circuits. *Brain Res Rev* 31:295–301.

Griffith JM, O'Neill JE, Petty F, et al. 1998. Nicotinic receptor desensitization and sensory gating deficits in schizophrenia. *Biol Psychiatry* 44:98–106.

Hyman SE, Arana GW, Rosenbaum JF. 1995. *Handbook of Psychiatric Drug Therapy*. Boston: Little Brown.

Jones EG. 1997. Cortical development and thalamic pathology in schizophrenia. *Schizophr Bull* 23:483–501.

Kandel ER, Schwartz JH, Jessel TM. 2000. *Principles of Neural Science*, 4th ed. New York: McGraw-Hill.

Kaplan HI, Sadock BJ, Grebb JA. 1994. *Synopsis of Psychiatry*, 7th ed. Baltimore: Williams and Wilkins.

Karayiorgou M, Gogos JA. 1997. A turning point in schizophrenia genetics. *Neuron* 19:967.

Kortla KJ, Weinberger DR. 1995. Brain imaging in schizophrenia. *Annu Rev Med* 46:113.

Lewis DA. 2000. Is there a neuropathology of schizophrenia? Recent findings converge on altered thalamic-prefrontal cortical connectivity. *The Neuroscientist* 6:208–218.

Lewis DA, Lieberman JA. 2000. Catching up on schizophrenia: natural history and neurobiology. *Neuron* 28:325–334.

Lidow MS, Williams GV, Goldman-Rakic PS. 1998. The cerebral cortex: A case for a common site of action of antipsychotics. *Trends Pharmacol Sci* 19:136–140.

Marek GJ, Aghajanian GK. 1998. The electrophysiology of prefrontal serotonin systems: Therapeutic implications for mood and psychosis. *Biol Psychiatry* 44:1118–1127.

Piomelli D, Giuffrida A, Calignano A, Rodriguez de Fronseca F. 2000. The endocannabinoid system as a target for therapeutic drugs. *Trends Pharmacol Sci* 21:218–224.

Schatzberg AF, Nemeroff CB. 1995. *Textbook of Psychopharmacology*. Washington DC: American Psychiatric Press.

Selemon LD, Goldman-Rakic PS. 1999. The reduced neuropil hypothesis: A circuit based model of schizophrenia. *Biol Psychiatry* 45:17–25.

Shenton ME, Kikinis R, Jolesz FA, et al. 1992. Abnormalities of the left temporal lobe and thought disorder in schizophrenia: A quantitative magnetic resonance imaging study. *New Engl J Med* 327:604–612.

Snyder SH. 1996. *Drugs and the Brain*. New York: Scientific American Library.

Taylor JR, Birnbaum S, Ubriani R, Arnsten AF. 1999. Activation of cAMP-dependent protein kinase A in prefrontal cortex impairs working memory performance. *J Neurosci* 19:RC23.

Willins DL, Berry SA, Alsayegh L, et al. 1999. Clozapine and other 5-hydroxytryptamine-2A receptor antagonists alter the subcellular distribution of 5-hydroxytryptamine-2A receptors in vitro and in vivo. *Neuroscience* 91:599–606.

Chapter 18

Sleep, Arousal, and Attention

KEY CONCEPTS

- Sleep, arousal, and attention are active processes mediated by specific brain regions.

- Sleep can be divided into two phases, non-REM and REM sleep, the latter being a unique state of arousal that is characterized by brain activity resembling that observed during the waking state.

- The physiologic functions of sleep are unknown.

- The initiation of non-REM sleep is controlled in part by neurons in the preoptic/anterior hypothalamic area; the initiation of REM sleep is controlled by cells in the pontine tegmentum.

- The suprachiasmatic nucleus is the primary pacemaker for the circadian rhythms of numerous biologic processes, such as temperature regulation and cortisol secretion, which interact in complex ways with the need for sleep.

- Circadian rhythms are due, in part, to the complex transcriptional regulation of "clock" genes that have been conserved throughout evolution.

- Sleep disorders are a primary cause of morbidity. A major advance in research on sleep is the finding that abnormalities related to the hypothalamic peptide orexin (also called hypocretin) may contribute to narcolepsy.

- Benzodiazepines are the most common treatment for insomnia.

- The parietal cortex and frontal cortex are particularly important in orienting and maintaining attention, which is a distributed process that involves many additional brain areas.

- Attention deficit and hyperactivity disorder (ADHD) is a heterogeneous syndrome, the etiology of which is unknown. Psychostimulant drugs, such as methylphenidate and amphetamines, currently are the most effective treatment for ADHD.

Before the beginning of the 20th century, sleep and arousal states were conceptualized as passive processes and were believed to reflect a continuous gradient of levels of consciousness ranging from coma to catatonic excitement. Moreover, it was believed that each level of arousal corresponded to the number of neurons that were actively engaged in processing information, in much the same way that the illumination from a light bulb varies depending on the amount of electric current it receives. During the second half of the 20th century, it was discovered that distinct cells in the brain stem and in the basal forebrain are active during periods of wakefulness and sleep. Discoveries such as these demonstrated that the passive model of sleep and arousal was simplistic and inaccurate.

The first part of this chapter presents a broad overview of the neurobiology of sleep and arousal states. It is important to mention that a consensus on the definition of arousal has yet to be obtained. Behavioral states, such as fear, anxiety, panic, freezing, and pleasurable excitement, and different sleep states, such as rapid eye movement (REM) and nonrapid eye movement (NREM) sleep, appear to be governed by disparate populations of neurons. Moreover, sleep is different from hibernation, coma, or stupor secondary to anesthesia. Certain behavioral phenomena that occur during sleep may employ some of the neural circuitry that contributes to behavioral states during waking hours. **Night terrors,** for example, involve a partial arousal out of deep NREM sleep, and patients who experience these phenomena have signs of extreme sympathetic activation such as tachycardia, mydriasis, and diaphoresis, despite the fact that they remain asleep. In contrast, patients with **REM behavior disorder** may have bouts of extreme violent behavior during REM sleep that are not accompanied by elevations in heart rate or blood pressure. Hence, states of arousal are heterogeneous and complicated and cannot be explained by a simple rheostat model.

The second part of this chapter focuses on attention. The neurobiologic mechanisms that control attention share several features with those that control the sleep–wake cycle and arousal. This is not surprising, because attention requires an awake and alert organism. However, attention differs from arousal in that attention refers to selective responsiveness to particular stimuli as opposed to the general state of enhanced reactivity that characterizes arousal.

HISTORICAL OVERVIEW

An early clue that sleep is not merely a passive state but an active process emerged with the finding that particular brain regions must be intact for sleep to occur. It was discovered, for example, that lesions involving the anterior hypothalamus create a state of chronic insomnia; this finding suggested that activity in this region is necessary for sleep. In contrast, lesions involving the posterior hypothalamus create a state of hypersomnolence.

The introduction of the electroencephalogram (EEG) permitted the noninvasive assessment of some aspects of sleep. In 1948 it was discovered that stimulation of reticular cells in the brain stem elicits EEG arousal that is independent of classic sensory afferent pathways. Subsequently, arousal began to be viewed as an intrinsic property of the brain mediated by specific areas rather than as an epiphenomenon that simply occurs in response to increased sensory input. This change in perspective roughly coincided with the discovery that alertness and arousal have a circadian rhythmicity that is independent of the number of hours an individual sleeps. Studies of sleep-deprived individuals indicated that alertness increases in the midmorning from a nadir that occurs late at night despite a longer period of continuous wakefulness. Such findings affirm that arousal is not a simple function of previous rest or sensory input.

Our understanding of the physiology of sleep and arousal grew with the increased use of EEGs in the evaluation of human sleep. In the late 1930s many features of EEG patterns in NREM sleep were identified. Shortly thereafter REM sleep and the ultradian NREM–REM sleep cycle were described. (An ultradian rhythm is a biologic rhythm that cycles more often than every 24 hours). REM sleep was determined to be associated with EEG activation, generalized muscle atonia with the exception of rapid eye movements, and fluctuating irregularities in heart rate and respiration.

During the late 1950s, cats with pontine lesions were reported to have undergone REM sleep without atonia. In these studies, which examined neural substrates of REM sleep, the lesioned cats walked and exhibited attack and defense behaviors while their EEGs showed every indication that they were in a REM state. Yet during REM sleep, the cats were unresponsive to external stimuli. These findings provided rich fuel for speculation about the function of REM and confirmed the active nature of this brain state. Histochemical studies of the brain stem suggested that REM is a complex state that is controlled by several neurotransmitter systems; these studies laid the groundwork for electrophysiologic experiments in the 1970s, which showed that the onset of REM is generated by cholinergic cells in the pontine tegmentum and that inputs from the noradrenergic locus ceruleus and serotonergic raphe nuclei inhibit REM. These findings in turn led to the development of an influential reciprocal interaction model of REM regulation, which is described later in this chapter. However, despite considerable advances in the neurobiology of NREM and REM sleep, the precise physiologic function of these two states remains unknown.

NORMAL HUMAN SLEEP

The EEG, which records summed electrical activity across many different brain regions through electrodes attached to the scalp, is the primary means by which stages of human sleep are monitored. An EEG recording of this summed electrical activity during a normal waking state is characterized by low-amplitude, mixed-frequency activity (Figure 18–1). The electrical activity of the brain is desynchronized because individual neurons are in many different states of activity. When a complex visual scene is being processed, for example, some neurons of the occipital cortex fire rapidly, some fire slowly, and others do not fire at all.

The onset of sleep is marked by the appearance of lower-frequency waves in the EEG recording (see Figure 18–1). The predominance of low-frequency activity indicates greater synchrony in neuronal firing and leads to a summed polarization and depolarization large enough to be recorded by the EEG. Different stages of sleep are generally classified according to EEG wave patterns. NREM sleep is composed of four stages. Stage 1 occurs during the transition between wakefulness and sleep and is defined by the presence of background theta (4- to 7-Hz) activity that comprises more than 50% of each 30-second epoch. Stage 2 is composed of a background rhythm of theta activity with superimposed burst–pause wave forms such as K-complexes (high-amplitude, slow-frequency electronegative waves followed by electropositive waves) and spindles (brief bursts of 7- to 14-Hz activity). Stages 3 and 4 are defined by the presence of slow-wave (0.1- to 4-Hz), or delta, sleep activity that comprises 20% and 50% of each epoch of sleep time, respectively. Slow-wave sleep is associated with a reduced metabolic rate and a decline in brain and body temperature. Electrophysiologic features of all four stages of sleep include increased firing of sleep-active centers in the anterior hypothalamus, hyperpolarization of thalamocortical neurons, and burst–pause activity driven by the reticular thalamic nucleus. Broad systemic features of stages 1–4 include behavioral quiescence, low muscle activity, reduced blood pressure, reduced heart and respiration rates, reduced cortisol and thyroid hormone levels, and increased growth hormone, testosterone, prolactin, insulin, and glucose levels.

REM sleep, which normally occurs only after a progression through sleep stages 1–4, is a unique state of arousal characterized by electrical brain activity, cerebral blood flow, and brain glucose metabolism similar to that of wakefulness. The onset of REM is represented in EEG recordings by a shift to desynchronized, low-amplitude electrical activity that also resembles that of the waking state. REM sleep is accompanied by a generalized muscular atonia that excludes the extraocular muscles and the diaphragm, clitoral or penile tumescence, phasic bursts of eye movements, and alternating acceleration and deceleration of heart and respiratory rates.

Electrophysiologic recordings during REM sleep have documented tonic cerebral activity, synchronized firing of hippocampal neurons in the theta frequency range, and phasic ponto-geniculo-occipital (PGO) spikes. Several areas in the limbic system, hypothalamus, and brain stem achieve their highest firing rate during REM, providing further evidence that sleep is not a quiescent state. Indeed, positron emission tomography (PET) studies in humans have shown that limbic structures such as the amygdala become metabolically active during REM sleep. Surprisingly, despite the pattern of cerebral activation, the threshold for arousal from REM sleep is higher than that from NREM sleep.

During the first half of the night, sleep is dominated by slow–wave sleep patterns (Figure 18–2). The first REM cycle occurs after approximately 90 minutes of NREM sleep, and tends to be brief in duration. During the latter half of the night, NREM cycles comprise stages of lighter NREM sleep, with little slow-wave sleep activity. Later REM sleep periods are longer and have more phasic REM activity, including eye movements. Intermittent awakenings are a part of normal sleep and may serve an adaptive function; for example, they may enable changes in posture to minimize circulatory pooling, or appraisals of the environment to guard against possible threats. Humans are unaware of most of these brief awakenings because they experience retrograde amnesia for several minutes after resuming sleep. A common misperception is that dreams occur only during REM. In fact, dreams occur during all stages of sleep but tend to be more dramatic, varied, and vivid in the latter part of the night during REM.

ONTOGENY OF SLEEP

Newborns spend 20 hours a day in sleep. These hours are characterized by an incomplete segregation between REM-like, or *active* sleep and NREM-like, or *quiet,* sleep. By 6 months of age, REM and NREM sleep can be reliably distinguished. During the first three years of life, humans begin to segregate sleep and waking until they

Awake – low voltage – random, fast

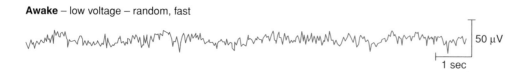

50 µV

1 sec

Drowsy – 8 to 12 cycles/s (cps) – alpha waves

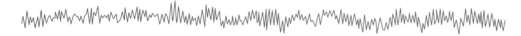

Stage 1 – 3 to 7 cps – theta waves

Theta waves

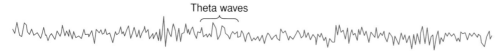

Stage 2 – 12 to 14 cps – sleep spindles and K complexes

Sleep spindles

K complex

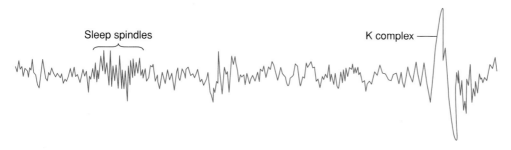

Delta sleep – $\frac{1}{2}$ to 2 cps – delta waves > 75 µV

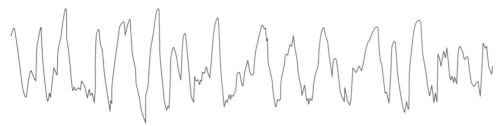

REM sleep – low voltage – random, fast with sawtooth waves

Sawtooth waves

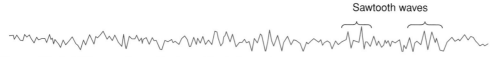

Figure 18–1. EEG recordings of brain activity during various stages of sleep. (Adapted with permission from Hauri P, Orr W. 1982. *Current Concepts: The Sleep Disorders.* Kalamazoo, MI: Upjohn.)

become two consolidated periods. During adolescence a precipitous drop in slow-wave sleep activity occurs, which coincides with a period of synaptic pruning in the cerebral cortex. With advancing age a gradual decline in total hours of sleep occurs together with an increase in the number of awakenings. The sixth and seventh decades of life are characterized by a decline in total slow-wave sleep activity, which is predominately related to a decline in EEG amplitude. Elderly people experience more awakenings, complain more often of insomnia, and shift more of their sleep time to the day in the form of naps. Several circadian rhythms, including the sleep–wake cycle, exhibit a decrease in amplitude and a phase advance during aging. Hence, older people have a propensity to fall asleep at earlier hours and to have more early morning awakenings. The decline in total sleep time in healthy older subjects is relatively modest, and the ability to experience a restoration of daytime vigor is intact. The prevalence of insomnia among the elderly appears to result from medical and neuropsychiatric disorders that adversely affect sleep.

FUNCTIONS OF SLEEP

The need to sleep is universal among mammals, birds, and reptiles and has been conserved in evolution. Despite the obvious disadvantages of sleep, such as reduced vigilance against predators, it is a behavior that is necessary to sustain life. In rats, total sleep deprivation or selective REM sleep deprivation results in death after a period of 2 to 3 weeks, which is comparable to the length of survival during starvation. The reason that sleep-deprived animals die is unknown but may relate to metabolic dysfunction; for example, sleep-deprived rats tend to lose weight, even though they eat more than rats that have not been deprived of sleep. More striking proof that sleep is a necessity has come from observations of marine mammals, who must remain awake constantly in order to surface every few minutes for air. It appears that these mammals sleep *unihemispherically;* that is, one cerebral hemisphere

exhibits sleep patterns detectable by EEG, while the other hemisphere remains awake. The persistence of sleeping behavior in animals that must maintain constant wakefulness is a powerful indication that sleep serves an essential function.

Despite intense scientific research, no theory has explained the function of sleep in a manner that holds true across species or across different levels of investigation. Questions regarding the amount of sleep that is needed, the stage of sleep that is most restorative, and the interventions that best promote healthy sleep remain unanswered. The popular belief that sleep is needed to restore the integrity of body functions makes some intuitive sense. Yet this theory is accompanied by a false assumption that sleep is an inactive state. Because quiet wakefulness and sleep differ very little in terms of energy expenditure, it is unlikely that sleep and its attendant reduction in vigilance was conserved in evolution simply to save energy. Furthermore, no compelling evidence suggests that tissue rebuilding or an increase in protein synthesis is associated with sleep. Many types of external and internal stimuli, including ambient temperature, darkness, food intake, exercise, and endogenous immune factors affect sleep, but none of these variables has provided clues to the core function of sleep.

Many hypotheses have been used to explain the functions of REM sleep, but these frequently focus on a particular feature of REM, such as PGO spikes, and ignore other features. One prominent and intriguing hypothesis is that REM is needed to enhance learning

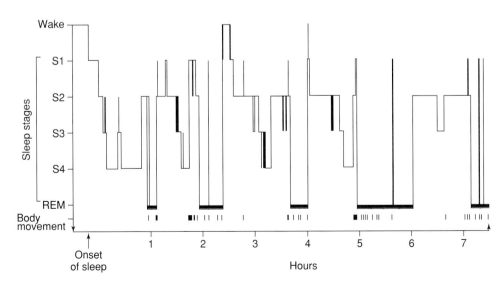

Figure 18–2. Sleep histogram shows a normal pattern of sleep in a young adult. Note that the time spent in REM increases as the night progresses. (Adapted with permission from Kryger MH, Roth T, Dement WC [eds]. 1994. *Principles and Practice of Sleep Medicine,* 2nd ed. Philadelphia: WB Saunders.)

or to discard irrelevant memory traces. However, evidence in support of such speculation is limited. Another interesting hypothesis, which arises from observed relationships between the proportion of sleep spent in REM by members of different species and their degree of maturity at birth, is that REM is needed for early neurodevelopment in altricial species characterized by marked immaturity at birth. However, this hypothesis does not adequately explain the persistence of REM in adulthood and the increased amount of REM sleep that occurs after sleep deprivation. Available hypotheses also fail to explain the functional significance of alternations between REM and NREM sleep cycles, although it appears that the length of these cycles in mammals correlates closely with brain size. Consequently, the function of sleep may relate to crucial molecular and cellular processes not yet adequately understood.

NEURAL SUBSTRATES OF SLEEP

NREM SLEEP

According to a simplified model of the neural control of NREM sleep, it is hypothesized that the hypersynchrony of thalamocortical rhythms emerges simultaneously with an active inhibition of arousal centers. Specifically, the onset of NREM sleep is driven by sleep-active cells in the preoptic–anterior hypothalamic (POAH) area that send extensive γ-aminobutyric acid (GABA)ergic projections to histaminergic neurons in the tuberomammillary nucleus of the posterior hypothalamus. This process results in the shutdown of the tonic activity of the tuberomammillary nucleus, which appears to be important for aborting sleep and sustaining wakeful arousal. Consistent with this model is the finding that POAH neurons and tuberomammillary neurons exhibit opposite patterns of activity during the sleep–wake cycle. In contrast to POAH neurons, which are active during sleep, tuberomammillary cells are persistently active during wakefulness but reduce their firing during NREM sleep and become inactive during REM sleep. The role of histaminergic neurons of the tuberomammillary nucleus in sleep–wake activity may explain how the older **H$_1$ histamine receptor antagonists,** which cross the blood–brain barrier, promote drowsiness and sleep.

Mesopontine cholinergic projection neurons in the ascending reticular activating system, which are discussed later in this chapter, also are inhibited by the onset of NREM sleep, by a mechanism that has yet to be determined. In the absence of tonic activity from the ascending reticular activating system and tuberomammillary nucleus, which promotes wakefulness, higher-frequency oscillations in the cortex disappear, giving

rise to the synchronous firing of a large thalamocortical neuronal ensemble. Thus the delta wave and spindling rhythms observed during NREM sleep most likely reflect intrinsic properties of thalamic neurons, which synchronize the large thalamocortical network. Because a large number of neurons fire in synchrony at this stage, EEG recordings detect high-amplitude waves. Transitions to waking or REM sleep occur when the slow hypersynchronized thalamocortical rhythm is broken up by the recruitment of multiple neuronal ensembles throughout the neocortex, which fire asynchronously at higher frequencies.

The brain structures involved in the control of NREM sleep are also crucial to thermoregulation. Some POAH neurons are thermosensitive; they respond to changes in temperature by activating broad thermoregulatory mechanisms. In fact, as indicated previously, NREM sleep is associated with a lowering of the set point for body temperature, a loss of body heat, and a decline in energy metabolism. Warm-sensitive cells in the POAH area appear to be sleep-active, whereas cold-sensitive cells are active during wakefulness. Consistent with these observations, warm-sensitive POAH neurons increase their firing rates during the transition from wakefulness to NREM sleep, whereas cold-sensitive neurons reduce their firing rates during the onset of sleep. Furthermore, warming of the POAH area induces NREM sleep, increases the length of NREM periods, and increases delta activity during slow-wave sleep. In contrast, POAH lesions result in chronic disruption of both NREM sleep and thermoregulation. Thus it appears that warm-sensitive neurons in the POAH area regulate the onset and maintenance of slow-wave sleep. Interestingly, passive heating of the body improves sleep continuity in patients with insomnia. Accordingly, sleep may function in part to regulate energy metabolism and conserve thermal energy.

REM SLEEP

Single-unit recordings, which are recordings of individual neurons, of sleeping animals have revealed that discrete areas in the brain stem are involved in the regulation of REM sleep. In contrast to the diffuse brain structures involved in NREM sleep, the neuroanatomy of REM-active structures is relatively circumscribed. As previously mentioned, the primary oscillator that drives REM sleep appears to be located among the cholinergic cells of both the pedunculopontine tegmental nucleus (PPT) and lateral dorsal tegmental nucleus (LDT), which together form the giant cell field of the pontine tegmentum (Figure 18–3). These cells are termed *REM-on cells* because they are extremely active

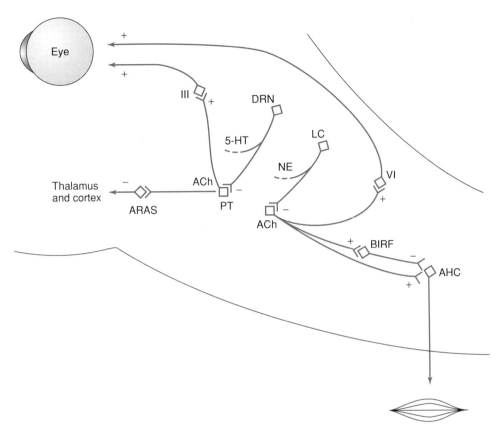

Figure 18–3. Some of the neural circuits that control REM sleep. Key areas of the brain involved in REM include the dorsal raphe nucleus (DRN), the locus ceruleus (LC), and the giant cell field of the pontine tegmentum (PT). PT cells (REM-on cells) are cholinergic and function to promote REM sleep. Firing of these cells activates the cortex by means of the anterior reticular activating system (ARAS), moves the eyes by means of oculomotor nuclei (cranial nerves III and VI), produces muscle twitches and changes in muscle tone by means of the bulbar inhibitory reticular formation (BIRF) and anterior horn cells (AHC) in the spinal cord, and causes cardiac and respiratory changes by means of the autonomic nervous system. The noradrenergic neurons of the LC and serotonergic neurons of the DRN (REM-off cells) suppress REM sleep by modifying these cholinergic outputs. NE, norepinephrine; 5-HT, serotonin; ACh, acetylcholine; +, excitatory; −, inhibitory. (Adapted with permission from Hauri P, Orr W. 1982. *Current Concepts: The Sleep Disorders.* Kalamazoo, MI: Upjohn.)

during REM sleep and during waking, but are almost inactive during NREM sleep. Not surprisingly, application of **cholinergic agonists** or **acetylcholinesterase inhibitors** to PPT or LDT cells activates REM sleep, whereas **muscarinic cholinergic antagonists** suppress REM sleep.

REM-on cells in the pontine tegmentum are reciprocally inhibited by serotonergic inputs from the dorsal raphe nucleus and by noradrenergic inputs from the locus ceruleus, which together with the cholinergic pontine tegmentum cells control the ultradian cycles of REM sleep. Cells in the raphe nuclei and the locus ceruleus are tonically active during waking, are less

active during NREM sleep, and are virtually silent during REM sleep. Consistent with the inhibition of REM-on cells by serotonergic and noradrenergic inputs, antidepressant drugs, which increase the availability of synaptic serotonin or norepinephrine (see Chapter 15), reduce REM sleep. It would seem likely that tricyclic antidepressants, which are also anticholinergic, reduce REM sleep by this mechanism as well.

Activity in the pontine tegmentum is responsible not only for initiating REM sleep but also for the physical manifestations of REM sleep. For example, cholinergic projections from the pons to the medulla and spinal cord regulate muscle atonia, most likely by hyperpolarizing motor neurons and associated interneurons. REM-associated cortical asynchrony, phasic eye movements, and cardiopulmonary accelerations and decelerations involve projections from the pons to the hypothalamus and thalamus. Moreover, the pons is the site at which PGO spikes originate and from which they propagate to the occipital cortex through the lateral geniculate nucleus of the thalamus.

Although discrete pontine structures appear to initiate most tonic and phasic elements of REM sleep, other structures appear to be involved in REM regulation. For example, a small number of neurons in the lateral hypothalamus, which express the neuropeptide orexin (also called hypocretin), appear to be critical for the regulation of REM sleep, as discussed in the section on narcolepsy in this chapter. In addition, inputs from the amygdala and other limbic structures can influence phasic REM activity. This finding may explain why stress and various stress-related disorders, such as depression, are associated with increased phasic REM activity. Furthermore, lesions caudal and rostral to pontine REM-on cells profoundly alter the characteristics of REM sleep; for example, such lesions can cause REM sleep without atonia, which can lead to the motoric expression of dreams. Such motoric activity in humans during sleep has been associated with nocturnal violence and injury from falls.

ASSOCIATION OF ADENOSINE WITH SLEEP

Several neurotransmitters and neuromodulators in addition to acetylcholine, serotonin, norepinephrine, histamine, and orexin/hypocretin influence sleep–wake activity. Dopaminergic systems, for example, dramatically promote wakefulness. Other modulators include prostaglandins, cholecystokinin, delta sleep-inducing peptide, interleukin-1, and adenosine. Particular attention has been focused on adenosine's involvement in mediating the sleep-inducing effects of prolonged wakefulness. Extracellular adenosine decreases during slow-wave sleep and increases after prolonged wakefulness. During sleep deprivation, adenosine levels in extracellular spaces increase, and recovery sleep leads to a decline in adenosine levels. Thus adenosine may serve to mark the duration of wakefulness and also may indicate an increased need for sleep.

The alertness associated with the use of **caffeine** and related methylxanthines appears to be mediated by their ability to block adenosine receptors (see Chapter 10). Although adenosine receptors are found in many regions of the brain, those in the cholinergic basal forebrain area, and particularly those in the substantia innominata, appear to regulate the effect of adenosine on sleep. The link between adenosine and sleep may be explained by the fact that adenosine is a breakdown product of adenosine triphosphate (ATP). Accordingly, increases in extracellular adenosine levels may indicate the expenditure of ATP, and in turn trigger sleep because such expenditure indicates a need for energy restoration; however, this theory remains highly speculative.

CIRCADIAN AND HOMEOSTATIC CONTROL OF THE SLEEP–WAKE CYCLE

As previously mentioned, sleep is partly controlled by a homeostatic drive that increases the propensity to fall asleep in response to sustained wakefulness. A student who has "pulled an all-nighter" may take an afternoon nap in response to a strong homeostatic drive resulting from an unmet need for sleep. However, the propensity to sleep is also affected by circadian variation. The student who stays awake to study may feel increasingly tired throughout the night, and yet may feel more alert at 8:00 AM than at 4:00 AM, despite the fact that by 8:00 AM four additional hours of sleep debt have accumulated.

Circadian variations in virtually all physiologic processes in plants and animals have been recognized for several centuries. Such circadian cycles prepare an organism to feed, avoid predators, and cope with environmental fluctuations, such as changes in light and temperature, during the day. To be useful, circadian cycles must correspond to environmental events. Environmental variables that entrain the circadian pacemaker are called zeitgebers (time givers). Light is the primary zeitgeber that helps an organism adapt to the light–dark cycle as it varies across the seasons. Other zeitgebers that entrain the circadian clock are temperature, food availability, and social cues.

Mammalian circadian rhythms are controlled by the suprachiasmatic nucleus (SCN), which is the primary pacemaker for neuroendocrine rhythms, the temperature cycle, and REM sleep periods. The SCN is located in the midline anterior hypothalamus immediately above the optic chiasm. Its importance is indicated by the elimination of circadian rhythms and the disorganization of sleep–wake patterns that occur when the SCN is lesioned.

In mammals, a connection between retinal ganglion cells and the SCN (the retinohypothalamic pathway) allows the latter to receive direct visual input that helps entrain circadian rhythms. The SCN also receives serotonergic input from the raphe nuclei and cholinergic inputs from the forebrain and brain stem. Moreover, it exerts control over circadian neuroendocrine and thermal rhythms through its projections to the paraventricular nucleus and to lateral and posterior areas of the hypothalamus. Although SCN cells are predominantly GABAergic, the peptide neurotransmitters somatostatin, vasopressin, and vasoactive intestinal peptide (VIP) also may be released by SCN neurons to modulate the activities of certain sleep- and wake-promoting cells.

Opposing interactions between the homeostatic sleep drive and the circadian pacing of sleep–wake activity can explain variability in daytime alertness and the timing of slow-wave sleep and REM sleep activity. For example, the homeostatic sleep drive becomes more forceful in response to sustained wakefulness (Figure 18–4), increasing the propensity to fall asleep with each successive waking hour. However, the circadian pattern of alertness and arousal can mask the homeostatic drive because the circadian peak of arousal occurs in the daytime and in the early evening before sleep. The net effect is that daytime vigilance and performance are well maintained throughout the day, with the exception of a reduction in alertness during midday, when napping is common. A rebound of alertness subsequently occurs during the early evening and, appropriately, a nadir of alertness occurs at night before the onset of sleep.

MOLECULAR CONTROL OF CIRCADIAN RHYTHMS

In the last decade of the 20th century several discoveries helped to elucidate the molecular basis of circadian timekeeping. The identification of the *clock* gene in mammals, the *period* and *timeless* genes in *Drosophila,* and the *frequency* gene in the fungus *Neurospora* illuminated conserved mechanisms for circadian regulation. The

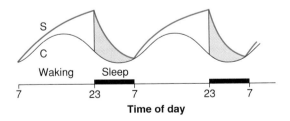

Figure 18–4. A two-process model of sleep regulation. The graph indicates the time course of the homeostatic process that promotes sleep (S) and the circadian process (C) that influences wakefulness. Awakening occurs at the intersection of S and C. (Adapted with permission from Kryger MH, Roth T, Dement WC [eds]. 1994. *Principles and Practice of Sleep Medicine,* 2nd ed. Philadelphia: WB Saunders.)

critical feature of the *clock* gene is a transcription–translation negative feedback circuit in which the cycle is initiated by stimulation of transcription of specific circadian genes, resulting in the accumulation of their proteins in the cytoplasm 4–8 hours later (Figure 18–5). These proteins are subsequently transported to the nucleus, where they directly or indirectly repress transcription of their own genes. Over the course of approximately 12 hours, these nuclear proteins are degraded. This permits resumption of transcription and the beginning of a new cycle. The activities of these pacemaker genes regulate multiple output genes, which in turn regulate the physiologic rhythms of several systems through a cascade of transcriptional control mechanisms. Ultimately, many genes exhibit circadian patterns of expression. Because some of these genes, including the one for growth hormone, have many diverse inputs that control their expression, the peaks and nadirs of expression do not strictly follow the patterns of the genes comprising the circadian machinery per se.

As most airplane travelers have experienced, circadian rhythms can shift to conform to new light–dark cycles, although they do not always shift as efficiently as one might wish. How do clock gene products, oscillating in their own time zone, adjust to a shifting of the light–dark cycle? The exact mechanisms that underlie such adjustment are unknown. However, the administration of bright light at times other than those predicted by the regular light–dark cycle can result in altered patterns of gene expression in SCN cells. This finding indicates that external stimuli can affect the expression of specific genes, which in turn may influence the production or activity of clock gene products.

Among the genes whose expression is altered in the SCN in response to changes in environmental lighting is that for c-Fos. As discussed in Chapter 6, c-Fos belongs to the Fos family of transcription factors, which are induced rapidly in a brain region-specific manner in response to many types of perturbations. c-Fos also has been used as a marker of neural activity involved in sleep–wake cycles outside the SCN. However, the roles that it may play in sleep–wake cycles are less well understood. c-Fos expression decreases throughout the brain during sleep, except in the SCN and intergeniculate leaflet (neural structures involved in circadian regulation) and in POAH neurons, whose activation during sleep is independent of circadian factors. Thus c-Fos is induced in wake-active cells during wakefulness and in sleep-active cells during sleep. In general, sleep deprivation induces c-Fos, whereas sleep recovery decreases c-Fos throughout the brain. Mice lacking the c-Fos gene experience insomnia, although they continue to have normal circadian temperature cycles. c-Fos is only

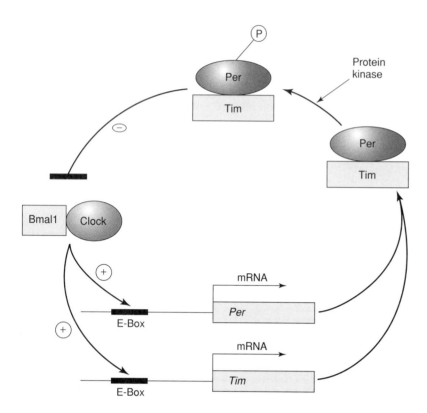

Figure 18–5. Molecular basis of circadian oscillators. Dimers of *Clock* and *Bmal1* bind DNA at sequences called E-boxes to activate the transcription of oscillator genes, including *per* and *tim* in *Drosophila,* and *per1, per2,* and *per3* in mammals. *Per* and *tim* proteins feed back, after a lag, to block their own activation. In *Drosophila* there is evidence of time-of-day-specific phosphorylation of per that may regulate turnover of these proteins.

one of many genes that are likely to act within the SCN and elsewhere to influence the sleep–wake cycle.

NEUROBIOLOGY OF AROUSAL

Wakefulness and arousal are controlled by multiple neural circuits from the brain stem and forebrain. Classic research conducted during the 1940s demonstrated that a key element in the regulation of alertness is the so-called ascending reticular activating system, which comprises two major circuits: a reticulothalamic-cortical pathway and a pathway from the reticular formation to the hypothalamus and basal forebrain (Figure 18–6). Recently, the concept of the ascending reticular activating system has been expanded to include the noradrenergic pathways from the locus ceruleus, serotonergic pathways from the raphe nuclei, dopamine pathways from the ventral tegmental area, and histamine pathways that originate in the tubero-mammillary nucleus of the hypothalamus. Because of these projections it is believed that cortical activation can occur even in the absence of thalamic input.

Cholinergic neurons in the basal forebrain and noradrenergic neurons in the locus ceruleus appear to perform essential functions related to the maintenance and control of arousal. As discussed in Chapters 8 and 9, both sets of neurons send diffuse projections throughout the cerebral cortex, and lesions in either area can result in coma and chronic slow-wave activity of the cortex. The locus ceruleus is a particularly intriguing area because not only do environmental stimuli with emotional salience, such as those that elicit fear, greatly increase the firing rate of neurons in this area, but direct pharmacologic stimulation of the locus ceruleus also increases cortical arousal.

One of the most powerful inducers of arousal is fear. This fact makes evolutionary sense because fear occurs in response to a potential environmental threat that requires increased vigilance and an appropriate response. A great deal is known about the neural circuits associated with fear, many of which appear to be linked to the amygdala (see Chapter 15). Projections from the amygdala to the hypothalamus, for example, most likely mediate the increases in heart rate and anxiety that occur during threatening conditions; those that extend from the amygdala to the vagus nerve mediate defecation and other immediate visceral responses to fear; and outputs to the paraventricular nucleus trigger the release of corticotropin releasing factor, which in turn triggers the release of peripheral cortisol, a hallmark of the stress response (see Chapters 13 and 15). Consistent with the amygdala's role in anxious arousal are reports of fear and anxiety in response to stimulation of this region of the brain in awake patients during surgery for epilepsy.

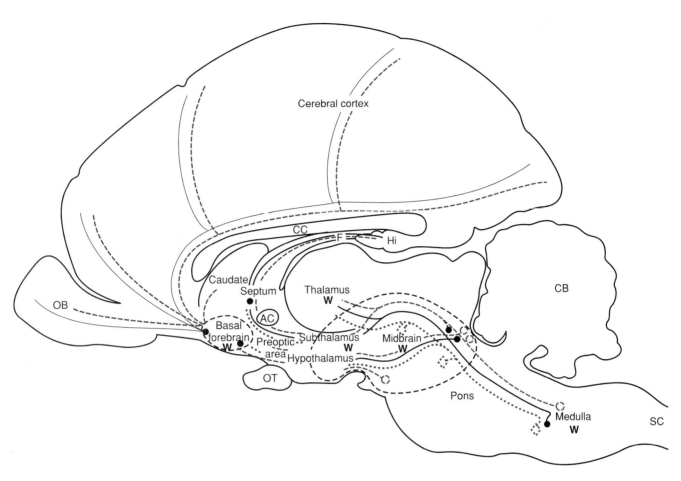

Figure 18–6. Areas of the brain that generate wakefulness. Indicated are regions in which electrical stimulation produces cortical activation and arousal, and those in which neurons exhibit higher rates of spontaneous activity during wakefulness than during slow-wave sleep (W); neurons of the reticular formation (*open diamonds*); catecholamine-containing neurons of the medulla, locus ceruleus, and substantia nigra–ventral tegmental area (*open circles*); and cholinergic neurons of the reticular formation and basal forebrain (*solid circles*). OB, olfactory bulb; AC, anterior commissure; Hi, hippocampus; F, fornix; CC, corpus callosum; OT, olfactory tubercle; CB, cerebellum; SC, spinal cord. (Adapted with permission from Kryger MH, Roth T, Dement WC [eds]. 1994. *Principles and Practice of Sleep Medicine*, 2nd ed. Philadelphia: WB Saunders.)

SLEEP DISORDERS

Difficulties related to sleep affect virtually all individuals at some point during their lives. Sleep disturbances can be categorized as primary sleep disorders or as sleep disorders associated with other neuropsychiatric or general medical conditions. The classification of sleep disorders that appears in the *Diagnostic and Statistical Manual of Mental Disorders*, fourth edition (*DSM-IV*) is presented in Table 18–1. This chapter focuses on primary sleep disorders, which are subdivided into dysomnias and parasomnias.

DYSOMNIAS

Dysomnias include primary insomnia, primary hypersomnia, narcolepsy, breathing-related sleep disorders, circadian rhythm sleep disorder, and other conditions. It is important to mention that most of these disorders are syndromes that are defined only by clinical signs and symptoms. The molecular and cellular underpinnings of these syndromes remain poorly understood.

Primary insomnia   This disorder, which is characterized by difficulty in initiating and maintaining sleep, causes significant psychological distress. It often is associated with a mood disorder, pain, or other medical condition. It can be a lifelong trait or may be acquired secondary to arousal caused by psychosocial stress. Primary insomnia can be measured objectively with polysomnography, which demonstrates an increased number of awakenings. Although the biology of insomnia is not well understood, it is increasingly viewed as a disorder of hyperarousal. Subjects with primary insomnia have an elevated 24-hour metabolic rate and a decreased propensity to sleep when given the opportunity to nap during sleep latency tests. Nonpharmacologic treatment that reduces arousal, including biofeedback, meditation, and relaxation therapy, are effective in the treatment of primary insomnia. Sleep hygiene also promotes healthy sleep through nonpharmacologic, common-sense measures; these include adherence to a stable sleep–wake schedule; a reduction in the use of caffeine and other stimulants; a reduction in the use of alcohol; regular exercise; and reduction of alerting stimuli in the sleep environment. Behavior modification therapy helps reduce the conditioned association between the sleep environment and wakeful arousal. Sleep restriction therapy and stimulus control behavior modification reduce the amount of awake time spent in bed. Patients who undergo sleep restriction therapy are instructed to get out of bed after a given period of wakefulness (approximately 15 minutes), and are advised not to return to bed until they feel tired enough to sleep. Thus the association between being in bed and going to

sleep is strengthened, and the association between being in bed and "tossing and turning" is weakened.

Primary hypersomnia   Patients who experience excessive somnolence are diagnosed with primary hypersomnia when other disorders of somnolence, such as narcolepsy and sleep apnea, have been ruled out. Subjects with this disorder appear to sleep longer during the day and have a greater propensity to fall asleep compared with normal controls. Primary hypersomnia is not well understood biologically but is believed to involve a disturbance of pathways that mediate wakeful arousal. Treatment primarily involves the use of psychostimulants, as discussed later in this chapter.

Narcolepsy   Narcolepsy was first described during the late 1800s. It is characterized by abnormal transitions between REM and NREM sleep during the night and across the sleep–wake cycle. Narcoleptic patients do not sleep more than normal individuals; however, they have intrusive episodes of REM sleep during the day and fragmented sleep at night. The characteristic symptoms of narcolepsy, which include pathologic sleepiness, sleep paralysis, hypnagogic hallucinations (hallucinations that occur with the onset or termination of sleep), and cataplexy, are caused by the sudden intrusion of REM sleep into wakefulness. Cataplexy is pathognomonic for narcolepsy and is characterized by the sudden loss of muscle tone during wakefulness. During a cataplectic attack, a narcoleptic may suddenly fall to the floor from a standing position and be unable to move even though fully conscious. Interestingly, cataplectic attacks often are elicited by positive emotional stimuli. The primary treatment for narcolepsy consists of **psychostimulants** or modafinil to counter the hypersomnolence and REM-suppressing drugs, such as **tricyclic antidepressants,** which reduce cataplexy. Nonpharmacologic treatment such as scheduled naps also are effective for treating daytime hypersomnolence.

Narcolepsy can be a heritable disorder, but in humans most cases are sporadic. In some families narcolepsy has been linked to a gene that is near the human leukocyte antigen (HLA) alleles DQB1 and DQA1 on chromosome 6. In a dog model of narcolepsy, transmission is autosomal recessive, which is clearly different from human transmission, and is due to loss-of-function mutations in the orexin/hypocretin receptor 2 gene. Disruption of the orexin/hypocretin gene in mice also causes a narcolepsy-like disorder. Orexin/hypocretin is a hypothalamic peptide that initially was believed to be involved in the control of feeding (see Chapter 13); yet its primary function may be to regulate sleep–wake cycles, and it may affect feeding only secondarily. Although a role for the orexin/hypocretin system in

Table 18–1 Categorization of Primary Sleep Disorders[1]

Dysomnias

Primary insomnia
Primary hypersomnia
Narcolepsy
Breathing-related sleep disorder
Circadian rhythm sleep disorder
    Delayed sleep phase type
    Jet lag type
    Shift work type
    Unspecified
Other dysomnias

Parasomnias
Nightmare disorder Sleep terror disorder Sleepwalking disorder Other parasomnias

[1] Sleep disorders related to other conditions such as neuropsychiatric disorders, general medical conditions, or drug abuse are classified as insomnia type, hypersomnia type, parasomnia type, and mixed type.
Based on American Psychiatric Association *Diagnostic and Statistical Manual of Mental Disorders*, 4th ed. Washington, D.C.

human narcolepsy remains unproven, preliminary findings suggest that narcolepsy may be associated with a loss of orexin/hypocretin-containing neurons in the hypothalamus. Along with the linkage of narcolepsy with HLA alleles, these results raise the interesting possibility that narcolepsy may be caused by an autoimmune-mediated destruction of orexin/hypocretin neurons. A search for small-molecule agonists at orexin/hypocretin receptors is under way and may lead to a possible treatment for narcolepsy. Another major goal of future research is to understand the neural circuitry through which orexin/hypocretin neurons regulate sleep.

Sleep apnea   Sleep apnea, a breathing-related sleep disorder, is a common, age-related condition characterized by oropharyngeal collapse during sleep. Such collapse causes sleep fragmentation, hypoxia, pulmonary and systemic hypertension, and cardiac arrhythmias. Obstructive sleep apnea can be caused by obesity or anatomic factors, such as micrognathia, that predispose patients to airway occlusion during sleep. Central sleep apnea is secondary to impaired central respiratory drive; it is associated with congestive heart failure and advanced age, and occurs in 30% of men older than 60 years of age. Treatment may involve behavior modification, including weight loss and sleep position therapy; the use of mechanical devices to eliminate airway collapse, such as continuous positive airway pressure; the use of dental appliances that adjust the position of the jaw and tongue; or surgery to enhance the size of the oropharynx.

Circadian rhythm sleep disorders   These disorders, which are caused by a misalignment between behavioral waking activity and the endogenous circadian cycle, are perhaps not properly classified as primary sleep disorders. They are chronobiologic disorders caused artificially by jet travel across multiple time zones, or by shift work that results in a rapidly changing sleep–wake cycle. Clinical manifestations of these disorders, which include sleepiness, insomnia, diminished attention, gastrointestinal discomfort, and fatigue, vary depending on the juxtaposition of the underlying circadian cycle and sleep–wake behavior.

PARASOMNIAS

Parasomnias are represented by **nightmares,** sleep or **night terrors, sleepwalking,** and other conditions that arise during stage-4 sleep. They are considered disorders only when their frequency, severity, or persistence disrupts the normal functioning of an individual. Excessive and severe nightmares are strongly associated with psychological trauma and often are

seen in the context of **posttraumatic stress disorder** (see Chapter 15). Night terrors and sleepwalking occur predominantly in children and involve a partial awakening out of slow-wave sleep. Children affected by night terrors experience extreme fear and sympathetic activation without fully awakening; consequently they are difficult to console, much to the consternation of alarmed parents. In most cases, night terrors represent a benign condition that a child is likely to outgrow. Sleepwalking similarly involves partial arousal from deep slow-wave sleep. Although this disorder typically is innocuous, the persistence of sleepwalking in adults can be associated with psychopathology, including schizophrenia and mood disorders. Medications that are effective in the treatment of these parasomnias have yet to be developed.

PHARMACOLOGY OF SLEEP–WAKE DISORDERS

BENZODIAZEPINES

Benzodiazepines became available in the late 1950s and rapidly replaced **barbiturates** as preferred sedative–hypnotics. Their wide acceptance resulted from their greater safety, including lower risks associated with overdose and abuse compared with those of barbiturates and related sedative–hypnotics such as **methaqualone, ethchlorvynol, meprobamate,** and **chloral hydrate;** benzodiazepines also are less likely to induce hepatic metabolism of other drugs. Yet like barbiturates and related sedative–hypnotics, benzodiazepine agents bind to and facilitate the functioning of $GABA_A$ receptors. Their mechanisms of action and general pharmacology are discussed in greater detail in Chapters 7 and 15. The chemical structures of representative benzodiazepines used as sedative–hypnotics are shown in Figure 18–7.

Benzodiazepines promote the onset of sleep and sleep continuity in the treatment of insomnia. They also are commonly used as anxiolytics (see Chapter 15). Much of the clinical art of benzodiazepine therapy for insomnia involves an understanding of the importance of drug half-life in determining appropriate drug therapy and minimizing adverse effects (Table 18–2). Long-acting benzodiazepines, such as **flurazepam** and **chlordiazepoxide,** have active metabolites with half-lives in excess of 200 hours; their use often interferes with daytime alertness and is associated with more errors while driving an automobile compared with the use of shorter-acting agents. In contrast, benzodiazepines with extremely short half-lives (2–4 hours), such as **triazolam,** are useful for promoting the onset of sleep, but may be of less benefit to those who have dif-

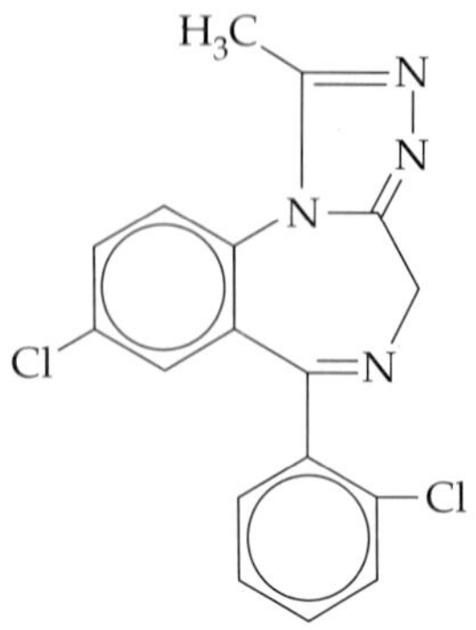

Triazolam

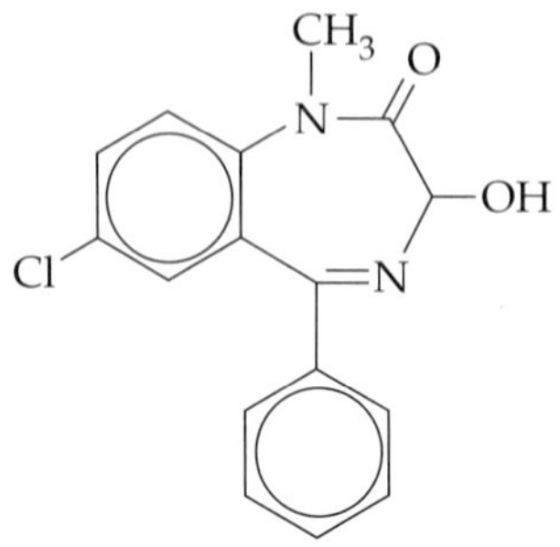

Temazepam

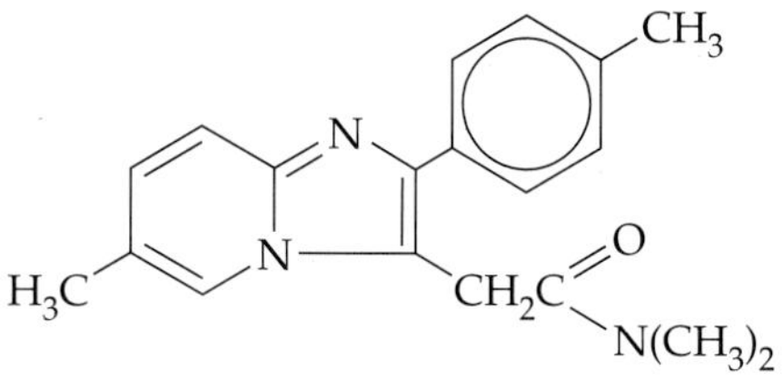

Zolpidem

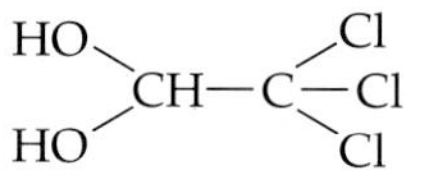

Chloral hydrate

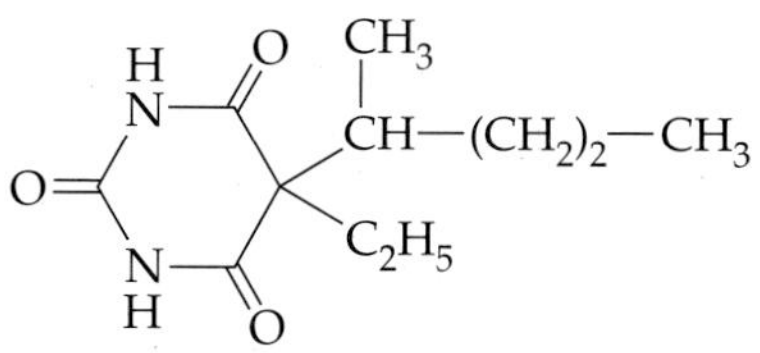

Pentobarbital

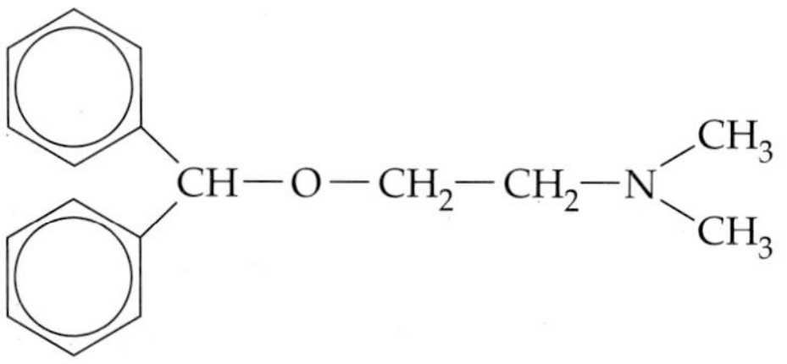

Diphenhydramine

Figure 18–7. Chemical structures of representative benzodiazepines and other drugs used to treat insomnia.

Table 18–2 Comparison of Representative Benzodiazepines for Insomnia Therapy

Drug	Half-Life	Advantages	Disadvantages
Estazolam	Intermediate		Some daytime sedation and performance decrements
Flurazepam	Long	Delayed rebound insomnia	Daytime sedation; high risk of falls and driving errors
Temazepam	Intermediate		Some daytime sedation and performance decrements
Triazolam	Short	No daytime sedation	Rebound insomnia
Zolpidem[1]	Short	No daytime sedation	Rebound insomnia

[1] Zolpidem does not have a benzodiazepine structure, but acts at the same site on the $GABA_A$ receptor as do the benzodiazepines (see Figure 18–7).

ficulty maintaining sleep. Short half-life agents can cause rebound insomnia and irritability during the latter half of the night, which can be viewed as a mild withdrawal syndrome that occurs in response to a single dose of the benzodiazepine. Repeated use of these agents can lead to more significant rebound insomnia and anxiety; however, the slow tapering of these agents can minimize the occurrence of a discontinuation syndrome. It is generally believed that sedative–hypnotic therapy should be limited to agents with short and intermediate half-lives. Although **zolpidem** is not chemically classified as a benzodiazepine (see Figure 18–7), it exerts the same mechanism of action. This agent also has a relatively short half-life but appears to be better tolerated than triazolam by some patients, perhaps because its half-life is slightly longer.

Benzodiazepines can be quite effective in the short-term treatment of insomnia; for example, they help relieve insomnia associated with jet lag, situational anxiety, and bereavement. However, these drugs are less effective when used to treat persistent insomnia, which remains a prevalent and troubling condition. As indicated in Chapter 15, the repeated use of benzodiazepines results in tolerance to their sedative effects. Benzodiazepines also can cause deleterious cognitive effects, particularly in elderly patients, who experience impairments in daytime alertness and in psychomotor performance even in response to short-acting drugs. Indeed, long-term use of benzodiazepines or related sedative–hypnotics is associated with an increased risk for hip fractures among the elderly. These drugs also have been proven to suppress the total amount of REM sleep and to alter the time spent in stages 1–4; thus sleep produced by a sedative-hypnotic may not be as physiologically useful as normal sleep.

Attempts to improve the long-term treatment of insomnia have addressed these various liabilities. If the mechanism of benzodiazepine tolerance were better understood (see Chapter 15), it might be possible to develop drugs that are not associated with this unwanted adaptation. One strategy, which remains speculative, might involve the use of partial agonists at the benzodiazepine site of the $GABA_A$ receptor; such drugs might be designed to cause sedation without producing tolerance. Another strategy might be to take advantage of the molecular diversity of $GABA_A$ receptor subunits. Because the sedative effects of benzodiazepines may be mediated by one particular $GABA_A$ receptor α subunit, such as the $α_1$ subunit (see Chapters 7 and 15), drugs might be developed that are selective for this subunit and therefore unlikely to cause the deleterious cognitive effects of previously mentioned agents. Such subunit-selective benzodiazepine-like drugs are not yet available but are in preclinical and clinical stages of development.

NONBENZODIAZEPINE SEDATIVE–HYPNOTIC AGENTS

Several nonbenzodiazepine classes of drugs are currently used to promote sleep (Table 18–3). Antihistamines (specifically H_1 receptor antagonists) are frequently used and in fact are the active ingredients in most over-the-counter sleep remedies. Examples of these medications include **diphenhydramine, dimenhydrinate, chlorpheniramine, hydroxyzine,** and **promethazine.** However, these drugs are less effective than benzodiazepines and are associated with more adverse daytime effects. Antihistamines also can adversely affect memory and psychomotor performance, even after the drugs are no longer detectable in the general circulation. Many people report the sensation of being "in a fog" for as many as 24 hours after taking an antihistamine. Such drawbacks have led to the development of newer antihistamines, such as **loratadine,** that do not enter the CNS and therefore do not produce CNS-related side effects. Such drugs are primarily used for the treatment of colds and allergies. Antihistamines that act on the CNS are believed to produce their sedative effects by blocking H_1 histamine receptors. Because the histaminergic neurons of the tuberomammillary nucleus of the hypothalamus are quiescent during sleep, antihistamines may cause more sedation during waking hours than promotion of sleep during the sleep cycle. As explained in Chapters 15 and 17, many tricyclic **antidepressants** and **antipsychotic** drugs have H_1 antagonist properties, which may explain the sedative effects of these agents. Another strategy for promoting sleep may involve the use of an H_3 receptor agonist. As described in Chapter 10, H_3 receptors are inhibitory autoreceptors on histaminergic neurons of the tuberomammillary nucleus. An agonist at these receptors, for example, **R-α-methylhistamine,** would be expected to reduce the activity of the neurons and thereby promote sleep. This approach has not yet been tested in humans.

Trazodone is marketed as an antidepressant, but is less effective in the treatment of depression than many other available agents (see Chapter 15). However, trazodone is sedating and is sometimes used to promote sleep. It improves sleep continuity and also subjective sleep quality. Although it is frequently recommended because of a putative lack of associated tolerance, data regarding its long-term efficacy have not been obtained. Although trazodone appears to be an agonist at several 5-HT receptors, its mechanism of action in promoting sleep remains undetermined.

There has been great interest in the melatonin system as a potential target for new sedative–hypnotic agents. Endogenous melatonin is synthesized exclusively in the pineal gland from tryptophan and serotonin (see Chapter 9). Its physiologic role in the control of circadian rhythms and sleep remains uncertain. Exogenous melatonin has been shown to help reset the circadian clock in some experimental situations (Box 18–1). It is commonly used to treat jet lag in individuals who travel across multiple time zones. Moreover, it has been used to help shift workers better adjust to new work hours, although its efficacy when used for these purposes has not been established in well-designed clinical trials. Its efficacy in the treatment of noncircadian insomnia also has not been supported by convincing evidence. Moreover, the safety of over-the-counter melatonin preparations in the United States has yet to be determined; indeed, even the composition of most of these preparations remains unknown because of the lack of regulatory oversight by the Food and Drug Administration. However, the dose commonly available in health food stores has been determined to produce a level of melatonin that is ten times greater than peak physiologic levels. Elevated concentrations of melatonin have been associated with endocrine disturbances such as amenorrhea in females and hypogonadism in males. Melatonin also can lead to the asynchrony of circadian physiology if used frequently at different times of the day. The pharmaceutical industry currently is attempting to develop agonists that are selective for various melatonin receptors (see Chapter 9); whether these drugs will prove to be safer and more effective than melatonin remains to be seen.

Because of the prevalence of insomnia, and the imperfect treatment offered by available medications, many individuals have turned to so-called **natural products** that are marketed to promote and improve sleep. These products include not only melatonin but also **herbal products** and hormones. As with melatonin, many of these products are not subject to regulation.

Table 18–3 Nonbenzodiazepine Therapy for Insomnia

Hypnotic	Advantages	Disadvantages
Antidepressants		
Amitriptyline	No tolerance	Anticholinergic delirium; increased risk of falls; daytime sedation
Doxepin	No tolerance	Increased risk of falls; daytime sedation
Trazodone	No tolerance	Increased risk of falls; daytime sedation
Antipsychotics		
Haloperidol	No tolerance; few anticholinergic effects	Extrapyramidal effects; increased risk of falls; limited sedation
Chlorpromazine	No tolerance	Extrapyramidal effects; increased risk of falls; anticholinergic delirium
Barbiturates	No pertinent advantages over benzodiazepines	High risk of addiction; dangerous withdrawal syndrome; overdose potential; daytime sedation
Antihistamines		
Diphenhydramine	No tolerance	Anticholinergic delirium; risk of falls; daytime sedation and memory impairment

Box 18–1 Circadian Regulation of Melatonin

Although a great deal is known about the regulation of endogenous melatonin, its physiologic function in humans has yet to be determined. In lower vertebrates, melatonin dramatically affects skin pigmentation: it lightens the skin by inducing pigment granule aggregation in melanocytes. This skin-lightening effect also occurs to a lesser degree in mammals. The reproductive systems and diurnal rhythms of some vertebrates, including some mammals, also are affected by melatonin. However, the significance of these effects in humans remains a matter of debate.

The nocturnal synthesis and release of melatonin, which is described in Chapter 9, is indirectly driven by the circadian oscillator in the suprachiasmatic nucleus (SCN). Interestingly, melatonin is released in the dark phase of all mammalian species, regardless of whether the animal is diurnal or nocturnal. In this respect, melatonin is very different from many factors that exhibit circadian cycles; for example, cortisol exhibits daytime peaks in diurnal species and nighttime peaks in nocturnal species. Among its many actions, the SCN induces nocturnal release of norepinephrine from sympathetic nerve endings that innervate the pineal gland. Released norepinephrine acts by means of β-adrenergic receptors to induce high levels of cAMP in the pineal gland. High levels of cAMP activate protein kinase A, which in turn induces transcription of the rate-limiting enzyme in melatonin synthesis, known as arylalkyamine-*N*-acetyltransferase (NAT). This norepinephrine-dependent diurnal variation in NAT transcription and melatonin synthesis is mediated by a switch between levels of phosphorylated CREB (p-CREB), the cAMP-dependent transcriptional activator (see Chapter 6), and inducible cAMP early repressor (ICER), the cAMP-dependent transcriptional inhibitor. p-CREB accumulates when darkness begins and declines as the amount of ICER rises. p-CREB mediates the induction of NAT transcription during the first half of the night, and ICER mediates the repression of transcription during the second half. This knowledge of melatonin regulation has aided our understanding of the molecular mechanisms that generate circadian oscillations, and should assist investigations aimed at better appreciating the physiologic function of melatonin in humans.

The public often believes that a natural product is unquestionably safe and likely to be efficacious. Yet the dangers of **digitalis,** originally derived as an herbal preparation from foxglove, and natural hormonal products such as insulin demonstrate that any drug powerful enough to have a desired effect may also have serious side effects. Moreover, reliance on natural products can prevent individuals from seeking medical attention, which in turn can cause serious disorders to remain undiagnosed. Insomnia, for example, can be a symptom of illnesses as diverse as depression and congestive heart failure. As with any pharmacologic treatment, treatment with natural products requires that manufacturers: 1) establish standardized preparations; 2) establish the safety and mechanism of action of these preparations in animals; and 3) establish safety and efficacy in humans. Just as identification and examination of the active ingredients in digitalis leaf led to the development of digoxin, it is hoped that the active ingredients in certain natural products can be identified so that their mechanisms of action can be studied and improved preparations can be formulated.

DRUGS THAT INCREASE ALERTNESS

The drugs used most commonly to promote wakefulness are **caffeine**—for example, in coffee, soda, and over-the-counter stimulants—and related substances such as **theophylline** in tea and **theobromine** in chocolate. Although these drugs have several mechanisms of action, their stimulant properties are most closely associated with antagonism of adenosine receptors, particularly that of A_1 and A_{2A} receptors (see Chapter 10). The medicinal use of these drugs is limited by side effects such as nausea, headache, and tremulousness, which are common at clinically relevant doses. More selective antagonists of adenosine receptors, which have yet to be developed, may offer the clinical benefits of these agents without such unpleasant side effects.

The most potent agents that promote wakefulness are amphetamine-like psychostimulants, including **D-amphetamine, methamphetamine, methylphenidate,** and **pemoline**. These drugs increase the synaptic levels of dopamine, serotonin, and norepinephrine primarily by blocking their uptake or promoting their release (see Chapters 8, 9, 15, and 16). Actions on the dopamine system are believed to be most important for the stimulant effects of these drugs. Amphetamines remain the treatment of choice for narcolepsy, and also are used to treat attentional disorders, as discussed later in this chapter. Although these drugs offer important symptomatic improvement in many patients, their use is associated with complications such as nighttime insomnia, tolerance, dependence, and in some cases addiction.

Modafinil, a (diphenyl-methyl)-sulfinyl-2-acetamide derivative, is another wakefulness-promoting drug approved by the United States Food and Drug Administration. It increases alertness and vigilance in normal individuals and in patients with narcolepsy, although it is clearly less efficacious than amphetamines. However, modafinil shows fewer cardiovascular side effects and less abuse potential compared with amphetamines. The mechanism of action of modafinil is unknown. The drug may act at the dopamine transporter, to which it binds with micromolar affinity, although some investigators have suggested that it acts by means of non-dopaminergic mechanisms.

Several antidepressants alter the sleep–wake cycle. Some of these drugs exhibit strong antagonism of H_1 histamine and muscarinic cholinergic receptors, which mediates the ability of these drugs to promote sleep independently of their antidepressant actions. However, several selective serotonin reuptake inhibitors (SSRIs) such as **fluoxetine** and **bupropion,** which has an amphetamine-like structure (see Chapter 15), exert the opposite effect in some patients and can lead to insomnia. Why some serotonin-acting antidepressants, such as trazodone, promote sleep, while others, for example, fluoxetine, disrupt sleep in a subset of patients, remains unknown but may be related to the different groups of 5-HT receptors that are activated by these medications.

Many distinct but interdependent neural pathways regulate the sleep–wake cycle. Because each of these pathways is subserved by distinct neurotransmitters, many pharmacologic agents can influence sleep patterns. The cellular and molecular mechanisms involved in the regulation of sleep and circadian rhythms require more investigation, but it is anticipated that the elucidation of these mechanisms will lead to new targets for the effective pharmacologic treatment of sleep disorders.

ATTENTION

The neurobiologic underpinnings of the sleep–wake cycle and arousal discussed in this chapter provide some background for the related topic of attention. Attention involves the proper allocation of resources to relevant stimuli. Accordingly, important stimuli receive a larger share of processing resources, including conscious awareness and neural representation, than do less important stimuli. At any given moment our nervous systems must process an enormous amount of information. Even a relatively quiet activity, such as reading a book in a library, may subject an individual to a wide range of sensory inputs, including the temperature of the room, the sensation of hunger or thirst, the sound of whispered conversation at other tables, and the sight of various objects. Nonetheless, it is possible to ignore distracting stimuli under such circumstances and to read for reasonably long periods of time. Furthermore, it is possible to maintain a state of alert-

ness in anticipation of important events while disregarding others; for example, an automobile driver may be completely oblivious to billboards that pass by but may quickly perceive and react to certain stimuli, such as stop signs, which are important to the task at hand.

This section explores the process by which the brain performs such selections. It examines the several brain regions that control attention and explains how they modify neural representations of sensory stimuli. It concludes with a discussion of the symptoms, possible causes, and treatment of a prevalent attention-related condition known as **attention deficit–hyperactivity disorder (ADHD).**

CORTICAL RESPONSIVENESS TO STIMULI

Two major processes are involved in directing attention. First, the brain maintains or promotes neural activity related to a particular stimulus or group of stimuli. Depending on the task undertaken by an individual, this activity may be anticipatory, which involves being alert for the appearance of particular environmental stimuli, or it may be focused, and thus require the ability to remain attuned to particular stimuli. Second, the brain filters out stimuli that compete with attended stimuli. Because the brain has limited processing power, the suppression of insignificant stimuli allows for better cognitive representation of important stimuli.

Studies have documented differences in the representation of attended and unattended stimuli at the cortical level. Such phenomena have been most thoroughly studied in the prestriate cortex, which is specialized to represent different features of visual stimuli. Research regarding attention has focused primarily on the visual system because this system is well characterized in primates and because the presentation of visual stimuli is straightforward. Although attentive processes occur in other sensory modalities—focusing on a telephone conversation, for example, may involve tuning out a radio playing in the background—and although these processes may be characterized by similarities, this chapter examines the well-studied field of visual attention for the sake of simplicity.

Neurons in some regions of the prestriate cortex respond mainly to colors, whereas neurons in other regions respond to particular shapes or to particular types of stimulus motion. Brain activity in these various prestriate regions has been compared in human PET imaging studies. In these investigations subjects viewed particular stimuli, such as a red square moving rightward, and were asked to attend specifically to the color, form, or motion of the stimulus in order to complete a task. Such selective attention is associated with the activation of corresponding prestriate regions. When a subject focuses on the *color* of a stimulus, activity is greatest in the area of the prestriate cortex specialized to represent this attribute, whereas attention to the *shape* of the same stimulus causes activity to shift to another area of the prestriate cortex. This phenomenon has been observed during attention to other types of stimuli as well; for example, increases in blood flow and other measures of neural activity have been reported in motor areas of subjects instructed to attend to motor actions, and in language areas of subjects attending to verbal tasks.

Attention to particular stimuli also may be accompanied by suppression of responses to unattended stimuli. When monkeys are required to respond to a change in color in a particular location, cells in another prestriate region stop responding to a stimulus in an unattended location. This finding demonstrates that attention involves decreased processing of irrelevant activity as well as augmented processing of attended stimuli.

Although attention to visual stimuli unquestionably modulates the activity of prestriate neurons, it does not seem to affect the activity of neurons in the primary visual or occipital cortex. Indeed, the latter group of neurons responds to stimuli even in fully anesthetized animals, whereas attentional modulation seems to be directed to higher level or associative cortices (see Chapter 17). This anatomic separation of function perhaps reflects an organism's need to maintain at least minimal awareness of unattended stimuli. Accordingly, it is useful to attend to the reading of a book, but such attention would be disadvantageous if it precluded attention to a fire starting in the corner of the room.

If attention is at least partly explained by greater cortical activity elicited by attended than unattended stimuli, what enables various cortical regions to respond more intensely to attended stimuli? This question is addressed in the section that follows.

ORCHESTRATION OF ATTENTIONAL PROCESSES

The control of particular aspects of attention by corresponding regions of the brain has been supported by several findings. Impairments caused by brain lesions, together with functional imaging studies that compare the activity of different areas of the brain during attentive and nonattentive tasks, have led to the recognition of regions that are selectively involved in attentional processes.

As briefly discussed in Chapter 17, the parietal cortex is an area of association cortex that is responsible for orienting attention to particular regions of space

(Figure 18–8). This function is best observed in patients with unilateral lesions of the parietal lobe. Such patients exhibit unilateral spatial neglect; that is, they ignore the visual hemifield that is contralateral to the side of the lesion. A patient with this type of lesion might write on only one side of a page (Figure 18–9), notice and eat food on only one half of a plate, and perhaps even fail to clothe and groom half of his or her body. Although such patients may not notice objects on the left side of their visual field without prompting, they become aware of these objects when they are cued to the objects' location. Thus these lesions produce attentional rather than visual field deficits. Single-cell recordings in monkeys and functional imaging studies in humans also reveal activation of regions of the parietal cortex during tasks that involve attending to particular regions of space.

The frontal and parietal cortices are selectively activated during sustained attention to a particular stimulus or location. This occurs during sustained attention not only to visual stimuli but also to somatosensory and auditory stimuli, suggesting that these brain areas might coordinate attention as a whole.

Although the frontal and parietal cortices appear to be involved in orienting and maintaining attention, other areas of the brain seem to modulate selective attention, or the allocation of processing resources to a particular stimulus in the presence of multiple distractors. Functional imaging studies indicate that the anterior cingulate gyrus and its adjacent frontal cortex are activated in tasks in which subjects must selectively attend to one feature of a stimulus rather than another—for example, to color rather than shape—or in tasks that require subjects to detect particular types of target stimuli among groups of target and nontarget stimuli. During the latter type of task, the anterior cingulate gyrus undergoes greater activation as the number and variety of nontarget stimuli increases, which perhaps reflects the need for greater selective attention in such a task. The anterior cingulate gyrus is also activated selectively in verbal attentional tasks; thus its function is not restricted to selective visual attention and indeed may encompass general selective attention. One theory is that the anterior cingulate gyrus is active under circumstances where there is competition for attentional resources.

As discussed in Chapter 17, working memory is responsible for enabling an individual to keep something in mind. Mediated primarily by the prefrontal cortex and other limbic cortical structures, working memory is closely related to attention and can be viewed as a type of executive function. Research has indicated that this type of memory can be manipulated pharmacologically and that it is influenced by drugs that act on the prefrontal cortex. It has been deter-

A

Parietal cortex
(spatial orientation)

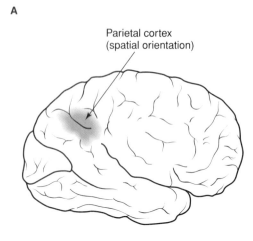

B

Cingulate gyrus (anterior)
(stimulus selection)

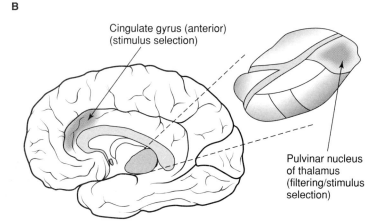

Pulvinar nucleus
of thalamus
(filtering/stimulus
selection)

Figure 18–8. Brain centers involved in attentional processes. **A.** The parietal cortex is selectively activated during tasks that require attention to particular regions of space. Unilateral lesions of parietal cortex can lead to unilateral neglect of the contralateral side; affected individuals fail to notice objects in the contralateral field of vision. **B.** The anterior cingulate gyrus and the pulvinar nucleus of the thalamus are selectively activated during selective attention, when particular stimuli must be singled out from a field of many distractors.

mined, for example, that small amounts of dopamine act on this area to enhance working memory, whereas large amounts exert the opposite effect; it is believed that D_1 and perhaps other dopamine receptor subtypes mediate these effects. Agonists at α_2-adrenergic receptors improve working memory under basal conditions and under conditions characterized by elevated dopaminergic transmission, such as stress. These findings led to the use of such drugs in the treatment of **ADHD**. The manipulation of working memory by these drugs and by ligands for other noradrenergic receptors is consistent with the involvement of the locus ceruleus in attentional states. This region of the brain provides virtually all noradrenergic innervation to the cerebral cortex. Moreover, as previously mentioned, it has been shown to profoundly regulate vigilance and attention.

The lateral pulvinar nucleus of the thalamus is strongly associated with stimulus filtering, or dampening responsiveness to unattended inputs. As the final gatekeeper for transmission of information to the cortex, the thalamus is ideally situated to perform such a

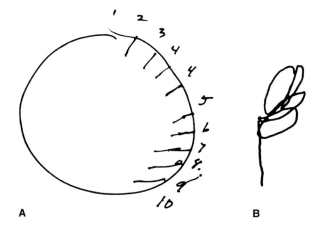

A   **B**

Figure 18–9. A patient with parietal lobe damage exhibits signs of unilateral neglect when asked to draw a clock (**A**) and a flower (**B**). (Adapted with permission from Waxman SG. 2000. *Correlative Neuroanatomy,* 24th ed, p. 269. New York: McGraw-Hill.)

function. The pulvinar nucleus is activated selectively during tasks in which stimuli must be selected from many similar stimuli. It is also activated selectively during crossmodal attention; for example, it is engaged when subjects must attend to auditory stimuli while ignoring visual stimuli.

It is important to recognize that the identification of brain regions involved in modulating attention has not explained how attention is controlled. Knowledge of the neuroanatomy of attention does not explain why one's attention might rapidly turn to a one hundred dollar bill on a sidewalk but not to a similarly shaped scrap of newspaper lying next to it. How does the brain decide what to attend to? Relevant circuits in the brain are believed to perform many tasks in addition to the modulation of cortical activity. Such circuits most likely also receive and integrate information from other circuits, including those that comprise the limbic system, the reticular activating system, and the primary and association cortices. They also may be responsible for determining the relative importance of such information. Information from other circuits, such as the visual features of a bill and knowledge of the importance of money, might be sufficient to shift one's attention from a previous object of interest to the unexpected appearance of a hundred dollar bill. Several models have been proposed to explain attentional processes in terms of both psychology and neural circuitry; the reader is referred to Suggested Reading for discussion of this work.

ATTENTION DEFICIT AND HYPERACTIVITY DISORDER

For most individuals, the ability to exercise selective attention is so automatic that it is difficult to imagine the consequences of impaired attention. However, a significant fraction of the population experiences a striking deficiency in the ability to maintain attention. Approximately 3% to 5% of school-aged children are affected by ADHD, which as its name suggests, is characterized by attention-related difficulties and behavioral symptoms such as impulsivity and overactivity. The incidence of ADHD is difficult to ascertain because objective diagnostic tests for this disorder have yet to be developed. Both the lack of laboratory diagnostic tools and a lack of pathophysiologic information have prompted concerns that ADHD may be underdiagnosed or overdiagnosed in different sectors of society.

Although ADHD initially was considered a childhood disorder that was believed to disappear by adulthood, research increasingly suggests that the symptoms of many children with ADHD persist into adulthood.

The following reports are from adults with ADHD and give some idea of the mental disruption that can be caused by this syndrome.[1]

I'm one of those people who are all of a sudden switching topics in a conversation....I was always the one everyone pointed to and said, "you're weird!" I feel like I'll never be on the same level everybody else is on.

In school it was hard for me to stay on the subject or to finish anything.... I couldn't take notes even if I really tried...if someone sneezed, I'd look at him and my mind would go off in a million directions. I'd look out the window, wondering why he had sneezed.

I feel ashamed. I'm frustrated as hell. I feel like I'm not a grownup yet. On days [that] I have to do paperwork, I make myself sit at my desk and try to get organized. . . . I pick up a bill, make it out, and start to put a stamp on it. But the stamps are next to the paper clip box and I think it should go in the desk, so I put it in the desk. And I see more pencils than I need, so I throw two of them out . . . then I start throwing out junk mail, and there are magazines on the desk, so I take them to the bookcase. In the bookcase there's an old magazine I don't need anymore so I throw that away. Then I realize the wastebasket is full, so I empty it. When I go outside to empty the wastebasket, I see that there's something going on in the kitchen, so I do something in there.

I can't seem to determine that, okay, this is the time to do one thing. My motivation is always crisis. What gets done is what has to get done. [I pay] the bills I have to pay so the insurance company and the light company don't shut off services. I'm always late for appointments. Bills get paid at the last moment, usually, like reports in school were done at the last minute. But if I had my druthers, I'd rather not file two extensions every year on my income tax.

Although ADHD typically is not as debilitating as disorders such as schizophrenia and Alzheimer disease, its impact on cognitive functioning is powerful enough to cause difficulties in social relationships, in school, and in work. Fortunately, when ADHD is properly diagnosed it usually is treatable. Moreover, our understanding of the biologic basis of this disorder, which is rudimentary but gradually improving, is likely to lead to improved diagnosis and more effective treatment.

NEUROBIOLOGIC MECHANISMS OF ADHD

ADHD most likely is not a single disease, but a syndrome that may be characteristic of any number of neural abnormalities. Individuals with ADHD display

[1]Weiss L. 1992. *Attention Deficit Disorder in Adults.* Dallas: Taylor Publishing Company.

considerable diversity in cognitive functioning and exhibit diverse symptoms. Such diversity may reflect distinct biologic abnormalities or merely variations in the expression of common abnormalities. The *DSM IV* formally recognizes three different types of ADHD: predominantly inattentive, predominantly hyperactive, and combined. Yet these formal categories have yet to be related to corresponding differences in etiology or pathophysiology.

Efforts to study the neurobiology of ADHD by means of neuroimaging are limited not only by the heterogeneity of the syndrome but also by the lack of tasks that reliably provoke symptoms. Preliminary structural imaging studies have implicated the frontal and cingulate cortex—brain structures previously discussed in relation to attention—in the mediation of ADHD. Preliminary imaging studies suggest that these areas of the brain are reduced in size and characterized by reduced metabolism in some individuals with this syndrome, compared with normal controls. The anterior basal ganglia, including the caudate nucleus and globus pallidus, also are reported to exhibit reduced size and activity in individuals with ADHD. These findings have led researchers to theorize that a deficit in the braking system represented by communication between the caudate–globus pallidus and thalamic output neurons (see Chapter 14) may result in ADHD symptoms such as impulsivity and hyperactivity.

Although abnormalities in attentional and motor control systems of the brain may be related to ADHD, the exact processing deficiencies that account for the symptoms of ADHD are unknown. Moreover the causes of related abnormalities in brain structure and function remain undetermined. Investigators have speculated that gestational hypoxia and some types of environmental stimuli may be associated with this disorder; however, considerable evidence suggests that ADHD is a heritable disorder. Indeed studies have indicated that monozygotic twins are 92% concordant for ADHD, whereas dizygotic twins are 33% concordant. Such findings provide compelling evidence that genetics strongly influences the development of ADHD, yet the specific gene(s) responsible for ADHD remain(s) unidentified.

Genetic association studies have weakly implicated two genes—one that encodes the dopamine transporter and one that encodes the D_4 dopamine receptor—in the predisposition for ADHD. Moreover, mutant mice that lack the dopamine transporter exhibit profound levels of hyperactivity; however, because these mice exhibit very high levels of sustained dopaminergic transmission and many related compensatory adaptations, such mutations may not produce a good model of ADHD. Mice that express lower than normal levels of the transporter also are hyperactive and are reported to be deficient in certain measures of habituation and perhaps attention. How might abnormalities in dopamine systems be responsible for ADHD? The explanation may lie in the manner in which attentional and motor systems are regulated by dopaminergic input. Activity in the anterior cingulate gyrus and frontal cortex, for example, is modified by dopaminergic inputs from the ventral tegmental area, as measured by working memory. Thus variations in proteins that control the dopamine system may compromise dopaminergic transmission to the cingulate and frontal cortices, and in turn may lead to abnormal activity in these areas. Such abnormal activity may compromise the ability to sustain attention and to attend selectively to a given stimulus in the presence of distractions. This hypothesis might account for the underactivity of the cingulate gyrus and frontal cortex that is common among individuals with ADHD. Underactivity in these regions also may lead to phenomena such as dendritic pruning, which in turn might account for the characteristically reduced size of these structures. However, it must be emphasized that adequate evidence to support the involvement of a dopamine-related gene in human ADHD has yet to be obtained. The models and theories described here have heuristic value but also indicate the need for further research.

TREATMENT OF ADHD

Amphetamines The most common treatment for ADHD is the administration of amphetamine-like drugs. **Methylphenidate** (Ritalin) is the drug most frequently prescribed for this disorder, but D-amphetamine, the active stereoisomer of amphetamine; **adderall,** a mixture of several amphetamine salts and stereoisomers; and **pemoline** also are commonly used (Figure 18–10). Pemoline is structurally unrelated to amphetamine but has very similar stimulant properties and may have a similar mechanism of action.

Although the administration of methylphenidate and amphetamines to children has been a subject of controversy, these drugs are safe and effective in the treatment of well-diagnosed ADHD. Symptomatic improvement associated with the use of any one of these drugs occurs in more than 70% of children with ADHD, provided that the chosen drug is titrated appropriately to meet individual needs. An NIH consensus conference concluded that there is little evidence of increased stimulant abuse among patients with ADHD who are treated with amphetamines; likewise, this conference found no indications of significant risks associated with these medications. Moreover, untreated individuals exhibit poor school performance and may be at increased risk for disciplinary or criminal problems and drug abuse. However, methylphenidate or amphetamine treatment is not without side effects, which can include insomnia, decreased appetite, stomachache, headache, and nervousness.

Another complication associated with the use of amphetamines in the treatment of ADHD is symptom rebound, or the reappearance and sometimes exaggeration of symptoms as the drugs are metabolized and cleared. The clinical action of both methylphenidate and D-amphetamine is of short duration (3–6 hours); thus the use of these agents can lead to the experience of two or three dips in the drug level each day unless an appropriate scheduling of doses is observed. Adderall and pemoline are advantageous in that they have a longer duration of action (4–10 hours); individuals with ADHD who take

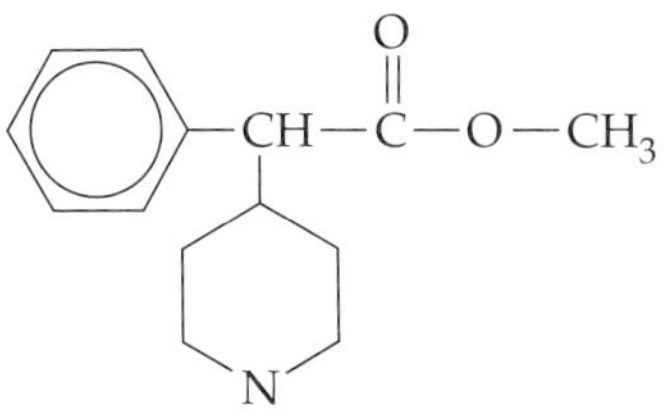

Methylphenidate

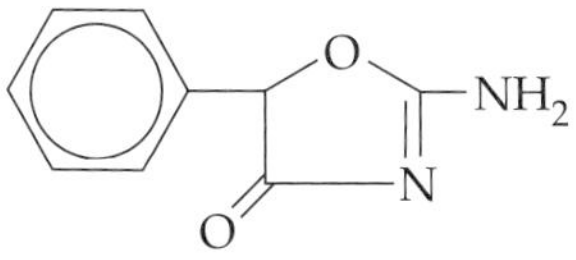

Pemoline

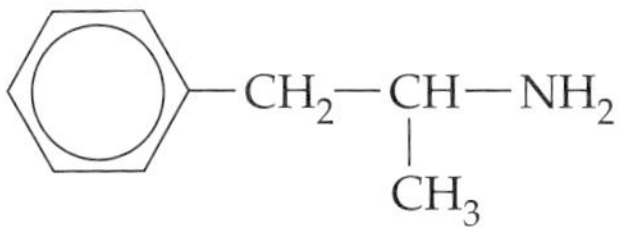

Amphetamine

Figure 18–10. Chemical structures of psychostimulants used to treat attention deficit and hyperactivity disorder (ADHD).

these drugs in the morning often can avoid experiencing these dips during the school or work day.

Although amphetamines are known to enhance monoaminergic transmission (see Chapters 8 and 9), the mechanism by which they alleviate the symptoms of ADHD remains a matter of speculation. Because of the multiple and widespread effects of amphetamines, it is difficult to demonstrate that a specific neurochemical change is responsible for ameliorating a particular symptom. A theoretically appealing possibility is that methylphenidate and amphetamines serve to boost dopaminergic transmission in the brain's attentional structures, as previously outlined in this chapter. However, the complexity of attentional and motor control systems and the multiple effects of amphetamines suggest that such a model is simplistic and incomplete.

Antidepressants   **Tricyclic antidepressants** and **bupropion** have shown some efficacy in the treatment of ADHD, but data from relevant clinical trials have been limited. In contrast, the SSRI antidepressants are not effective in the treatment of this disorder. The tricyclic agents inhibit the reuptake of norepinephrine and serotonin; in contrast, bupropion inhibits the reuptake of dopamine, although other actions also may be responsible for its clinical utility (see Chapter 15). These antidepressants offer an advantage over amphetamines in that they have relatively long courses of action and tend to produce fewer rebound effects.

Despite such advantages, antidepressants continue to be a second-line treatment for ADHD because they do not appear to treat the cognitive and attentional symptoms of this disorder as well as amphetamines. Moreover, side-effect profiles reveal that tricyclics and bupropion can be more disruptive than amphetamines. Bupropion causes a rash in approximately 17% of children who take it and also is associated with a risk for seizures. In addition to their previously discussed anticholinergic and antihistaminic side effects, tricyclic antidepressants can be cardiotoxic in children and also can cause seizures. Nevertheless, tricyclic antidepressants and bupropion are alternative treatment for individuals who cannot take amphetamines.

Other agents   As previously mentioned, α_2-adrenergic agonists are among the agents most recently introduced for the treatment of ADHD. Such agents, including **clonidine** and **guanfacine,** are of some benefit in a subset of patients with this disorder. Although these drugs are not associated with serious side effects, their use is limited somewhat by their tendency to produce sedation. Guanfacine, however, is usually less sedating than clonidine.

SELECTED READING

Arnsten AF. 1997. Catecholamine regulation of the prefrontal cortex. *J Psychopharmacol* 11:151–162.

Aston-Jones G, Rajkowski J, Kubiak P, et al. 1996. Role of the locus ceruleus in emotional activation. *Prog Brain Res* 107: 379–402.

Barkley RA. 1997. Behavioral inhibition, sustained attention, and executive functions: Constructing a unifying theory of ADHD. *Psychological Bull* 121:65–94.

Boivin DB, Duffy JF, Kronauer RE, Czeisler CA. 1996. Dose-response relationships for resetting of human circadian clock by light. *Nature* 379:540–542.

Castellanos FX. 1997. Towards a pathophysiology of attention deficit–hyperactivity disorder. *Clin Pediatrics* 36:381–393.

Challman TD, Lipsky JJ. 2000. Methylphenidate: its pharmacology and uses. *Mayo Clin Proc* 75:711–721.

Chemelli RM, Willie JT, Sinton CM, et al. 1999. Narcolepsy in orexin knockout mice: Molecular genetics of sleep regulation. *Cell* 98:437–452.

Coull JT. 1998. Neural correlates of attention and arousal: Insights from electrophysiology, functional neuroimaging, and psychopharmacology. *Prog Neurobiol* 55:343–361.

Czeisler CA. 1995. The effect of light on the human circadian pacemaker. *Ciba Found Symp* 183:254–290.

Dement WC. 1998. The study of human sleep: A historical perspective. *Thorax* 53(suppl):S2–S7.

Desimone R. 1996. Neural mechanisms for visual memory and their role in attention. *Proc Natl Acad Sci USA* 93: 13494–13499.

Dijk DJ, Duffy JF. 1999. Circadian regulation of human sleep and age-related changes in its timing, consolidation, and EEG characteristics. *Ann Med* 31:130–140.

Goldman LS, Genel M, Bexman RJ, Slanetz PJ. 1998. Diagnosis and treatment of attention deficit–hyperactivity disorder in children and adolescents. *JAMA* 279:1100–1107.

Jones BE. 1994. Basic mechanisms of sleep–wake states. In Kryger MH, Roth T, Dement WC (eds): *Principles and Practice of Sleep Medicine*, 2nd ed, pp 145–162. Philadelphia: WB Saunders.

Kastner S, Ungerleider LG. 2000. Mechanisms of visual attention in the human cortex. *Annu Rev Neurosci* 23:315–341.

King D, Takahashi JS. 2000. Molecular genetics of circadian rhythms in mammals. *Annu Rev Neurosci* 23:713–742.

Kornhauser JM, Ginty DD, Greenberg ME, et al. 1996. Light entrainment and activation of signal transduction pathways in the SCN. *Prog Brain Res* 111:133–146.

Lin L, Faraco JU, Li R, et al. 1999. The sleep disorder canine narcolepsy is caused by a mutation in the hypocretin (orexin) receptor 2 gene. *Cell* 98:365–376.

Lowrey PL, Shimomura K, Antoch MP, et al. 2000. Positional syntenic cloning and functional characterization of the mammalian circadian mutation tau. *Science* 288: 483–492.

Maronde E, Pfeffer M, Olcese J, et al. 1999. Transcription factors in neuroendocrine regulation: Rhythmic changes in pCREB and ICER frame melatonin synthesis. *J Neurosci* 19:3326–3336.

McCarley RW, Strecker RE, Porkka-Heiskanen T, et al. 1997. Modulation of cholinergic neurons by serotonin and adenosine in the control of REM and non-REM sleep. In: *Sleep and Sleep Disorders: From Molecule to Behavior*, pp. 63–79. Tokyo: Academic Press.

Nishino S, Ripley B, Overeem S, et al. 2000. Hypocretin (orexin) deficiency in human narcolepsy. *Lancet* 355:39–40.

Peyron C, Faraco J, Rogers W. et al. 2000. A mutation in a case of early onset narcolepsy and a generalized absence of hypocretin peptides in human narcoleptic brains. *Nature Med* 6:991–997.

Porkka-Heiskanen T, Strecker RE, Thakkar M, et al. 1997. Adenosine: A mediator of the sleep-inducing effects of prolonged wakefulness. *Science* 276:1265–1268.

Posner MI, Driver J. 1992. The neurobiology of selective attention. *Curr Opin Neurobiol* 2:165–169.

Posner MI, Petersen SE. 1990. The attention system of the human brain. *Annu Rev Neurosci* 13:25–42.

Rechtschaffen A. 1998. Current perspectives on the function of sleep. *Perspect Biol Med* 41:359–390.

Siegel JM. 1994. Brain stem mechanisms generating REM sleep. In Kryger MH, Roth T, Dement WC (eds). *Principles and Practice of Sleep Medicine*, 2nd ed, pp 125–144. Philadelphia: WB Saunders.

Steriade M. 1996. Arousal: Revisiting the reticular activating system. *Science* 272:225–226.

Steriade M, McCarley RW. 1990. *Brain Stem Control of Wakefulness and Sleep*. New York: Plenum Press.

Swanson J, Castellanos FX, Murias M, et al. 1998. Cognitive neuroscience of attention deficit hyperactivity disorder and hyperkinetic disorder. *Curr Opin Neurobiol* 8: 263–271.

Todd RD. 2000. Genetics of attention deficit/hyperactivity disorder: are we ready for molecular genetic studies? *Am J Med Genet* 96:241–243.

Weiss L. 1992. *Attention Deficit Disorder in Adults*. Dallas: Taylor Publishing Company.

Weitz CJ. 1996. Circadian timekeeping: Loops and layers of transcriptional control. *Proc Natl Acad Sci USA* 93:14308–14309.

Wilsbacher LD, Takahashi JS. 1998. Circadian rhythms: Molecular basis of the clock. *Curr Opin Gen Dev* 8:595–602.

Chapter 19

Pain

KEY CONCEPTS

- Pain has both a localizing somatic sensory component and an aversive affective component. Nociception is the form of somatic sensation that detects noxious and tissue-damaging stimuli.

- Nociception is mediated by peripheral afferent nociceptors, which are free endings of neurons that have their cell bodies in dorsal root ganglia and form synapses with other neurons in the spinal cord or brain stem.

- Many mediators released by damaged tissues and invading inflammatory cells directly activate peripheral afferent nociceptors. In addition, a subset of mediators, such as prostaglandins and leukotrienes, act indirectly by lowering the threshold for activation of nociceptors in an area extending beyond that of tissue injury. This sensitization process protects the wounded area but may also contribute to pain and disability.

- Nonsteroidal antiinflammatory drugs act by blocking prostaglandin-mediated sensitization, specifically by inhibiting the enzyme cyclooxygenase that is required for the synthesis of prostaglandins from arachidonic acid.

- Peripheral afferent nociceptors and the neurons on which they synapse in the dorsal horn of the spinal cord express many types of receptors,

- which represent possible targets for the development of analgesic drugs.

- Glutamate is a major neurotransmitter by which peripheral afferent nociceptors communicate with dorsal horn neurons. These nociceptors also release a large number of neuropeptide modulators that play an important role in pain.

- The dorsal horn of the spinal cord is an important site of integration for both ascending nociceptive information and descending antinociceptive influences.

- Opiate drugs selectively suppress nociception, but not other sensory modalities, by binding to endogenous opioid receptors in descending analgesic pathways.

- In addition to their actions on descending analgesic pathways, morphine-like opiates have central effects that diminish the affective response to pain.

- Damage to neurons in nociceptive pathways can lead to severe chronic pain syndromes.

- Plasticity within the dorsal horn, mediated by NMDA receptors, may be key in the initiation of chronic pain syndromes by increasing the excitability of neurons in nociceptive pathways.

The neurophysiologic term *nociception* refers to the detection of noxious stimuli or stimuli that are capable of damaging tissue. However, nociception is not identical to pain; pain represents the complex physiologic, behavioral, and subjective response to nociceptive inputs. Acute pain, which for example, may result from stepping on a nail, and chronic pain, which may accompany subsequent infection and inflammation, both begin with the activation of nociceptive pathways by a noxious stimulus. Both types of pain serve a survival function by leading to the behavioral and reflexive protection of injured tissue that permits healing. However, chronic pain can become autonomous; that is, it can occur independently of the tissue injury that initiates it. In almost all cases, autonomous pain results from injury to the pain pathways of the nervous system themselves and is termed *neuropathic pain*. Pain divorced from ongoing tissue damage or inflammation is maladaptive and represents a serious clinical problem. The subjective experience of all types of pain and the initiation of pain-related behaviors are influenced by the context in which nociception occurs, the affected individual's level of stress, and the significance the individual assigns to the sensation.

Pain can be separated into two components, both of which involve dedicated projection systems from the spinal cord or brain stem. One component is a modality of somatic sensation. It permits the localization of pain and enables discrimination among different types of painful sensations. The second component is affective; it activates circuits in the brain that produce negative emotion, brain stem systems that increase arousal, and regions of the hypothalamus and amygdala that initiate responses to stress. Because of the somatosensory aspects of pain, an individual can report its approximate location and describe its qualities, such as pricking or burning. Because of its powerful affective component, pain interrupts ongoing behaviors and demands attention; it also powerfully motivates learning and thereby suppresses behaviors that put an organism in harm's way. This affective component gives pain its survival value, but also can produce suffering and disability when pain is chronic.

Among the many different drugs that have been produced to relieve pain, the most important with regard to clinical use are **nonsteroidal antiinflammatory drugs** (**NSAIDs**) and **opiates**. Opiates offer the most potent pain relief available but have major drawbacks. First, although they are effective in the treatment of acute pain, they do not adequately relieve chronic neuropathic pain. Second, they have many side effects, including respiratory depression and constipation. Third, among the most serious drawbacks associated with their long-term use are the development of tolerance to their analgesic effects, dependence, and addiction (see Chapter 16). Because of these disadvantages, substantial efforts have gone into the search for alternatives to opiates in the treatment of pain.

PROCESSING OF PAIN-RELATED INFORMATION BY THE PERIPHERAL NERVOUS SYSTEM

PRIMARY AFFERENT NOCICEPTORS

The clinical significance of pain varies, depending on its anatomic origin. Although musculoskeletal pain, such as that from arthritis, and visceral pain, including pain from ischemia, distention, malignant infiltration, or torsion of an organ, are responsible for many chronic pain syndromes, the nociceptive afferent nerve endings in the skin have been the most thoroughly studied because of their accessibility.

Cutaneous receptors involved in nociception, often called *nociceptors*, are free nerve endings. Among receptors involved in somatic sensation, nociceptors are the least differentiated. They transduce mechanical, thermal, or chemical tissue-damaging stimuli into a train of action potentials that are transmitted along their axons to the spinal cord or to homologous regions of the brain stem. As with all afferent nerves involved in somatic sensation, the cell bodies of peripheral nociceptors are located in dorsal root ganglia (Figure 19–1). Nociceptive neurons of dorsal root ganglia synapse in the dorsal horn of the spinal cord on local interneurons and on projection neurons, which carry nociceptive information primarily to the brain stem, thalamus, and hypothalamus.

Peripheral nerves contain several different types of axons that carry sensory information; the greater the diameter and thickness of myelination of the axons, the greater their conduction velocity. The axons of cutaneous afferent nerves belong to one of three main classes. The largest and most heavily myelinated axons that originate from the skin are called A_β fibers. A_α axons, which are thicker, innervate muscles and joints; these axons are involved in proprioception, or the transmission of sensory information related to posture, motion, and position. A_β fibers include cutaneous mechanoreceptors, which are free nerve endings that respond to light touch and the bending of hairs. Primary nociceptive neurons have small-caliber axons, which are classified as A_δ or C fibers (Table 19–1; Box 19–1). A_δ fibers are thinly myelinated, and C fibers are unmyelinated. Because C fibers lack myelination, their conduction is quite slow (<2 m/s) compared with that of A_δ fibers (approximately 20 m/s).

A nociceptive neuron must distinguish between innocuous and noxious stimuli. Nociceptors accomplish this either because they have high thresholds for stimu-

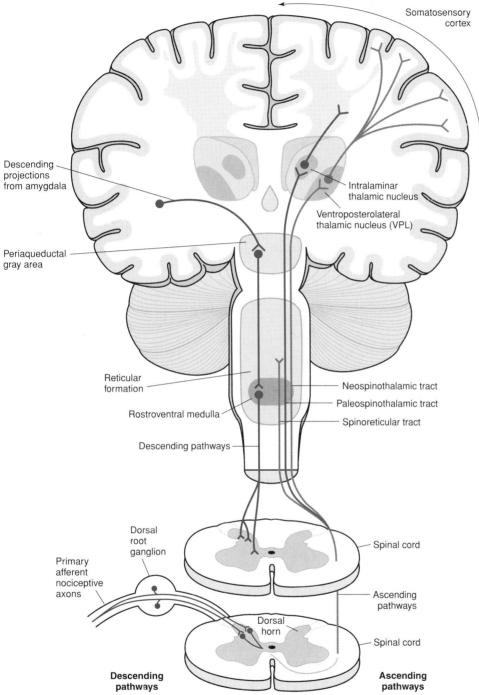

Figure 19–1. Major nociceptive pathways. A primary afferent nociceptive neuron synapses in the superficial layers of the dorsal horn. Axons of dorsal horn neurons cross the midline and ascend into the spinoreticular or spinothalamic tracts (*right*). The spinothalamic tract comprises the neospinothalamic and paleospinothalamic tracts. In the neospinothalamic tract, second-order neurons synapse in the ventroposterolateral nucleus of the thalamus (VPL), and third-order neurons project to the primary somatosensory cortex. In the paleospinothalamic tract, second-order neurons synapse in the intralaminar thalamic nuclei and project to the association cortex and regions of the brain that control emotion. Descending analgesic systems believed to originate with cortical neurons and neurons of the amygdala carry survival-relevant information (*left*). Such descending analgesic systems are mediated in part by the periaqueductal gray area (PAG). A projection from the PAG to the rostrolventral medulla that descends to the dorsal horn mediates opiate-dependent descending analgesia.

Box 19–1 First and Second Pain

When a distal part of an individuals's extremity receives an acute high-intensity stimulus, such as a kick in the shin, two distinct sensations are experienced. The first sensation arrives swiftly and is sharp and brief; the second sensation, which arrives belatedly, typically burns, is described as more unpleasant, and tends to be more prolonged. The first sensation, or *first pain*, is caused by rapidly conducting A_δ fibers, whereas the more aversive *second pain* is caused by slowly conducting C fibers.

Indeed, differences in the subjective perceptions of first and second pain are directly related to physiologically significant differences in the conduction velocities of A_δ and C fibers. Imagine accidentally placing a finger tip into a cup of scalding coffee. If the distance from finger tip to spinal cord were 1 meter, an A_δ fiber conducting at 20 m/s would deliver the message to the CNS in 0.05 seconds. A C fiber conducting at 0.5 m/s would require 2 seconds to deliver the same message. Under such circumstances, the response of A_δ fibers leads to a rapid spinal reflex that causes the finger to be withdrawn and rescued from further harm. In contrast, the response of C fibers is slow enough to permit serious tissue damage.

Efforts to alleviate pain require an understanding of the differences between these two types of fibers. A_δ fibers are relatively sensitive to pressure but are relatively insensitive to low doses of local anesthetics. Conversely, C fibers are more sensitive to local anesthetics (see Table 19–1). Because of such differences it is possible to selectively suppress the firing of A_δ fibers, for example, by inflating a blood pressure cuff around a limb, and the firing of C fibers, for example, by an appropriate injection of local anesthetic. The blocking of A_δ fibers by such means suppresses the sharp first pain that occurs in response to an acute noxious stimulus, but may cause the delayed second pain to be experienced as stronger and more aversive. These findings suggest that A_δ fiber stimulation may reduce C fiber-mediated nociception. The mechanism responsible for this phenomenon is not known, but it is possible that the effectiveness of **acupuncture** and other forms of analgesia that protect against the perception of apparently painful stimuli may involve such interactions between A_δ and C fibers.

---

lation or because they are capable of coding the intensity of a stimulus in the frequency of impulses relayed centrally, so that stimuli that produce the highest firing rates are determined to be noxious (Figure 19–2). A_δ nociceptors, or high-threshold mechanoreceptors, respond to noxious mechanical stimuli, especially sharp objects; approximately half of them—mechanothermal nociceptors—also respond to noxious thermal stimuli. The majority of C fibers in cutaneous nerves have higher thresholds than those of myelinated axons, and respond nonselectively to noxious mechanical, thermal, and chemical stimuli. Thus they are known as polymodal nociceptors.

Activation of C fibers is mediated by a wide range of endogenous chemicals that are released in response to damaged tissue or inflammation. These fibers tend to respond only indirectly to exogenous chemicals, through

the mediation of tissue damage. However, they do respond to the exogenous chemical **capsaicin,** a product of the capsicum family of peppers. Capsaicin directly stimulates an ion channel, vanilloid receptor subtype 1 (V_1R), that is activated in vivo by noxious heat and by H^+ ions. The actions of capsaicin and the regulation of V_1R are described in Box 19–2.

Primary nociceptive neurons express many receptors in addition to V_1R. Ligand-gated channels expressed on these neurons include AMPA and NMDA glutamate receptors, γ-aminobutyric acid $(GABA)_A$ receptors, nicotinic acetylcholine receptors (nAChRs), 5-HT_3 receptors, and P_{2X3} receptors. As explained in Chapter 10, ligand-gated channels activated by adenosine triphosphate (ATP) are called P_{2X} receptors, whereas G protein-coupled receptors activated by ATP are designated P_{2Y}. Of seven known P_{2X} receptors, only P_{2X3} appears to be

Table 19–1 Characteristics of Primary Nociceptive Fibers

	A_δ Fibers	C Fibers
Diameter	2–5 μm	0.2–1.5 μm
Conduction velocity	6–30 m/s	0.5–2 m/s
Myelination	Thinly myelinated	Unmyelinated
Time to conduct 1 meter	Approximately 0.05 sec	Approximately 2.0 sec
Responsiveness to stimuli	High-threshold mechanoreceptors, mechanothermal receptors	Polymodal
Blocked by	Pressure	Low doses of local anesthetics

Box 19–2 The Capsaicin Receptor

Capsaicin, a major component of many spicy hot foods, is also a powerful experimental tool in the study of pain. Many individuals who have touched their eyes after cutting chili peppers without gloves can attest to the intense burning pain that capsaicin can produce. Moreover, in developing animals capsaicin has been proven to kill unmyelinated

V_1R is a heat-gated nonselective cation channel that is believed to mediate responses of small-diameter sensory neurons to moderate (43°C) thermal stimuli. V_1R is also activated by H^+, which may be generated by several types of tissue damage. Thus it can directly elicit pain or produce sensitization of nociceptors. Further insight into the physi-

$$CH_3O-\underset{HO}{\overset{}{\bigcirc}}-CH_2-NH-\overset{O}{\overset{\|}{C}}-(CH_2)_4-CH=CH-CH\overset{CH_3}{\underset{CH_3}{}}$$

Capsaicin

dorsal root ganglion neurons, and in mature animals it has been used to produce models of cutaneous pain without tissue damage. Therapeutically, capsaicin creams are used as analgesics because they desensitize nociceptive nerve terminals (nociceptors).

The capsaicin receptor has been designated as vanilloid receptor subtype 1 (V_1R). A vanilloid moiety is a shared feature of capsaicin and **resiniferatoxin,** another natural plant product that is a potent ligand at this receptor. The identification and characterization of the V_1R receptor have been particularly interesting because the natural ligand for this receptor appears to be noxious heat. Indeed,

ologic function of V_1R has come from mice that lack this receptor. V_1R knockout mice show normal responses to noxious mechanical stimuli, but reduced responses to noxious thermal stimuli. They also show less of the hypersensitivity to heat that is normally seen in the context of inflammation.

A structurally related receptor, V_1RL, does not respond to capsaicin, H^+, or moderate heat; however, it does respond to high temperatures, with a threshold of approximately 52°C. V_1RL is expressed in many neuronal cell types in addition to sensory neurons, but its precise physiologic role remains unknown.

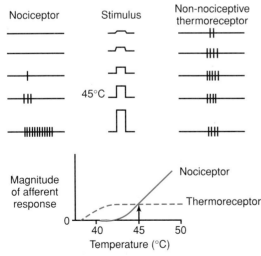

Figure 19–2. Physiologic recordings from two cutaneous primary sensory neurons. Action potentials from both are compared as the intensity of a stimulus increases (*top to bottom*); 45° C is the threshold for tissue damage. The nociceptor (*left*) has a higher threshold, but exhibits an increasing firing rate once within the noxious range. The thermoreceptor, which detects non-noxious heat, has a low threshold and exhibits no change in firing rate as the stimulus intensity increases.

expressed in sensory neurons and in the spinal cord neurons of humans. P_{2X} also is expressed in cardiac cells. G protein-coupled receptors expressed on primary nociceptive neurons include B_2 bradykinin, eicosanoid, histamine, 5-HT_1 and 5-HT_2, $GABA_B$, α_2-adrenergic, somatostatin, neuropeptide Y, and μ, δ, and κ opioid receptors. As discussed later in this chapter, a subset of these neurons also express TrkA, the neurotrophin receptor that binds nerve growth factor (NGF). This panoply of receptors permits primary nociceptive neurons to respond to a wide range of mediators. Tissue damage, for example, causes the release of K^+ and H^+ ions and ATP. In the region of an injury, serotonin is released from platelets, and histamine from tissue mast cells. Bradykinin, one of the most potent activators of nociception, is produced from plasma kininogen by the actions of kallikreins, enzymes that are activated rapidly at the site of an injury (Box 19–3).

SENSITIZATION

Sensitization is a clinically significant aspect of pain. Certain diffusible chemical mediators, including

Box 19–3 Bradykinin

Bradykinin is one of the most potent pronociceptive, or *algesic*, substances known. It is capable of eliciting intense pain and burning sensations when administered to humans. The term *bradykinin* (*brady*, slow; *kinin*, movement) refers to the substance's ability to produce a slow-onset contraction of smooth muscle in the gut in vitro. Bradykinin is a peptide composed of 9 amino acids and is closely related to kallidin, a peptide composed of 10 amino acids. Both peptides are derived from kininogen, a propeptide. Two forms of kininogen are generated in vivo by means of alternative splicing.

Kininogens are converted into bradykinin and kallidin through the actions of kallikrein enzymes, which are primarily concentrated in plasma but also can be found in smaller quantities in tissues. Kallikreins are inactive in their basal state; they become activated when they are cleaved by factor VII, a protease that also plays a role in blood clotting cascades (see Chapter 21). Factor VII is activated in response to contact with collagen and other negatively charged substances revealed during tissue injury. After they are formed, bradykinin and kallidin promote pain and inflammation; thus factor VII is primarily responsible for the coordinated response of blood clotting, pain, and inflammation that occurs after tissue is damaged. Bradykinin and kallidin exhibit very short half-lives because they are rapidly degraded by a variety of plasma and tissue proteases.

The actions of these peptides are mediated by means of two subtypes of G protein-coupled receptors, termed B_1 and B_2 (see Chapter 10). Of these two subtypes, B_2 receptors are more strongly related to the perception of acute pain and the precipitation of acute inflammation; B_1 receptors may contribute to chronic pain and inflammation. Both receptors appear to be coupled primarily to G_q and are believed to produce their physiologic effects through the activation of the phospholipase C-phosphatidylinositol cascades described in Chapter 5. The activation of these receptors also leads to the stimulation of phospholipase A_2, which catalyzes the formation of arachidonic acid and the generation of a host of prostaglandins and other eicosanoid mediators; however, the mechanism by which B_1 and B_2 receptors cause such stimulation is poorly understood. Activation of these receptors also can lead to the release of substance P, calcitoningene-related peptide, and other substances from primary sensory neurons, which further contributes to pain and inflammation.

The principal involvement of the bradykinin system in nociception and in the inflammatory response has spurred intense interest in the possible therapeutic use of agents directed at this system. Thus far antagonists of B_1 and B_2 receptors and inhibitors of kallikrein have been developed; however, despite their efficacy in animal models, the clinical utility of such agents has been disappointing to date. The possibility that the degradation of bradykinin and kallidin may be inhibited by certain drugs used in the treatment of **hypertension** is also under investigation. It is believed that **angiotensin-converting enzyme (ACE) inhibitors** such as **captopril** may inhibit such degradation in addition to inhibiting angiotensin-converting enzyme. Furthermore, it has been proposed that related increases in bradykinin and kallidin may contribute to some of the clinical actions of these medications.

---

arachidonic acid metabolites such as prostaglandins and leukotrienes, do not activate nociceptors directly; rather, they sensitize the nociceptors to subsequent stimulation. Sensitized nociceptors usually extend beyond the borders of tissue damage, and exhibit a decreased threshold for firing such that previously innocuous stimuli may be experienced as painful (Figure 19–3). This phenomenon is termed *allodynia*. When inflammation is present, for example, stimulation of A_β fibers may produce pain, an increased and prolonged firing of nociceptors occurs in response to noxious stimuli. The result is an exaggerated response to noxious stimuli referred to as *hyperalgesia*. Heightened sensitivity in response to somatic sensory stimuli presumably serves an adaptive purpose and leads an organism to protect an injured part. Tissue injury and sensitization in the peripheral nervous system also can lead rapidly to sensitization in the dorsal horn of the spinal cord, which is reflected in a further increase in responsiveness to sensory inputs.

The sources of sensitizing mediators are varied. Prostaglandins and leukotrienes are released from damaged tissue. Other sensitizing mediators, such as interleukin-1, may be released from invading inflammatory cells. Bradykinin activates nociceptors directly, as previously mentioned, and sensitizes them indirectly by increasing the synthesis of prostaglandins. The trophic factor NGF also may contribute to sensitization. During development, NGF is required for the generation of nociceptive neurons. Transgenic mice with null mutations in the genes that encode NGF or its receptor TrkA lack most small-caliber primary sensory neurons, nearly all of which are nociceptive neurons, and consequently are hypoalgesic (see Chapter 11). In mature animals, NGF is expressed in inflamed tissues and appears to contribute to hyperalgesia. The potential involvement of a trophic factor in pain suggests that remodeling of peripheral or central nociceptive terminals may contribute to the persistence of pain after nociceptive

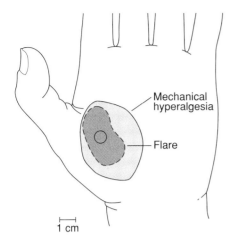

Figure 19–3. Sensitization of tissue. A burn (*solid dark circle*) produces an area of reddening, or a flare (*dashed line*), that extends beyond the injury and is caused by increased blood flow. An even larger area (*solid line*) is characterized by enhanced sensitivity to subsequent stimulation, which reflects the sensitization of nociceptive neurons. When such sensitization occurs in the immediate vicinity of an injury, it is sometimes referred to as primary hyperalgesia; when it occurs within an extended area, it often is referred to as secondary hyperalgesia.

inputs cease, perhaps by maintaining a sensitized state or inducing spontaneous activity or both.

NEUROGENIC INFLAMMATION

The biology of inflammation is beyond the scope of this book. However, the phenomenon of neurogenic inflammation is particularly relevant to the concepts addressed in this chapter. Neurogenic inflammation occurs in response to chemical mediators of nociception that arise not only from damaged tissues and invading inflammatory cells but also from nociceptive neurons themselves. After tissue damage occurs, free nerve endings may release pronociceptive substances, which activate adjacent nociceptors and contribute to both pain and inflammation. The best established pronociceptive substance derived from nerve endings is substance P (Figure 19–4). Substance P causes vasodilation and extravasation of plasma proteins from capillaries, which contributes to the edema associated with inflammation and to the generation of bradykinin from kininogen. Moreover, substance P triggers the release of histamine from tissue mast cells. Because NK_1 is the major receptor for substance P, neurogenic inflammation is markedly attenuated by NK_1 receptor antagonists. It also is reduced in knockout mice that lack the gene that encodes substance P. Another putative mediator of neurogenic inflammation is calcitonin gene-related peptide (CGRP), although its precise function is not well characterized. Neurogenic inflammation has been associated with **migraine, rheumatoid arthritis,** and other diseases.

PROCESSING OF PAIN-RELATED INFORMATION BY THE CNS

DORSAL HORN OF THE SPINAL CORD

The gray matter of the spinal cord is a complex structure composed of lamina that in turn consist of

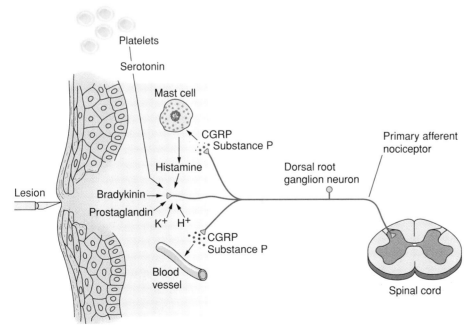

Figure 19–4. Chemical mediators of primary nociceptive neuronal activation and neurogenic inflammation. Tissue injury causes the release of bradykinin and the activation of cyclooxygenases, which in turn leads to the generation of prostaglandins, and other mediators, such as K^+ and H^+. Bradykinins and prostaglandins activate and sensitize neurons. Substance P, released in retrograde fashion from free nerve endings, acts on local blood vessels to extravasate fluid and protein. This process mediates a neurogenic component of the inflammatory process. Substance P also triggers the release of histamine from mast cells. (Adapted with permission from Kandel ER, Schwartz JH, Jessell TM. 2000. *Principles of Neural Science,* 4th ed. New York: McGraw-Hill.)

neurons of different sizes and densities. According to one widely used model, this gray matter is divided into 10 laminae (Figure 19–5). Laminae I–VI make up the dorsal horn, with lamina VI discernible only in the cervical and lumbar enlargements of the cord. Based on the appearance of freshly cut sections, lamina II often is referred to as the substantia gelatinosa. Primary nociceptive neurons synapse in the dorsal horn of the spinal cord on neurons in laminae I, II, IV, and V. (Axons from the face and head synapse in the trigeminal

nucleus in the brain stem.) Within these laminae, the primary nociceptive neurons synapse on both projection neurons, which relay information to the brain stem, hypothalamus, and thalamus, and local circuit neurons, including both excitatory and inhibitory interneurons. Local circuit neurons not only process afferent information but also convey nociceptive information to the autonomic nervous system and to motor neurons involved in local withdrawal reflexes. Diverse inputs may converge on a single dorsal horn cell. Such

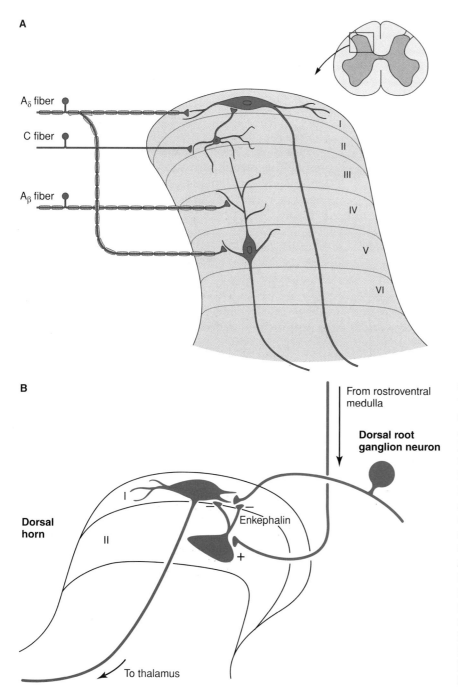

Figure 19–5. Laminae of the dorsal horn of the spinal cord. **A.** One of several possible synaptic arrangements of A_δ and C fibers. A_δ fibers synapse on projection neurons in lamina I. These neurons receive indirect input from C fibers that synapse on interneurons in lamina II. Lamina V neurons are projection neurons that receive direct inputs from both A_δ fibers and C fibers that carry information about innocuous stimuli (not shown). (Adapted with permission from Kandel ER, Schwartz JH, Jessell TM. 2000. *Principles of Neural Science,* 4th ed. New York: McGraw-Hill.) **B.** Descending analgesia in the dorsal horn. Projections from the rostrolventral medulla synapse on enkephalinergic interneurons in lamina II. These interneurons in turn synapse on dorsal horn neurons in lamina I, inhibiting their firing and thereby interrupting the flow of nociceptive information.

inputs include those from descending antinociceptive pathways, which are discussed in a subsequent section of this chapter. Consequently, the dorsal horn is not a simple relay station but an important site of integration for both nociceptive and antinociceptive information.

The existence of multiple inputs on individual dorsal horn neurons may help to explain the phenomenon of *referred pain*. Such pain, which is frequently observed in clinical practice, arises in viscera but is experienced as emanating from the body surface. Pain that originates in particular deep structures tends to correspond to the same sites of referred pain in all individuals. The pain of cardiac ischemia, for example, is commonly experienced as running from the chest down the left arm. Likewise, pain that originates in the diaphragm is often referred to the shoulder. These and other types of referred pain are most likely caused by the convergence of axons of visceral and cutaneous nociceptive neurons on the same neurons in the dorsal horn of the spinal cord. When a single neuron in the dorsal horn receives both visceral and cutaneous inputs, higher processing centers of the brain cannot distinguish the source of pain. Why these higher centers tend to interpret such pain as coming from the body surface rather than from viscera remains unknown.

NEUROTRANSMITTERS AND RECEPTORS IN THE DORSAL HORN

Stimulation of afferent A_δ and C fibers evokes fast excitatory postsynaptic potentials in dorsal horn neurons, which appear to be mediated by glutamate, the major neurotransmitter used by dorsal root ganglion neurons. These fast responses to glutamate are mediated by both AMPA and NMDA receptors. Certain projection neurons with cell bodies in the dorsal horn, which are described as nociceptive-specific, exhibit high electrophysiologic thresholds. Others, which are referred to as wide dynamic range (WDR) neurons, receive inputs from both nonnociceptive and nociceptive neurons and respond to stimuli of increasing intensity with a corresponding increase in their rate of firing.

High-intensity stimulation of primary nociceptive neurons produces additional slow excitatory postsynaptic potentials in dorsal horn neurons, which most likely are caused by the release of various neuropeptides or other substances. Indeed, primary nociceptive neurons contain a complex array of neuropeptides (Figure 19–6), among which the most abundant are CGRP and the tachykinins, substance P and neurokinin A (see Chapter 10). Substance P is synthesized in some C fiber neurons and is co-released with glutamate; CGRP is found in subsets of both A_δ and C fiber neurons. Investigators long believed that substance P played a central role in

pain and in neurogenic inflammation. However, mice with disruption of the gene encoding substance P exhibit only subtle differences in pain behavior compared with wildtype mice. In response to noxious thermal stimulation, for example, these knockout mice exhibit a deficit in pain response only over a relatively narrow temperature range; in fact they exhibit a threshold for response to noxious thermal stimuli and responses to very high temperatures that are identical to those of wildtype mice. Furthermore, **NK$_1$ receptor antagonists** have not been impressive as analgesics in clinical trials, although they do show potential as anxiolytics and antidepressants (see Chapter 15) and as antiemetics. Such findings do not indicate that substance P is unimportant in the mediation of pain; rather it appears that other mediators can fill the role of substance P when it is absent or when its receptor is blocked.

NK$_1$ receptors are found in lamina I of the dorsal horn and in deeper layers, including laminae III and V. Interestingly, the densest substance P innervation is not in lamina I, but in lamina II, the substantia gelatinosa, a layer that is nearly devoid of NK$_1$ receptors. This finding represents a striking example of the apparent mismatch between peptides and their receptors discussed in Chapter 10, and recognition of this mismatch has given rise to the theory that peptides must diffuse extrasynaptically and sometimes for long distances to reach their targets. The binding of substance P to NK$_1$ receptors and the physiologic consequences of such binding can be readily visualized with fluorescently labeled antibodies directed against the NK$_1$ receptor. Such visualization is possible because after binding substance P, the receptors are rapidly internalized and later recycled to the surface, giving the cell a markedly altered appearance. (Details regarding the molecular mechanisms of such receptor trafficking are discussed in detail in Chapter 8.) This type of visualization has led to some interesting observations. Short-term mechanical and thermal stimuli lead to the internalization of receptors in lamina I but not in lamina V. Only persistent stimulation causes receptors as deep as those in lamina V to be internalized. This finding is consistent with the belief that the intensity and persistence of stimulation are key regulators of the release of substance P and other neuropeptides from nerve endings in the dorsal horn. Moreover, these factors most likely determine the target neurons in the spinal cord that can be reached by these neuropeptides.

The plasticity of dorsal horn neurons is believed to be an important factor in pain. As previously mentioned, the sensitization of cutaneous nociceptors can cause the sensitization of dorsal horn neurons. Evidence suggests, for example, that nerve injury leads to neuropathic pain because it triggers an NMDA recep-

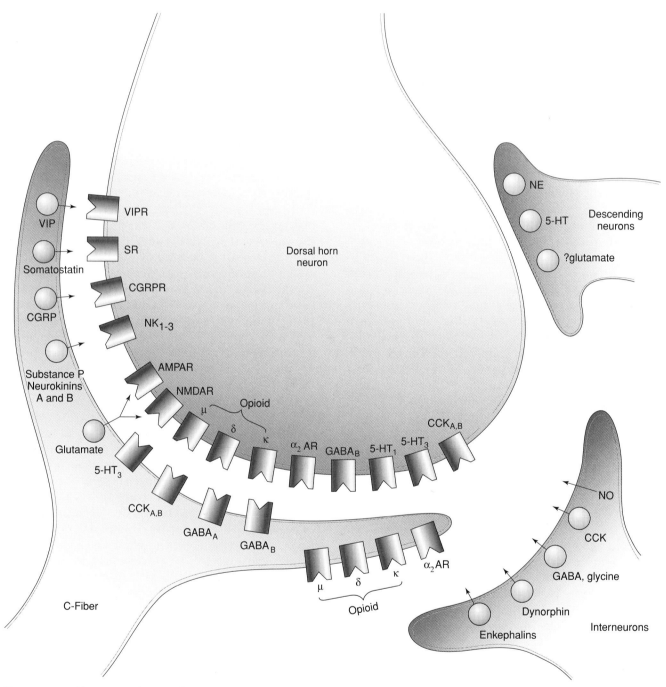

Figure 19–6. Neurotransmitters and receptors on synapses in the dorsal horn. Composite figures represent neurotransmitters and receptors expressed on a presynaptic terminal of a C fiber; a dendrite of a dorsal horn projection neuron; a presynaptic terminal of a neuron that descends from the locus ceruleus (if noradrenergic) or other brain stem sites, which may be serotonergic or glutamatergic; and a presynaptic terminal of an interneuron. SR, somatostatin receptors; α_2AR, α_2-adrenergic receptor.

tor-mediated, long-lasting increase in the excitability of dorsal horn neurons. Concerns about such plasticity have led to some changes in surgical practice. Based on animal experimentation, it is known that general anesthesia does not inhibit physiologic responses to periph-eral tissue injury in the dorsal horn, even though the subject is incapable of feeling pain. Consequently, some surgeons have begun the practice of injecting a **local anesthetic** into the skin of a patient before cutting the skin and its nerves, even when the patient is under general anesthesia. Local anesthetics, by blocking voltage-gated Na^+ channels (see Chapter 3), block the ability of nociceptors and their axons to send a barrage of action potentials to the dorsal horn. Thus it has been hypothesized that such preemptive analgesia may decrease the incidence of postoperative neuropathic pain.

MULTIPLE PATHWAYS TO THE BRAIN

Axons of projection neurons from the dorsal horn cross the midline and ascend into the anterolateral quadrant of the spinal cord (see Figure 19–1). However, a small but significant number of axons remain ipsilateral. These uncrossed axons may contribute to the return of pain after unilateral neurosurgical lesions of the anterolateral spinal cord have been made to alleviate intractable pain. Most of the nociceptive neurons that ascend into the anterolateral quadrant terminate in the reticular formation of the brain stem (spinoreticular tract) and in the thalamus (spinothalamic tract). The spinoreticular tract, which originates largely in laminae VII and VIII of the spinal cord, lacks precise topographical information in that the reticular neurons receive dorsal horn inputs that represent wide receptive fields. The reticular neurons send projections to many brain regions, among which is a prominent input to the thalamus (the reticulothalamic tract). Consistent with this wiring pattern is the theory that the spinoreticular tract contributes to general aspects of pain perception; for example, it may alert an individual to the onset of pain.

Neurons in the spinothalamic tract originate in laminae I and V–VII. A related projection extends from laminae I and V of the dorsal horn to the midbrain (spinomesencephalic tract). A major target of this spinomesencephalic tract is the periaqueductal gray matter (PAG) of the midbrain. Neurons of the PAG represent an important site of convergence between ascending axons that carry sensory information from the spinal cord and descending axons that arise from neurons in brain structures involved in the processing of emotion, such as the amygdala (see Chapter 15). Although the PAG receives nociceptive input from the spinal cord, it is not a pain relay nucleus because destruction of the PAG does not alter pain threshold. Rather, the PAG appears to play an important role in the brain's endogenous system of analgesia, which is described later in this chapter. Other nociceptive neurons project to the hypothalamus and amygdala, where they most likely mediate some of the autonomic, affective, and neuroendocrine responses to pain.

Neurons that project from the dorsal horn (or from the trigeminal nucleus) to the thalamus segregate into two divisions. In the *lateral division* of the spinothalamic tract, axons that relay information from the trunk and extremities terminate in the ventroposterolateral (VPL) nucleus of the thalamus, and axons that relay information from the trigeminal system terminate in the ventroposteromedial (VPM) nucleus of the thalamus. In the *medial division,* axons terminate mostly in the intralaminar nuclei of the thalamus.

Because the lateral division is phylogenetically recent it is often called the *neospinothalamic tract* (see Figure 19–1). It is somatotopically organized and is responsible for the localizing and discriminative aspects of pain. Consistent with this function, the dorsal horn neurons of laminae I and V, from which the neospinothalamic tract originates, have small receptive fields that permit accurate localization of nociceptive stimuli. The VPL and VPM nuclei of the thalamus receive inputs from all modalities of somatic sensation. Less than 10% of the neurons in these thalamic nuclei respond to nociceptive stimuli; the majority respond to touch and proprioceptive inputs from dorsal column neurons that reach the thalamus by way of the medial lemniscus. VPL and VPM neurons, including those that receive nociceptive inputs, project somatotopically to the primary somatic sensory cortex of the parietal lobe.

Because the medial division of the spinothalamic tract is phylogenetically old it is often called the *paleospinothalamic tract.* Unlike VPL and VPM neurons, whose projections are restricted to somatosensory cortex, intralaminar thalamic neurons have widespread cortical projections, which include major projections to association cortex such as prefrontal cortex. The paleospinothalamic tract, like the spinoreticular tract, lacks precise somatotopic organization. The dorsal horn neurons from which it originates, which are typically found in laminae that lie deeper in the spinal cord than those that give rise to the neospinothalamic tract, have large and complex receptive fields; indeed, the receptive fields of some of these cells comprise the entire body. Such large receptive fields are consistent not with the precise localization of pain but with more generalized responses. Thus it is believed that the paleospinothalamic tract, like spinoreticular, reticulothalamic, and spinohypothalamic projections, is involved in the affective and alerting aspects of pain.

How nociceptive information is understood as pain has yet to be determined. Before this mystery can be unraveled, more must be learned about the relationship among cerebral association cortices and the ventral striatum and amygdala (see Chapters 15 and 16), all of which receive input from the paleospinothalamic tract and subcortical circuits and process emotion. Similar gaps in knowledge of the neural circuitry that underlies complex behaviors have been evident in many other chapters of this book. Indeed, a major goal of neuroscientific research is to elucidate the neural circuits that are involved in complex functions of the brain.

ENDOGENOUS MECHANISMS OF ANALGESIA

ENDOGENOUS OPIOIDS AND RELATED PEPTIDES

Many neurotransmitters are involved in endogenous analgesic pathways, but the most important of these are a family of endogenous peptides with opiate-like activity. As explained in Chapter 10, the endogenous opioid peptides that are well-characterized are products of three large precursors—preproopiomelanocortin (POMC), preproenkephalin, and preprodynorphin—each of which is encoded by a separate gene. A fourth precursor, preproorphanin FQ–nociceptin, encodes the ligand for the orphanin FQ–nociceptin receptor (Figure 19–7). The ligand for this receptor originally was given two names—orphanin FQ and nociceptin—by the two groups that discovered it, and a single name has yet to be agreed upon. Despite significant homologies with opioid peptides, orphanin FQ–nociceptin lacks classic opiate-like activity, and may even promote nociception, as explained later in this chapter. Two additional putative opioid peptides, endomorphin 1 and 2, also have been described (see Figure 19–7). In vitro, these peptides bind to the μ opioid receptor with greater affinity and selectivity than that of any other endogenous peptide. However, their status as endogenous signaling

Met-enkephalin	Y G G F M
Leu-enkephalin	Y G G F L
Dynorphin A	Y G G F L R R I R P K L K W D N Q
α-Endorphin	Y G G F M T S E K S Q T P L V T
Orphanin FQ	F G G F T G A R K S A R K L A N Q
Endomorphin 1	Y P W F
Endomorphin 2	Y P F F

Figure 19–7. Amino acid sequences of selected endogenous opioid peptides and orphanin FQ–nociceptin. As described in Chapter 10, the major opioid products of proopiomelanocortin (endorphins), proenkephalin (enkephalins), and prodynorphin (dynorphins) contain a conserved Tyr-Gly-Gly-Phe (YGGF) motif followed by Met or Leu. The endomorphins, which may represent additional endogenous opioid peptides, but which are less well-established, share the N-terminal tyrosine residue but lack the rest of this conserved motif. Orphanin FQ (also known as nociceptin) is the only member of the family that lacks an N-terminal tyrosine. Based on current three-dimensional models, opiate alkaloids derived from the opium poppy, such as morphine, and their synthetic congeners mimic the structure of the N-terminal tyrosine that characterizes most opioid peptides.

peptides will remain uncertain until their precursor is identified.

Based on molecular cloning studies, three types of opioid receptors—μ, κ, and δ—have been recognized. Pharmacologic studies have suggested that subtypes of these receptors may exist (e.g., μ_1, μ_2, and κ_1–κ_3 receptors), but such subtypes have not been definitively confirmed by molecular cloning. Of unknown physiologic significance is the observation that μ, κ, and δ receptors can form heterodimers, which exhibit ligand binding and functional properties different from individual receptors. Should this type of phenomenon occur in vivo, it might explain some of the receptor subtypes identified pharmacologically. Other posttranscriptional modifications, for example, RNA splicing or the covalent modification of receptor proteins, also may contribute to the pharmacologic heterogeneity reported to be characteristic of opioid receptors. Such posttranscriptional modifications would be consistent with the observations that all known μ, δ, or κ receptor subtypes are lost in mice that lack the μ, δ, or κ receptor gene. β-Endorphin, a processing product of POMC, has high affinity for both the μ and δ receptors; met- and leu-enkephalin, processing products of proenkephalin, exhibit the highest affinity for the δ receptor but also can bind to μ and κ; and dynorphin and other products of the prodynorphin gene have the greatest affinity for the κ receptor but also can bind to μ and δ. In vivo, not only the affinity of various ligands for receptors but also the proximity of peptides to receptors determines which peptide stimulates which receptor.

Another receptor that was cloned based on its homology to the δ opioid receptor was originally described as an opioid-like orphan receptor until its ligand, orphanin FQ–nociceptin, was found. This receptor currently is known as the orphanin FQ–nociceptin (OFQN) receptor. Despite its homology to the δ opioid receptor, the OFQN receptor does not significantly bind opioid ligands, including the nonselective opioid antagonist naloxone. Accordingly, unlike the opioid receptors, the cellular effects of orphanin FQ–nociceptin are naloxone-insensitive.

All of the opioid receptors, as well as the OFQN receptor, are seven transmembrane domain receptors linked to heterotrimeric $G_{i/o}$ proteins. As mentioned in Chapter 5, $G_{i/o}$-coupled receptors inhibit the electrical firing of neurons through the opening of inwardly rectifying K^+ channels and the closing of voltage-gated Ca^{2+} channels. They also inhibit cAMP formation, and in turn may exert inhibitory or excitatory effects on neurons, depending on the types of channels they express. Opioids generally inhibit the firing of their target neurons.

DESCENDING ANALGESIC PATHWAYS

Because severe pain can disorganize behavior and in turn interfere with the ability to escape danger, mechanisms that suppress pain at times of extreme emergency have significant survival value. Some of the most striking examples of such phenomena have been observed during combat situations. According to a report during World War II, for example, two thirds of infantrymen who were severely wounded during a particular battle denied that they experienced pain and refused morphine. The stimuli that activate descending analgesic systems in such situations include acute stress and pain, but the threshold for activation appears to be high under most circumstances. If the threshold for the activation of these systems were not high, pain would lose its survival value.

One of the most dramatic laboratory demonstrations of the modification of afferent nociceptive information by descending pathways occurred during studies in which electrical stimulation of the PAG of rats was used to produce profound analgesia. The fact that **naloxone,** a nonselective opioid receptor antagonist, partially inhibits such stimulation-produced analgesia suggested that electrical stimulation of the PAG is effective because it releases endogenous substances that act on opioid receptors. Consistent with this theory is the observation that microinjection of morphine directly into the PAG also produces analgesia. Historically, these experiments were influential in the search for the endogenous opioid peptides previously described. Local stimulation and locally applied morphine also produce effective analgesia at sites in the rostral ventral medulla, a region of the brain that includes the nucleus raphe magnus, the nucleus gigantocellularis, and the adjacent reticular formation. Stimulation-produced analgesia also has been demonstrated in humans.

In sharp contrast to local anesthetics, which produce numbness, both stimulation-produced analgesia and morphine are modality-specific with regard to somatic sensation; that is, they suppress only nociception, and do not affect touch, proprioception, and the sensation of temperature. This specificity can be confirmed electrophysiologically: nociceptive neurons in lamina V of the dorsal horn are inhibited by stimulation-produced analgesia or opiates, but nonnociceptive neurons in lamina III are unaffected by either type of analgesia.

The best-characterized descending analgesic pathway involves a projection from the PAG to the rostral ventral medulla, which in turn projects to the dorsal horn by means of the dorsolateral funiculus of the spinal cord. The cutting of fibers that descend in the dorsolateral funiculus blocks analgesia produced by electrical stimulation of the PAG. High levels of endogenous opioid peptides and opioid receptors are found within the PAG, rostral ventral medulla, and dorsal horn, and neurons of both the PAG and rostral ventral medulla can be activated by opioids. Because opioid receptors generally produce inhibitory effects on neuronal firing, the ability of endogenous opioid peptides or opiate drugs to activate neurons within the PAG, rostral ventral medulla, and other brain regions is dependent on an anatomic arrangement whereby opioid receptors inhibit GABAergic (inhibitory) interneurons in these brain regions. Activation of PAG neurons by descending projections—for example, from the amygdala—activates neurons in the rostral ventral medulla. Neurons of the rostral ventral medulla that project to the dorsal horn activate enkephalinergic interneurons that are located in the dorsal horn. The neurotransmitter involved in opioid-mediated descending analgesia was long believed to be serotonin from the nucleus raphe magnus (see Chapter 9). Indeed, serotonergic neurons do project to the dorsal horn but do not appear to be directly involved in opioid responses. Rather, they appear to play a more complex modulatory role. This theory is consistent with the clinical observation that selective serotonin reuptake inhibitors (SSRIs), such as **fluoxetine,** lack analgesic properties.

Within the rostral ventral medulla three physiologic classes of cells project to the dorsal horn. "On" cells are excited by noxious stimuli and inhibited by opioids; "off" cells are inhibited by noxious stimuli and excited by opioids; and neutral cells do not respond to noxious stimuli or opioids. The "off" cells are involved in the classic descending analgesic circuit, and glutamate may be the critical neurotransmitter that conveys descending analgesic information to the dorsal horn. Serotonin is found in neutral cells. Orphanin FQ–nociceptin appears to inhibit opiate-activated descending analgesic outflow from the rostral ventral medulla, and may be responsible for similar activity in the PAG.

Within the dorsal horn, enkephalin-containing interneurons appear to inhibit dorsal horn neurons at the origin of the spinothalamic tract by making direct postsynaptic contact with them. Indirect evidence suggests that presynaptic inhibition of primary nociceptive neurons by opioid-containing interneurons also occurs, but anatomic evidence for this arrangement is lacking. Presynaptic inhibition also may be accomplished by an opioid peptide other than enkephalin—for example, by dynorphin—or may result from paracrine-like nonsynaptic actions of enkephalin released from distant nerve terminals, in accordance with the mismatch theory mentioned earlier in this chapter.

ANALGESIC MEDICATIONS

OPIATES

Several classes of opiate drugs are important analgesics (Figure 19–8). Opiates often are called narcotics because of their potent sedative effects. However, the term *narcotic* also has a legal definition in the United States, which is used for regulation purposes by the Food and Drug Administration and the Drug Enforcement Agency. For legal purposes the term *narcotics* is applied to both opiate and nonopiate drugs with substantial abuse liability. The production, distribution, and prescription of these drugs is closely monitored and regulated. Some of these drugs, such as heroin, have no legally acceptable use outside of research in the United States.

Morphine-like opiates comprise the most important class of compounds used in the treatment of severe acute pain and severe cancer pain. These drugs bind preferentially to the μ opioid receptor, which appears to be the most significant opioid receptor involved in both supraspinal and spinal analgesia. The μ Receptors are located in areas known to be involved in descending analgesia, including the PAG, rostral ventral medulla,

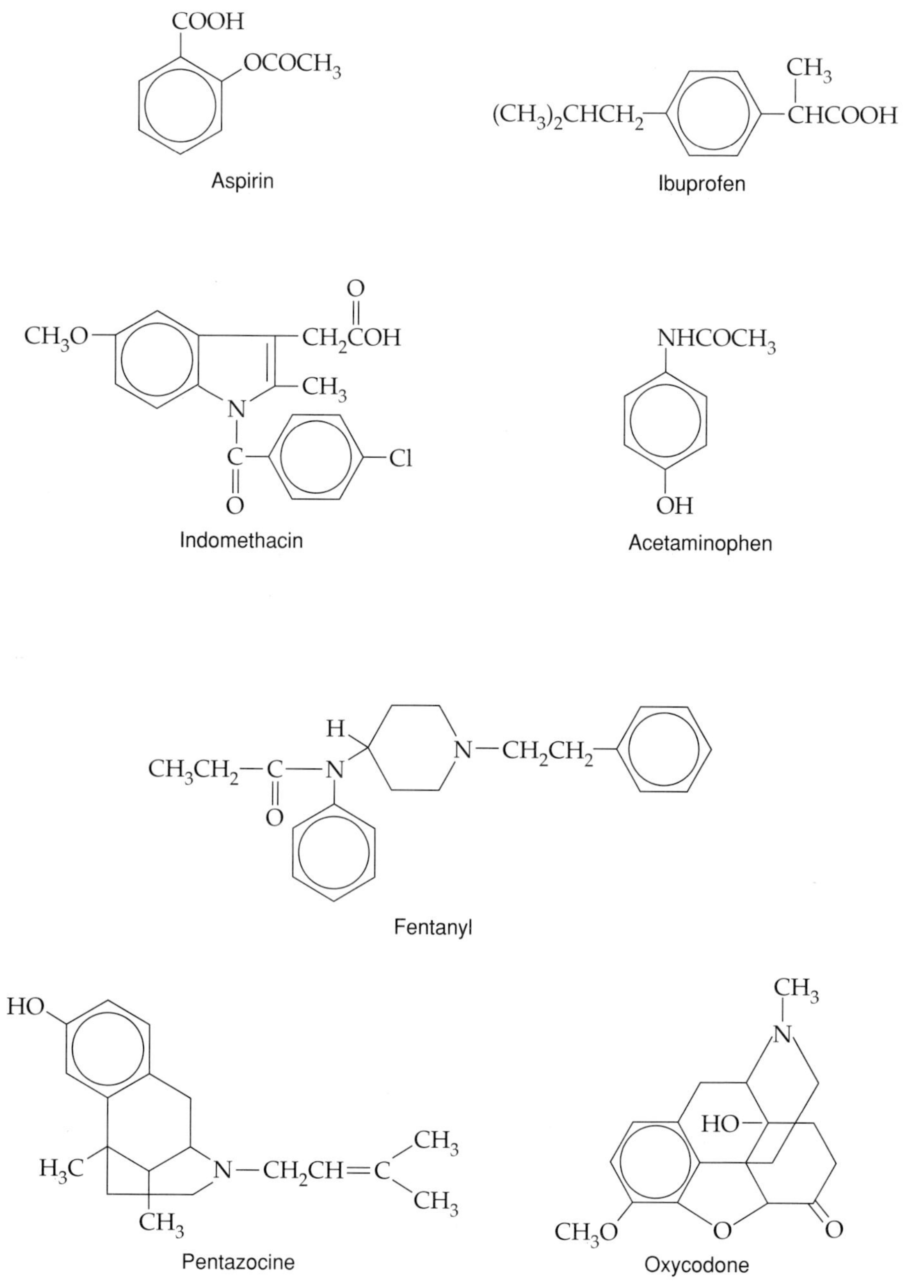

Figure 19–8. Chemical structures of representative analgesics. (See Chapter 16 for the structure of morphine.)

and dorsal horn of the spinal cord. They also are found in regions such as the ventral tegmental area (VTA) of the midbrain and the ventral striatum, where they are responsible for the reinforcing effects of opiates, and in the locus ceruleus, which mediates many somatic aspects of physical dependence on opiates (see Chapter 16).

The usefulness of morphine-like drugs is limited by their side effects, such as constipation and respiratory depression, and the risks associated with their use, including dependence and addiction. A side effect of morphine-like opiates is prominent miosis, or pupillary constriction, a clinical sign that is used to diagnose cases of opiate overdose. Repeated use of these drugs also results in tolerance to their analgesic effects. Considerable progress has been made in understanding the molecular adaptations that contribute to tolerance at the cellular level (see Chapter 16), but which of these adaptations is responsible for analgesic tolerance at the behavioral level remains unknown.

A very large number of morphine-like opiates are available clinically (Table 19–2). These drugs differ primarily in terms of their pharmacokinetic properties, particularly with regard to their suitability for oral administration, and their relative affinity for the μ receptor. **Codeine** and **oxycodone** are examples of low-potency μ agonists; both are effective when administered orally and are commonly combined with **aspirin** or **acetaminophen** (e.g., **Percocet**). **Dilaudid** and **fentanyl** are examples of very-high-potency μ agonists; the former is suitable for oral administration, whereas the latter is suitable for parenteral or transdermal administration. As previously discussed, the use of each of these μ agonists is associated with tolerance and physical dependence and the risk for addiction. The use of partial agonists at the μ receptor, such as **buprenorphine,** may be associated with fewer liabilities; it is believed that such agents sufficiently activate the receptor to induce some analgesia but are not strong enough to in-

duce the molecular adaptations that underlie tolerance and dependence. Partial agonists also may carry a lower risk for abuse because higher doses of the drug do not lead to greater behavioral effects. Many patients have benefited from the use of such partial agonists.

Benzomorphan opiate drugs, such as **pentazocine,** exhibit a high affinity for κ opioid receptors (see Table 19–2). Like many opiates, κ receptor agonists produce sedation and miosis. Although, in contrast to μ agonists (see Chapter 16), they are often aversive, resulting in negative emotional effects, they can be abused and can produce addictive behaviors. κ Receptors are found in the dorsal horn of the spinal cord, in deep cortical layers, and in many other brain regions. Many κ agonist drugs possess properties of μ receptor antagonists and may precipitate withdrawal symptoms in individuals who are dependent on morphine-like drugs. Despite their aversive properties, κ agonists frequently are used instead of μ agonists for obstetric analgesia, to reduce the risk of respiratory depression in the newborn.

Considerable effort has been aimed at the development of small-molecule δ agonists during the past two decades; however, only peptides, which lack substantial clinical utility, remain available ligands with a high affinity for the δ opioid receptor. δ Receptors are concentrated not only in the limbic system and in the dorsal horn of the spinal cord but also in regions of the brain that have no clear association with pain. Like κ opioid receptors, δ receptors appear to mediate analgesia at the level of the dorsal horn. These receptors also mediate hypotension and miosis.

Opiate antagonists also have clinical utility. **Naloxone,** a nonselective antagonist with a relative affinity of μ > δ > κ, is used to treat heroin and other opiate overdoses. Such treatment often is life saving, because opiate overdose can be fatal when it results in severe respiratory depression. A longer-acting nonselective antagonist, **naltrexone,** is used in some rapid withdrawal protocols for dependent heroin addicts. Because opiate antagonists precipitate a severe withdrawal syndrome in dependent individuals, they typically are used with drugs that inhibit somatic withdrawal symptoms, such as **clonidine,** an α₂-adrenergic receptor agonist (see Chapter 16). Naltrexone is also used to help prevent relapse in detoxified individuals who have been addicted to opiates or alcohol. The chemical structures of these opioid antagonists can be found in Chapter 16.

Opiates such as morphine also may be effective analgesics when administered directly into an inflamed area of the body, such as a joint. This effect can be blocked by concomitant administration of naloxone. However, local application of morphine cannot be used effectively to produce systemic (spinal or supraspinal) analgesia. It is believed that opioid receptors in in-

Table 19–2 Classification of Representative Opiate Drugs

μ Receptor Agonists

Codeine	Diacylmorphine (heroin)
Fentanyl	Hydrocodone
Hydromorphone	Levorphanol
Meperidine	Methadone
Morphine	Oxycodone

Partial μ Receptor Agonist

Buprenorphine

κ Receptor Agonists and μ Receptor Antagonists

Butorphanol	Dezocine
Nalbuphine	Pentazocine

flamed tissue are expressed or up-regulated on peripheral nerve endings. Invading immune cells may be a source of endogenous opioids under such circumstances; indeed, the release of opioid peptides from immune cells in response to cytokines has been observed. Although the peripheral administration of opioids appears promising, therapeutic applications remain experimental.

A variety of drugs have been used as adjuncts to opiate therapy to minimize the use of opiates or to increase the efficacy of lower doses of opiates. However, the effectiveness of most of these drugs is not well established, with the exception of D-amphetamine (see Chapter 16), which has been shown to effectively decrease opiate doses and thus unwanted sedation in patients with severe cancer pain. **Tricyclic antidepressants** (see Chapter 15) and **anticonvulsants,** including **carbamazepine, phenytoin, valproic acid,** and **clonazepam** (see Chapter 21), can be used in conjunction with opiates or, in the treatment of neuropathic pain, as alternatives to opiates. Other drugs used as adjuvants include **antihistamines,** for example, H_1 antagonists such as **hydroxyzine;** the α_2-adrenergic agonist **clonidine; benzodiazepines; antipsychotic** drugs; **local anesthetics;** and the $GABA_B$ agonist **baclofen.**

NONSTEROIDAL ANTIINFLAMMATORY DRUGS

NSAIDs, including **ibuprofen, aspirin, indomethacin,** and many related compounds, have analgesic actions as well as antiinflammatory and antipyretic effects (see Figure 19–8). In contrast, **acetaminophen,** the active ingredient in **Tylenol,** is an effective analgesic and antipyretic that is not associated with significant antiinflammatory activity. Interestingly, **glucocorticoids,** which are perhaps the most potent antiinflammatory agents known, are neither analgesic nor antipyretic. As previously mentioned, NSAIDs produce analgesia primarily by decreasing sensitization. They do so by inhibiting the enzyme cyclooxygenase, the first enzyme in the pathway that catalyzes the generation of prostaglandins, leukotrienes, and other eicosanoids from arachidonic acid (Figure 19–9; see Chapter 5). NSAIDs also have been reported to act directly in the spinal cord, where they block hyperalgesia induced by the stimulation of glutamate and substance P receptors. The mechanism responsible for this action is not yet known. Although NSAIDs can be very effective in treating low-intensity pain, and indeed are commonly used for this purpose, they have little effect on acute, high-intensity pain.

As discussed in Chapter 13, there are two major isoforms of cyclooxygenase: COX1 and COX2. NSAIDs are nonselective inhibitors of both isoforms. COX2 appears to be the more important target for the antiinflammatory and analgesic effects of these drugs, because COX2 is induced in tissues in the context of inflammation and pain. One of the major side effects of NSAIDs is ulceration of the gastric and duodenal mucosa, which is caused by inhibition of COX1 and loss of the protective effects of prostaglandins on the epithelium of the gut. This side effect led to the introduction of selective COX2 inhibitors, potent antiinflammatory and analgesic medications that lack the deleterious effects on the gut associated with older agents. **Rofecoxib** and **celecoxib** are examples of selective COX2 inhibitors that are used clinically. Unlike aspirin and other nonselective NSAIDs, COX2 inhibitors do not impair platelet aggregation and thus cannot be used prophylactically to protect against **myocardial infarction** or **stroke** (see Chapter 21).

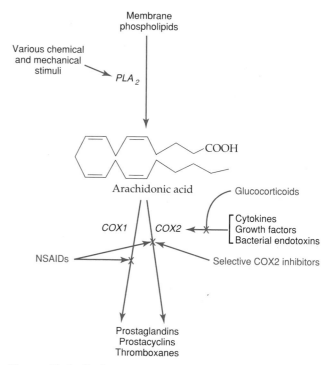

Figure 19–9. Cyclooxygenase pathways. Cyclooxygenase 1 (COX1) is constitutively expressed; cyclooxygenase 2 (COX2) is induced at the site of inflammation by cytokines, growth factors, and other endogenous mediators, as well as by exogenous substances such as bacterial endotoxins. The induction of COX2 protein can be blocked by glucocorticoids, powerful antiinflammatory agents that act by a variety of mechanisms. Aspirin and other nonselective NSAIDs block the enzymatic activity of both isoforms of cyclooxygenase; however, because they inhibit COX1 activity in the gut, their use is accompanied by a risk of peptic ulcer. Because COX2 is induced at sites of inflammation, selective COX2 inhibitors are effective antiinflammatory agents that have fewer side effects than nonselective inhibitors. PLA_2, phospholipase A_2.

NONOPIOID, NON-NSAID ANALGESICS

The limitations of opiates and NSAIDs have spurred intense interest in the development of analgesics with novel mechanisms of action. Many of the chemical mediators outlined earlier in this chapter represent potential targets for new drugs, although some, including bradykinin and substance P antagonists, have proven disappointing to date.

Among the drugs that remain promising are nicotinic cholinergic receptor (nAChR) agonists. The antinociceptive activity of **nicotine,** the defining nAChR agonist, has long been recognized (see Chapter 9). **Epibatidine,** an nAChR agonist isolated from the skin of Ecuadorian frogs, is a more potent analgesic than nicotine. However, epibatidine acts nonselectively; it stimulates not only neuronal nAChRs, but also nAChRs found at autonomic ganglia and at the neuromuscular junction (see Chapter 12). Thus the analgesic effects of epibatidine are accompanied by muscular paralysis, seizures, and hypertension. During the 1990s, agonists selective for nAChRs expressed in the CNS have been synthesized. **ABT-594** is one such compound. It has a high affinity and reasonable selectivity for nAChRs composed of $\alpha_4\beta_2$ subunits, which together with α_7 homo-oligomers, are the predominant nAChRs in the CNS of rodents and perhaps of humans. Knockout mice lacking the gene that encodes either the α_4 or β_2 subunit of the nAChR display reduced antinociceptive responses to nicotine. In initial tests, ABT-594 and morphine had equivalent analgesic properties in three pain models: acute pain, in which a thermal model was used; persistent pain; and neuropathic pain. Moreover, ABT-594 reportedly does not produce tolerance or dependence after repeated administration.

In preliminary experiments, lesions of serotonergic neurons in the nucleus raphe magnus have blocked the analgesic actions of nicotinic drugs. These and related studies raise the interesting possibility that nAChR agonists exert their analgesic effects at a supraspinal level by means of serotonergic or other projections of the rostral ventral medulla. However, because transmitters other than serotonin may be critical in conveying information related to descending analgesia from the rostral ventral medulla to the dorsal horn, additional investigations will be needed to determine the mechanism by which nicotinic receptors produce analgesia.

Descending noradrenergic projections from the locus ceruleus or from related noradrenergic nuclei in the dorsal pons inhibit dorsal horn neurons, and thereby contribute to descending analgesia. The role of norepinephrine in descending analgesia may explain the analgesic effects of **tricyclic antidepressants,** including those of selective norepinephrine reuptake inhibitors such as **desipramine** (see Chapter 15), which often are effective in the treatment of neuropathic pain. Although many individuals with chronic neuropathic pain experience depression, the analgesic effects of these agents are clearly independent of their antidepressant effects, because the analgesic effects occur at lower doses and after shorter periods of treatment. In contrast to tricyclic antidepressants, SSRIs appear to lack analgesic properties. Norepinephrine exerts its antinociceptive effects by means of α_2-adrenergic receptors on dorsal horn neurons. Consequently, α_2-adrenergic receptor agonists such as **clonidine** may be effective in potentiating the analgesic effects of opiates.

Cannabinoids, the active ingredients in **marijuana,** also have analgesic properties. As discussed in Chapters 16 and 17, there are two known subtypes of cannabinoid receptors: CB_1, which is expressed in the brain, and CB_2, which is found only in peripheral tissues. CB_1 appears to be the more important receptor for mediating the analgesic effects of cannabinoids. Knockout mice lacking CB_1 receptors have diminished responses on several tests of nociception. Based on preliminary experiments, CB_1 receptor-mediated antinociception requires an intact descending analgesic pathway in the rostral ventral medulla but appears to be independent of opioid activity. The potential role of the CB_2 receptor in analgesia is less clear. Because CB_2 receptors are found on certain activated inflammatory cells, it has been hypothesized that these receptors might be useful targets of drugs designed to decrease inflammation, but such hypotheses have yet to be confirmed.

Although there has been considerable interest in the use of cannabinoids as analgesic medications, the clinical use of these agents has been limited because of concerns about their potential for abuse. However, it has been speculated that non-cannabinoid agonists of the CB_1 receptor, given the right pharmacokinetic properties and delivery system, might offer effective analgesia without an accompanying tendency to produce addiction.

CLINICAL PAIN SYNDROMES

Mild to moderate acute pain is generally treated with NSAIDs, and severe acute pain, such as that which occurs after trauma or surgery, is usually treated with opiates. A short course of opiates, when used to treat acute pain, is not associated with an addiction risk. The risk for addiction in the context of chronic pain remains a matter of considerable debate. Indeed, concerns about tolerance, physical dependence, and addiction make the use of opiates in the treatment of serious chronic pain syndromes a difficult clinical decision. Such concerns are not relevant for terminally ill patients. However, despite widely distributed treatment guidelines, inappropriate fears related to addiction have led to a generalized underuse of opiates in the treatment of cancer pain and other types of severe pain experienced toward the end of life.

A detailed discussion of pain syndromes is beyond the scope of this book. The sections that follow address the topics of neuropathic pain and pain associated with migraines because of the large amount of available information concerning their pathophysiology and treatment, respectively.

NEUROPATHIC PAIN

Damage to neurons in nociceptive pathways generally causes some loss of normal pain sensation. However, after a delay, such damage can result in severe neuropathic pain. Neuropathic pain can be produced by several disease processes that injure neurons or lead to cell death, such as painful **neuropathies;** viral infections, including **HIV** or **postherpetic** neuralgia; and **cancer.** Painful **diabetic neuropathy** is associated with retrograde loss of A_δ and C fibers. Postherpetic neuralgia, or **shingles,** is caused by the reactivation of a latent varicella-zoster virus, or chicken pox virus. This type of virus can remain dormant in primary sensory neurons for decades and become reactivated by unknown mechanisms. Shingles generally affects a single spinal nerve or cranial nerve branch and thus affects a single dermatome. Because of damage to the nerve, persistent and sometimes severe neuropathic pain may result. Neuropathic pain also may be caused by amputation (phantom limb pain); spinal cord injury; nerve avulsion; nerve compression, for example, from spinal disk disease; and stroke, such as thalamic pain from a lesion in the ventroposterolateral nucleus. Neuropathic pain also may be idiopathic; for example, trigeminal neuralgia (also called tic douloureux) produces severe lancinating pain in a trigeminal nerve distribution. This disorder, the cause of which is not known, is often treated with the anticonvulsant **carbamazepine** or with a **tricyclic antidepressant.** Carbamazepine's mechanism of action in the treatment of this disorder is unclear.

Patients with neuropathic pain may experience spontaneous pain, such as persistent burning; dysesthesias, such as pins and needles, numbness, or tingling; or unprovoked paroxysms of lancinating pain that subjectively appear to be from the deafferented region. In addition, such patients experience a marked decrease in pain threshold so that previously innocuous stimuli are painful (allodynia), or responses to noxious stimuli are exaggerated (hyperalgesia). Neuropathic pain is believed to be initiated and maintained by abnormal barrages of high-intensity action potentials from injured nervous tissue. Such barrages likely cause plastic changes

in the dorsal horn and in higher centers, which in turn may lead to the recurrence of pain even after surgical interruption of the damaged nerves or central structures. Indeed, because they produce deafferentation, surgical lesions placed to relieve pain may themselves result in delayed-onset neuropathic pain.

A new term that is being proposed for some types of neuropathic pain is *complex regional pain syndromes.* These pain syndromes are characterized by complex symptoms that generally extend beyond pain itself. Complex regional pain syndrome type 1, traditionally called *reflex sympathetic dystrophy,* generally occurs after a soft tissue injury without an identifiable nerve injury. In complex regional pain syndrome type 2, traditionally called *causalgia,* a definable nerve injury is present. The role of the sympathetic nervous system in reflex sympathetic dystrophy is variable. Following a tissue injury, the pain of reflex sympathetic dystrophy is more severe than would be expected and spreads to affect a larger region than expected. The pain has an intense burning quality, is associated with extreme local tenderness, and may be accompanied by signs of excess sympathetic nervous system activity such as increased sweating and vasoconstriction. When this syndrome involves a limb, the limb is often held so still that secondary complications, such as edema, muscle atrophy, or osteoporosis, develop. One mechanism hypothesized for this syndrome is ephaptic transmission (cross-talk between axons in the absence of synapses) that occurs between axons of primary afferent nociceptive neurons and those of efferent sympathetic neurons. When sympathetic signs are present, treatment of pain syndromes often involves regional sympathetic blocks achieved with the injection of **local anesthetics** (see Chapter 3) or α_1 antagonists such as **prazosin** or **phenoxybenzamine** (see Chapter 12). In one clinical trial in which dystonia was present in patients with reflex sympathetic dystrophy, intrathecal administration of the $GABA_B$ receptor agonist baclofen relieved this complication. Satisfactory treatment of neuropathic pain is one of the greatest unmet clinical needs. Opiates can partially alleviate neuropathic pain, but as previously discussed, their long-term use poses the risk of addiction. NSAIDs and tricyclic antidepressants also have not proven to be adequately effective in the treatment of neuropathic pain. Consequently, patients with neuropathic pain syndromes often remain in pain, and therefore experience considerable social and occupational disability.

MIGRAINE

Migraine is a paroxysmal syndrome characterized by headache and a variety of other symptoms. The headache is classically described as severe, throbbing, and unilateral, and often is accompanied by nausea, vomiting, photophobia, and malaise. Such symptoms often are preceded by an aura, such as visual scotomata or flashing lights. However, the clinical presentation of migraine is highly variable and may not include several of these attributes.

The causes of migraine remain controversial. It was long believed that cerebral vasoconstriction produced the aura associated with the disorder and that subsequent vasodilation produced the headache and related symptoms. Blood flow changes have been documented in human subjects with migraine, but these have been relatively small in magnitude and generally have been difficult to correlate with symptoms of migraine. According to an alternative hypothesis, migraine may result from a spreading depression of cortical electrical activity. In animal models, noxious stimuli have produced depressed cortical electrical activity that is initially focal and that subsequently spreads across the involved hemisphere; such activity may be followed by reduced cerebral blood flow. However, convincing evidence that these events occur in humans with migraine has yet to be obtained.

Considerable attention has been given to possible environmental causes of migraines. Some affected individuals appear to experience migraine in response to specific foods. Common precipitants are chocolate, peanuts, and red wines. However, most patients cannot identify specific factors that precipitate their migraines. Stress and fatigue are sometimes considered causative factors, but these states can be subjective in nature and thus are too vague to offer any useful insight. Indeed, stress and fatigue exacerbate most neuropsychiatric syndromes.

For mild to moderate migraine, treatment consists of a mild analgesic, such as aspirin, acetaminophen, or an NSAID, sometimes used in conjunction with an antiemetic. Ergot alkaloids, such as **ergotamine** or **dihydroergotamine**, also are commonly used. Ergot alkaloids have complex pharmacologic properties and act as agonists or antagonists of 5-HT$_1$ and 5-HT$_2$ receptors, dopamine receptors, and adrenergic receptors, in addition to their other effects (see Chapter 12). Mixtures of **butalbital** (a barbiturate derivative), **caffeine,** and **aspirin** or **acetaminophen**—for example, **Fiorinal** and **Fioricet,** which are often combined with **codeine**—are longtime standard therapies for migraine and continue to be widely prescribed. The effectiveness of these mixtures has yet to be explained.

A major breakthrough in the treatment of more severe migraines came with the introduction of triptan drugs. These agents act as agonists at 5-HT$_{1B/D}$ receptors. As explained in Chapter 9, these receptors function as inhibitory autoreceptors on presynaptic serotonergic nerve terminals; the 5-HT$_{1B}$ receptor is expressed in

Figure 19–10. Chemical structure of sumatriptan.

rodents, and the 5-HT$_{1D}$ receptor is expressed in humans. The mechanisms by which activation of these receptors alleviates the symptoms of migraine remain obscure. **Sumatriptan** was the first agent of this class to be introduced clinically (Figure 19–10). It was effective only by parenteral administration, and its use was complicated by a risk of cardiac side effects in some patients. More recently, alternative formulations of sumatriptan and several other orally effective triptan derivatives have become available; examples include **zolmitriptan, naratriptan, rizatriptan,** and **eletriptan.**

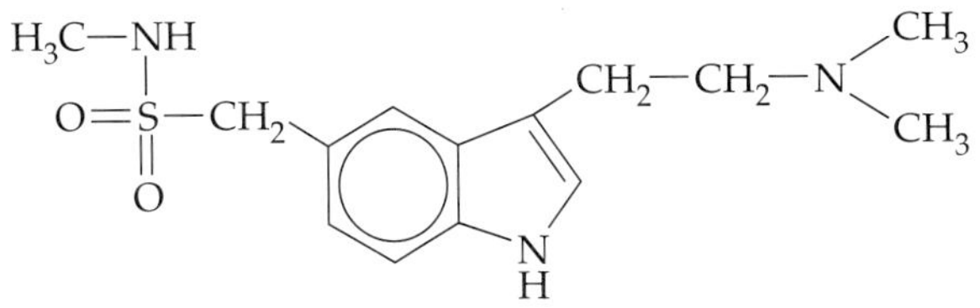

Migraine is a chronic illness; thus long-term prophylaxis may be indicated for patients who experience frequent or particularly severe recurrences. However, medications currently available for prophylaxis are ineffective for many patients. **Amitriptyline** and other **tricyclic antidepressants,** the β-adrenergic antagonist **propranolol,** and L-type Ca^{2+} channel blockers, such as **verapamil,** have been used with moderate success. The anticonvulsant **valproate** is a newer candidate for migraine prophylaxis, although its mechanism for migraine prevention remains unknown (see Chapter 21). **Magnesium** is also being tested for possible use in the prevention of migraine. It is a general inhibitor of neuronal excitability that works by stabilizing cell membranes. Such attributes are believed to explain its usefulness in the treatment of **eclampsia,** or **toxemia,** a life-threatening condition of heightened neuronal excitability that occurs during childbirth. Further investigation is needed to determine magnesium's efficacy in migraine prophylaxis.

SELECTED READING

Akil H, Mayer DJ, Liebeskind JC. 1976. Antagonism of stimulation-produced analgesia by naloxone, a narcotic antagonist. *Science* 191:961–962.

Bannon AW, Decker MW, Holladay MW, et al. 1998. Broad-spectrum, non-opioid analgesic activity by selective modulation of neuronal nicotinic acetylcholine receptors. *Science* 279:77–81.

Basbaum AI. 1999. Distinct neurochemical features of acute and persistent pain. *Proc Natl Acad Sci USA* 96:7739–7743.

Basbaum AI, Woolf CJ. 1999. Pain. *Curr Biol* 9:R429–R431.

Beecher HK. 1946. Pain in men wounded in battle. *Ann Surg* 123:96.

Bley KR, Hunter JC, Eglen RM, Smith JAM. 1998. The role of IP prostanoid receptors in inflammatory pain. *Trends Pharmacol Sci* 19:141–147.

Calixto JB, Cabrini DA, Ferreira J, Campos MM. 2000. Kinins in pain and inflammation. *Pain* 87:1–5.

Cao YQ, Mantyh PW, Carlson EJ, et al. 1998. Primary afferent tachykinins are required to experience moderate to intense pain. *Nature* 392:390–397.

Caterina MJ, Leffler A, Malmberg AB, et al. 2000. Impaired nociception and pain sensation in mice lacking the capsaicin receptor. *Science* 288:306–313.

Caterina MJ, Rosen TA, Tominaga M, et al. 1999. A capsaicin-receptor homologue with a high threshold for noxious heat. *Nature* 398:436–441.

Caterina MJ, Schumacher MA, Tominaga M, et al. 1997. The capsaicin receptor: A heat-activated ion channel in the pain pathway. *Nature* 389:816–824.

Civelli O, Nothacker HP, Reinscheid R. 1998. Reverse physiology: Discovery of the novel neuropeptide orphanin FQ–nociceptin. *Crit Rev Neurobiol* 12:163–176.

Darland T, Heinricher MM, Grandy DK. 1998. Orphanin FQ–nociceptin: A role in pain and analgesia, but so much more. *Trends Neurosci* 21:215–221.

Davis JB, Gray J, Gunthorpe MJ, et al. 2000. Vanilloid receptor-1 is essential for inflammatory thermal hyperalgesia. *Nature* 405:183–187.

Deleu D, Hanssens Y. 2000. Current and emerging second-generation triptans in acute migraine therapy: a comparative review. *J Clin Pharmacol* 40:687–700.

Ding Y, Cesare P, Drew L, et al. 2000. ATP, P2X receptors and pain pathways. *J Autonomic Nerv Sys* 81:289–294.

Gao K, Chen DO, Genzen JR, Mason P. 1999. Activation of serotonergic neurons in the raphe magnus is not necessary for morphine analgesia. *J Neurosci* 18:1860–1868.

Gillespie CS, Sherman DL, Fleetwood-Walker SM, et al. 2000. Peripheral demyelination and neuropathic pain behavior in periaxin-deficient mice. *Neuron* 26:523–531.

Gomes I, Jordan BA, Gupta A, et al. 2000. Heterodimerization of μ and δ opioid receptors: a role in opiate synergy. *J Neurosci* 20:RC110(1–5).

Hughes J, Smith TW, Kosterlitz HW, et al. 1975. Identification of two related pentapeptides from the brain with potent opiate agonist activity. *Nature* 258:577–580.

Mantyh PW, Allen CJ, Ghilardi JR, et al. 1995. Receptor endocytosis and dendrite reshaping in spinal neurons after somatosensory stimulation. *Science* 268:1629–1632.

Marubio LM, Arroyo-Jimenez M, Codero-Erausquin M, et al. 1999. Reduced antinociception in mice lacking neuronal nicotinic receptor subunits. *Nature* 398:805–810.

McClesky EW, Gol MS. 1999. Ion channels of nociception. *Annu Rev Physiol* 61:835–856.

Meng ID, Manning BH, Martin WJ, Fields HL. 1998. An analgesia circuit activated by cannabinoids. *Nature* 395:381–383.

Mezey E, Toth ZE, Cortright DN, et al. 2000. Distribution of mRNA for vanilloid receptor subtype 1 (VR1), and VR1-like immunoreactivity, in the central nervous system of the rat and human. *Proc Natl Acad Sci USA* 97:3655–3666.

Mitchell JM, Lowe D, Fields HL. 1998. The contribution of the ventromedial medulla to the antinociceptive effects of morphine in restrained and unrestrained rats. *Neuroscience* 87:123–133.

Mogil JS, Yu L, Basbaum AI. 2000. Pain genes? Natural variation and transgenic mutants. *Annu Rev Neurosci* 23:777–811.

Snider WD, McMahon SB. 1998. Tackling pain at the source: New ideas about nociceptors. *Neuron* 20:629–632.

Stein C. 1995. The control of pain in peripheral tissue by opioids. *N Engl J Med* 332:1685–1690.

Wall PD, Melzack RE. 1994. *Textbook of Pain*. Edinburgh: Churchill Livingston.

Woolf CJ, Doubell TP. 1994. The pathophysiology of chronic pain: Increased sensitivity to low threshold Aβ fiber inputs. *Curr Opin Neurobiol* 4:525–534.

Woolf CJ, Safieh-Garabedian B, Ma QP, et al. 1994. Nerve growth factor contributes to the generation of inflammatory sensory hypersensitivity. *Neuroscience* 62:327–331.

Yaksh TL. 1999. Spinal systems and pain processing: Development of novel analgesic drugs with mechanistically defined models. *Trends Pharmacol Sci* 20:329–336.

Zimmer A, Zimmer AM, Baffi J, et al. 1998. Hypoalgesia in mice with a targeted deletion of the tachykinin 1 gene. *Proc Natl Acad Sci* 95:2630–2635.

Chapter 20
Memory and Dementias

KEY CONCEPTS

- Declarative memory, which is the memory of facts and events, and nondeclarative memory—which includes all other forms of memory, such as procedural memory and habits—are the two broad categories of memory.

- Structures in the medial temporal lobe, such as the hippocampus, are particularly important for the temporary storage of declarative memories.

- Long-lasting changes in synaptic efficacy (synaptic plasticity) are thought to be important mechanisms for storing memories.

- The most extensively studied form of synaptic plasticity is long-term potentiation (LTP) in the hippocampus, which is triggered by strong activation of NMDA receptors and the consequent large rise in postsynaptic calcium concentration.

- Long-term memory storage requires gene transcription and new protein synthesis as does a long-lasting form of LTP.

- Long-term depression, a long-lasting decrease in synaptic strength, also occurs at most excitatory

synapses and may contribute to the formation of memories.

- Strong emotions enhance memory formation, likely because of the associated activation of monoaminergic and cholinergic neurotransmitter systems.

- The pathologic hallmarks of Alzheimer disease, the most common cause of severe memory impairment in the elderly, are senile plaques, neurofibrillary tangles, dystrophic neurites, and neuronal loss.

- The development of Alzheimer disease may be due to the improper biochemical processing of amyloid precursor protein (APP) and the subsequent accumulation of β amyloid.

- Inherited forms of Alzheimer disease have been linked to mutations in APP or in proteins called presenilins, which alter the processing of APP.

- Currently there is no effective treatment for Alzheimer disease, although a number of pharmacologic strategies for preventing the buildup of β amyloid appear promising.

*Right now I'm wondering, have I done or said anything
amiss? You see, at this moment everything looks clear to me,
but what happened just before? That's what worries me.
It's like waking from a dream. I just don't remember.*

*Amnesiac H.M., who lost the ability to consolidate
events into conscious memory after undergoing
neurosurgery to correct epilepsy.*

Our ability to learn and remember is such an integral
part of our lives that it is difficult to imagine functioning with any significant memory impairment. Memory
permeates existence, from the mundane (Where did I
park the car? Where did I put my keys?) to the profound (Who am I? What are my beliefs? Where did I
learn them?). It is only a slight exaggeration to say that
our memories are *who we are*. Although each of us was
born with intrinsic tendencies, including inherent apti-
tudes and personality traits, the manner in which the
environment has shaped our flexible neuronal connections determines the languages we speak, the stories we
tell to others, and our personal belief systems. Unfortunately, like all biologic processes, the ability to store
and recall memories is prone to failure. Memory depends on the precise functioning of healthy neurons.
Age, trauma, malnutrition, and genetic factors can diminish our ability to store and recall information, and
severe forms of memory impairment can lead to profound tragedy. Individuals with **Alzheimer disease,** for
example, often lose the ability to perform everyday

functions and may even fail to recognize their closest
friends and relatives. This chapter considers the biologic processes that underlie learning and memory and
disorders of memory, such as the dementias, and also
examines possible approaches to alleviating memory
impairment.

MEMORY

DECLARATIVE AND NONDECLARATIVE MEMORY

Learning and memory are closely related to one
another, but the terms are not interchangeable. Learning refers to the process by which behavior can be
changed as a result of experience or practice. Memory
refers to the ability to recall things that have been
learned. There are several different types of memory. A
child who has just mastered the ability to ride a bicycle,
a college student who has memorized an equation, and
a war veteran who experiences uncontrollable panic in
response to loud, sudden noises have stored different
types of information. Psychologists and neuroscientists
recognize two major classes of memory, which are described as *declarative* and *nondeclarative* (Figure 20–1).
Declarative memory, which also is known as *explicit
memory,* refers to the process that enables us to recall
facts or events. Memorizing the Gettysburg Address, recalling the names of the people you have met through-

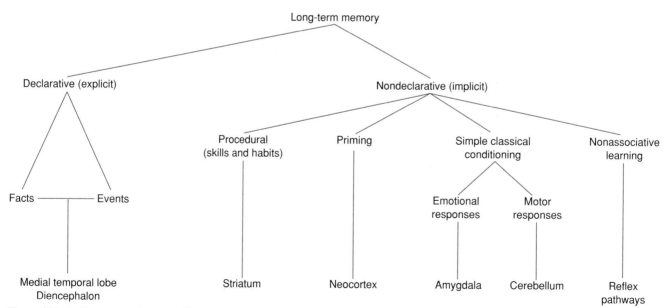

Figure 20–1. Taxonomy of mammalian memory systems. This categorization of the
different types of memory recognized by psychologists and neuroscientists indicates the
brain structures and neural connections believed to be especially important for each kind
of memory. (Adapted with permission from Milner B, Squire LR, Kandel ER. Cognitive
neuroscience and the study of memory. 1998. *Neuron* 20:445.)

out your life, and remembering where you parked your car this morning involve declarative memory. This type of memory also may be thought of as *conscious memory* or as memory that is capable of being verbalized. In contrast, nondeclarative memory can be thought of as subconscious or unable to be verbalized. Nondeclarative memory is used broadly and may refer to a variety of learning processes, including those that involve procedural skills, conditioning, priming, and the forming of habits.

Procedural memory is a type of nondeclarative memory that is used to learn skilled behavior; it is used, for example, when an individual learns to type or to play tennis. Procedural memory is distinct from a declarative memory of the actual training episode; for example, typing is distinct from remembering when you learned how to type. Another type of nondeclarative memory is used during the process of *conditioning*, which involves learning to respond appropriately to stimuli through experience or practice. Examples of this phenomenon include *classic conditioning*, which in Pavlov's experiment involved the process by which a dog learned to salivate at the sound of a tone that predicted the appearance of food, and *fear conditioning*, which describes the process by which a rodent learns to freeze at the sound of a tone that predicts an unpleasant experience such as a mild electric shock.

Nondeclarative memory also underlies *priming*, or the ability to detect or identify objects as a result of recent encounters. Priming, which can be thought of as a subconscious memory of an event that is capable of influencing later actions, can be demonstrated in experiments. In one such experiment, subjects are shown a list of multiple-syllable words. Subsequently they are shown a list of three-letter word stems. Afterward they are asked to transform the word stems into words, for example, cot into *cot*tage or *cot*ton. When a multisyllable word from the first list contains a word stem from the second list, subjects have a much stronger than average tendency to extend the single-syllable word, such as cot, to form a multisyllable word they have recently seen, such as cotton, regardless of whether they consciously remember having seen the longer word. The formation of *habits*, or the gradual acquisition of behavioral tendencies that are specific to a set of stimuli, also involves nondeclarative memory. Habit learning is exhibited during *operant conditioning*, as when an animal learns to perform a task to obtain some reward, such as food or a drug of abuse.

It is important to mention that memory is not arbitrarily assigned to declarative and nondeclarative categories; nor were these categories established merely on the basis of introspection and conjecture. These two memory processes are recognized because they can be experimentally distinguished and are mediated by distinct neural substrates.

THE MEDIAL TEMPORAL LOBE SYSTEM

In 1953, a patient referred to as H.M. underwent a bilateral resection of the medial structures of the temporal lobe—including the anterior two thirds of the hippocampus, the posthippocampal gyrus, and the amygdala—as a desperate measure to treat intractable epilepsy. This surgery had tragic consequences that caused H.M. to become one of the best known neurologic patients. After his operation, H.M. had severe *anterograde amnesia;* that is, he lost his ability to store new memories. Although he could recall the names of people he had known for many years before his operation, he could not remember the names of individuals he met postoperatively, including those of nurses and doctors whom he would meet repeatedly over a period of several months. In addition to his inability to form new memories, H.M. lost memories of events that had occurred up to a decade before his surgery. Yet his ability to recall more remote events remained intact.

Fourteen years after the onset of his amnesia, doctors gave this description of H.M.'s mental condition:

> He fails to recognize people who are close neighbors or family friends but who met him after the operation. . . . Although he gives his date of birth unhesitatingly and accurately, he always underestimates his own age and can only make wild guesses as to the current date. . . . During nights at the Clinical Research Center, H.M. would ring for the night nurse, asking her apologetically if she would tell him where he was and how he came to be there. He clearly realized that he was in a hospital but seemed unable to reconstruct any of the events of the previous day. . . . His experience seems to be that of a person who is just becoming aware of his surroundings without fully comprehending the situation, because he does not remember what went before. . . . H.M. was given protected employment in a state rehabilitation center . . . he was given rather monotonous work. . . . It is characteristic that he cannot give any description of his place of work, the nature of his job, or the route along which he is driven each day to and from the center.

H.M. was extraordinarily impaired in his ability to remember facts and events that occurred after his surgery. Yet his I.Q. test scores rose after the surgery (from 104 to 118), an improvement that might be attributed to postsurgical control of his seizures. Moreover, H.M. retained some memory capacity; for example, if he concentrated and did not encounter any distractions, he was able to remember facts, such as short strings of digits, for approximately 15 minutes. However, as soon as he was distracted, such facts would vanish from his memory. Thus H.M. did have the ability to store facts for brief periods of time in what is sometimes called *working memory*, or memory for immediately preceding events, such as the memory of a telephone number that lasts just long enough to place a call (see Chapter 17). However, he appeared unable to transfer a fact from working memory to *long-term memory*, which enables facts to remain accessible for long periods of time.

Despite his difficulty in storing facts, H.M. was capable of learning. Striking proof of his ability to learn was reflected in his performance on a test of procedural learning. During this test he was asked to trace an object while viewing his hand in a mirror. Although such a task is tricky because objects and movements are reversed by a mirror, it can be accomplished with practice. H.M. learned to perform this task as quickly and as well as control subjects. However, after repeating the task he was completely unable to recall whether he had ever previously performed the task. H.M.'s improvement came as a surprise to the scientists who conducted the test, and demonstrated that procedural learning can occur independently of declarative learning.

The characteristics of H.M.'s amnesia indicate that declarative memory, but not procedural or other types of nondeclarative memory, is critically dependent on at least one of the brain structures that had been removed during H.M.'s surgery. However, only H.M. and a small number of other patients have had similar lesions and deficits. Moreover, prospective studies on the role of these various structures in humans cannot be conducted for obvious reasons. Thus our knowledge of the brain structures that are crucial for declarative learning has been drawn from animal experiments, particularly experiments on nonhuman primates. At first it may seem problematic to attribute declarative learning to a monkey that cannot make declarations to human experimenters. However, it is possible to distinguish "learning what" (declarative memory) from "learning how" (nondeclarative memory) in primates and in smaller-brained animals such as rats. One method of testing declarative memory in animals involves the use of the "delayed nonmatching to sample task." During this task, a test subject is shown an object that is subsequently taken away. Next, two objects—a new object and the original object—are presented. To receive a reward, the subject must choose the object that has *not* been seen before; to choose correctly, the subject must be able to retain a declarative memory of the original object between the two presentations. Normal monkeys perform this task well. Monkeys with bilateral medial temporal lobe lesions perform at chance levels, except when the intervals between presentations are short. Studies that have attempted to determine how monkeys with different lesions perform declarative tasks such as these have indicated that the crucial structures under-

lying the ability to store declarative memories are the hippocampus proper, the dentate gyrus, the subicular complex, and the entorhinal cortex (Figure 20–2). Animal studies have revealed that a lesion restricted to any of these regions has a significant impact on declarative memory. Importantly, these findings are consistent with what has been learned from the small number of human patients with lesions restricted to medial temporal lobe structures; for example, two patients who suffered bilateral damage restricted to the CA1 region of the hippocampus experienced declarative memory deficits similar in nature to, but less severe than, those experienced by H.M.

Does the medial temporal lobe store our declarative memories? The answer is that it probably does not, at least not permanently. As previously mentioned, H.M. did not lose all of his declarative memories. He was able to recall his name and his date of birth, and he appeared to have accurate and normal memories of events that had occurred 10 or more years before his operation. Results of animal experiments are consistent with H.M.'s experience. In one type of experiment, animals are trained in a task, and at varying times

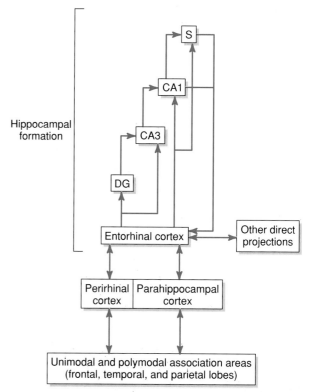

Figure 20–2. The medial temporal lobe memory system. Some of the interconnections among the structures of this system and connections between the medial temporal lobe and the neocortex are shown. S, subiculum; DG, dentate gyrus. (Adapted with permission from Milner B, Squire LR, Kandel ER. 1998. Cognitive neuroscience and the study of memory. *Neuron* 20:445.)

thereafter undergo bilateral damage to the hippocampal formation. Retention of the task is then assessed shortly after the surgery. These studies reveal that such damage causes a retrograde amnesia of days to months depending on the time interval between the training and the surgery. For example, in animals that are trained a month before hippocampal ablation, postoperative memory is identical to that of control animals. However, those that receive training only a few days before hippocampal damage exhibit exceedingly poor memory for the training.

Experiments such as these and observations of human amnesiacs have led investigators to postulate that structures in the medial temporal lobe coordinate a process by which memories or associations are gradually imprinted on the cerebral cortex. How this occurs has not been determined, but it is believed that inputs from the medial temporal lobe to specific cortical regions gradually reorganize synaptic connections in the cortex until memories are somehow stored and available for recall. Thus when introduced to someone new, we associate a particular face with a sound (Ms. Jones). The medial temporal lobe is responsible for ensuring that the visual and auditory–verbal inputs connect as a single consolidated event. A second encounter with Ms. Jones most likely would cause the medial temporal lobe system to prompt the recall of her name from verbal memory. Over time, corticocortical, visual–verbal connections may prompt one another directly, without the need for medial temporal lobe support. Thus H.M. was able to recall the names of his parents and his childhood friends (the memories had been *corticalized*), but was unable to learn the names of people he met after his surgery because he did not have the medial temporal system to establish and support the link between faces and names.

In contrast to declarative memory, nondeclarative memory does not appear to be supported by a particular center in the brain. Instead, nondeclarative memory represents the gradual modification of neural circuits that are themselves components of the pathway that underlies corresponding behavior. This process is best established for procedural memory. H.M.'s ability to learn the mirror-drawing task did not require participation of the medial temporal lobe system; rather, the learning related to the task most likely took place among the neurons in the visual and motor systems—the very neurons that directed the task. Similarly, other types of nondeclarative memory most likely involve the particular brain systems responsible for their execution. Fear conditioning, for example, depends on modulation of the amygdala, whose activation elicits emotional responses such as fearfulness and aggression (see Chapter 15), whereas several addictive behaviors depend on the

modulation of ventral striatal circuits, such as the nucleus accumbens, which mediate the reinforcing effects of drugs of abuse (see Chapter 16).

SYNAPTIC PLASTICITY: HOW DO NEURONS REMEMBER?

Whether we examine declarative or nondeclarative memory, we must address two important questions: What happens to neurons while new memories are forming? How do their synaptic responses and electrical properties change? In an era in which electrophysiologic, cellular imaging, and molecular biologic techniques are being developed as fast as uses can be found for them, the mystery of the precise changes that take place within and between neurons during memory formation has become one of the most popular topics in neuroscience.

In an effort to identify the possible cellular mechanisms that underlie memory it is useful to consider a classic investigation of nondeclarative learning mentioned earlier in this chapter, the experiments of Ivan Pavlov. Pavlov's dogs were taught to associate the appearance of food with the ringing of a bell; their anticipation was measured by salivation that occurred in response to the ringing of the bell. This type of learning, classic conditioning, has been detected in almost all species studied, including invertebrates, and has significant survival value because it allows organisms to predict the presence of important environmental features, including the presence of food or predators, based on associated cues, such as scents and sounds. It is this type of learning that causes a house cat to run toward the sound of an electric can opener.

What neural changes might underlie such behavioral changes? It appears that neurons that receive important predictive input, such as the sound of the bell, must become efficacious at driving the neurons that are responsible for the corresponding output, such as salivation or other responses to food. According to the most straightforward theory, sensory neurons send a very weak message to neurons that orchestrate behavioral responses, such as response to food, and this input increases in strength after repeated associations, for example, between the sound of a bell and the appearance of food. This model of behavioral change was first suggested by Ramón y Cajal in the early twentieth century, and in 1949 was postulated by Donald Hebb as follows: "... when an axon of cell A ... excites cell B and repeatedly or persistently takes part in firing it, some growth process or metabolic change takes place in one or both cells so that A's efficiency as one of the cells firing B is increased." If we postulate that cell A fires in response to the sound of a bell but only weakly excites cell B, which fires when food is present, Hebb's hypothesis explains how the firing of cell A (the bell neuron) might gradually elicit a strong response from cell B (a food response neuron), if bell ringing and food presentation are paired frequently enough.

LTP AND MEMORY FORMATION

Several studies have shown that synapses can indeed undergo the types of changes postulated by Hebb. In 1973, Bliss and Lomo reported that synapses in the mammalian CNS are capable of undergoing a Hebbian-like increase in efficacy. They demonstrated that low-frequency stimulation of perforant path axons of the hippocampus in rabbits elicits a relatively stable depolarizing synaptic response in the postsynaptic neurons of the dentate gyrus (Figure 20–3A). However, when high-frequency stimulation is repeatedly applied to per-

forant path axons, and in turn postsynaptic dentate neurons are strongly depolarized, subsequent stimulation of these axons leads to a postsynaptic response that is much larger in magnitude than the response observed before high-frequency stimulation. Importantly, this increase in synaptic efficacy persists over a long period of time; a single episode of high-frequency perforant path stimulation can lead to an increase in synaptic efficacy that lasts for hours, and repeated episodes of tetanic stimulation cause increases that last for weeks.

The finding that synapses exhibit an activity-dependent long-lasting increase in their strength resonated with theoretical expectations. Moreover, it disclosed a biologic phenomenon with properties seductively similar to declarative memory itself: the repetition of a single event (high-frequency stimulation) was proven to initiate a neural change that could persist for weeks. This phenomenon, currently known as long-term potentia-

A

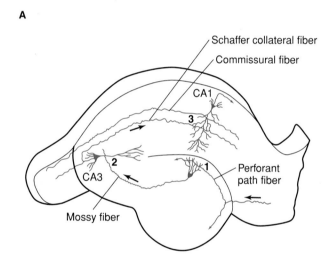

B

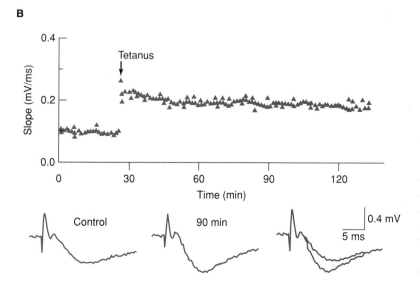

Figure 20–3. **A.** Diagram of the major excitatory pathways (**1, 2, 3**) in the hippocampus. **B.** Long-term potentiation (LTP) obtained from a hippocampal slice preparation. Schaffer collateral and commissural fibers were stimulated to generate a synaptic response in CA1 pyramidal cells; after baseline recordings were obtained for 30 minutes, a high-frequency train of stimuli (tetanus) was given. This tetanus elicited a stable, long-lasting increase in the size of the postsynaptic response. Sample extracellular synaptic responses are shown below the graph. (Adapted with permission from Nicoll RA, Kauer JA, Malenka RC. 1988. The current excitement in LTP. *Neuron* 1:97.)

tion (LTP) (see Figure 20–3B), exhibits two important properties that make it an attractive candidate for the synaptic mechanism that underlies the storage of new information: *input-specificity* and *associativity*. Because it exhibits input specificity, LTP occurs only at synapses that are stimulated by a given pattern of afferent activity, and not at adjacent, unstimulated synapses on the same postsynaptic cell (Figure 20–4). When a limited number of synapses on a given cell are modified by afferent activity, the storage capacity of a neural circuit is dramatically increased. The property of associativity refers to the fact that the generation of LTP requires coincident presynaptic and postsynaptic activity. Importantly, a weak input that is incapable of significantly depolarizing the cell is potentiated only if it is active at the same time that the postsynaptic cell is depolarized by a strong input (see Figure 20–4).

LTP can be elicited in each of the three principal pathways of the hippocampus (see Figure 20–3A) and at glutamatergic synapses in many other brain regions. Although the most prevalent and most extensively studied form of LTP is input-specific and associative, LTP is not identical at all synapses. At some synapses LTP is nonassociative; for example, in the mossy fiber pathway of the hippocampus it does not require coincident presynaptic and postsynaptic activity. Rapid firing of the presynaptic element alone is sufficient to produce LTP in these synapses. However, because this form of LTP has been found only at a few synapses, it is not discussed further in this chapter.

Induction of LTP   Since the major form of LTP is input-specific and associative, it is coincidence dependent: a synaptic input, either weak or strong, can be potentiated only if it is active when the postsynaptic cell is depolarized. However, if an input is active when the postsynaptic cell is not strongly depolarized, potentiation does not occur. Likewise, potentiation does not occur if the postsynaptic cell is depolarized but the input is not active. Because a neuron in the CNS generally has hundreds to thousands of inputs, and several of these inputs must be active at once in order to cause significant depolarization of the neuron, the firing of a single input does not generally depolarize the neuron to the extent required for the generation of LTP.

How a neuron can discriminate between coincident activity and noncoincident activity and determine whether potentiation will occur has been elegantly explained (Figure 20–5). As mentioned in Chapter 7, there are two major classes of ionotropic glutamate receptors in the CNS: AMPA and kainate receptors, which generally conduct Na^+ and K^+ but not Ca^{2+}, and NMDA receptors, which are permeable to Na^+, K^+, and Ca^{2+}. The AMPA receptor requires only the binding of glutamate to pass current, and thereby carries current whenever the presynaptic cell is active (releasing glutamate), regardless of the state of the postsynaptic cell. In contrast, the NMDA receptor acts as a coincidence detector: it requires both presynaptic activity (glutamate release) and postsynaptic depolarization in order to pass current. At normal resting (hyper-

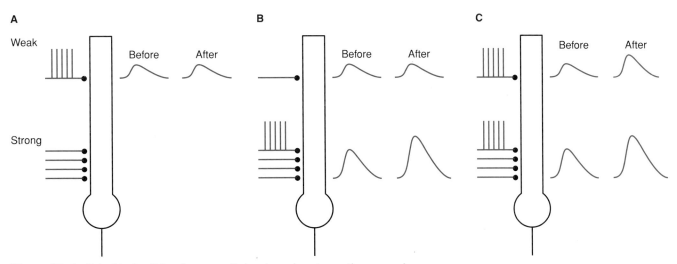

Figure 20–4. Coincident activity of presynaptic inputs and postsynaptic neurons is required to induce long-term potentiation (LTP). **A.** Repetitive activation of a weak presynaptic input does not trigger LTP because it does not elicit sufficient depolarization of the postsynaptic cell. **B.** Repetitive activation of a strong input, which depolarizes the postsynaptic cell, triggers LTP at synapses of the strong, but not the weak, input. **C.** If a weak input is active at the same time that the postsynaptic cell is depolarized, for example, by repetitive activation of a strong input, LTP is triggered at the weak input. (From Nicoll RA, Kauer JA, Malenka RC. 1988. The current excitement in LTP. *Neuron* 1:97.)

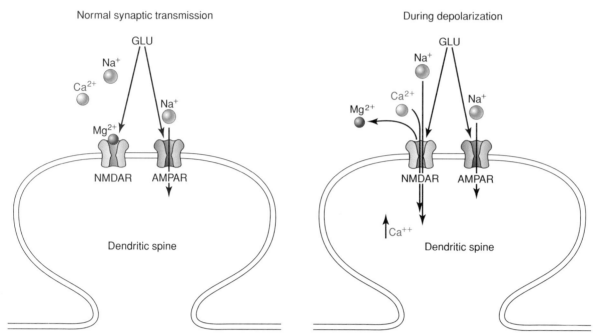

Figure 20–5. The NMDA receptor acts as a coincidence detector to trigger long-term potentiation (LTP) in a CA1 hippocampal pyramidal neuron. During normal synaptic transmission, glutamate (GLU) is released from the presynaptic terminal and binds to both AMPA and NMDA receptors. Current flows through the AMPA receptor but not through the NMDA receptor, because the NMDA receptor channel is blocked by Mg^{2+}. Depolarization of the postsynaptic cell removes the Mg^{2+} block of the NMDA receptor, and allows Na^+ and Ca^{2+} to flow into the cell. The subsequent increase in Ca^{2+} in the dendritic spine is necessary to trigger events leading to LTP. Thus the NMDA receptor serves to detect coincident activity from different synaptic inputs. (Adapted with permission from Malenka RC. 1995. LTP and LTD: Dynamic interactive processes of synaptic plasticity. *The Neuroscientist* 1:35.)

polarized) potentials, the NMDA receptor does not conduct current even after binding glutamate, because extracellular Mg^{2+} ions block the channel. However, when the postsynaptic membrane is depolarized, as during the induction of LTP, Mg^{2+} is expelled from the channel and the NMDA receptor is free to pass current. Thus, coincident activity—the release of glutamate from the presynaptic terminal and the depolarization of the postsynaptic cell—is required for the NMDA receptor to function.

NMDA receptor channel opening, with the resulting influx of Ca^{2+}, is the critical event in the induction of LTP. With repeated activation of NMDA receptors during adequate postsynaptic depolarization, Ca^{2+} builds in the dendritic spine to a high level and activates the signaling mechanisms responsible for LTP. Thus LTP occurs only at stimulated synapses because NMDA receptors must be activated by synaptically released glutamate so that they can permit Ca^{2+} influx. The properties of the NMDA receptor also explain the associative induction of LTP: the depolarization provided by a strong input helps to depolarize the adjacent synapses activated by

weak inputs. Consistent with this explanation, LTP can be generated when low-frequency afferent stimulation is paired with postsynaptic depolarization by an intracellular recording electrode.

A great deal of experimental evidence supports the requirement of NMDA receptor activation and Ca^{2+} influx for the induction of associative LTP. For example, blockade of the NMDA receptor, with antagonists such as **APV** (see Chapter 7), prevents the induction of LTP, and mouse mutants that lack functional NMDA receptors do not exhibit LTP. Moreover, when the postsynaptic cell is filled with a Ca^{2+} chelator that prevents a rise in Ca^{2+}, LTP induction is prevented, and when Ca^{2+} is directly increased in postsynaptic cells, synaptic transmission is enhanced, thereby mimicking LTP.

How is a rise in postsynaptic Ca^{2+} linked to the molecular mechanisms that result in an increase of synaptic strength? The multiple potential targets of Ca^{2+} in neuronal second messenger systems (see Chapter 5) suggest numerous possibilities. Several different protein kinases have been suspected of playing important roles in the induction of LTP, but the strongest evidence implicates Ca^{2+}/calmodulin-dependent protein kinase II (CaMKII) and protein kinase C (PKC). When injected into CA1 pyramidal cells, inhibitors of these enzymes block LTP, and both CaMKII and PKC have been shown to be activated by the tetanic stimulation that elicits LTP. Moreover, injection of an activated fragment of CaMKII into hippocampal CA1 cells leads to a synaptic enhancement that mimics LTP. However, the precise roles of these kinases and other second messenger systems in the induction of LTP must still be determined.

Although the intracellular signaling cascade responsible for the induction of LTP remains only partially understood, it is possible to investigate the downstream mechanisms by which LTP might be expressed and maintained. Protein kinases may affect synaptic transmission in numerous ways, but reasonably strong evidence suggests that phosphorylation of AMPA receptor subunits by CaMKII, protein kinase A, or another protein kinase enhances the conductance of the AMPA receptor-channel complex and, in so doing, enhances synaptic transmission. It also is possible that LTP involves the regulated insertion of AMPA receptor complexes into the postsynaptic membrane. Although this theory has not been proven, intriguing evidence supports it; for example, when inhibitors of membrane fusion such as *N*-ethyl-maleimide (**NEM**) or **botulinum toxin B** are injected into the postsynaptic cell, LTP is diminished. Furthermore, visualization of AMPA receptors that have been tagged with green fluorescent protein (GFP) reveals that the receptors are delivered to synapses during LTP.

An alternative hypothesis is that the expression of LTP is presynaptic—that is, LTP is caused by an increase in presynaptic neurotransmitter release. Because the induction of LTP clearly depends on postsynaptic events, these hypotheses require the existence of retrograde messengers that are released from the postsynaptic cell and that diffuse across the synaptic cleft to modify presynaptic function. The best known candidate for such a retrograde messenger is the gas nitric oxide (NO), which is produced by nitric oxide synthase (NOS) (see Chapter 5); however, evidence that supports its involvement in LTP is controversial.

Persistence of LTP   The enzymatic alteration of preexisting synaptic proteins, for example, by means of phosphorylation, may be sufficient to change synaptic efficacy for relatively short periods of time. The maintenance of LTP for days or weeks, however, is likely to involve additional mechanisms. Considerable evidence currently suggests that the prolonged enhancement of synaptic strength requires the activation of particular genes and new protein synthesis. The critical gene products are unknown, but they may include increased

expression of glutamate receptor proteins or altered expression of protein kinases, protein phosphatases, or cytoskeletal elements that contribute to the modification of synaptic structure, as explained later in this chapter. The cAMP pathway and its regulation of the transcription factor CREB (see Chapters 5 and 6) have been strongly implicated in the long-term maintenance of LTP and in the maintenance of long-term memory in animals. In diverse invertebrate and vertebrate species, for example, manipulations that decrease functioning of the cAMP pathway or CREB have been shown to impair certain memory tasks, whereas manipulations that enhance functioning are reported to exert the opposite effect.

Alterations in synaptic morphology also may contribute to the long-lasting nature of LTP; for example, if LTP involves the insertion of AMPA receptors into the dendritic spine plasma membrane, cytoskeleton-based structural changes might support this membrane in a relatively permanent manner. Accordingly, LTP may consist of the building of bigger dendritic spines or even an increased number of spines. This theory is interesting because it could explain how a long-lasting enhancement of synaptic strength might remain synapse-specific. However, this hypothesis does not appear to explain how altered gene expression, which occurs in the nucleus of the cell body at what can be a tremendous distance from a modified synapse, leads to the maintenance of potentiation only in previously stimulated synapses, and not in the neuron's thousands of other synapses. One possibility is that the modification of preexisting synaptic proteins that occurs immediately after the induction of LTP might somehow tag these synapses so that the newly synthesized proteins generated through the stimulation of gene transcription are targeted to these synapses and not to adjacent synapses on the same cell.

LTP and its relationship to memory   Although LTP displays characteristics that might be expected of a memory mechanism, attempts to design and perform experiments that link LTP directly to real memory processes have proven difficult. Based on the hypothesis that LTP underlies learning and memory, two major predictions can be made. First, the prevention of LTP should be able to prevent or at least disrupt the establishment of memories. Consistent with this prediction, genetic manipulations in mice that lead to the absence of the NMDA receptor in pyramidal cells in the CA1 region of the hippocampus result in profound deficits in spatial learning. Conversely, mutant mice with enhanced NMDA receptor function in this brain region, achieved through the overexpression of $NMDAR_{2B}$ receptor subunits, which increases receptor-mediated currents (see Chapter 7), perform better than wildtype mice in certain memory tasks. These findings strongly suggest that spatial learning requires NMDA receptor function, specifically in the excitatory synapses on CA1 pyramidal cells.

Second, if LTP underlies learning and memory, it also should occur during the formation of memories. However, its presence during memory formation is not easy to demonstrate: is it possible to isolate the few neural connections that are responsible for a learning event from trillions of connections? Nonetheless, LTP-like phenomena have been observed to occur in parallel with learning in a fear conditioning paradigm. As described in Chapter 15, conditioned fear is produced in experimental animals when a neutral tone is paired with an electric shock. This fear conditioning is mediated by the amygdala, which receives glutamatergic auditory inputs, and these glutamatergic synapses undergo NMDA receptor-dependent LTP. Furthermore, the blocking of NMDA receptors in the amygdala prevents the development of the conditioned fear response. A subsequent critical experiment, in which auditory-evoked responses in the amygdala were recorded while an animal underwent a conditioning procedure, demonstrated that fear conditioning induces LTP in the auditory pathway to the amygdala (Figure 20–6). Together, these findings make an impressive case for a connection between memory processes and LTP.

OTHER FORMS OF SYNAPTIC PLASTICITY

Although evidence to support connections between LTP and memory must be considered limited, LTP remains the synaptic mechanism most commonly thought to mediate learning and memory. However, other forms of synaptic plasticity may play equally important roles. These include several different forms of so-called long-term depression (LTD), a generic term used to describe a long-lasting, activity-dependent decrease in synaptic strength (Figure 20–7). Evidence suggests, for example, that a form of LTD observed in the cerebellum is critically important for mediating certain types of motor learning. LTD also may be important for reversing LTP because without such a mechanism, LTP would be likely to completely saturate synaptic strength at large numbers of synapses and thereby limit the storage capacity of any given neural circuit. Indeed, computational models of neural networks have demonstrated that the ability to bidirectionally modify synaptic strength, that is, utilizing both LTP and LTD, greatly increases the power of these circuits to store and retrieve information.

Most synapses that express NMDA receptor-dependent LTP also express a form of homosynaptic LTD that

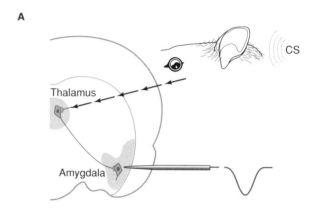

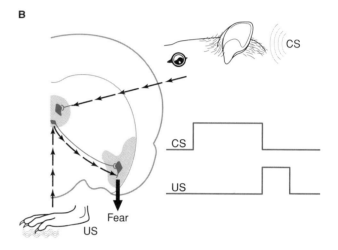

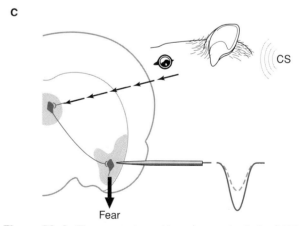

Figure 20–6. The occurrence of long-term potentiation (LTP) during fear conditioning. **A.** An auditory conditioned stimulus (CS) evokes a synaptic response (generated by way of the thalamus) in the amygdala. **B.** The CS is paired with a foot shock, which is referred to as the unconditioned stimulus (US). **C.** After repeated training (pairing of the CS and US), the CS causes a larger synaptic response in the amygdala and is capable of eliciting fear. (Adapted with permission from Malenka RC, Nicoll RA. 1997. Learning and memory: Never fear, LTP is hear. *Nature* 390:552.)

appears to be related to a reversal of at least some of the modifications that are responsible for LTP. Like LTP, this form of LTD also requires activation of NMDA receptors and is believed to be triggered by a modest rise in postsynaptic Ca^{2+}, in contrast to the high level of Ca^{2+} required to trigger LTP. One manner in which different levels of increase in postsynaptic Ca^{2+} may activate different biochemical cascades, which in turn may decrease or increase synaptic strength, is represented in Figure 20–8. This model involves a tug of war between protein kinase and protein phosphatase activity. An attractive feature of this model is that the kinase (CaMKII) and the phosphatase (PP1) both act on the same set of substrates, including the AMPA receptor itself.

Although synaptic plasticity (LTP and LTD) is the best understood mechanism by which neuronal responsiveness can be regulated, there is evidence that *nonsynaptic plasticity* may also be important, particularly for more generalized forms of learning and memory, such as emotional memory versus memory of a specific event. Nonsynaptic plasticity comprises changes in the electrical excitability of neurons that are generalized to many synapses or perhaps the entire cell and not localized to a particular dendritic spine. For example, altered levels of expression of ion channels in a neuron or even changes in the subtypes of ion channels expressed in response to some stimulus would be expected to either increase or decrease that neuron's excitability by a host of inputs. Similarly, general growth or retraction of dendritic arborizations would have significant effects on neuronal responsiveness that would not be limited to

specific synapses. It is easy to imagine how such nonsynaptic plasticity might mediate changes in the responsiveness of neurons to certain types of environmental exposures, for example, tolerance or sensitization to a drug of abuse, which can be viewed as a type of memory. Further work is needed to determine whether nonsynaptic plasticity also contributes to memory of nonpharmacologic—for example, behavioral—environmental stimuli.

A detailed understanding of the physical changes in the nervous system that are responsible for learning and memory will require a great deal of additional research. However, the elucidation of some of the basic mechanisms underlying LTP and LTD and other mechanisms of plasticity has focused attention on what for many decades was believed to be an intractable problem. Thus it seems likely that major discoveries are on the horizon and that during the next decade new pharmacologic agents will be developed to facilitate learning and memory by acting directly on corresponding molecular targets.

BEYOND LTP: WHY WE REMEMBER WHAT WE REMEMBER

None of us has the ability to remember everything. An important goal is to understand the factors that play a role in our tendency to remember facts or learn associations. Extreme emotion can enhance memory. Almost all Americans who were old enough when the events occurred can recall their whereabouts when they heard

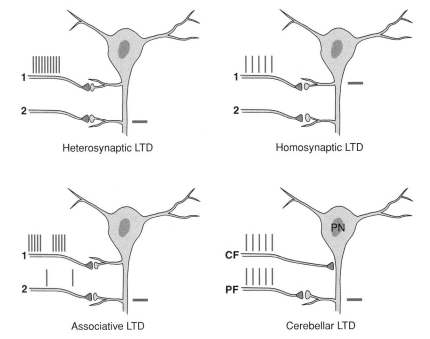

Figure 20–7. Several different forms of long-term depression (LTD). Heterosynaptic LTD is induced at quiescent synapses when adjacent synapses on the same cell are strongly activated. Homosynaptic LTD is induced at synapses that are repetitively activated at a low frequency. Associative LTD is induced when synapses are activated out of phase with strong activation of adjacent synapses. Cerebellar LTD occurs at the parallel fiber (PF)–Purkinje cell synapse when climbing fibers (CF), the other major input to Purkinje cells, are simultaneously activated. PN, Purkinje neuron. (Adapted with permission from Linden DJ. 1994. Long-term synaptic depression in the mammalian brain. *Neuron* 12:457.)

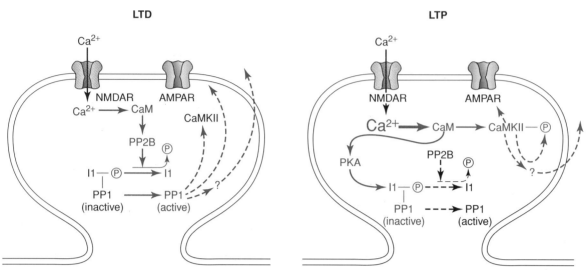

Figure 20–8. Signaling cascades responsible for long-term depression (LTD) and long-term potentiation (LTP). During modest synaptic activity, a small rise in Ca^{2+}, in conjunction with calmodulin (CaM), preferentially activates the Ca^{2+}/CaM-dependent protein phosphatase calcineurin, also known as protein phosphatase 2B (PP2B) (see Chapter 5). Calcineurin subsequently dephosphorylates inhibitor 1 (**I1**), a protein whose phosphorylation (P) inhibits protein phosphatase 1 (PP1). Because dephosphorylated I1 is incapable of inhibiting PP1, the activity of PP1 increases. PP1 subsequently acts on several substrates, including CaMKII and the AMPA receptor itself. In contrast, during LTP a larger rise in Ca^{2+} (bound to CaM) preferentially activates CaMKII. An increase in Ca^{2+}/CaM, presumably through the activation of adenylyl cyclases, also results in the activation of protein kinase A (PKA), which phosphorylates I1 and in turn decreases PP1 activity. An attractive feature of this model is that calcineurin has a higher affinity for Ca^{2+}/CaM compared with CaMKII; thus calcineurin is preferentially activated by smaller rises in Ca^{2+}. (Adapted with permission from Malenka RC. 1995. LTP and LTD: Dynamic interactive processes of synaptic plasticity. *The Neuroscientist* 1:35.)

that President Kennedy was shot or when they learned that the space shuttle Challenger exploded. This type of declarative memory, which is enhanced by strong emotion, is often called *flashbulb memory*. In general, the stronger the associated emotion when a memory is encoded, the more vivid the memory is. This cognitive enhancement of declarative memory, which is hippocampal dependent, also requires an intact amygdala. Preliminary evidence suggests that such enhancement can be inhibited, without associated amnesia, by **β-adrenergic antagonists**. This observation is consistent with the well-established promotion of certain forms of LTP in the hippocampus by β-adrenergic receptor activation, which involves stimulation of the cAMP pathway.

Strong emotion also produces amygdala-dependent emotional memories (see Chapter 15). This form of nondeclarative memory can be observed even in individuals with hippocampal lesions who have no conscious recall of the circumstances under which the memory was acquired. Emotional memories are usually activated by cues that are reminiscent of the original stimulus and that produce physiologic and behavioral responses appropriate to the emotion. In the case of fear,

such responses include activation of the sympathetic nervous system and may result in a freezing response in prey species. Conversely, in strongly rewarding situations, responses elicited by emotional memory lead to approach behavior and physiologic preparation for activities such as eating, drinking, or sex.

Both the declarative and nondeclarative components of memories when encoded in the context of strong emotional stimuli have survival value: a vivid memory of a dangerous situation helps an organism avoid similar situations in the future, and memory of a rewarding situation helps an organism obtain future rewards. However, emotional memory can be maladaptive in some situations; for example, when it is activated under the pathologic circumstances that characterize **posttraumatic stress disorder** (**PTSD;** see Chapter 15) or **drug addiction** (see Chapter 16). Most research on the neural substrates of emotional memory has focused on the amygdala in studies of aversive stimuli and on the ventral striatum in studies of reinforcing stimuli. Currently, a major challenge is to understand how these subcortical structures interact with more traditional memory structures, such as the hippocampus and neocortex, to produce fully integrated emotional memories, and how such circuits malfunction in pathologic conditions.

Attention and alertness also play a significant role in memory. Someone intently watching a lecture is likely to have a better recall of the information presented than an audience member who is daydreaming. Likewise, someone who is well rested is likely to remember better than someone who is groggy. The neurobiology of these facets of memory is discussed in Chapter 18.

PHARMACOLOGIC REGULATION OF MEMORY

Many neurotransmitter systems influence both memory performance and the generation of LTP in the hippocampus. Among the neurotransmitters with the greatest influence on memory is acetylcholine. In both humans and animals, muscarinic cholinergic antagonists, such as **atropine** and **scopolamine,** produce memory deficiencies at low doses and a more profound disruption of memory and consciousness, known as **delirium** (Box 20–1), at higher doses. In the mammalian brain, cholinergic nuclei—most notably the nucleus basalis, or Meynert's nucleus, in the basal forebrain—project heavily to the neocortex and hippocampus (see Chapter 9). The release of acetylcholine by these nuclei generally promotes depolarization or rhythmic firing of postsynaptic neurons through the activation of muscarinic and nicotinic cholinergic receptors. **Carbachol,** for example, is an agonist of muscarinic receptors that produces rhythmic, synchronized firing of hippocampal CA1 cells. This synchronized firing occurs at a frequency of approximately 5–7 Hz and is described as a *theta rhythm.* The precise role of theta rhythm in memory storage is not completely understood; however, when it is induced in a hippocampal slice preparation, weak stimuli that ordinarily do not produce potentiation can evoke LTP when they are applied in synchronization with the theta rhythm. It is believed that the role of cholinergic activity may be to decrease the threshold of neural activity necessary for learning. Nicotinic receptors are similarly implicated in hippocampal function, and in the formation of memory.

Acetylcholine is believed to serve a critical function in certain memory disorders. **Alzheimer disease,** for example, decimates cholinergic neurons and overall cholinergic activity in the brain, as is reflected by measures of choline acetyltransferase, the rate-limiting enzyme in acetylcholine synthesis (see Chapter 9). Cholinergic agents, most notably **acetylcholinesterase inhibitors,** are currently used to treat the symptoms of Alzheimer disease; however, given the pervasive and degenerative nature of the illness, it is not surprising that these agents have shown very limited efficacy.

Many other neurotransmitter systems involved in the functioning of memory-related circuits are expected to be exploited in the future to modulate learning and memory. A major goal of pharmaceutical research is to develop so-called **cognitive-enhancing agents**. Such drugs might be used not only to treat memory impairments in patients with Alzheimer disease and in nondemented elderly individuals but also to enhance memory performance in normal individuals. Several drugs are under consideration for these uses, based on research involving animal models of cognitive function (Box 20–2). **Benzodiazepines,** especially potent and short-acting agents such as **midazolam** and **triazolam,** can disrupt the encoding of declarative memories. In fact, such drugs are used preoperatively to decrease patient recall of unpleasant events surrounding surgery. The effects of these agents on memory suggest that weak partial **inverse-agonists** at the benzodiazepine site of γ-aminobutyric acid $(GABA)_A$ receptors (see Chapters 7 and 15) might serve to enhance memory. The use of full inverse agonists, of course, would present problems because of the risk of seizures. Partial agonists or weak positive allosteric regulators of various **glutamate** receptors (discussed later in this chapter), antagonists at various **adenosine** receptors (see Chapter 10), and agonists at **dopamine** D_1 receptors (see Chapters 8 and 17) are also under consideration. Moreover, pharmacologic manipulation of certain memories may be possible in the future; for example, as previously indicated, it appears that β-adrenergic antagonists such as **propranolol** may be useful in preventing memories of traumatic events (see Chapter 15).

DISORDERS OF MEMORY

Many disorders are associated with cognitive impairment (Table 20–1). Among these are metabolic diseases, for example, altered serum levels of Na^+, K^+, or Ca^{2+}; endocrinopathies, such as thyroid- and cortisol-related disorders; and autoimmune diseases, including collagen vascular disorders such as lupus erythematosus. Despite our knowledge of the molecular abnormalities involved in these disorders, we know surprisingly little about how each of these pathologic processes leads to the dysfunction of specific neural circuits and to memory impairment. Moreover, treatment of the cognitive symptoms of these disorders is generally directed at their underlying causes and not at the neural mechanisms underlying the associated abnormalities in cognition per se. For example, cognitive dysfunction caused by Cushing disease is treated by reducing cortisol secretion, and that caused by lupus erythematosus is treated with immunosuppressive agents. Other common

Box 20–1 Delirium and Dementia

Cognitive impairments often are assigned to one of two broad categories: delirium and dementia (see table). Delirium refers to an acute disruption in cognition that is accompanied by symptoms that fluctuate and typically are short-lived. Common features of delirium include a reduced level of consciousness, such as drowsiness or stupor; disorientation; attentional difficulties; and perceptual abnormalities, such as hallucinations or illusions. The prototypical example of delirium is a drug-induced toxic state. In contrast, dementia refers to a long-term condition characterized by cognitive impairments that tend to be progressive and often permanent. Some of the causes of dementia are listed in Table 20–1. The cardinal feature of dementia is a profound loss of short- and long-term memory. However, it must be emphasized that considerable overlap exists between these states, since many people with severe dementia show many of the symptoms categorized under delirium.

Delirium typically is reversible when the precipitating insult is removed. Among the many causes of delirium are abnormalities in serum electrolytes and acid–base balance; metabolic abnormalities, including renal failure, liver failure, and vitamin deficiencies; endocrinopathies, such as abnormal functioning of the adrenal cortex, thyroid, and parathyroid glands; and infections such as encephalitis and meningitis.

Drugs and toxins also are important causes of delirium. The prototypical state of delirium is caused by muscarinic cholinergic antagonists, such as **scopolamine** and **atropine** (see Chapter 9). Numerous psychotropic medications, including many commonly prescribed **antidepressants** and **antipsychotic** drugs, have muscarinic cholinergic antagonist

properties. Some patients, particularly the elderly, are especially vulnerable to the effects of these agents and can develop delirium as a side effect. Many drugs of abuse, including **alcohol, sedative-hypnotics, opiates, phencyclidine,** and **stimulants** can cause a state of intoxication that, when extreme, can present as delirium. Moreover, withdrawal from these drugs can cause delirium (see Chapter 16). Numerous medications used in general medical practice also can be associated with delirium. Some common offending agents include **theophylline** (used to treat asthma), **dilantin** and other **anticonvulsants** (see Chapter 21), **cimetidine** and other histamine H_2 antagonists (used in therapy for heartburn and peptic ulcer disease), and **digitalis** and other drugs used to treat cardiac dysrhythmias.

	Delirium	Dementia
Course	Acute	Chronic
Symptoms	Fluctuating	Persistent
Level of consciousness	Reduced	Alert
Orientation	Impaired	Variable
Attentional deficit	Prominent	Variable
Thought processes	Disorganized	Variable
Perceptual abnormalities	Present	Variable
Sleep–wake cycle	Disrupted	Variable
Memory	Impaired (particularly recent memory)	Impaired (short- and long-term memory)

causes of memory impairment involve physical disruption of the brain, such as that caused by surgery, trauma, or stroke (see Chapter 21); treatment of these cognitive impairments focuses on the general strategies for improving memory outlined previously in this chapter.

Individuals with **Korsakoff syndrome,** like those with medial temporal lobe damage, suffer from anterograde amnesia. Also referred to as **Wernicke-Korsakoff syndrome,** this disorder is caused by **thiamine** deficiency and occurs mainly in alcoholics who obtain most of their calories from alcohol. Individuals with this syndrome also experience extensive retrograde amnesia, which can span several decades prior to the onset of their disease. Affected individuals often exhibit disorientation with regard to time and place, and they may compensate for their memory loss with confabulation, that is, they may fill a memory gap with a falsification that they accept as correct. The damaged neural systems generally believed to be responsible for this disorder are the mammillary bodies of the hypothalamus and parts

of the dorsomedial thalamus. Yet the exact role of these structures in the storage and retrieval of memories is poorly understood. Peripheral neuropathies also are a common finding. How thiamine deficiency results in damage to these specific neuronal cell types is not known. Treatment with thiamine can prevent further deterioration, and if therapy is initiated early enough, the condition often can be ameliorated or reversed.

Korsakoff syndrome illustrates an important consideration with regard to common causes of memory impairment. Namely, it appears that impaired memory is commonly related to neuronal loss, whether such loss occurs from surgery, stroke, trauma, or neurodegeneration. Thus the treatment of these various conditions is quite difficult because the death of neurons currently cannot be reversed. Effective therapies ultimately must involve preventing the disease process that results in neuronal injury. The remainder of this chapter is devoted to a discussion of Alzheimer disease and related dementias, which involve neural-specific pathologic

Box 20–2 Animal Studies of Learning and Memory

Much of what we know about memory processes has been derived from studies of animal behavior. A number of tests, including the delayed nonmatch to sample test, the Morris water maze, the Barnes maze, and the radial arm maze, have been used to investigate the molecular, cellular, and anatomic substrates of memory in animals. The following discussion is not meant to provide a comprehensive list of these tests, but rather a condensed overview of some of the techniques for studying learning and memory in the laboratory.

Invertebrate models

Several invertebrate species have been studied to learn how neural circuitry changes during simple conditioning. Among the most commonly studied is the sea slug (*Aplysia californica*), which has approximately 20,000 neurons. These cells are clustered into ganglia that each comprise approximately 2000 neurons. Many of these neurons are large enough to be seen by the naked eye and are excellent targets for electrophysiologic study. Each ganglion is responsible for a particular set of behaviors, such as gill movements and the release of reproductive hormones. *Aplysia* is capable of many types of conditioning: it can habituate to innocuous stimuli, sensitize to noxious stimuli, and even associate one stimulus with another. *Aplysia* can, for example, learn to associate a mild tactile stimulus with an electric shock to the tail; after conditioning, it exhibits a defensive response upon sensing the mild stimulus that predicts the shock. Many laboratories have taken advantage of *Aplysia's* relatively simple nervous system to trace the exact molecular and cellular changes in neural functioning that occur during different forms of conditioning.

Emotional memory

Advances in the neurosciences have enabled the study of neural circuit changes during various forms of conditioning in mammals. In one particularly well-studied model, a rat or mouse hears a tone and subsequently receives a mild foot shock. After only one or two pairings of the tone and the foot shock, the animal responds to the tone as if it were afraid; for example, it stops moving (freezes), its hair stands up (piloerection), and its heart rate increases. This phenomenon signifies conditioned fear (see Chapter 15). Unlike declarative learning, conditioned fear is not affected by hippocampal lesions; rather this type of fear appears to be most dependent on the amygdala, another structure of the limbic system. As discussed in this chapter, conditioned fear is believed to involve NMDA receptor-dependent long-term potentiation (LTP).

Declarative memory

The *delayed nonmatch to sample test* is perhaps the most straightforward measure of declarative memory. Animals that undergo this test, typically monkeys, are shown a single stimulus, such as a toy or a colored light, that is subsequently hidden from view. After a given period of time, animals are presented with two stimuli: the previously displayed stimulus, and a novel stimulus, such as a different toy or a different colored light. To receive a reward, animals must choose the novel stimulus. Successful performance of this task requires the ability to remember the first stimulus. This test has been used widely to determine the regions of the temporal cortex that are critical for declarative memory.

Various specialized mazes have been devised to assess spatial memory in animals. The use of these mazes is preferable to the use of traditional tunnel-type mazes because they more clearly separate spatial memory from other types of memory; animals can learn to perform in a tunnel maze by remembering a series of movements even when spatial memory is impaired. At the beginning of each spatial memory trial, animals (typically rats or mice) are placed at random locations and must find their way to a goal using only the memory of spatial cues, the visual landmarks placed around the maze. Motor memory cannot be used to navigate these specialized mazes.

The **Morris water maze** consists of a circular pool of cloudy water in which there is a hidden, slightly submerged, platform. A rat or mouse placed in the water, because it dislikes swimming, typically swims until it finds the platform, which it can use to escape. This maze is used to test an animal's ability to remember the location of the platform, which is measured in terms of how quickly and directly the animal swims to the platform.

The **Barnes maze** comprises a large disc that contains several peripheral holes, placed in an open, lighted area. Most of these holes lead nowhere, but one is connected to a cubbyhole. This connection allows the mouse to escape from the open field, and mice prefer dark enclosures to open fields. This maze is used to test the animal's ability to remember the location of the escape hole.

A slightly different type of task used to evaluate spatial, declarative learning is the **radial arm maze**. This maze consists of eight arms that extend radially from a center start area. Food is placed at the end of each arm. The task of the animal is to find the food as efficiently as possible, which means making no more than one visit to each arm. Normal rats and mice visit each arm of the maze only once. Animals with declarative memory deficiencies visit many arms repeatedly, indicating that they cannot remember whether they have already retrieved food from those arms.

These tests have been used to determine the anatomic substrates necessary for spatial memory, which in all cases appear to be the hippocampus and adjacent temporal lobe structures. More recently, they have been used to study genetically altered strains of mice to determine the role of specific genes in learning and memory.

Table 20–1 Selected Causes of Dementia

Cardiovascular
Large strokes
Multi-infarct dementia (multiple small strokes)

Infectious
HIV dementia
Viral encephalitis
Creutzfeldt-Jakob disease
Abscesses (fungal, bacterial)
Neurosyphilis

Metabolic[1]
Vitamin deficiencies
Starvation

Endocrinopathies[1]
Hyperthyroidism or hypothyroidism
Hypercortisolism or hypocortisolism
Diabetes mellitus

Neurodegenerative disorders
Alzheimer disease
Frontotemporal dementias (e.g., Pick disease)
Down syndrome
Huntington disease[2]
Parkinson disease[2]
Wilson disease[2]

Drugs and Toxins[1]
Alcohol and other drugs of abuse
Heavy metals

Other
Tumors
Trauma
Multiple sclerosis and other demyelinating diseases

[1]Dementia requires chronic exposure.
[2]See Chapter 14.

processes and pose some of our greatest public health challenges.

ALZHEIMER DISEASE AND RELATED DEMENTIAS

Let me tell you about the mother I knew.... She was an independent, willful, and witty child. Just as she could toss out phrases and be clever, she could toss on clothes and be beautiful. She graduated from the University of Colorado with a degree in journalism and became a newspaper reporter, a wife, a girl scout leader, a visiting nurse volunteer, and a truly remarkable mother.

We used to sail together. When the wind would pick up and the boat would heel way over, we balanced together on the rail with our toes tucked onto the centerboard trunk; we leaned out way over the water, daring the water to curl up and get us. And we laughed and whooped when the wind backed around and tossed us into the cabin.

My mother went on to get a master's degree in education and to become a teacher at a bilingual high school on the lower east side of Manhattan. It was a few years after that that she became slightly confused. In time she was reduced to a clerical position at her school, and eventually she had to leave her job.

What I called madness began as forgetfulness: her keys, her phone number at the house we shared. What I called madness developed into a severe depression and vast memory lapses, confusion, and loss of her previous articulate nature. She groped for words like a partially blind person reeling in the half light of dusk....

I remember saying to my mother, "Hi Mom, how are you?" and she said "What day is it?" and I said, "Oh, Mom, I have the flu," and she said, "What day is it? What time is it?"

During the progression of her disease, she became frightened, angry, paranoid, hostile, and incompetent. She became completely dependent on the aid of others. She could not be left alone. She became repetitive, confused, agitated. She stopped reading. Now she can no longer form complete sentences. She speaks rapid gibberish. She has no memory, and she has to be bathed, fed, and dressed. She lives in a nursing home where total care is provided.

My mother is 57 years old. She seems terribly young to be so terribly ill.

Marion Roach (from Kalicki AC [ed]. 1987. Confronting Alzheimer Disease. Owings Mills, MD: Rynd Communications.)

Alzheimer disease is characterized by a gradual decline in cognition over a period of many years. It generally presents late in life, typically after the age of 60. Less commonly, the disease may begin in midlife. Among the earliest symptoms of Alzheimer disease is memory impairment. Patients begin to have difficulty retaining new information for more than a few minutes. Affected individuals may develop a tendency to become lost when walking or driving. As cognitive impairment progresses, patients may become increasingly unable to perform daily tasks; for example, they may experience difficulty in preparing meals, taking regular medications, or managing finances. However, these patients usually retain the ability to perform basic self-care, such as bathing and dressing, until the later stages of the disease. In addition to cognitive decline, mood changes involving depression, irritability, and anxiety often occur.

As Alzheimer disease advances, the ability to learn new information is increasingly compromised. Access to distant memories, which is relatively intact in the initial stages of the disease, begins to diminish. As cognition declines, patients may begin to experience delusions and hallucinations (see Chapter 17). Patients also may become aggressive, even toward their caretakers. The end stage of Alzheimer disease is generally characterized by a complete loss of independence. The patient may be unable to bathe, dress, or eat without extensive assistance. Moreover, some patients may experience impairment of their mobility because of extreme cognitive impairment or because of the effects of the disease on motor cortices. Because of the degree of cognitive impairment that eventually develops and the extensive support required by Alzheimer patients, the disease exacts an enormous toll from not only affected individuals but also the friends and family members who care for them and society at large.

Once considered a rare disorder, Alzheimer disease has become a major public health problem, in part because the human life span has been extended by modern medicine. Alzheimer disease afflicts approximately 4 million Americans, most of them elderly. Among individuals older than 65 years of age, 6% to 8% have Alzheimer disease; among persons aged 85 and older, the prevalence of Alzheimer disease is approximately 30%. As the number and percentage of elderly persons increases steadily, the prevalence of Alzheimer disease almost certainly will rise. It is estimated that by the year 2030 more than 64 million people in the United States will be older than 65 years of age, and much of this population will be older than 85. Thus the overall impact of Alzheimer disease during the next 30 years is likely to be tremendous.

Many other disorders also are characterized by dementia. Next to Alzheimer disease, the most common is **multi-infarct dementia**. This disorder, which often is associated with the loss of fine motor control in addition to memory impairment, is caused by multiple small, or lacunar, strokes (see Chapter 21). The pathophysiology of multi-infarct dementia is fundamentally different from that of Alzheimer disease, even though the symptoms can be quite similar. Another cause of dementia is **Pick disease,** and related "tauopathies" such as **frontotemporal dementia with parkinsonism (FTDP)**. Because it is pathophysiologically related to Alzheimer disease, FTDP is discussed further in subsequent sections of this chapter. **Parkinson disease** and **Huntington disease** also lead to dementia, apparently by means of distinct neurodegenerative processes (see Chapter 14).

PATHOLOGY

Even cursory inspection reveals that the brain of a patient with mid- to late-stage Alzheimer disease is noticeably different from that of a normal person of the same age. The diseased brain appears shrunken compared with the normal brain, and has wider gyri, larger ventricles, and less overall mass. However, the pathologic hallmarks of Alzheimer disease, and clues as to its etiology, can be observed only at the microscopic level. These

hallmarks include the presence of various plaques and other abnormal structures. *Senile plaques* are dense, extracellular deposits that are composed primarily of the 39- to 43-amino-acid amyloid β protein (Aβ), the biochemistry of which is discussed later in this chapter. Two types of senile plaques—*diffuse plaques* and *neuritic plaques*—have been identified. Diffuse plaques are extracellular deposits of Aβ; most of these are formed by the 40-amino-acid form of the peptide ($A\beta_{40}$). *Neuritic plaques* also consist of extracellular masses of Aβ, but are distinguished from diffuse plaques by the presence of dystrophic dendrites and glia. Moreover, the Aβ in neuritic plaques is generally filamentous and consists of both 40- and 42-amino-acid lengths of Aβ ($A\beta_{40}$ and $A\beta_{42}$). $A\beta_{40}$ and $A\beta_{42}$ peptides self-assemble into filaments in vitro, and filamentous Aβ is much more toxic to cultured neurons in vitro compared with nonfilamentous Aβ. The toxicity of filamentous Aβ most likely explains why filamentous plaques, unlike nonfilamentous plaques, tend to be associated with dystrophic neuronal processes in neuritic plaques.

Intracellular accumulations of abnormally phosphorylated helical filaments known as *neurofibrillary tangles* also are hallmarks of Alzheimer disease. The major constituent of the tangles is the microtubule-associated protein tau, which is present in normal brain tissue. It is believed that the accumulation of tau occurs as a result of its abnormal phosphorylation and that tau accumulation disrupts microtubule stability or function. Dystrophic neuronal processes which generally occur in the vicinity of senile plaques, and neuronal loss, which appears to be associated primarily with areas containing plaques, also are characteristic of this disease.

For reasons that currently are unclear, plaques tend to develop preferentially in the hippocampus, in the temporal and frontal lobes of the cerebral cortex, in other association cortices, and in cholinergic nuclei such as the nucleus basalis. Primary sensory cortices and subcortical brain regions tend to be spared. Indeed, this pattern might be expected in a disease whose earliest symptoms include impaired memory and decline of cognitive function.

The significance of the defining pathologic features of Alzheimer disease has been the topic of intense research. Among the most important questions that investigators have attempted to answer are those related to causality. Do abnormal accumulations of Aβ promote neural damage? Or do accumulations of Aβ merely occur as a side effect of neuronal death? Is the phosphorylation of tau a key step in neurodegeneration? Or is tau abnormally phosphorylated because neurons are already damaged?

Although these questions remain subjects of debate, a growing body of evidence suggests that the gradual buildup of Aβ peptides is a causative and requisite factor in the development of Alzheimer disease. The accumulation of Aβ in the cerebral cortex is an early and invariant event in the development of this disease. Moreover, disorders that lead to the oversecretion of the amyloid precursor protein (APP) result in Alzheimer disease or Alzheimer disease-like syndromes. Examples include **Down syndrome** (**trisomy 21**) and the overexpression of various forms of Aβ peptides in several lines of transgenic mice. Most importantly, recent findings regarding the molecular and genetic basis of Alzheimer disease strongly support speculation that Aβ—particularly its extracellular deposition and its aggregation into filaments—is the key culprit in the development of Alzheimer disease.

Evidence also indicates that abnormalities in tau can be pathogenic. These findings have been drawn from studies of FTDP, at least one variant of which is caused by a mutation in the tau gene, as discussed later in this chapter. FTDP and related tauopathies are associated with very large numbers of neurofibrillary tangles but is not associated with senile plaques. Yet despite the absence of senile plaques, profound neuronal loss is characteristic of this form of dementia.

GENETIC AND MOLECULAR MECHANISMS

Two primary risk factors for Alzheimer disease have long been recognized: genetics, which entails either a family history or the presence of trisomy 21, and old age. Although most patients with Alzheimer disease are elderly, there are inherited forms of the disease in which symptoms appear in middle age. The exact age at which these latter forms of the disease emerge varies among different families. Familial forms of Alzheimer disease follow autosomal dominant inheritance patterns. Indeed, autosomal dominant mutations in any of three known genes can cause early-onset Alzheimer disease, as discussed later in this chapter. FTDP, a familial disease whose onset typically occurs during middle age, more closely resembles early-onset Alzheimer disease.

When symptoms of Alzheimer disease appear in individuals older than 60 years of age, the disease does not occur in a distinctly mendelian inheritance pattern. Nonetheless, family studies have revealed that between 25% and 50% of relatives of patients with Alzheimer disease eventually are afflicted with the disease themselves, compared with approximately 10% among control groups. Although recent studies have revealed genes that modify the risk for Alzheimer disease and the age at which the disease emerges, other factors are important in determining whether or not an individual will develop the disease.

ROLE OF APP AND Aβ

Initial insight into the genetic causes of Alzheimer disease was obtained from studies of early-onset forms of the disease. The first advance occurred with the discovery of a significant link between Alzheimer disease in some families and the region of chromosome 21 that codes for APP, whose products include Aβ peptides. Further evidence consistent with a role for APP in Alzheimer disease is that patients with Down syndrome (Trisomy 21) have an extra copy of the APP gene and generally develop early-onset Alzheimer disease.

The cellular functions of APP in healthy individuals remain unknown despite intensive research. APP is a transmembrane protein that is expressed in many tissues, including the brain. It has multiple splice variants, the longest of which (APP770) contains 770 amino acid residues. It has a short half-life and is metabolized rapidly by proteases by means of two pathways, which are designated α and β. The β pathway, which leads to the production of Aβ (Figure 20–9), involves cleavage of APP by protease β-secretase between residues 671 and 672, and subsequent cleavage by γ-secretase near residue 712. The location of the second cleavage is not precise. When it occurs at residues 712–713, a 40-amino-acid protein termed *short Aβ*, or $A\beta_{40}$, is produced. When it occurs after residue 714, the resultant product is long Aβ, either $A\beta_{42}$ or $A\beta_{43}$. The biochemical events underlying the production of Aβ, and the mechanisms that determine which Aβ forms are produced, have yet to be determined. The α pathway involves cleavage by α-secretase between APP residues 687 and 688, which are located within the Aβ domain. Thus cleavage of APP by means of the α pathway precludes the generation of Aβ peptides. A product of the α pathway is the p3 peptide, whose physiologic function is largely unknown.

Five different mutations of the APP gene have been determined to lead to early-onset Alzheimer disease. The biochemical effects of these mutations on APP processing have been studied extensively (see Figure 20–9; Table 20–2). All of these mutations lead to the production of excessive long Aβ, either through overall increased production of Aβ, or through increased production of $A\beta_{42–43}$. As previously indicated, the production of $A\beta_{42–43}$ is noteworthy because it is abundant in neuritic plaques, where it is associated with dystrophic neuronal processes, and it is the species of Aβ with the greatest tendency to aggregate into fibril form. These findings, together with discoveries of other genes associated with this disease, have led to the hypothesis that Alzheimer disease is caused by excessive extracellular $A\beta_{42–43}$, which forms insoluble filaments that ultimately lead to neural damage.

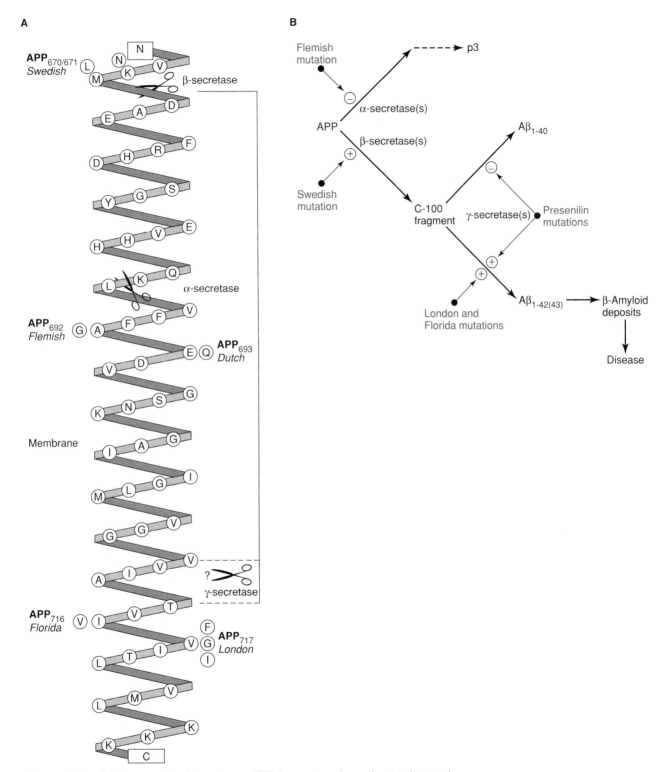

Figure 20–9. A. Diagram of the Aβ portion of APP shows sites of genetic mutations and sites of cleavage by β-,α-, and γ-secretases. **B.** Initial steps in the cascade leading from APP to Aβ. (Adapted with permission from Hardy J. 1997. Amyloid, the presenilins, and Alzheimer disease. *Trends Neurosci* 20:154.)

Table 20–2 Known Routes to Alzheimer Disease

Mutation	Biochemical Cause	Molecular Effect
Down syndrome	More APP production	More $A\beta_{1-42(43)}$ and more $A\beta_{1-40}$
$APP_{670/671}$ (Swedish)	Potentiation of β-secretase	More $A\beta_{1-42(43)}$ and more $A\beta_{1-40}$
APP_{692} (Flemish)	Inhibition of α-secretase	More $A\beta_{1-42(43)}$
APP_{716} (Florida)	Alteration of site of γ-secretase cut	More $A\beta_{1-42(43)}$
APP_{717} (London)	Alteration of site of γ-secretase cut	More $A\beta_{1-42(43)}$
PS1 mutations	Subtle alteration of APP processing	More $A\beta_{1-42(43)}$
PS2 mutations	Subtle alteration of APP processing	More $A\beta_{1-42(43)}$

How does $A\beta_{42-43}$ harm neurons? The application of aggregated, or filamentous, $A\beta$ is toxic to cultured neurons; this finding suggests a direct toxic effect of $A\beta$ aggregates in vivo. Moreover, $A\beta$ amyloid deposits are subject to attack by microglia, which may regard the plaques as unwanted foreign bodies. Under other circumstances, such as those associated with infection, microglial activity may be beneficial because microglia release cytokines and other mediators that can fight infection (see Chapters 2 and 11). However, these mediators do not destroy amyloid plaques, and if they are released over extended periods of time, they may ultimately damage neurons. $A\beta$-initiated neurotoxic and inflammatory processes may in addition cause the generation of free radicals, which are also damaging to neurons (see Chapter 21). The hypothetical scheme by which these pathologic processes may lead to familial forms of Alzheimer disease is represented in Figure 20–10. Because the more common nonfamilial forms of Alzheimer disease involve similar pathologic findings, they may be caused by related mechanisms.

ROLE OF PRESENILINS

Mutations in APP were the first genetic abnormalities to be linked to the inheritance of early-onset Alzheimer disease. However, germline mutations in two other genes—*presenilin 1* (PS1) and *presenilin 2* (PS2)—account for the majority of autosomal dominant cases of early-onset Alzheimer disease. PS1 and PS2 are membrane-associated proteins that are predicted to contain between 7 and 9 transmembrane segments and to have a long hydrophilic loop between the sixth and seventh transmembrane domains (Figure 20–11).

How might mutations in presenilins increase the risk for developing Alzheimer disease? Consistent with the previously described hypothesis, evidence has indicated that mutations in the presenilins lead to alterations in APP processing, which ultimately result in the production of more $A\beta_{42-43}$. For example, fibroblasts from individuals carrying mutant presenilin produce high levels of $A\beta_{42-43}$. Transgenic animals that overexpress mutant (but not wildtype) presenilin 1 also produce more $A\beta_{42-43}$ than normal mice. Moreover, cells transfected with mutant presenilin secrete significantly increased levels of $A\beta_{42-43}$. Although the exact biochemical function of the presenilins is unknown, research in the late 1990s suggests that presenilin 1 is itself either the γ-secretase or an essential cofactor for γ-secretase activity. Alternatively, presenilins may play an important role in the trafficking of APP to the appropriate cellular compartment for processing by γ-secretase.

One clue to the activity of the presenilins at the molecular level, albeit a clue difficult to relate to Alzheimer disease, has emerged from analysis of presenilin 1 knockout mice, which die during embryogenesis. This prenatal lethality may be explained by the need for presenilins in Notch signaling. Notch is a protein involved in the cell–cell interactions that specify cell fate during early stages of development. Findings drawn from the study of presenilin 1 knockout mice highlight an important point: the functional roles of a protein during development and during adulthood may be quite different. Presumably the evolution of various organisms led to the use of the same protein for different purposes, which may vary according to tissue type and the developmental stage of the organism.

ROLE OF ApoE

Apolipoprotein E (ApoE) is a 34-kDa protein that plays an important role in cholesterol transport, uptake, and redistribution. The three common alleles of ApoE (ϵ_2, ϵ_3, and ϵ_4) are inherited in a co-dominant fashion. The inheritance of each copy of the ϵ_4 allele tends to increase the risk and decrease the age of onset of Alzheimer disease. Conversely, each ϵ_2 allele results in lower risk and increased age of onset in most populations studied to date. Thus ϵ_2 is protective (Figure 20–12). Based on these observations, it has been proposed that in the general population the ApoE gene is an important modifier of the risk for common (nonfamilial) forms of Alzheimer disease; in fact, it may account for up to half of the genetic risk of developing the disease in some populations.

How might a lipoprotein have such a profound influence on the risk of developing Alzheimer disease? The most likely answer is that ApoE promotes amy-

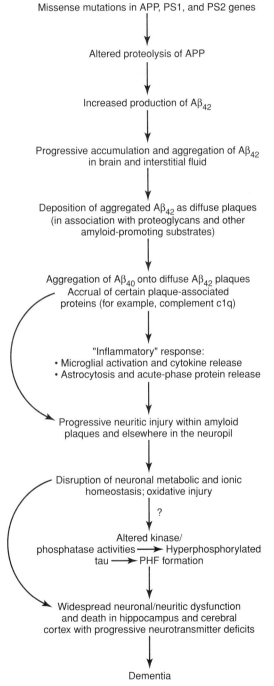

Missense mutations in APP, PS1, and PS2 genes

↓

Altered proteolysis of APP

↓

Increased production of Aβ$_{42}$

↓

Progressive accumulation and aggregation of Aβ$_{42}$ in brain and interstitial fluid

↓

Deposition of aggregated Aβ$_{42}$ as diffuse plaques (in association with proteoglycans and other amyloid-promoting substrates)

↓

Aggregation of Aβ$_{40}$ onto diffuse Aβ$_{42}$ plaques Accrual of certain plaque-associated proteins (for example, complement c1q)

↓

"Inflammatory" response:
• Microglial activation and cytokine release
• Astrocytosis and acute-phase protein release

↓

Progressive neuritic injury within amyloid plaques and elsewhere in the neuropil

↓

Disruption of neuronal metabolic and ionic homeostasis; oxidative injury

↓ ?

Altered kinase/phosphatase activities ⟶ Hyperphosphorylated tau ⟶ PHF formation

↓

Widespread neuronal/neuritic dysfunction and death in hippocampus and cerebral cortex with progressive neurotransmitter deficits

↓

Dementia

Figure 20–10. Hypothetical pathogenic processes in Alzheimer disease. (Adapted with permission from Selkoe DJ. 1999. Translating cell biology into therapeutic advances in Alzheimer disease. *Nature* 399[suppl]:A23.)

loidogenesis, or the generation of an Aβ-containing plaque. This process might occur either because the lipoprotein seeds a reaction that augments amyloid production, or because it stabilizes the aggregate form of Aβ, or both. Three principal lines of evidence support the hypothesis that ApoE promotes amyloidogenesis. First, unlike wildtype mice, mice that lack the gene for ApoE are protected against amyloid deposition. Second, in vitro experiments have demonstrated that ApoE can indeed increase deposition of Aβ and enhance the ability of Aβ to form fibrils. Of the three ApoE alleles, ε$_4$ promotes the greatest amount of fibril formation—a finding that is consistent with the genetic and epidemiologic data previously presented. Third, transgenic mice that overexpress various forms of Aβ develop more plaques when they also overexpress ApoE$_4$ (the protein product of ε$_4$).

Although a great deal of experimental evidence supports the hypothesis that ApoE$_4$ increases the risk for Alzheimer disease by promoting amyloid deposition and fibrillation, different hypotheses about the role of ApoE in Alzheimer disease have been proposed. It has been hypothesized, for example, that ApoE$_2$ binds to amyloid and facilitates its removal from the extracellular space, whereas ApoE$_4$ is less effective in this capacity. It also has been postulated that ApoE$_2$ and ApoE$_3$ may bind the microtubule-associated tau protein, and thereby prevent its hyperphosphorylation, whereas ApoE$_4$ performs this tau-protecting function less effectively. Although the validity of these alternative hypotheses must be tested, both hypotheses hold that ApoE acts as an amyloid deposit-enhancing agent.

ROLE OF OTHER GENES

Mutations in the gene for α$_2$-macroglobulin (α$_2$M) have tentatively been linked to an increased risk for developing late-onset Alzheimer disease. Normal α$_2$M is a serum pan-protease inhibitor that may function to help inactivate proteases that might have toxic effects on neurons and other cell types. A more direct role in controlling the amount of Aβ deposition is suggested by the presence of α$_2$M in neuritic plaques, its ability to bind directly to Aβ, and the finding that cells take up and degrade the α$_2$M–Aβ complex. The binding of α$_2$M to Aβ may further promote Aβ clearance or its sequestration from the extracellular space. Moreover, α$_2$M prevents the formation of Aβ fibrils in vitro. Thus polymorphisms in α$_2$M may make the protein less efficient in clearing Aβ and in preventing fibril formation. The various alleles of ApoE may interact synergistically with α$_2$M mutations to promote the development of Alzheimer disease, perhaps because the transport of the

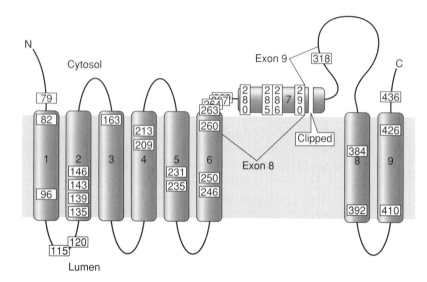

Figure 20–11. Proposed structure of presenilin 1. Sites of many mutations that have been linked to early-onset Alzheimer disease are indicated. The numbers in boxes refer to the amino acid residues affected in these mutations. Presenilin 2 is highly homologous to presenilin 1. (Adapted with permission from Hardy J. 1997. Amyloid, the presenilins, and Alzheimer disease. *Trends Neurosci* 20:154.)

α_2M–Aβ complex into cells requires the same receptor that ApoE uses to enter cells. Accordingly, ApoE$_4$ or other forms of ApoE may compete with the α_2M–Aβ complex for binding to the ApoE receptor and transport into cells that clear debris from the extracellular space.

Despite the importance of tau in the formation of neurofibrillary tangles, thus far no mutation in tau has been associated with Alzheimer disease. However, mutations in tau are found in families with FTDP. It is believed that these mutations enhance tau's ability to be phosphorylated, and in turn lead to the hyperphosphorylated state of the protein that is characteristic of the disease. The brains of patients with FTDP exhibit widespread neurofibrillary tangles in the absence of significant Aβ deposits—a finding that suggests that the development of neuritic plaques is not a consequence of the formation of neurofibrillary tangles. Current genetic and biologic evidence suggests instead that alterations in tau in the context of Alzheimer disease occurs as a consequence of Aβ accumulation. Thus the hyperphosphorylation of tau and the generation of neurofibrillary tangles may represent a common final pathogenic mechanism that leads to the development of Alzheimer disease, FTDP, and related dementias (see Figure 20–10); however, this theory remains conjectural.

Perhaps it is most appropriate to think of these dementias as a collection of heterogeneous genetic disorders that result in similar patterns of end-stage neuronal death by means of related pathophysiologic mechanisms. Mutations in presenilins and APP are involved in familial forms of Alzheimer disease, and mutations in tau are involved in FTDP. Although specific alleles of ApoE are important contributors to common forms of Alzheimer disease, it is not known whether the remaining risk factors are mutations in other genes not yet identified or environmental exposures. Identification of these determinants should facilitate the development of definitive treatment of these dementias as well as preventive measures.

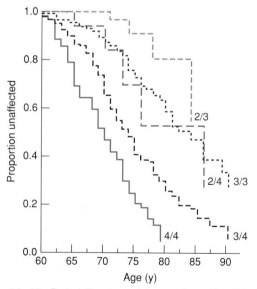

Figure 20–12. Probability of remaining unaffected by Alzheimer disease as a function of ApoE genotype. Note that an increased incidence and decreased age of onset of the disease occurs among individuals with two copies of ApoE$_4$, whereas those with even one copy of ApoE$_2$ are relatively protected. The numbers on the curves designate alleles. (Adapted with permission from Strittmatter WJ, Roses AD. 1996. Apolipoprotein E and Alzheimer disease. *Annu Rev Neurosci* 19:53.)

TREATMENT

Available therapies for Alzheimer disease are not particularly effective. Consequently, intense research efforts in the pharmaceutical industry and in academic settings have been devoted to examining the etiology of Alzheimer disease and related dementias to develop agents that will prevent or retard the disease process. Currently used agents include drugs that increase cholinergic neurotransmission and antiinflammatory mediations. Moreover, several strategies are aimed at developing drugs that are designed to target molecules involved in suspected disease processes themselves, such as Aβ formation.

Cholinergic agents   Because cholinergic neurons of the nucleus basalis are among those on which Alzheimer disease has the most impact, and because cholinergic activity regulates memory processing, enhancement of cholinergic functioning has been regarded as a promising strategy for improving cognitive function in patients with Alzheimer disease. The earliest attempts to increase cholinergic functioning involved the administration of precursors of acetylcholine, **choline** and **lecithin,** which provides a source of choline. Although a similar strategy has proven effective for other neurodegenerative diseases, namely the use of L-dopa to improve the functioning of individuals with **Parkinson disease** (see Chapter 14), multiple studies found that cholinergic precursors were not effective in the treatment of Alzheimer disease.

Other approaches aimed at enhancing cholinergic function have involved the inhibition of acetylcholinesterase activity and the use of cholinergic agonists (see Chapter 9 for a general discussion of cholinergic systems). Two acetylcholinesterase inhibitors are currently approved for the treatment of Alzheimer disease in the United States: **tacrine** and **donepezil** (Figure 20–13). These agents do not reverse the course of the disease but can produce small and usually short-term cognitive improvements in some patients. However, these agents appear to have a marginal effect on the overall quality of life for patient and caregivers. The use of cho-

linergic agonists has been hampered by the lack of clinically tor agonists are undergoing clinical trials. Among these are subtype-specific muscarinic agonists, such as **xanomeline,** which has selectivity for M_1 receptors. Unfortunately, early reports indicate that these agents may be no more effective than tacrine and donepezil.

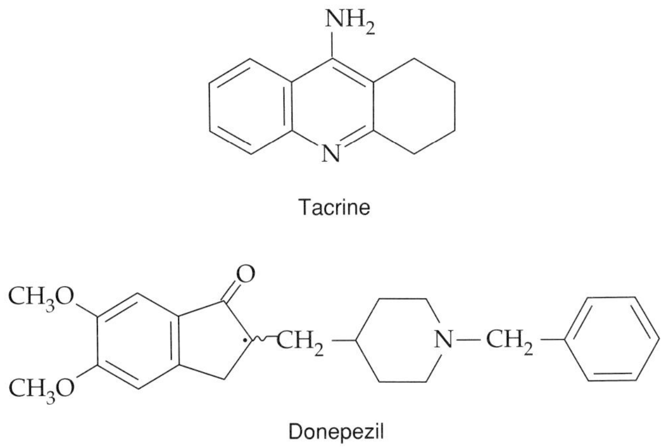

Antiinflammatory agents and antioxidants   The buildup of Aβ into plaques appears to result in local microglial and astrocytic activation, with concomitant release of cytokines and acute-phase proteins. Thus inflammatory processes are implicated in the neurodegeneration that is characteristic of Alzheimer disease. Consistent with this suspicion, large epidemiologic studies have suggested that patients who have taken nonsteroidal antiinflammatory drugs (**NSAIDs**) on a regular basis—for example, for arthritis—have a reduced risk of developing Alzheimer disease. The Baltimore Longitudinal Study of Aging, for example, reported a reduced relative risk of 0.40 for individuals who used NSAIDs for 2 years, compared with controls who did not use NSAIDs. These drugs are inhibitors of cyclooxygenase, a key enzyme in arachidonic acid signaling (see Chapters 5 and 19). Because some studies have not confirmed this association, prospective trials will be required to confirm or refute whether NSAIDs are effective in preventing this disease.

A related treatment strategy currently under investigation involves the use of antioxidants and free-radical scavengers. Activated microglia secrete hydrogen peroxide, superoxides, and hydroxyl radicals; these are useful in combating foreign cells or organisms but can damage neurons. Thus it is possible that antioxidants and free-radical scavengers may serve a protective function in Alzheimer disease and in other neurodegenerative diseases. Indeed, results of a therapeutic trial of **vitamin E (α-tocopherol)** suggest that this substance may cause a slower clinical progression of Alzheimer disease.

Estrogen and neurotrophic factors   During the mid-1990s, a wave of reports suggested a correlation between estrogen replacement and a decreased risk of developing Alzheimer disease in postmenopausal women. That estrogen replacement might forestall the onset of Alzheimer disease is a biologically plausible idea. Estrogen is also reported to increase synaptic spine density in hippocampal neurons of artificially postmenopausal (ovariectomized) rats. However, all human studies have been retrospective. Thus whether women who chose to take estrogen replacement therapy made additional lifestyle changes, such as adopting a balanced diet or engaging in adequate exercise, that might reduce the risk of developing Alzheimer disease is unknown. Ultimately, double-blind, placebo-controlled trials of

Figure 20–13. Structures of tacrine and donepezil.

randomly assigned subjects will be required to determine whether estrogen replacement therapy is an effective means of reducing the risk for this disease in elderly women.

Because neurotrophic factors promote the survival of neurons, they also are under consideration for use in the treatment of neurodegenerative diseases (see Chapter 11). However, these agents do not readily cross the blood–brain barrier. Moreover, because senile plaques are associated not only with neuronal death but also with abnormal sprouting and growth of neuronal processes, neurotrophic factors may not provide adequate treatment of Alzheimer disease. Yet further clinical investigation of their efficacy is warranted, given their known potency in supporting neuronal survival.

Inhibition of Aβ production and tau phosphorylation

The development of agents that alter the production of Aβ, with the intent of slowing overall Aβ formation or perhaps specifically preventing the production of the harmful $Aβ_{42-43}$ form, represents an exciting approach to treatment. Agents that inhibit β- or γ-secretase activity, as well as agents that inhibit the aggregation of Aβ into insoluble deposits, currently are being tested in mouse models of Alzheimer disease. The use of agents that increase α-secretase activity, or directly modulate the physiologic activity of presenilins, may represent alternative pharmacologic strategies. Agents such as cyclin-dependent kinase 5 or glycogen synthase kinase 3 (see Chapters 5 and 15), which inhibit the protein kinases responsible for the hyperphosphorylation of tau that is characteristic of Alzheimer disease and FTDP, may prove to be similarly effective.

Other therapeutic strategies

Further knowledge about the mechanisms by which ApoE and $α_2M$ act may lead to methods of controlling senile plaque deposition. For example, because individuals with the $ε_2$ allele of ApoE have a lower risk of developing Alzheimer disease, an active effort is under way to develop methods of delivering $ApoE_2$ to the brain. Two recent studies have suggested that **statins,** developed to control serum cholesterol, may prevent Alzheimer disease.

Several drugs that interact with specific glutamate receptor subtypes have been used in phase II clinical trials to enhance cognitive performance with limited success. As mentioned earlier in this chapter, LTP is a cellular mechanism believed to be involved in learning and memory. Because LTP is typically triggered by the activation of NMDA receptors, investigators have proposed that agents that enhance NMDA receptor function, such as **D-cycloserine,** a partial agonist (see Chapter 7), might be beneficial. However, early clinical trial results have been discouraging. A similar strategy has involved the use of agents that enhance the function of AMPA receptors. These receptors help trigger LTP by providing the requisite depolarization and are themselves modified during LTP. One class of such agents is represented by small benzamide compounds termed **ampakines.** These compounds enhance excitatory synaptic responses by slowing the deactivation rate of AMPA receptors and have been reported to enhance memory function in animal models. However, their clinical usefulness in the treatment of Alzheimer disease remains to be established. **Nootropics,** a class of agents postulated to enhance cognition and currently in use in Europe, include **piracetam, pramiracetam, oxiracetam,** and **aniracetam.** Aniracetam, like ampakines, enhances synaptic responses by altering the kinetics of AMPA receptors. The exact mechanisms of action of the other nootropics remain unknown; however, they may involve enhanced release of acetylcholine, dopamine, or norepinephrine. Data regarding the clinical efficacy of these compounds have been contradictory, but current phase III trials in the United States should assist in determining their usefulness.

Drugs designed to enhance synaptic transmission are likely to represent mere stop-gap measures in the treatment of Alzheimer disease and related dementias because they do not address the pathologic processing of APP and the hyperphosphorylation of tau. Thus, especially when used alone, they are unlikely to slow the progression of these diseases. However, the development of such agents is worthwhile because any enhancement of cognitive function, even for a limited period of time, may improve the quality of life of affected individuals and their caregivers. Furthermore, such drugs may be of value to elderly individuals without Alzheimer disease who experience moderate memory loss.

Future treatment and prevention

Ultimately scientists hope to attain a complete understanding of the molecular biology of Alzheimer disease and related dementias so that treatment might be aimed at the causes of these diseases. The rapid progress in our understanding of the molecular basis of memory should facilitate the development of novel compounds designed to improve memory performance and cognitive function. Moreover, it is hoped that the identification of individuals with an inherited predisposition to dementia will lead to much earlier interventions. Indeed, research suggests that a preventative approach might work; for example, the immunization of mice with Aβ before the onset of detectable neuropathology has prevented the formation of plaques and neuritic dystrophy in mouse models of Alzheimer disease. These findings and many others suggest that future editions of this book will include proven therapies for the dementias in place of promising avenues of research.

SELECTED READING

Andertson B, Dayanandan R, Killick R, Lovestone S. 2000. Does dysregulation of the Notch and wingless/Wnt pathways underlie the pathogenesis of Alzheimer's disease? *Mol Med Today* 6:54–59.

Bales KR, Verina T, Dodel RC, et al. 1997. Lack of apolipoprotein E dramatically reduces amyloid-β-peptide deposition. *Nature Genetics* 17:263–264.

Bartus RT. 2000. On neurodegenerative diseases, models, and treatment strategies: lessons learned and lessons forgotten a generation following the cholinergic hypothesis. *Exp Neurol* 163:495–529.

Blacker D, Wilcox MA, Laird M, et al. 1998. Alpha-2 macroglobulin is genetically associated with Alzheimer disease. *Nature Genetics* 19:357–360.

Cahill L, McGaugh JL. 1998. Mechanisms of emotional arousal and lasting declarative memory. *Trends Neurosci* 21:294–299.

Davis KL. 1998. Future therapeutic approaches to Alzheimer disease. *J Clin Psychiatry* 59(suppl)11:14–16.

Hardy J. 1997. Amyloid, the presenilins, and Alzheimer disease. *Trends Neurosci* 20:154–159.

Hebb DO. 1949. *The Organization of Behavior: A Neuropsychological Theory.* New York: Wiley.

Heutink P. 2000. Untangling tau-related dementia. *Human Mol Genet* 9:979–986.

Hutton M, Lendon CL, Rizzu P, et al. 1998. Association of missense and 5′-splice-site mutations in tau with the inherited dementia FTDP-17. *Nature* 393:702–705.

Kalicki AC (ed). 1987. *Confronting Alzheimer Disease.* Owings Mills, MD: Rynd Communications.

Lee VM-Y, Trojanowski JQ. 1999. Neurogenerative tauopathies: human disease and transgenic mouse models. *Neuron* 24:507–510

Luscher C, Nicoll RA, Malenka RC. 2000. Synaptic plasticity and dynamic modulation of the postsynaptic membrane. *Nature Neurosci* 3:545–550.

Malenka RC. 1995. LTP and LTD: Dynamic and interactive processes of synaptic plasticity. *Neuroscientist* 1:35–42.

Malenka RC, Nicoll RA. 1999. LTP: A decade of progress? *Science* 285:1870–1874.

Milner B, Corkin S, Teuber HL. 1968. Further analysis of the hippocampal amnesic syndrome: 14-year follow-up study of HM. *Neuropsychologia* 6:215–34.

Milner B, Squire LR, Kandel ER. 1998. Cognitive neuroscience and the study of memory. *Neuron* 20:445–468.

Morrison-Bogorad M, Phelps C, Buckholtz N. 1997. Alzheimer disease comes of age. *JAMA* 277:837–840.

National Institute on Aging. 1996. *Progress Report on Alzheimer Disease, 1996.* Washington, DC: NIH Publication 96–4173.

Neve RL, Robakis NK. 1998. Alzheimer's disease: a re-examination of the amyloid hypothesis. *Trends Neurosci* 21:15–19.

Nicoll RA, Kauer JA, Malenka RC. 1988. The current excitement in LTP. *Neuron* 1:97–103.

Price DL, Tanzi RE, Borchelt DR, Sisodia SS. 1998. Alzheimer disease: Genetic studies and transgenic models. *Annu Rev Genet* 32: 461–493.

Routtenberg A Cantallops I, Zaffuot S. et al. 2000. Enhanced learning after genetic overexpression of a brain growth protein. *Proc Natl Acad Sci USA.* 97:7657–7662.

Scoville WB, Milner B. 1957. Loss of recent memory after bilateral hippocampal lesions. *J Neurol Neurosurg Psychiatry* 10:11–21.

Selkoe DJ. 1997. Alzheimer disease: Genotypes, phenotype, and treatment. *Science* 275:630–631.

Selkoe DJ. 1999. Translating cell biology into therapeutic advances in Alzheimer disease. *Nature* 399(suppl):A23–A31.

Selkoe DJ. 2000. Notch and presenilins in vertebrates and invertebrates: implications for neuronal development and degeneration. *Curr Opin Neurobiol* 10:50–57.

Shie SH, Hayashi Y, Petralia RS, et al. 1999. Rapid spine delivery and redistribution of AMPA receptors after synaptic NMDA receptor activation. *Science* 284:1811–1816.

Small GW. 1998. Treatment of Alzheimer disease: Current approaches and promising developments. *Am J Med* 104: 32S–38S.

Squire LR, Kandel ER. 1999. *Memory: From Mind to Molecules.* New York: WH Freeman.

Stewart WF, Kawas C, Corrada M, Metter EJ. 1997. Risk of Alzheimer disease and duration of NSAID use. *Neurology* 48: 626–632.

Strittmatter WJ, Roses AD. 1996. Apolipoprotein E and Alzheimer disease. *Annu Rev Neurosci* 19:53–77.

Tanzi RE, Parson AB. 2000. *Decoding Darkness: The Search for the Genetic Causes of Alzheimer's Disease.* New York: Perseus Book Group.

Trojanowski JZ, Clark CM, Schmidt ML, et al. 1997. Strategies for improving the postmortem neuropathological diagnosis of Alzheimer disease. *Neurobiol Aging* 18:S75–S79.

van Leuven F. 2000. Single and multiple transgenic mice as models for Alzheimer's disease. *Prog Neurobiol* 61: 305–312.

Wellington CL, Hayden MR. 2000. Caspases and neurodegeneration: on the cutting edge of new therapeutic approaches. *Clin Genet* 57:1–10.

Yan R, Bienkowski MJ, Shuck ME, et al. 1999. Membrane-anchored aspartyl protease with Alzheimer's disease beta-secretase activity. *Nature* 402:533–537.

Chapter 21
Seizures and Stroke

KEY CONCEPTS

- When the supply of oxygen to the brain is disrupted, a complex series of biochemical events takes place leading to neuronal injury. Such events are triggered by the depolarization of neurons and increases in extracellular glutamate concentration—a process called excitotoxicity.

- A large increase in intracellular calcium and overactivation of calcium-dependent enzymes are important factors in causing neuronal damage during excitotoxicity.

- Formation of free radicals and genetically programmed cell death, called apoptosis, may also contribute to neuronal damage during strokes.

- Despite increased understanding of the biochemical processes underlying excitotoxicity, the best therapy for stroke remains rapidly restoring the brain's blood supply and preventing the formation of clots and emboli.

- A seizure is caused by the abnormal synchronous firing of large ensembles of neurons.

- Epilepsy refers to any neurologic disorder that is characterized by recurrent seizures.

- Seizures can be classified as focal, which indicates that the initial abnormal firing is limited to a specific area in one hemisphere, or general, which indicates that a large population of neurons in both hemispheres is involved immediately at the start of the seizure.

- Seizures are thought to occur because of a change in the brain's delicate balance of excitatory and inhibitory synaptic processes. This change can be caused by a large number of different brain insults, including tumors, strokes, and head injury.

- Many forms of epilepsy have a genetic component, although the inheritance of epilepsy is rarely simple.

- Most anticonvulsants work by modifying the behavior of sodium channels or calcium channels or by enhancing GABA-mediated inhibitory synaptic transmission.

Vertebrate neurons are exquisitely specialized for the functions they perform. As explained in previous chapters, a single neuron may receive information from and relay information to thousands of other neurons; consequently the nervous system is capable of remarkably complex functions. Moreover, the brisk flux of ions across neural membranes permits extremely rapid interneuronal signaling. However, this specialization comes at a cost. A tremendous amount of energy is required to maintain ionic gradients across the membranes of the approximately 100 billion neurons that comprise the human brain. Although the brain represents only 2% of the body's total mass, it uses approximately 20% of the body's oxygen supply, and blood flow to the brain accounts for about 15% of total cardiac output. *Ischemia,* or insufficient blood supply, results in oxygen and glucose deprivation and in the buildup of potentially toxic metabolites such as lactic acid and CO_2. Interruption of blood flow to the brain can lead to complete loss of consciousness within 10 seconds, the approximate amount of time required to consume the oxygen contained in the brain.

When neurons are deprived of the nourishment they require, they quickly become unable to maintain their resting potentials, and thus are prompted to fire. Their firing triggers the release of neurotransmitters, which in turn promotes depolarization in neighboring neurons. Such activity sets the stage for a destructive cycle of neuronal activation, neurotransmitter release, and further activation. Prolonged periods of neuronal activation can lead to the disruption of ionic gradients, massive Ca^{2+} influx, cellular swelling, activation of cellular proteases and lipases, and eventually widespread neuronal death. Ischemia of only a few minutes' duration can result in permanent brain damage.

Stroke, or ischemia of brain tissue caused by obstruction or hemorrhage, is the focus of the first half of this chapter. The exquisite vulnerability of neurons to energy deprivation caused by stroke results in vast medical, economic, and personal costs. In the United States alone, roughly 550,000 strokes occur each year. Approximately 150,000 of these strokes are fatal, which makes stroke the third-leading cause of death in the United States. Survivors of stroke often are beset by serious long-term disabilities, including paralysis and disruption of higher cognitive functions such as speech. Individuals with such disabilities may be unable to resume work and other daily activities, and often require extensive long-term care by health care professionals or friends and family.

The second half of this chapter is devoted to seizure-related disorders such as **epilepsy.** Seizures are characterized by uncontrolled firing of sets of neurons in the brain and can have devastating consequences. Like stroke, seizure disorders are common: they affect approximately 2.5 million individuals in the United States, many of whom are children. Fortunately, the treatment of seizures has steadily improved with the introduction of safer and more effective anticonvulsant agents.

STROKE

The term *stroke,* or cerebrovascular accident (CVA), broadly refers to neurologic symptoms and signs that result when blood flow to brain tissue is interrupted. The two primary types of stroke are occlusive and hemorrhagic. An *occlusive* stroke is caused by the blockage of a blood vessel. Vascular occlusion, which generally restricts blood flow to a discrete area of the brain, results in neurologic deficits and in a loss of functions controlled by the affected region. Occlusive strokes typically are caused by embolic, atherosclerotic, or thrombotic occlusion of cerebral vessels. A *hemorrhagic* stroke is caused by bleeding from a vessel. Epidural, subdural, and subarachnoid bleeding often results from head trauma or the rupture of an aneurysm. In addition to the damage caused by the loss of blood supply to affected areas of the brain, hemorrhages can cause damage by increasing intracranial pressure. Moreover, through mechanisms that are not completely understood, subarachnoid hemorrhage can cause reactive vasospasm of cerebral surface vessels, which in turn can lead to a further reduction in blood supply.

Intraparenchymal hemorrhage may be caused by acute elevations in blood pressure or by a variety of disorders that weaken blood vessels. Chronic hypertension is the most common predisposing factor, but coagulation disorders, brain tumors that promote the development of fragile blood vessels, and the use of cocaine or amphetamines—both of which cause rapid elevation of blood pressure—are among the risk factors for intraparenchymal hemorrhages. Intraparenchymal hemorrhaging can lead to the formation of blood clots (hematomas) in the cerebrum, cerebellum, or brain stem, which in turn may limit the blood supply to nearby brain regions and exacerbate the injurious effects of a stroke.

BASIC MECHANISMS OF EXCITOTOXICITY

When blood flow to brain tissue ceases, conduits through which oxygen and nutrients enter and potentially toxic metabolites exit are severed. Interference with these conduits triggers many biochemical changes in the affected area of the brain. Predictable changes in the extracellular environment rapidly lead to a large number of detectable cellular disruptions: ion gradients dissipate, ion channels open and shut, Ca^{2+} pours into cells, numerous second messenger systems are activated, and many biochemical signals are produced in unusually high concentrations. Many of these biochemical changes are quite harmful to neurons and contribute to the neuronal death that results from prolonged ischemia. However, some of the sequelae of ischemia may have little effect on neuronal survival and some may even have neuroprotective effects, that is, responses to ischemic insult that neurons produce in self-defense. Accordingly, strategies designed to minimize infarct related neural damage must be based on a clear understanding of how each ischemia-related process affects neuronal survival.

Experimentally, a process is demonstrated to promote neural damage if interference with the process significantly decreases neural damage. It is widely believed, for example, that Ca^{2+} entry into neurons significantly contributes to ischemia-related toxicity because removal of Ca^{2+} from the extracellular medium greatly reduces hypoxic damage to neurons in culture. Consequently, antagonists of both NMDA receptors and voltage-gated Ca^{2+} channels are effective in preventing excitotoxic damage in the laboratory, and their use in the treatment of acute stroke has been tested in clinical trials.

Although the significance of many ischemia-related occurrences is not yet completely understood, the series of events that occur during an ischemic episode are outlined in the sections that follow (Figure 21–1).

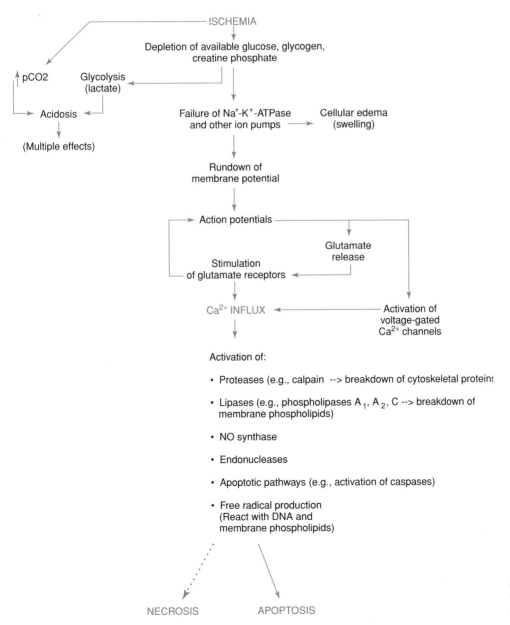

Figure 21–1. Events that lead to cell death, including apoptosis and necrosis, after ischemia.

DEPLETION OF ENERGY STORES

Under normal conditions, the brain uses oxygen and glucose to produce adenosine triphosphate (ATP) through the processes of oxidative phosphorylation and glycolysis. As previously mentioned, a complete interruption of brain blood flow can deplete the brain's supply of oxygen within 10 seconds. In the absence of oxygen, oxidative phosphorylation ceases, and anaerobic glycolysis becomes the only source of ATP for neurons. Anaerobic glycolysis supplies less than 10% of the ATP garnered from complete oxidation of glucose and leads to the production of lactic acid. Moreover, without incoming blood to supply glucose, neurons must rely on the glycolytic processing of preexisting stores of glucose and glycogen. During ischemia, these reserves are depleted within 2 to 3 minutes. Phosphocreatine stores also are consumed during this time; thus ischemia can lead to the depletion of neuronal ATP within minutes. Because the basal metabolic activity of neurons is so great, such depletion rapidly leads to serious consequences.

FAILURE OF ION PUMPS

One of the most important consequences of the loss of available ATP is the failure of ATP-dependent ion pumps and the subsequent dissipation of membrane potential. As discussed in Chapter 3, the maintenance of neuronal resting membrane potential is ultimately dependent on Na^+-K^+-ATPase, which exports Na^+ and imports K^+ against their concentration gradients at the cost of ATP. Although very large neurons can maintain a negative resting potential for some time after the inhibition of Na^+-K^+-ATPase, small and highly branched neurons of the mammalian brain are extremely vulnerable to Na^+-K^+-ATPase inhibition because of their very large surface-area-to-volume ratio. Consequently, many neurons of the CNS depolarize rapidly after ATP depletion.

The cessation of Na^+-K^+-ATPase activity has other consequences in addition to depolarization. Many ion pumps, including the Na^+–Ca^{2+} exchanger, are dependent on the transmembrane Na^+ gradient for their activity. As this gradient declines, so does the activity of these exchange systems; subsequently, further disruptions of ionic equilibrium occur. Moreover, many ATP-dependent ion pumps, such as ATP-dependent Ca^{2+} pumps, are disabled when neuronal energy stores are depleted.

DEPOLARIZATION AND FIRING

Failure of the Na^+-K^+-ATPase pump leads to cellular depolarization and eventually to the firing of action potentials. As such firing escalates, further depolarization occurs, causing an increased rundown of ionic gradients and the release of neurotransmitter. Released neurotransmitter (excitatory neurotransmitter such as glutamate) can trigger neighboring neurons to depolarize and fire action potentials, further extending the injurious chain of events.

Neural damage during ischemia also can be caused by the failure of neurotransmitter transporters, particularly of those that transport glutamate. As explained in Chapter 7, glutamate transporters, which are expressed by glial and neural cells, assist in terminating the actions of synaptically released glutamate by removing glutamate from the synaptic cleft. This reuptake process depends on ATP; thus when ATP stores in the brain become depleted in response to ischemia, the functioning of these transporters is compromised. Subsequently, higher-than-normal levels of glutamate accumulate in synapses and cause activation of glutamate receptors for abnormally long periods of time.

INCREASES IN INTRACELLULAR Ca^{2+}

Under normal conditions, concentrations of cytosolic Ca^{2+} are under extremely tight regulation. In a neuron at rest, these concentrations are approximately 100 nM, whereas extracellular Ca^{2+} concentrations are approximately 1 mM. With extracellular Ca^{2+} approaching concentrations that are about 10,000 times greater than cytosolic concentrations, there is normally a tremendous driving force for Ca^{2+} to enter the neuronal cytoplasm. The great effort that a neuron expends in maintaining a low cytosolic Ca^{2+} concentration is compromised during ischemia (Figure 21–2). Ca^{2+} that enters the cytosol is removed by a variety of mechanisms, including the ATP-dependent Ca^{2+} pumps and Na^+–Ca^{2+} exchangers previously mentioned. Both of these pumps are ultimately ATP-dependent because ATP-dependent maintenance of the Na^+ gradient is required for the effective performance of the Na^+–Ca^{2+} exchanger; indeed, as the Na^+ gradient dissipates, it may even reverse and cause Ca^{2+} to be pumped into the cell. Depolarization also can lead to the opening of various voltage-gated Ca^{2+} channels, and glutamate release from neighboring cells can induce the entry of Ca^{2+} through NMDA receptors.

ACTIVATION OF ENZYMES BY Ca^{2+}

Increases in neuronal Ca^{2+} may be the ultimate cause of ischemia-related neuronal death. When Ca^{2+} entry is restricted in vitro, for example, through the removal of Ca^{2+} from the extracellular medium or through the blockage of certain Ca^{2+}-conducting ion channels, neurons are protected against excitotoxic damage. More-over, neuronal subpopulations that express atypical, Ca^{2+}-conducting AMPA receptors exhibit heightened vulnerability to **kainate**-induced toxicity. Kainate is a glutamate receptor agonist that causes massive depolarization of neurons, which in turn causes neuronal death.

Why does a high cytosolic Ca^{2+} concentration induce neuronal death? This question remains under investigation, but there are several clues to the answer. One clue lies in the fact that Ca^{2+} functions as a signaling molecule (see Chapter 5). Under normal conditions, a small rise in cytoplasm Ca^{2+} concentrations signals to the neuron that an important event has occurred; for example, it may signal the depolarization and activation of voltage-dependent Ca^{2+} channels, or the activation of second messenger systems that have triggered the release of Ca^{2+} from intracellular stores. As described in previous chapters, many neuronal enzymes, and hence

many neural processes, are poised to respond to this signal. It is possible that excessive activation of these various enzymes and processes, caused by inappropriate Ca^{2+} levels in cells, may contribute to neuronal stress and death.

Among the many enzymes that are suspected to play a role in Ca^{2+}-mediated neuronal damage are *Ca^{2+}-activated proteases,* particularly calpain, which can produce widespread cellular damage. Calpain breaks down the cytoskeletal proteins spectrin and microtubule-associated protein 2 (MAP2). Destruction of these proteins leads in turn to severe cytoskeletal damage. *Phospholipases,* such as phospholipase A_2 (PLA$_2$), also can be activated by Ca^{2+}. PLA$_2$ targets membrane phospholipids and hydrolyzes the bond between the fatty acid portions and the polar head groups. When activated en masse, phospholipases may disrupt membrane integrity by changing the numbers and proportions of phospho-

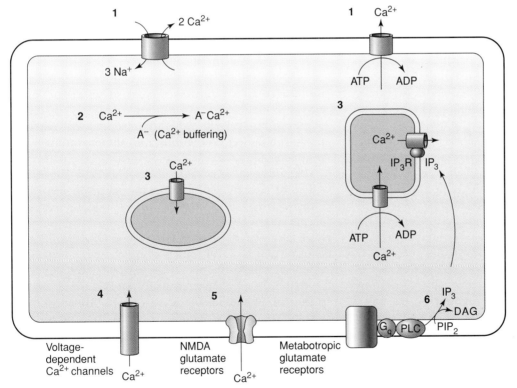

Figure 21–2. Ca^{2+} homeostasis in neurons. **1.** Ca^{2+} is removed from the cytoplasm by Ca^{2+}–Na^+ exchangers and adenosine triphosphate (ATP)-dependent pumps. **2.** Ca^{2+} is buffered by intracellular anions (A$^-$). **3.** Subsequently it is sequestered in organelles, such as mitochondria and endoplasmic reticulum, in an ATP-dependent fashion. During ischemia, Ca^{2+} pumps fail because of the lack of ATP. **4.** Decreases in membrane potential lead to Ca^{2+} entry through voltage-dependent Ca^{2+} channels. Release of glutamate by neighboring cells permits Ca^{2+} entry through NMDA and other Ca^{2+}-conducting glutamate receptors (**5**) and activates G_q-coupled metabotropic glutamate receptors (**6**), which increase the formation of inositol triphosphate (IP$_3$) and the release of Ca^{2+} from internal stores. ADP, adenosine diphosphate; PLC, phospholipase C; PIP$_2$, phosphatidylinositol bisphosphate; IP$_3$R, IP$_3$ receptor; DAG, diacylglycerol.

lipids in the neuronal membrane. Moreover, the resulting free fatty acids, which include arachidonic acid, are metabolized by cyclooxygenases and lipoxygenases to yield numerous biologically active products, such as prostaglandins (see Chapter 5). The highly reactive $\bullet O_2^-$ radical is formed as part of these reactions.

Nitric oxide synthase (NOS), which is activated upon binding to Ca^{2+}–calmodulin complexes, produces gaseous nitric oxide (NO) from arginine. As explained in Chapter 5, NO is an important messenger molecule; among its other actions, it activates guanylyl cyclase, which catalyzes the formation of cGMP. NO also can inhibit many cellular enzymes, particularly those containing iron–sulfur complexes. Many enzymes that contain iron–sulfur complexes, such as mitochondrial NADH–ubiquitone oxidoreductase and NADH–succinate oxidoreductase, are crucial to metabolism. Other reactions of the NO molecule—especially its reaction with oxygen to yield peroxynitrite—also may be important in neuronal demise because they may lead to the formation of free radicals.

The importance of NOS activation in neuronal injury has been tested through the use of specific NOS inhibitors, such as **L-nitroarginine**. Initial studies produced inconsistent results: NOS inhibitors displayed neuroprotective effects in some experiments, especially in experiments conducted in cell culture, and produced either no effect or a detrimental effect in others. These conflicting results most likely were attributable to the multiple roles and sources of NO in the brain. Three different isoforms of NOS exist, each of which is the product of a distinct gene. Neuronal NOS (nNOS) is expressed exclusively in neurons, endothelial NOS (eNOS) originally was identified in endothelial cells, and inducible NOS (iNOS) originally was identified in certain immune system cells. Some neurons may express eNOS and iNOS in addition to nNOS. NO produced by eNOS acts as an endothelial relaxing factor: it promotes the relaxation of the smooth muscle surrounding arterioles and leads to vasodilation and increased blood flow.

Gene knockout technology has helped to elucidate the roles of the various NOS isoforms in neuronal injury. Compared with their wildtype counterparts, mice deficient in the nNOS gene typically have smaller infarct volume after an experimentally induced ischemic stroke. This finding suggests that nNOS activity may be detrimental to neuronal survival during ischemia. However, mice deficient in the eNOS gene tend to have greater than normal infarct volumes after experimentally induced stroke, which indicates that eNOS has neuroprotective activity. (Infarct volume refers to the amount of necrotic tissue resulting from the stroke.) Most likely, eNOS exerts its beneficial effect by promoting the reperfusion of the ischemic area. Interestingly, iNOS knock-

out mice, like nNOS knockout mice, display diminished infarct volume after ischemic stroke; it is speculated that a decreased inflammatory response may reduce infarct size in these mice.

The multiple effects of NO on ischemic injury provide an excellent lesson in the complexity of the brain's response to ischemia. Other events that take place during ischemia, such as Ca^{2+} entry into cells, also may have multiple and varied effects, and these actions must be carefully examined if effective therapies are to be devised. If, for example, NOS inhibition can be developed as a clinical treatment for ischemic neuronal injury, such inhibition most likely will have to be carefully targeted to nNOS or perhaps iNOS.

ACIDOSIS

Interruption of blood supply to the brain leads to both increased CO_2 tension—due to decreased CO_2 removal—and increased lactate accumulation caused by forced glycolysis in the absence of aerobic respiration. These two events result in acidosis. Ischemia-related acidosis can be severe; indeed, pH values in an ischemic region often approach 6.0. Acidosis affects cellular function in multiple ways, including the promotion of free radical formation; inhibition of the Na^+–Ca^{2+} exchanger; decomposition of nicotinamide-adenine dinucleotide, which is essential for oxidative phosphorylation; and inhibition of neurotransmitter reuptake.

Despite our knowledge of these effects, the significance of acidosis to the ultimate death or survival of ischemic neurons is unclear. In fact, acidosis may have certain neuroprotective functions. Neurons exposed to high levels of glutamate in vitro undergo injury at a neutral pH; however, much of this damage is avoided when such experiments are performed at an acidic pH of 6.6. Although many plausible explanations for the protective effect of acidosis exist, one of the most likely involves the pH sensitivity of the Ca^{2+}-conducting NMDA receptor. At acidic pH, NMDA currents are drastically reduced, which may in turn significantly reduce Ca^{2+} accumulation in challenged neurons.

FORMATION OF FREE RADICALS

In vitro studies have demonstrated that excitotoxicity is frequently associated with the production of large numbers of free radicals. Free radicals are molecules with an unpaired electron in an outer shell; this unpaired electron causes the molecule to be very unstable and highly reactive. Among other reactions, free radicals can peroxidize membrane fatty acids, and in turn can cause alterations in membrane fluidity and integrity.

They also can oxidize protein sulfhydryl ($-SH$) groups, a process that impairs the functioning of the affected proteins. Moreover, free radicals can lead to strand scission, or breakage, of DNA, which causes the destruction of genetic material. A strong free radical "hit" that is powerful enough to overcome a cell's built-in defenses against free radical damage almost certainly can inflict substantial or even fatal damage on a neuron.

Many of the ischemia-related events previously described can lead to a flood of free radical formation. Loss of membrane integrity caused by osmotic swelling or overactivation of phospholipases, for example, may cause mitochondrial contents, including oxygen radicals (oxygen-reactive species), to leak into the cytosol. Activation of PLA_2 by Ca^{2+} leads to the production of arachidonic acid, which subsequently is metabolized to yield a variety of products, including $\bullet O_2^-$. Activation of NOS by Ca^{2+} increases levels of NO, which can react with oxygen or O_2^- to yield peroxynitrite (ONOO); ONOO decomposes with the production of $\bullet OH$, a highly toxic free radical.

Among the many possible sources of free radicals, the most significant in mediating ischemic damage has yet to be determined. Regardless of the source, many experiments have shown that free radical scavengers protect against excitotoxicity in vitro. However, only a small number of free radical scavengers have been investigated in clinical studies of stroke, and these have shown little beneficial effect. Such scavengers may effectively reduce ischemic injury only when given soon after the occurrence of a stroke; thus further studies are warranted.

APOPTOSIS

Neuronal death from ischemia has long been attributed to *necrosis*. Necrotic neurons and the organelles they contain swell until their membranes eventually burst. Necrosis is exactly what might be expected of a cell undergoing failure of active transport, membrane integrity, and osmotic stability, all of which ultimately result in disintegration.

After ischemic insult, many of the brain's neurons also undergo *apoptosis*, or programmed cell death. Apoptotic neurons are characterized by chromatin aggregation, exocytosis of membrane-bound cytoplasmic fragments (apoptotic bodies), and progressive loss of cell volume. Apoptosis is generally recognized as a series of steps undertaken by a doomed cell in order to prevent necrosis. Necrosis, as previously indicated, is accompanied by the leakage of cytoplasmic and organelle contents into the extracellular space; such leakage can be toxic to neighboring cells and can promote inflammatory processes. In contrast, during apoptosis this potentially

dangerous material is packaged in vesicles, which can be safely taken up into surrounding cells—most likely glia—by endocytosis. Unlike necrosis, which is a passive process, cell death by apoptosis results from the execution of specific and well-regulated genetic programs. In many biologic systems, inhibition of protein synthesis—for example, with **cycloheximide**—can prevent apoptosis.

Apoptosis may result in the death of neurons only moderately affected by ischemic injury. It may, for instance, affect neurons that undergo a mild or short-lived ischemic event, such as those in a peri-infarct area, which is the area between severely ischemic and normal tissue. In cortical cell cultures treated with very high levels of NMDA or NO and superoxide, neuronal death is generally observed to be necrotic; however, with lower levels of NMDA or NO–superoxide, apoptosis occurs. These findings suggest that severely damaged neurons quickly undergo necrosis before apoptosis can occur, whereas in moderately damaged neurons apoptotic processes may be initiated.

Apoptosis involves, among many other processes, the breakdown of double-stranded DNA into nucleosomal segments. This breakdown makes it possible for apoptosis to be observed because the resulting segments can be visualized as DNA "laddering" on an electrophoretic gel. Histologically, apoptosis can be distinguished from necrosis with the use of a technique called "terminal tranferase-mediated dUTP-biotin nick end-labeling" (TUNEL). This technique involves the end-labeling of DNA in tissue sections with the enzyme terminal deoxynucleotidyltransferase.

Apoptosis is characterized by altered ratios of members of the Bcl family of proteins: pro-apoptotic family members such as Bax increase, while anti-apoptotic members such as Bcl-2 and Bcl-xL decrease (see Chapter 11). Also increased are levels of p53, a nuclear tumor-suppressor protein that promotes apoptosis. Moreover, apoptosis, but not necrosis, involves the activation of a family of enzymes called *caspases*, of which twelve members have been identified. Caspases are aspartate-specific cysteine proteases. Under basal conditions, caspases are zymogens, which means that they exist as inactive pro-enzymes until they are activated by proteolytic cleavage. After they are activated, caspases cleave numerous types of proteins that trigger biochemical cascades that lead to cell death. Much remains to be learned about the activation of caspases and the cellular consequences of such activation (see Chapter 11), but one important consequence is the release of cytochrome *c* from the inner mitochondrial membrane. After it enters the cytoplasm, cytochrome *c* interacts with apoptosis-activating factor APAF3 to promote the cleavage and activation of caspase 3. Activation of caspase 3 then triggers the cleavage and activation of several other caspases, which leads ultimately to several features of apoptosis, including fragmentation of DNA.

Would interference with apoptotic processes decrease the area of infarction caused by stroke? Overexpression of the anti-apoptosis bcl-2 gene or knockout of the pro-apoptosis bax and p53 genes reduces infarction in rodent brains subjected to focal ischemic insults. These findings indicate that reductions in apoptosis may indeed be neuroprotective. Studies involving rat models of focal ischemia have revealed that infarct volumes are reduced to a greater extent with the administration of cycloheximide and NMDA receptor antagonists compared with the administration of either drug alone. Caspase inhibition also is being explored, but which of the many known forms of the enzyme would be an ideal drug target remains undetermined. **Caspase inhibitors** currently available consist of small peptides that do not readily cross the blood–brain barrier or enter cells. Major efforts are under way to develop small molecule inhibitors that might overcome such limitations.

It is important to emphasize that therapies directed against apoptosis must be developed with caution. Under some circumstances interference with apoptosis may worsen stroke-related damage. If neurons were to undergo necrosis instead of apoptosis, for example, increased damage to healthy neighboring neurons might result.

TREATMENT OF STROKE

Despite our growing knowledge of the mechanisms that underlie ischemic neuronal death, our ability to treat stroke remains limited. Among the treatment strategies currently available, the best are geared toward prevention through the maintenance of cardiovascular health, restoration of blood supply with drugs such as aspirin and thrombolytic agents, and the slowing of metabolism with hypothermia. Although none of these therapies have capitalized on the sophisticated studies that have investigated the biochemical events underlying neuronal cell death, efforts to prevent stroke nevertheless have been successful. The incidence of stroke has been reduced markedly by preventive measures aimed at controlling hypertension and hypercholesterolemia. Moreover, prophylactic use of small doses of drugs that inhibit platelet function, such as **aspirin** and **ibuprofen,** has proven to be effective in reducing the risk of occlusive stroke at the cost of slightly increasing the risk of hemorrhagic stroke. **Estrogen** replacement therapy in postmenopausal women and other measures associated with beneficial cardiovascular effects also may prove to decrease the incidence of stroke.

One reason that stroke prevention is so important is that current stroke therapies are pitted against an unforgiving opponent: time. By the time an individual becomes aware of the occurrence of a stroke, travels to a hospital, and is diagnosed, hours often have elapsed. Even in current clinical trials, several hours usually elapse between the onset of stroke and the administration of treatment. As previously emphasized, serious neural damage can occur within minutes of an ischemic event. Barring round-the-clock observation of all individuals at risk for stroke, the effectiveness of treatment in humans is unlikely to approach that of laboratory animals because in the laboratory, researchers have the luxury of administering therapy during or immediately after an ischemic insult.

THE PERI-INFARCT AREA: AN IMPORTANT TREATMENT TARGET

Many of the approaches to treatment discussed in the sections that follow involve actions that occur primarily in the peri-infarct area and serve to salvage neurons that would otherwise be destined to die within hours or days after a stroke. The peri-infarct area constitutes compromised but potentially salvageable tissue between the severely ischemic core and adequately perfused brain tissue. Although potentially salvageable, the peri-infarct area is quite vulnerable because it is subject to high levels of excitotoxic neurotransmitters and free radicals, waves of cellular depolarization, and inflammatory processes.

RESTORING BLOOD SUPPLY

After an occlusive stroke, blood supply can be restored with anticoagulants and thrombolytic agents, which dissolve the clots that impede the normal flow of blood. Thrombolytic agents have been found to improve the outcome of this type of stroke in recent clinical trials. However, these agents must be used with great caution because they increase the risk of hemorrhage. Consequently, the presence of hemorrhagic stroke must be ruled out—typically by means of computed tomography or magnetic resonance imaging—before anticoagulant and thrombolytic agents are used. Even occlusive strokes are accompanied by a small but real risk of hemorrhage.

Thrombolytics   **Urokinase, streptokinase, prourokinase,** and **tissue plasminogen activator** (**tPA**) are proteins that promote the conversion of the proenzyme plasminogen into plasmin, an enzyme that degrades fibrin, a key structural protein in most blood clots (Figure 21–3; Table 21–1). Currently, tPA is the only thrombolytic substance approved for use in the United States. The clinical trials that demonstrated its efficacy showed that intravenously delivered tPA reduced the disability of patients with acute ischemic stroke who were treated within the first 3 hours of the onset of symptoms. Although tPA-treated patients did have an increased incidence of brain hemorrhage, overall mortality at 3 months was the same in treatment and control groups.

In contrast to tPA, streptokinase has been ineffective in three different clinical trials. These findings may be related not only to differences between the two thrombolytic agents, in that streptokinase has a longer half-life and a slightly different mode of action, but also to

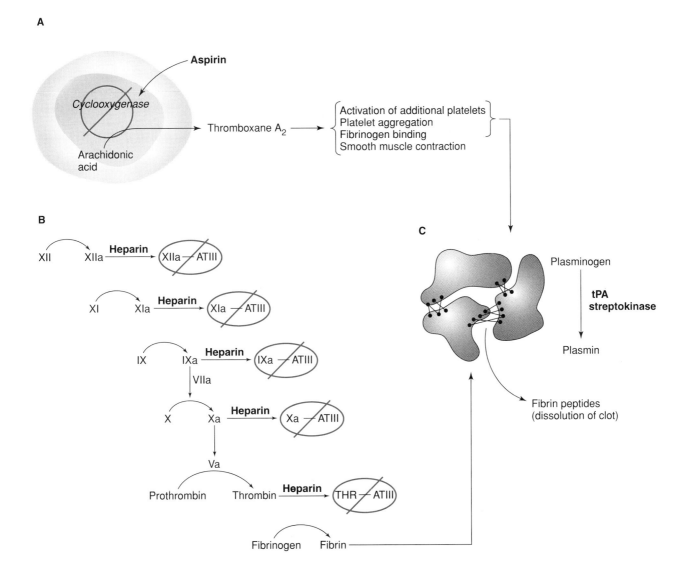

= inactive form

Figure 21–3. Mechanisms of action of anticoagulants and thrombolytics. **A.** Platelets are activated by molecules exposed during tissue injury. Aspirin inhibits cyclooxygenase, which catalyzes the formation of thromboxane A_2, a key intermediary in the clotting process (see Chapter 5). **B.** During the clotting cascade, a chain of precursor proteins activate one another, a process that results in amplification of the signal. Heparin catalyzes the binding of antithrombin III (ATIII) to several of the activated clotting proteins denoted by roman numerals; the antithrombin-bound clotting factors are inactive. **C.** Thrombolytics such as tissue plasminogen activator (tPA) and streptokinase catalyze the conversion of the inactive precursor plasminogen to the active enzyme plasmin, which catalyzes the breakdown of fibrin polymers. Fibrin is a key component of the clot; it is produced from its precursor fibrinogen through catalysis by thrombin, a major product of the clotting cascade.

Table 21–1 Treatment of Stroke

Category	Name	Action/Type of Agent	Clinical Efficacy
Anticoagulation and thrombolysis	Aspirin	Inhibits synthesis of thromboxane A$_2$, inhibiting platelet aggregation	Modest
	Heparin	Activates antithrombin III, which inhibits clotting factor proteases	Modest
	Nadroparin	Heparin-like anticoagulants	Being tested
	Orgaron		Being tested
	tPA	Converts plasminogen to plasmin, which cleaves thrombin	Modest
	Urokinase		Being tested
	Streptokinase		None
Glutamate receptor blockade	Aptiganel	NMDA receptor channel blocker	None
	Dextrorphan		None
	Dextromethorphan		None
	Magnesium		Being tested
	NPS 1506		Being tested
	Remacemide		Minimal
	ACEA 1021 (licostinel)	NMDA glycine-site antagonist	None
	GV 150526		Being tested
	Eliprodil	NMDA polyamine-site antagonist	None
	YM872	AMPA receptor antagonist	Being tested
	ZK-200775 (MPQX)		None
Voltage-gated Ca^{2+} channel blockers	Nimodipine	Reduces Ca^{2+} influx	None
	Lifarizine		?
	Flunarizine		None
Na$^+$ channel blockers	Lubeluzole	Reduces excitability and glutamate release	?
	Riluzol		?
	Phenytoin		None
Voltage-dependent K$^+$-channel agonist	BMS-204352	Reduces Ca^{2+} influx	Being tested
Enhancement of inhibitory neurotransmission	Clormethiazole[1]	GABA receptor agonist	Being tested
Free radical scavengers/ antioxidants	Pergorgotein	Reduces free-radical-mediated injury	?
	Tirilazad		None
	Ebselen		Minimal
Neural repair	Citicholine	Phospholipid precursor	?
	Trofermin	bFGF receptor agonist	Minimal

[1]Clormethiazole enhances the action of GABA at GABA$_A$ receptors, although its exact mechanism of action is unknown.
None—either a clinical trial of the drug was completed and no efficacy was found or the clinical trial had to be stopped because of adverse side effects.
?—either no data on clinical efficacy are available or the clinical data are preliminary.
tPA, tissue plasminogen activator.

the design of the streptokinase studies. Specifically, the time that elapsed before treatment was much greater in the streptokinase studies than in the successful tPA trial. Prourokinase was proven to be somewhat beneficial in early clinical trials, but more studies will be required before this agent can be considered efficacious. Urokinase is currently unavailable because of production difficulties.

Anticoagulants   **Heparin** is a heterogeneous mixture of sulfated mucopolysaccharides. It is found in

mast cells and in the extracellular matrix of most tissues. It has a molecular mass of 750–1000 kDa and is composed of long polymers of glycosaminoglycan chains that are attached to a core protein (Figure 21–4). Because of its structure, heparin is not effective after oral administration and must be given parenterally. It inhibits clot formation by enhancing the activity of antithrombin III, a protein that forms equimolar complexes with the various proteases activated during the clot formation process (see Figure 21–3). By binding directly to antithrombin III, heparin causes a conformational change in the protein that enhances its binding to the clotting factor proteases. Because heparin works by inhibiting the formation of clots, rather than by degrading existing clots, its use typically is considered a preventive measure against the recurrence of stroke. Patients treated with heparin for 1–2 weeks after an initial episode of stroke show a significant improvement in their condition compared with patients who receive a placebo. However, this improvement in overall outcome may not persist long after the treatment period.

As discussed in Chapter 5, **aspirin** (see Figure 21–4) inhibits cyclooxygenase, which in platelets catalyzes the conversion of arachidonic acid to thromboxane A_2, among other products. Thromboxane is a critical intermediate in the recruitment of platelets necessary for the clotting cascade. Aspirin administered to patients during hospital admission for stroke produces a small but significant net benefit: its use prevents death or disability in approximately 13 per 1000 affected individuals compared with placebo. Other cyclooxygenase inhibitors, including some nonsteroidal antiinflammatory drugs (NSAIDs), may have similar activity. **Ticlopidine** is another antiplatelet agent in current use. It acts by inhibiting the binding of fibrinogen to activated platelets through interactions with glycoproteins on platelet membranes.

Patients who do not respond to aspirin and related compounds often are treated with **warfarin** (see Figure 21–4). Warfarin is a synthetic derivative of a related compound in sweet clover, which was found in the early

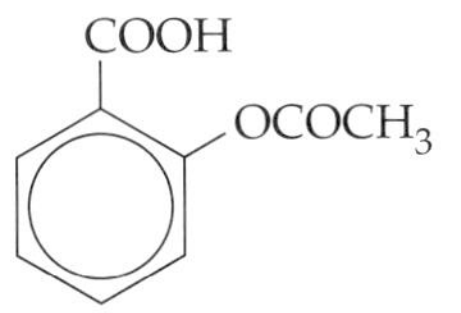

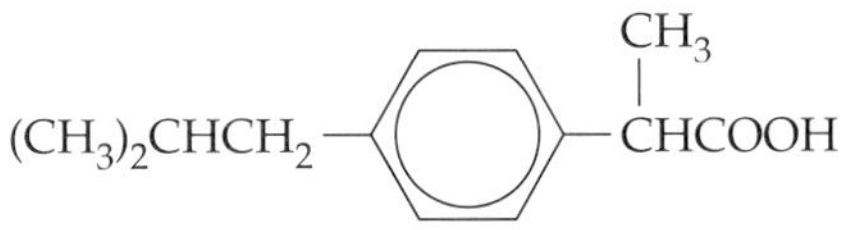

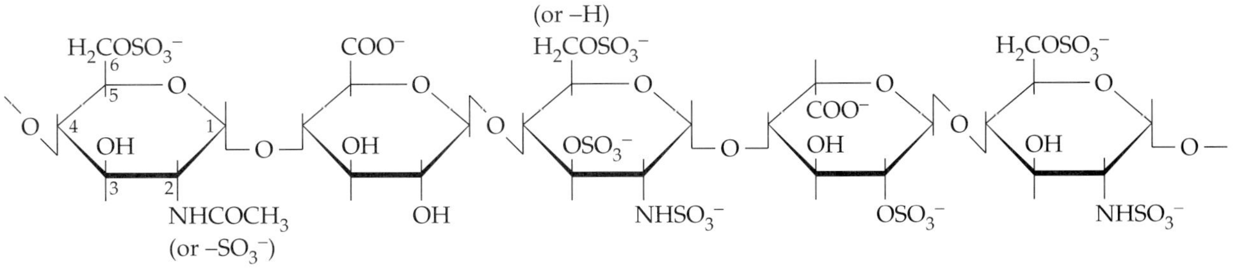

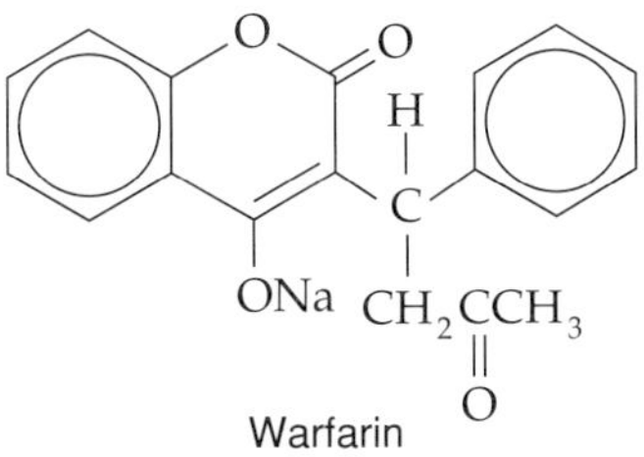

Figure 21–4. Chemical structures of representative antiplatelet and anticoagulant drugs.

20th century to promote bleeding. Warfarin acts as a **vitamin K** antagonist. Vitamin K is a required cofactor for the enzymes that activate several clotting factors, including II, VII, IX, and X. Warfarin prevents the reduction of oxidized vitamin K into its active form. Warfarin and related compounds are the most potent oral anticoagulants known; indeed, they are so potent that severe hemorrhage is a significant side effect of their use. (This effect, at high doses, is exploited in warfarin's use as a rat poison.) Patients who take warfarin must have regular blood tests to ensure that their bleeding times are within safe boundaries.

Aspirin, warfarin, and other oral anticoagulants are used not only to treat stroke but also to prevent transient ischemic attacks (**TIAs**), which are brief periods of brain ischemia that resolve without a lasting neurologic deficit. These attacks are believed to be caused by transient occlusions of the cerebral vasculature. The symptoms of TIAs are similar to those of stroke, except that they resolve within minutes to hours of onset.

MINIMIZING Ca^{2+} INFLUX INTO CELLS

Because Ca^{2+} appears to be critically involved in promoting the biochemical processes that lead to neuronal destruction, the reduction of Ca^{2+} influx might be considered a promising strategy in the treatment of stroke. However, the effectiveness of drugs that reduce the influx of Ca^{2+} into neurons (see Table 21–1) has yet to be demonstrated in clinical trials. **NMDA receptor antagonists** exhibit a robust protective effect on neurons in culture but have not proven to be effective in humans. Even if they were effective, many of these antagonists have **phencyclidine**-like adverse effects, such as psychosis and dissociation (see Chapter 17), that severely limit the dose that can be used. Inhibitors of voltage-dependent Ca^{2+} channels (see Chapter 3) such as **nimodipine,** an L-type Ca^{2+} channel blocker, and **flunarizine,** a T-type Ca^{2+} channel blocker, have been investigated as potential therapies for stroke but thus far have not been shown to improve the functional outcome of patients after ischemic stroke. Similarly, antagonists of voltage-dependent Na$^+$ channels, such as **phenytoin,** which can be very effective in the treatment of seizure disorders, have failed to improve clinical outcomes of stroke.

REDUCING FREE RADICAL DAMAGE

Free radical scavengers are agents that are oxidized by oxygen-reactive species without deleterious effects to the cell. **Tirilazad,** a nonglucocorticoid steroid that inhibits lipid peroxidation, has been shown to reduce infarct area in animals treated within 10 minutes of complete focal ischemia. However, tirilazad has no effect on functional outcome when administered to humans approximately 4 hours after stroke. **Ebselen,** another free-radical scavenger, was reported to produce a very modest reduction in damaged tissue when given 6–12 hours after acute occlusion of the middle cerebral artery in one clinical study. Other antioxidants, such as **vitamin E (α-tocopherol)**, are being considered for prophylactic use to limit the free radical damage that occurs after stroke.

PROMOTING NEURAL RECOVERY

Another approach to stroke therapy is to promote the self-repair of damaged neurons or the growth of healthy neurons to help compensate for the loss of neurons destroyed during an ischemic attack. Two general strategies can be used to this end. A nutritive strategy involves ensuring that neurons have the molecules they need for repair and growth, and a signaling strategy involves providing the chemical signals that instruct neurons to grow. The first strategy has been attempted with administration of the phospholipid precursor **citicholine,** for which a small beneficial effect on outcome has been claimed, as measured by functional recovery and examination of mental status. Citicholine is a key intermediate in the biosynthesis of phosphatidylcholine, an important component of the neural cell membrane. **Neurotrophic factors** such as basic fibroblast growth factor (bFGF; see Chapter 11) also are being considered for restorative therapy. In animal stroke models, bFGF reduces infarct volume when given shortly after the onset of focal ischemia. Although bFGF did not reduce infarct size when given 24 hours after experimentally induced stroke, it did improve outcome as measured by behavioral tests. This neurotrophic factor and others have yet to be assessed in human clinical trials.

Despite all of the advances in our understanding of neural injury related to stroke, the best-established way to ensure long-term recovery of function is through rehabilitation. Research involving laboratory animals has provided insight into how rehabilitation might work at the neurobiologic level (Box 21–1). The results of such research raise the possibility that neurobiologic mechanisms may be exploited in the future to ensure maximal return of function after stroke.

SEIZURES AND EPILEPSY

A seizure is a paroxysmal derangement of cerebral function caused by excessive and generally synchronized activity of a group of neurons. Seizure activity can occur in many different regions of the brain, and its physical manifestations vary according to the region in which it

Box 21–1 Neurobiologic Basis of Rehabilitation

Stroke patients with large initial deficits often can exhibit striking improvement. The length of the recovery process (typically 1–2 years) suggests that events other than the resolution of edema and inflammation are responsible for improvement in function. In some cases, restoration of blood flow through the development of collateral circulation may contribute to the regaining of function. However, several lines of evidence indicate that neurons undergo anatomic and functional changes that significantly assist in functional improvement after a stroke. In rats, for example, increased expression of the growth-cone-associated protein GAP-43 and of the synaptic vesicle protein synaptophysin have been detected near experimentally induced infarct areas. *Growth cones* are specialized endings of growing axons before they form mature synapses. Increased expression of GAP-43 also has been noted in the periphery of infarcted human brain tissue examined at autopsy. Interestingly, dendritic sprouting has been observed contralateral to cortical lesions produced by electrocauterization in rats. This finding suggests that recovery of function may occur as the corresponding, contralateral area of the brain assumes the function of its injured counterpart.

The occurrence of compensatory neural remodeling after stroke has been demonstrated experimentally. Electrophysiologic experiments have revealed a reassignment of function after ischemic infarct in squirrel monkeys: when small infarcts are produced in the area of the motor cortex that corresponds to the hand, new areas of the cortex, previously responsible for movements of the arm and shoulder, slowly gain the ability to control hand motions. This topographical reorganization of neuronal function required that the monkeys perform tasks that necessitated the use of their debilitated hand. Thus frequent activation may stimulate the growth of remaining neuronal processes responsible for control of the hand into arm-and-shoulder territory. Alternatively, such activation may increase the potency of a small number of "hand neurons" that preexisted in the arm and shoulder space.

Similar reassignment of function likely takes place in the human brain. Positron emission tomography and magnetic resonance imaging studies indicate that adjacent or contralateral brain regions may indeed work to compensate for damaged tissue. Verbal tasks typically cause activation of speech areas in the left hemispheres of normal subjects; however, in some recovered aphasic patients, increased activation of homologous areas in the right hemisphere have been observed. Is this an indication that the right hemisphere can undergo changes that allow compensation for the damaged left hemisphere? Unfortunately, current experiments have not conclusively answered this question. It is possible, for example, that speech centers in the right hemispheres of certain aphasics participated in verbal tasks to an unusual degree before the onset of stroke. However, in light of anatomic and physiologic data from animal models, dendritic and axonal growth and other forms of neural plasticity are mechanisms worth investigating in stroke patients. Knowledge of the molecular and cellular events that influence such rearrangement may eventually lead to techniques for aiding the recovery of stroke victims. Moreover, because shifts of function depend on the use of an affected area after stroke, it is likely that aggressive physical or speech therapy will continue to be a critical tool in promoting recovery after stroke.

---

occurs. Thus the term *seizure* may refer to a 3-second lapse of consciousness that is barely noticeable to the affected individual or to witnesses of the event. The same term also applies to a grand mal tonic–clonic seizure that causes an individual to tense for several seconds before experiencing a jerking of his or her entire body.

Approximately one individual in 20 experiences a seizure at some point during his or her lifetime. In most cases a seizure can be traced to a specific insult, such as head trauma, high fever, or alcohol withdrawal. Approximately 1 individual in 200 can be described as **epileptic,** or as having a propensity for recurring seizures. Inherited vulnerabilities, focal brain injury, or chronic illness can produce lower seizure thresholds in epileptic individuals, who generally require medication to control their seizures.

Because there are many varieties of seizures, there are many types of epilepsy. Patients who visit epilepsy clinics typically include those who are receiving successful therapy and have not had a seizure for years, those who have difficulty maintaining employment because of poorly controlled seizures, those with seizures that consist of lapses of consciousness and odd behavior such as lip smacking, individuals who have experienced generalized tonic–clonic attacks, children who experience 5-second lapses of attention that occasionally interfere with their ability to concentrate in class, and mentally retarded spastic quadriplegics who must wear protective helmets because of their uncontrolled falling attacks. The impact of a tendency toward seizure varies. Some epileptic patients are inconvenienced only by their need for daily medication, whereas others can be nearly incapacitated by their condition. The effectiveness of treatment also can be highly variable. Some types of epilepsy, including juvenile absence epilepsy, are eminently treatable; other types, especially those related to gross developmental disorders, cannot be adequately treated. Moreover, some patients readily tolerate pharmacotherapy, while others experience distressing side effects such as fatigue, forgetfulness, and medical complications.

The treatment of seizures, along with our understanding of their biologic basis, has undergone slow, steady progress during the last decade. New anticonvulsant drugs, such as **gabapentin** and **lamotrigine,** are improving seizure control and reducing side effects for many patients. The genetic factors that underlie seizure vulnerability are increasingly well understood, and the physiology of certain types of seizures is slowly being elucidated. Moreover, the molecular events that contribute to epileptogenesis in previously healthy neuronal tissue are beginning to be discovered. Although epilepsy remains a serious disorder for many, effective treatment continues to be developed.

GENERATION OF A SEIZURE

In a normal, conscious state, the net neuronal activity recorded by an electroencephalogram (EEG) reveals few waves and no large shifts in polarity (see Chapter 18). Such activity does not indicate that the brain is quiet; rather it indicates that neuronal activity is asynchronous. To maintain balance, posture, and fine motor control, for example, some cortical motor neurons may fire action potentials while others are hyperpolarized.

At the onset of a seizure, the EEG changes (Figure 21–5). Events that may include dramatic upward and downward shifts of polarity begin to appear. Such events indicate that a large number of neurons are firing and repolarizing in synchrony; the summation of their activity produces a noticeable effect on the EEG recording. This type of synchrony can be accompanied by abnormalities in movement, sensation, or consciousness. If synchronous firing occurs in cortical motor neurons, for example, twitching and jerking of affected body parts may replace the fine gradations of muscle activity needed to maintain balance, posture, and smooth, controlled motion. When synchrony occurs in other brain regions, the result may be strange sensations, such as the perception of a particular odor, confusion, or the loss of consciousness.

What causes this change from normal neuronal activity to abnormal synchronized firing of large ensembles of neurons? Many factors can set the stage for a seizure. Abnormal synchronized activity often arises from a particular area in the brain, referred to as a *seizure focus.* Brain imaging and electroencephalography often can be used to identify seizure foci, which may be associated with areas of neuronal degeneration or with an abnormality such as a tumor. A decrease in the overall level of inhibitory transmission in the brain also can precipitate a seizure. Such decreases can occur after the administration of γ-aminobutyric acid (GABA) antagonists, or during withdrawal from repeated exposure to GABA agonists such as alcohol or benzodiazepines. Moreover, events that do not cause seizures in most people, such as hyperventilation or flashing lights, may precipitate seizures in vulnerable individuals.

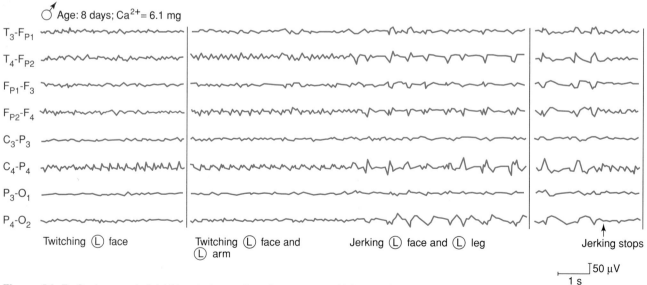

Figure 21–5. Scalp-recorded right hemisphere seizure in a neonate with hypercalcemia. Note that the onset of large shifts in potential correspond to the progression of the seizure. L, left. (Adapted with permission from Wyllie E. 1997. *The Treatment of Epilepsy: Principles and Practice,* 2nd ed. Baltimore: Williams and Wilkins.)

Box 21–2 Rasmussen Encephalitis: An Autoimmune Disorder?

During the early 1990s, experimenters attempting to generate antibodies to the external portion of the GluR3 receptor, an AMPA receptor subunit (see Chapter 7), noticed that two of the three rabbits they had immunized with the GluR3 protein began to have recurrent seizures. The brains of these two rabbits exhibited pathology similar to that seen in **Rasmussen encephalitis,** a rare syndrome characterized by seizures, progressive dysfunction, and inflammatory histopathology that typically is confined to a single cerebral hemisphere. The onset of this syndrome usually occurs between 2 and 10 years of age and is followed by progressive atrophy and dysfunction.

Until recently, treatment of Rasmussen encephalitis has been frustratingly ineffective. The pathogenesis of this syndrome had not been determined, and typical anticonvulsant drugs provided little benefit. However, because of the serendipitous finding regarding the GluR3 protein, investigators currently believe that the ultimate cause of Rasmussen encephalitis is an autoimmune response to this protein. Serum from individuals with Rasmussen encephalitis does indeed exhibit immunoreactivity against GluR3, unlike serum from control subjects. Moreover, plasma exchange has been demonstrated to reduce seizure frequency and

increase cognitive function in many patients. Although GluR3 autoimmunity appears to be the cause of Rasmussen encephalitis, how the disease starts and progresses, why circulating GluR3 antibodies are produced, and how antibodies slip past the blood–brain barrier after they are generated has yet to be established.

The generation of GluR3 antibodies may be explained by an autoimmune response that occurs after a disruption of the blood–brain barrier or by a response to a bacterial protein that is homologous to GluR3. Subsequently, GluR3 antibodies may access the brain and initiate seizures, possibly by triggering an immune response that injures affected neurons. Studies have indicated that some GluR3 antibodies are capable of activating GluR3-containing AMPA receptors; thus these antibodies may generate seizures by direct activation of glutamate receptors. After a seizure is triggered, a damaging cycle may ensue, involving seizure-induced disruption of the blood–brain barrier, increased entry of GluR3 antibodies, recurring seizures, and further neural injury. Regardless of the exact mechanism of progression, the discovery of the autoimmune basis of Rasmussen encephalitis is likely to advance the treatment of this once baffling condition.

Although the exact chain of events that trigger individual seizures may be poorly understood, the tendency of neurons to fire in synchrony is related to their extensive interconnectedness. Neurons in different regions of the brain, as well as those within single regions, often have extensive reciprocal connections with one another; for example, glutamatergic neurons in the thalamus project to glutamatergic neurons in the cortex, which in turn project to neurons in the thalamus. After they emerge, waves of activity can become self-sustaining and can even propagate from one region of the brain to another.

CLASSIFICATION OF SEIZURES

Seizures can be broadly categorized as *focal* (partial) or *generalized*. As their name suggests, focal seizures are characterized by clinical and electroencephalographic changes that indicate an initial activation of neurons in a relatively small, discrete region of the brain, whereas generalized seizures are characterized by initial involvement of both hemispheres and widespread neuronal activation. These two broad classifications comprise dozens of subtypes of seizures that have distinct clinical manifestations and involve particular brain regions. A detailed description of seizure types can be found in the Suggested Reading.

Seizure classification aids in the selection of optimal treatment regimens. However, one individual can undergo multiple seizures of varying types; indeed, a single seizure event can involve more than one type of seizure. Focal seizures, for example, commonly evolve into a generalized seizure as activity spreads from the seizure focus to other areas of the brain. The identification of such progression in seizure activity also helps to determine an optimal treatment regimen (Box 21–2).

As previously mentioned, the clinical manifestations of *focal seizures* reflect the region of brain in which they occur; for example, a focal seizure in sensory cortex may produce an odd sensory experience, such as a noxious smell or a clicking sound. Other types of focal seizures include aphasic/phonatory, somatosensory, and adversive seizures. *Aphasic/phonatory seizures* result in a sudden inability to speak, write, or read. Related seizure foci often are found in the temporal, inferior frontal, or inferior parietal cortex. *Somatosensory seizures* cause paresthesias often referred to as pins and needles, or hot or cold sensations, with corresponding seizure foci often found in somatosensory cortex. *Adversive seizures* result in sudden movements of the head and eyes to the contralateral side of the seizure focus, and related foci often are found in the frontal lobe or precentral gyrus.

Box 21–3 Complex Partial Seizures

Complex partial seizures can be amazingly intricate. An example of their complexity is illustrated in the details of one such seizure experienced by a teenaged girl. Mary's seizure caused her to display a series of behaviors while exhibiting only partial awareness of the environment. At the beginning of the seizure, Mary suddenly began to raise and lower the tilting top of her desk in class. When the teacher asked her to stop, Mary looked at the teacher blankly and began to fumble with the buttons on her sweater. When the teacher walked toward Mary to find out what was wrong, Mary put out her arms as though to ward off the teacher. Mary subsequently stood up and wandered aimlessly around the classroom. After a few minutes she stopped, looked around as though puzzled, returned to her desk, put her

head down, and fell asleep. Mary had little memory of what had happened except for an awareness that she had behaved strangely; she was embarrassed by the episode and was reluctant to return to school.

After examining Mary, her doctor was convinced that Mary had experienced many other such lapses. An EEG revealed frequent sharp-wave discharges from Mary's right temporal lobe. After she adopted a regimen that included regular use of **carbamazepine,** Mary stopped experiencing seizures. The details of Mary's complex partial seizure disorder explain why such symptoms are sometimes misconstrued as conduct problems. (Gumnit RJ. 1995. *The Epilepsy Handbook: The Practical Management of Seizures.* New York: Raven Press.)

Focal motor seizures are characterized by clonic twitching of the contralateral muscles consequent to a localized epileptic discharge from the motor cortex. The muscles involved depend on the affected area of the brain. The motor activity can be moderate (inconspicuous twitching) or extreme (massive jerking of the affected muscles). Focal motor seizures spread from the focus to neighboring areas of motor cortex; for example, the seizure may spread from one twitching area of the body to the next until the entire half of the body shows clonic activity. Focal motor seizures also may progress into full-blown grand mal attacks.

Complex partial seizures are focal seizures characterized by an impairment of consciousness and can arise from virtually any area of cortex that subserves a complex function such as speech, emotion, or memory. These seizures can produce a variety of effects, including auditory or visual hallucinations, feelings of familiarity (déjà vu) or strangeness (jamais vu), or automatisms such as lip smacking or chewing motions. Although complex partial seizures involve impaired consciousness, the affected individual often continues to interact with the environment, in ways that are sometimes bizarre (Box 21–3).

The behaviors and experiences that occur during a complex partial seizure are usually initiated in higher-level association cortices (see Chapter 17), which may explain why resulting behaviors are complex, including automatisms such as chewing or picking at clothes, rather than gross, for example, tonic–clonic movements of an appendage. The involvement of high-level auditory and visual association cortices most likely explains the occurrence of hallucinations during some complex partial seizures. The temporal lobe is a particularly common

focus for complex partial seizures. **Temporal lobe epilepsy** is often associated with complex partial seizures involving aphasia and sensations of jamais vu or déjà vu. The hippocampus, which is critical for learning and memory (see Chapter 20), is believed to be the source of many temporal lobe epilepsies, which in some cases are associated with atrophy of the hippocampus and reorganization of dentate granule cell axons.

Generalized seizures are those that provide no evidence of a localized onset. The exact cause of most generalized seizures is unknown. Although a focal seizure can spread or generalize, there are many instances in which the entire cortex seems to give rise to seizure activity all at once. Many generalized seizures are associated with developmental disorders.

Tonic seizures are characterized by an extension of the extremities and a rigid stretching of the body. These attacks are most common in children with **Lennox–Gastaut syndrome**. This syndrome is characterized by a slow spike-and-wave complex on EEG recordings, impaired cognitive function, and multiple types of seizure, including atonic drop attacks. Lennox–Gastaut syndrome typically becomes evident between 1 and 10 years of age, and often is refractory to anticonvulsant medications. The cause of this syndrome remains unknown; however, it has been associated with brain malformations, hypoxic–ischemic brain injury, encephalitis, meningitis, and tuberous sclerosis. Because Lennox–Gastaut syndrome generally appears at a very early age, it may result as a consequence of various types of insults to the developing brain. A heritable susceptibility also may be a factor in the acquisition of this syndrome: a family history of epilepsy is evident in 3 to 27% of cases.

Atonic seizures are accompanied by a sudden loss of muscle tone, which is sometimes preceded by a myoclonic jerk; if standing, the affected individual typically falls to the ground. These attacks generally last only a few seconds, and do not involve a loss of consciousness. A patient generally can recover immediately after an atonic seizure; however, a risk of injury is present during the fall, and many affected individuals must wear protective gear such as helmets to prevent fall-related injuries. *Clonic seizures* involve repetitive muscle twitching; such attacks can last as long as 1 minute. *Myoclonic seizures* are rapid involuntary muscle contractions; the term *myoclonic* is used to denote a single twitch event, which is distinct from repetitive, or clonic, twitching. Myoclonic seizures are sometimes referred to as myoclonic jerks.

Grand mal (tonic–clonic) seizures are associated with immediate profound coma and orderly sequences of motor activity. This activity comprises distinct tonic phases (arms in semi-flexion and legs extended) that are followed by a clonic phase (full-body spasms with intermittent relaxations). EEGs exhibit massive fast spiking during the tonic phase and bursts of polyspikes interrupted by slow waves during the clonic phase. Such seizures are frequently preceded by focal seizures.

Generalized absence seizures, or *petit mal seizures,* are characterized by a brief lapse of consciousness (approximately 10 seconds or less) accompanied by an EEG recording of a spike-and-wave discharge of approximately 3 Hz (Figure 21–6). The earliest clinical description of a generalized absence seizure appeared in 1705, in a report by the French physician Poupard: "At the approach of an attack the patient would sit down in a chair, eyes open, and would remain there immobile and would not afterward remember falling into this state. If she had begun to talk and the attack interrupted her, she took it up again at precisely the point at which she stopped and she believed she had talked continuously." Although this description gives the essence of an absence seizure, additional phenomena such as mild atonia, automatisms, and mild tonic or clonic components may occur in some patients. The 3-Hz spike-and-wave pattern that accompanies an absence seizure almost certainly reflects a widespread phase-locked oscillation between excitation (spike) and inhibition (wave) in mutually connected thalamocortical neuronal networks. As discussed in previous chapters, the thalamus is the relay and processing station that receives input from sensory neurons and delivers input to the cortex. Thalamic neurons shift between oscillatory and tonic firing modes. Alertness and conscious awareness are characterized by a desynchronized firing of thalamic neurons, which reflects faithful and detailed transmission of information from sensory organs to the cortex. When the firing pattern of thalamocortical neurons shifts to a synchronized, oscillatory mode, the firing threshold of thalamic neurons is raised and signal transmission to the cortex is reduced. This reduced signal transmission corresponds to a reduced conscious awareness. As discussed in Chapter 18, widespread EEG recording of discernible waves is associated with synchronized neural activity and subconscious states such as non-REM sleep.

What determines whether thalamocortical neurons are in a tonic or oscillatory state? The activity of a group of neurons in the nucleus reticularis thalami (NRT) appears to assist in such determination. GABAergic neurons of the NRT project densely to one another and to almost all thalamic relay nuclei. They also receive excitatory, glutamatergic inputs from the collaterals of both thalamocortical axons and corticothalamic axons (Figure 21–7). During periods of synchronized EEG activity, NRT neurons exhibit firing in rhythmic bursts, whereas during wakefulness, they exhibit tonic single-spike firing. The cellular event that is responsible for the oscillatory (rhythmic burst) modes of NRT neurons is the low-threshold (T-type) Ca^{2+} spike. The T-type Ca^{2+} channel is activated experimentally by small-amplitude depolarizing steps from a hyperpolarized potential (see Chapter 3). Owing to its activation–inactivation properties, the inward current produced by T-channels is negligible at resting membrane potential. It can be activated only when a neuron has experienced prior hyperpolarization and is subsequently depolarized to the threshold voltage for T-channel activation (approximately -50 mV). In the NRT, the necessary hyperpolarization is provided by $GABA_B$ receptor-mediated currents that are generated by adjacent NRT neurons. A small depolarization can subsequently activate the T current, leading to a burst of Ca^{2+}-generated action potentials. This activity in turn leads to the release of GABA onto thalamic, cortical, and neighboring NRT neurons. T-type channels subsequently are inactivated over time, and the activation of $GABA_B$ receptors by inputs from neighboring NRT neurons hyperpolarizes the cell. This hyperpolarization counters the inactivation of T-channels, and the cycle begins anew.

Although this model explains how rhythmic firing can occur, the circumstances that cause cells to shift from tonic firing to rhythmic burst firing are unknown. Absence seizures often can be precipitated by hyperventilation; thus subtle changes in blood pH may somehow modify the properties of NRT cells so that oscillatory firing is favored. However, absence attacks also occur without an apparent trigger.

The basic mechanisms responsible for absence seizures elegantly explain the actions that underlie their pharmacologic treatment. **Ethosuximide** currently is the drug of choice in the treatment of absence seizures. At clinically relevant concentrations, ethosuximide diminishes T-channel currents in NRT neurons; it is believed that this action quells the 3-Hz spike-and-wave activity that characterizes the absence seizure. Interestingly, absence seizures are among the few types of seizure that are actually made worse by the administration of GABA agonists. Drugs that promote GABAergic transmission such as **vigabatrin** may enhance the ability of NRT neurons to adopt an oscillatory firing mode by enhancing $GABA_B$-mediated hyperpolarization of NRT cells.

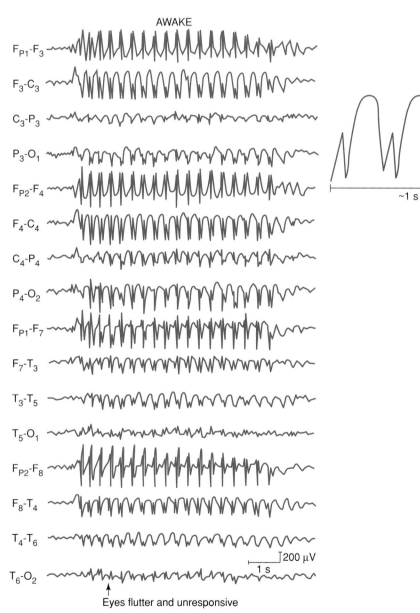

Figure 21–6. Absence seizure recorded in a 7-year-old girl. The 3-Hz spike-and-wave activity occurs simultaneously across the entire cortex. Less than a second after the beginning of this activity, the girl becomes unresponsive. *Inset,* expansion of the 3-Hz spike and wave. (From Wyllie E. 1997. *The Treatment of Epilepsy: Principles and Practice,* 2nd ed. Baltimore: Williams and Wilkins.)

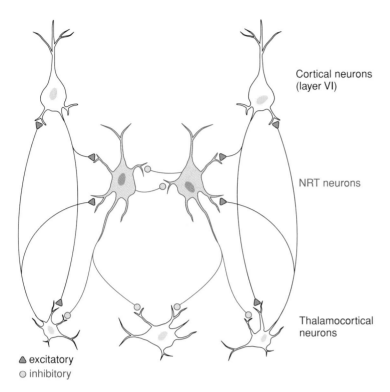

Cortical neurons
(layer VI)

NRT neurons

Thalamocortical
neurons

△ excitatory
○ inhibitory

Figure 21–7. Thalamocortical circuitry believed to be involved in absence seizures. Note that nucleus reticularis thalami (NRT) neurons are excited by both cortical and thalamic inputs and inhibited by one another. The NRT also provides inhibitory input to the thalamus.

WHAT CAUSES EPILEPSY?

Had epilepsy never existed, it would have been discovered eight times over the past year by those intent on knocking out mouse genes one at a time.

Noebels, 1996

What causes the tendency to experience seizures? The causes of epilepsy are too numerous to list. Many knockout mice experience spontaneous seizures, and the various forms of human epilepsy that appear to have a genetic basis have been traced to many different genes. Moreover, as previously indicated, epilepsy frequently occurs after brain trauma or infection.

Because neurons are extensively and often reciprocally interconnected, it has been theorized that any excitatory activity can propagate and perpetuate itself across a brain or brain circuit. In healthy individuals, inhibitory circuitry generally limits the degree to which any neural signal is propagated, either spatially or temporally. Thus any condition that upsets the delicate balance between excitation and inhibition is likely to cause a seizure. The sections that follow discuss a few of the many different ways such imbalance can occur.

GENETIC INFLUENCES

More than 20 strains of knockout mice exhibit spontaneous seizures, as do several strains of mice in which particular proteins have been overexpressed (Table 21–2). Spontaneous seizures are seen, for example, in mice that lack the genes for ion channels, such as the delayed rectifier K^+ channel mKv1.1; for neurotransmitter receptors, such as GluR2 and serotonin 5-HT$_{2C}$; for enzymes, such as Ca^{2+}/calmodulin kinase II; and for transcription factors. That such a wide variety of gene products can influence seizure susceptibility is not surprising. Ion channels and neurotransmitter receptors influence the excitability of neurons directly; enzymes, which modify neurotransmitter receptors and ion channels, influence neuronal excitability in many ways; DNA-binding proteins influence the repertoire of proteins expressed by neurons, which might in turn affect excitability. Moreover, these proteins might influence epileptogenesis in a more complex manner; for example, they might alter developmental processes so that abnormal neural circuits are produced.

GluR2 mutant mice provide an interesting situation in which an ion channel abnormality is believed to promote epileptogenesis. As neonates, GluR2 mutant mice are seizure-free, but in the beginning of the third postnatal week they exhibit spontaneous recurrent seizures. All GluR2 mutant mice die by the twentieth postnatal day. As discussed in Chapter 7, the wildtype GluR2 subunit makes AMPA receptors impermeable to Ca^{2+}. This property requires posttranscriptional editing of GluR2 mRNA. GluR2 expressed early in development is not edited and therefore does not reduce Ca^{2+} permeation of AMPA receptors, whereas GluR2 expressed after birth is edited and does limit Ca^{2+} permeability. The sequence of the GluR2 gene in the GluR2 mutant mouse is altered so that this posttranscriptional editing cannot occur properly; thus increased Ca^{2+} permeation of AMPA receptor channels occurs. The absence of seizures in neonatal mutant mice, and the gradual increase in seizure severity during the ensuing 3 weeks, suggests two plausible scenarios that are not mutually exclusive. First, the effect of the mutation, with subsequent seizure activity, becomes apparent only after RNA editing of GluR2 would normally occur, when the editing is required to dampen Ca^{2+} fluxes into neurons. Alternatively, the increased Ca^{2+} influx caused by abnormal AMPA receptors promotes neural changes at some point during development, which increases the excitability of the affected circuits. Such changes may self-perpetuate as excitability increases, and in turn may allow even more opportunities for Ca^{2+} to enter affected neurons.

Many cases of human epilepsy appear to have a genetic component, although the inheritance of epilepsy is rarely simple (mendelian). Numerous human epilepsy syndromes have been mapped to specific chromosomes and, in a few cases, the specific genes have been identified. These types of epilepsy are listed in Table 21–3. All known epilepsy-causing mutations in humans affect channels or receptors; thus they represent deficits that would be expected to directly affect neuronal excitability.

NEURAL DEATH, NEUROGENESIS, AND NEURAL SPROUTING: KEYS TO EPILEPTOGENESIS?

In addition to the large number of genetic abnormalities that can lead to epilepsy, trauma, such as a blow to the head, can cause epilepsy in humans as well as in experimental animals. Seizure-inducing trauma is generally associated with discrete anatomic changes, which have been most intensively studied in the hippocampus, a particularly epileptogenic area of the brain. In animal models, seizure-inducing trauma is associated with selective loss of inhibitory interneurons of the dentate hilus, and also with an increase in the number of excitatory dentate granule cell axons (mossy fibers). Loss of hilar cells and sprouting of mossy fibers are also a prominent aspect of the pathologic changes observed in human temporal lobe epilepsy.

These observations raise several questions. The loss of hilar inhibitory interneurons is consistent with the imbalance of excitation and inhibition that might be expected to lead to seizures. However, why do hilar interneurons die in greater numbers than excitatory neurons? More-

Table 21–2 Mouse Genes Linked to an Epileptic Phenotype

Gene	Protein	Age of Onset	Postnatal Lethality
Spontaneous seizures			
Deletions			
5-HT$_{2C}$	Serotonin receptor	<5 weeks	+
Synapsin I, II	Synaptic vesicle proteins	>2 months	−
CaMKIIα	Ca^{2+}/calmodulin protein kinase		−
TNAP	Nonspecific alkaline phosphatase	2 weeks	+
Centromere BP-B (ins)	Brain-specific DNA binding protein	3–4 months	−
mKv1.1	K^+ channel	2 weeks	+
Weaver (spon)	G protein–gated inward rectifier (GIRK2)	Adult	+
GluR2	Q/R site editing of glutamate receptor subunit	2 weeks	+
Overexpression			
GAP–43	Neural growth-associated protein	>4 weeks	−
Pip	Myelin protected protein	<4 weeks	+
No seizures, but increased			
threshold for epileptogenesis			
Tyn	Tyrosine kinase receptor		−
tPA	Tissue plasminogen activator		−
BDNF (−/+)	Brain–derived neurotrophic factor		−

Reproduced with permission from Noebels JL. 1996. *Neuron* 16:241.

Table 21–3 Molecular Genetics of Idiopathic Epilepsies

Epilepsy Syndrome	Linkage	Gene
Epilepsies with simple inheritance		
Benign familial neonatal convulsions	20q	KCNQ2[2]
	8q	KCNQ3[2]
Benign familial infantile convulsions	19q	?
	16	?
Autosomal dominant nocturnal frontal lobe epilepsy	20q	CHRNA4[3]
	15q[1]	?
Familial partial epilepsy with auditory features	10q	?
Familial partial epilepsy with variable foci	2q[1]	?
Epilepsies with complex inheritance		
Juvenile myoclonic epilepsy	6p	?
	15q[1]	?
Idiopathic generalized epilepsy, unspecified	8q[1]	?
Idiopathic generalized epilepsy, unspecified	3p[1]	?
Persisting absence with later myoclonic epilepsy	1p[1]	?
Persisting absence with tonic–clonic seizures	8q[1]	?
Generalized epilepsy with febril seizures	2q[1]	?
	19q	SCN1B[4]
Benign rolandic epilepsy	15q[1]	?
Febrile seizures	8q[1]	?
	19p[1]	?

[1]Single report to date so linkage should be regarded as tentative.
[2]KCNQ2 and KCNQ3 are novel neuronal potassium channel genes.
[3]CHRNA4 is the gene for the alpha-4 subunit of the neuronal nicotinic acetylcholine receptor.
[4]SCN1B is the gene for the beta-1 sodium channel subunit.
? Unknown.
Reproduced with permission from Berkovic SF, Scheffer IE. 1999. *Curr Opin Neurol* 12:177–182.

over, what mechanisms underlie the increased number of mossy fibers, and what are the consequences of this sprouting? An increase in mossy fibers may result from the sprouting of existing dentate granule cells or it may be related to an increase in the total number of dentate granule cells. The proliferation of dentate granule cells, which is moderate during adulthood, has been found to increase after trauma (see Chapters 2 and 11).

The ultimate effects of the increase in mossy fiber density are uncertain. It is possible that mossy fiber sprouting contributes to epileptogenesis by increasing excitatory input to hippocampal circuits. Alternatively, mossy fibers may selectively synapse onto remaining hilar interneurons in an attempt to return the overall level of inhibition to its normal level. Mossy fiber proliferation may be manipulated by means of pharmacologic and molecular interventions. The NMDA receptor antagonist **MK-801** retards seizure development and mossy fiber sprouting, as does elimination of the gene for the transcription factor c-Fos. Neurotrophic factors most likely play a role in mossy fiber proliferation, and research into the effects of neurotrophins such as brain-derived neurotrophic factor (BDNF) on mossy fiber sprouting has begun to yield interesting results. If mossy fiber sprouting is proven to contribute directly to the development of seizures, these findings might be exploited to inhibit epileptogenesis.

TREATMENT OF EPILEPSY

Despite advances in our understanding of the etiologies of seizure disorders, the development of new and effective forms of epilepsy treatment and prevention has been rather limited. Most individuals with recurrent seizures continue to be treated with anticonvulsant drugs that have been available for many years (Figure 21–8).

Almost all anticonvulsants work by directly modifying neural excitability through alterations either in ion channels or in the availability of amino acid neurotransmitters. The key to seizure prevention is interference with rapid, synchronized firing of neurons. The ideal anticonvulsant drug must prevent the excessive, synchronized discharges that occur during a seizure without impeding normal neuronal function. Most anticonvulsants can be divided into three general categories

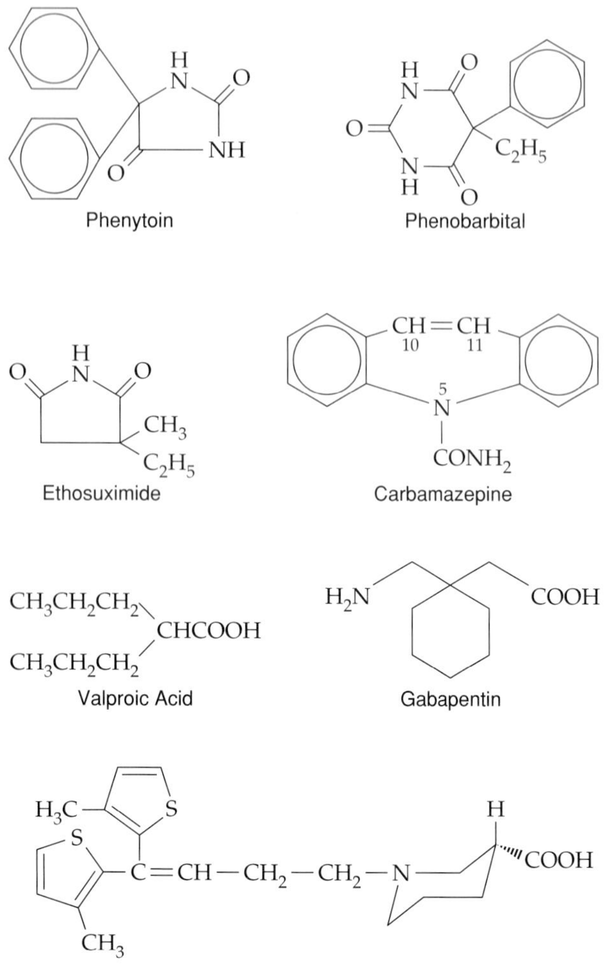

Phenytoin

Phenobarbital

Ethosuximide

Carbamazepine

Valproic Acid

Gabapentin

Tiagabine

Figure 21–8. Chemical structures of commonly used anticonvulsants.

according to their mechanisms of action: agents that act on Na^+ channels, those that affect GABAergic transmission, and those that act on Ca^{2+} channels. Drugs that selectively stabilize the inactive state of Na^+ channels thereby decrease a nerve's ability to fire rapid bursts of action potentials. Drugs that enhance inhibitory GABAergic transmission are able to increase GABA availability or to enhance the effect of GABA on GABA receptors. The activities of drugs that inhibit Ca^{2+} channels were discussed earlier in this chapter; inhibitors of T-type Ca^{2+} channels are especially effective against general absence seizures.

Although most anticonvulsant drugs have at least one of these mechanisms of action, many appear to affect other aspects of neurotransmission. Some anticonvulsant drugs, for example, are believed to reduce glutamatergic neurotransmission by altering glutamate metabolism or by blocking glutamate receptors directly.

DRUGS THAT ENHANCE Na^+ CHANNEL INACTIVATION

Phenytoin, carbamazepine, oxcarbazepine, lamotrigine, topirimate, and **felbamate** all enhance Na^+ channel inactivation, although some of these substances produce additional effects that may contribute to their anticonvulsant activity. Because these drugs bind to and stabilize Na^+ channels that are inactivated, their binding is dependent on the opening of Na^+ channels, which leads to the inactivated state. Stabilization of the inactivated state of the voltage-gated Na^+ channel has the ultimate effect of reducing sustained high-frequency firing of action potentials (Figure 21–9). Drugs with this mechanism act specifically on rapidly firing neurons, and the ability of neurons to fire one or a few action potentials is little affected.

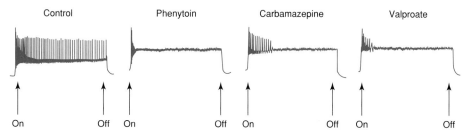

Figure 21–9. Effects of three anticonvulsant drugs on sustained high-frequency firing of action potentials by cultured neurons. In control neurons, a depolarizing pulse leads to repetitive firing of action potentials. In the presence of phenytoin, carbamazepine, or valproate, the number of action potentials is drastically reduced. (Adapted with permission from Katzung BG. 1998. *Basic and Clinical Pharmacology,* 7th ed. Originally published by Appleton and Lange. Copyright © 1998 by The McGraw-Hill Companies, Inc.)

Valproate is another use-dependent Na$^+$ channel blocker, although it is weaker in this regard than drugs such as phenytoin and carbamazepine. However, valproate exerts other effects as well. Not only is it a Ca^{2+} channel blocker, but based on the results of many studies, it also may be able to increase levels of GABA in the brain.

Interestingly, several of these anticonvulsant agents, particularly valproate and carbamazepine, are used clinically in the treatment of **bipolar disorder.** The mechanism by which these drugs exert such mood-stabilizing effects is a matter of considerable debate (see Chapter 15).

DRUGS THAT ENHANCE INHIBITORY GABAERGIC TRANSMISSION

Benzodiazepines and **barbiturates** bind to distinct sites on the GABA$_A$ receptor and increase the receptor's affinity for GABA, thereby increasing its chloride conductance (Figure 21–10; see Chapters 7 and 15). These agents, such as **phenobarbital,** are not as frequently prescribed for epilepsy as they once were. They often produce unwanted sedative effects in patients, who may complain of tiredness, forgetfulness, and con-

fusion. Moreover, patients are subject to rapid tolerance to the anticonvulsant effects of benzodiazepines with repeated administration. However, several newer anticonvulsants with different mechanisms of action may be more effective and are better tolerated.

Vigabatrin, a relatively new anticonvulsant medication, is a synthetic structural analogue of GABA that acts as a specific inhibitor of GABA transaminase, an enzyme critical to the breakdown of GABA in the nerve terminal. As might be expected, patients who take vigabatrin have increased levels of GABA in their cerebrospinal fluid; thus vigabatrin may exert its anticonvulsant action by increasing the overall availability of GABA.

Tiagabine is an inhibitor of the GABA transporter that removes released GABA from the synaptic space and returns it to the nerve terminal for recycling or catabolism (see Chapter 7). By inhibiting the GABA transporter, tiagabine most likely acts to increase the time that GABA remains in the synaptic cleft after its release. In hippocampal CA1 cells, tiagabine increases the duration of inhibitory postsynaptic currents—an action that is consistent with its ability to produce a prolonged effect of GABA at inhibitory synapses.

Gabapentin is a GABA analogue; however, it has not been proven to bind to the GABA receptor or affect

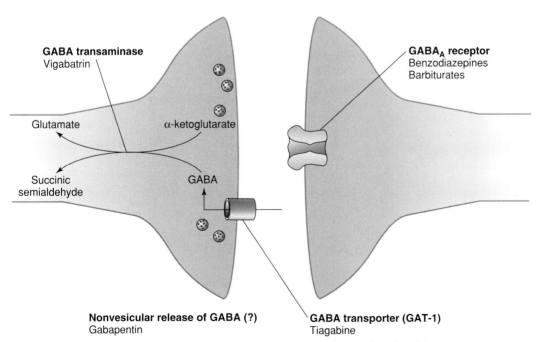

Figure 21–10. Actions of various anticonvulsant drugs that act at γ-aminobutyric acid (GABA) synapses. Vigabatrin inhibits GABA transaminase, and in turn prevents the breakdown of GABA. Tiagabine inhibits GABA reuptake. Benzodiazepines and barbiturates enhance the function of GABA$_A$ receptors. Gabapentin's mechanism of action remains unknown; however, it may promote the nonvesicular release of GABA from synaptic terminals.

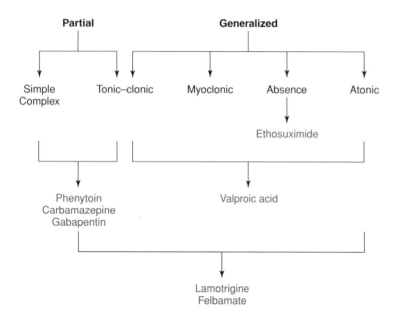

Figure 21–11. Specificity of anticonvulsant drugs in the treatment of partial and generalized seizures.

GABA metabolism or reuptake. Nonetheless, gabapentin increases total GABA concentration in the cerebrospinal fluid of patients who receive it. It has been suggested that gabapentin increases GABA availability by stimulating the release of nonvesicular pools of GABA. It also may stimulate GABA synthesis by a mechanism that has yet to be identified.

RHYME AND REASON: DETERMINING THE APPROPRIATE DRUG

Clinical trials and experience, rather than an understanding of the pathophysiology of epilepsy and the mechanisms of anticonvulsant medications, have provided the best guidelines for determining the epileptic drug that is most effective in controlling each type of seizure. Valproic acid, for example, is effective in controlling primary generalized epilepsy of the absence, myoclonic, or tonic–clonic type. Valproic acid is less effective in the treatment of partial seizures, for which phenytoin and carbamazepine are the drugs of choice. As previously mentioned, the T-channel blocker ethosuximide is most useful in treating generalized absence seizures; this finding is consistent with what is known about the processes that underlie this type of seizure. In general, agents that are effective in controlling partial seizures appear to produce relatively effective use-dependent Na^+ channel blockade compared with drugs that are most useful for treating generalized seizures. Conversely, drugs effective in controlling generalized seizures tend to be better Ca^{2+} channel blockers (Figure 21–11).

SELECTED READING

Andrews PI, McNamara JO. 1996. Rasmussen's encephalitis: An autoimmune disorder? *Curr Opin Neurobiol* 6:673–678.

Berkovic SF, Scheffer IE. 1997. Genetics of human partial epilepsy. *Curr Opin Neurol* 10:110–114.

Berkovic SF, Scheffer IE. 1999. Genetics of the epilepsies. *Curr Opin Neurol* 12:177–182.

Chinese Acute Stroke Trial Collaborative Group. 1997. CAST: Randomised placebo-controlled trial of early aspirin use in 20,000 patients with acute ischemic stroke. *Lancet* 349: 1641–1649.

Choi DW. 1996. Ischemia-induced neuronal apoptosis. *Curr Opin Neurobiol* 6:667–672.

Chollet F, DiPiero V, Wise RJ, et al. 1991. The functional anatomy of motor recovery after stroke in humans: A study with positron emission tomography. *Ann Neurol* 29:63–71.

Coughlin SR. 2000. Thrombin signalling and protease-activated receptors. *Nature* 407:258–264.

Dawson VL, Dawson TM. 1998. Nitric oxide in neurodegeneration. *Prog Brain Res* 118:215–229.

Dirnagl U, Iadecola C, Moskowitz MA. 1999. Pathobiology of ischaemic stroke: An integrated view. *Trends Neurosci* 22: 391–397.

Dugan LL, Choi DW. 1994. Excitotoxicity, free radicals, and cell membrane changes. *Ann Neurol* 35:S17–S21.

European Cooperative Acute Stroke Study (ECASS). 1995. Intravenous thrombolysis with recombinant tissue plasminogen activator for acute hemispheric stroke. *JAMA* 274:1017–1025.

Green AR, Hainsworth AH, Jackson DM. 2000. GABA potentiation: a logical pharmacological approach for the treatment of acute ischaemic stroke. *Neuropharmacology* 39: 1483–1494.

Gumnit RJ. 1995. *The Epilepsy Handbook: The Practical Management of Seizures.* New York: Raven Press.

Hicken SL, Grotta J. 1998. Neuroprotective therapy. *Semin Neurol* 18:485–492.

International Stroke Trial Collaborative Group. 1997. The International Stroke Trial (IST): A randomized trial of aspirin, subcutaneous heparin, both, or neither among 19,435 patients with acute ischemic stroke. *Lancet* 349: 1569–1581.

Koroshetz WJ, Moskowitz MA. 1996. Emerging treatments for stroke in humans. *Trends Pharmacol Sci* 17:227–233.

Kristian T, Siesjo BK. 1998. Calcium in ischemic cell death. *Stroke* 29:705–718.

Lee J-M, Zipfel GJ, Choi DW. 1999. The changing landscape of ischaemic brain injury mechanisms. *Nature* 399(suppl): A7–A14.

Leifer D. 1998. Neuronal plasticity and recovery from stroke. *The Neuroscientist* 4:68–70.

Lester JA, Karschin A. 2000. Gain of function mutants: Ion channels and G protein-coupled receptors. *Annu Rev Neurosci* 23:89–125.

Lipton P. 1999. Ischemic cell death in brain neurons. *Physiol Rev* 79:1431–1568.

MacDonald RL, Greenfield LJ. 1997. Mechanisms of action of new antiepileptic drugs. *Curr Opin Neurol* 10:121–128.

Majerus PW, Broze GJ Jr, Miletich JP, Tollegsen DM. 1996. Anticoagulant, thrombolytic, and antiplatelet drugs. In Hardman JG, Limbird LE (eds): *Goodman and Gilman's The Pharmacological Basis of Therapeutics*, 9th ed, pp. 1341–1359. New York: McGraw-Hill.

Matchar DB, Duncan PW. 1994. Cost of stroke. *Stroke Clinical Updates* 5:9–12.

McNamara JO. 1999. Emerging insights into the genesis of epilepsy. *Nature* 399(suppl):A15–A22.

Moshe SL. 2000. Mechanisms of action of anticonvulsant agents. *Neurology* 55(suppl):S32–S40.

National Institute of Neurological Disorders and Stroke-PA Stroke Study Group. 1995. Tissue plasminogen activating factor for acute ischemic stroke. *New Engl J Med* 333: 1581–1587.

Nijhawah D, Honarpour N, Wang X. 2000. Apoptosis in neural development and disease. *Annu Rev Neurosci* 23: 73–87.

Noebels JL. 1996. Targeting epilepsy genes. *Neuron* 16:241–244.

Nudo RJ, Wise BM, SiFuentes F, Milleken GW. 1996. Neural substrates for the effects of rehabilitative training on motor recovery after ischemic infarct. *Science* 272:1791–1794.

Parent JM, Lowenstein DL. 1997. Mossy fiber reorganization in the epileptic hippocampus. *Curr Opin Neurol* 10:103–109.

Rossi DJ, Oshima T, Attwell D. 2000. Glutamate release in severe brain ischaemia is mainly by reversed uptake. *Nature* 403:316–321.

Sabatini U, Toin D, Pantano P, et al. 1994. Motor recovery after early brain damage: A case of brain plasticity. *Stroke* 25:514–517.

Snead OC. 1995. Basic mechanisms of generalized absence seizures. *Ann Neurol* 37:146–157.

Steinlein OK. 1999. The genetic basis of epilepsy: Mutant alleles of ligand- and voltage-gated ion channels. *The Neuroscientist* 5:295–301.

Wilder BJ. 1995. The treatment of epilepsy: An overview of clinical practices. *Neurology* 45(suppl):S7–S11.

Wyllie E (ed). 1997. *The Treatment of Epilepsy: Principles and Practice*, 2nd ed. Baltimore: Williams and Wilkins.

INDEX

UNIVERSITY OF WOLVERHAMPTON
LEARNING RESOURCES